P9-DNA-406

RADIOLOGY

An Illustrated History

RADIOLOGY

An Illustrated History

Ronald L. Eisenberg, M.D.

Chairman of Radiology
Highland General Hospital
Oakland, California
Clinical Professor of Radiology
University of California
at San Francisco and Davis

Formerly, Professor and Chairman of Radiology
Louisiana State University School of Medicine
Shreveport, Louisiana

with 979 illustrations

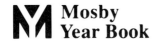 **Mosby Year Book**

St. Louis   Baltimore   Boston   Chicago   London   Philadelphia   Sydney   Toronto

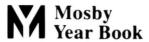

Mosby
Year Book

Dedicated to Publishing Excellence

Editor: Anne S. Patterson
Assistant Editor: Anne Gunter
Project Manager: Carol Sullivan Wiseman
Designer: Susan Lane

Printed in the United States of America

Mosby-Year Book, Inc.
11830 Westline Industrial Drive
St. Louis, Missouri 63146

Library of Congress Cataloging in Publication Data

Eisenberg, Ronald L.
    Radiology : an illustrated history / Ronald L. Eisenberg.
      p.   cm.
    Includes bibliographical references and index.
    ISBN 0-8016-1526-7
    1. Radiology—History.   2. Radiography, Medical—History.
    [DNLM: 1. Radiology—History.   2. Technology, Radiologic—history.
WN 11.1 E36r]
RC78.E55 1991
616.07′57′09—dc20
DNLM/DLC
for Library of Congress   91-35008
                                               CIP

92 93 94 95 96 VT/W/W 9 8 7 6 5 4 3 2 1

Preface

Almost four years ago, while on sabbatical at the University of California in San Diego, I was complaining to John Amberg that I could not think of a topic for my next book. He suggested that, in view of the upcoming one-hundredth anniversary of Roentgen's epochal discovery of x-rays, I should consider writing a history of radiology. On returning home, I began reading about the fascinating history of our specialty and decided that I would devote most of my literary efforts for the next several years to producing a lavishly illustrated history of radiology.

The book opens with the predecessors of Roentgen, who developed the principles of electricity and magnetism, and continues with the exciting discoveries of x-rays and radium. This is followed by a description of the early days of radiology, the historic firsts, and the initial application of x-rays to diagnostic problems. Section Two details some of the technical developments (plates and film, power generators, tubes, and cones and grids) that transformed radiology from an experimental curiosity to a valuable diagnostic tool. This section concludes with a sobering chapter dealing with the unexpected dangers of radiation, the tragic deaths of many of the most eminent pioneers, and the development of effective radiation protection. Section Three is devoted to clinical radiology and the development of organ-related specialization. Whenever possible, archival material is included, illustrating the earliest examples of diagnostic procedures that have faded into oblivion or are still used today. Section Four is modality oriented, depicting the development of conventional tomography, vascular radiology, nuclear medicine, and the cross-sectional techniques of ultrasound, computed tomography, and magnetic resonance imaging. Section Five describes the evolution of interventional procedures and the use of x-rays and radium for therapeutic purposes. Section Six then traces the development of radiology organizations, journals, and education. The whimsical finale delves into the lighter side of radiology with an assortment of anecdotes and cartoons.

This book has two major purposes—to give radiologists an understanding of the rich tradition of their specialty and to offer other physicians and the lay public an insight into the historic developments that have propelled radiology from the obscure province of engineers and photographers to one of the most rapidly growing fields in medicine.

Ronald L. Eisenberg

Acknowledgments

Of the many individuals who have contributed to this book, space limitations permit listing only a few. The guiding force who introduced me to the wonderful world of history was Nancy Knight, Ph.D., the Curator of the Center for the American History of Radiology at the American College of Radiology. She possessed the unique ability to make history come alive and enabled me to feel that the authors of the classic texts in radiology had become personal friends. Once my quest for illustrations began, I visited several major museums and libraries where I was given access to a treasure trove of material. Special thanks go to C. Neil Brown and Tim Boon at the Science Museum and Wellcome Collection in London; Ulrich Hennig at the German Roentgen Museum in Remscheid-Lennep; Walter Rathjen and Alto Brachner at the Deutsches Museum in Munich; Richard Wolfe at the Countway Library in Boston; Jan Lazarus at the National Library of Medicine in Bethesda; and Dorothea Nelhybel at the Burndy Library in Norwalk, Connecticut. I greatly appreciate the many superb photographs graciously provided to me by Jack Cullinan of Eastman Kodak and Gene Medford of General Electric. I am grateful to Chuck Mitchell of the University Medical Center in Jacksonville, Florida, for sparking my interest in radiology-related stamps that led to their inclusion in the chapter openers. Thanks should also go to the many radiologists and other physicians who permitted me to reproduce the marvelous illustrations from their books, articles, and exhibits.

I greatly appreciate the assistance of Betty DiGrazia for typing the manuscript and Toiee Murray for reproducing articles from dusty journals in the library. Special thanks should go to Pam Ashley, Rose Powell, and Lisa Ebarb of the LSUMCS Library who spent hours poring over microfiches to find and order old books and journals through inter-library loan. Thanks should also go to Ron Aldin, Glen Bundrick, and Stan Carpenter of the Medical Communications Department at LSU who made the glossy photographs from these often crumbling tomes.

Ronald L. Eisenberg

To the pioneers of Radiology
and their medical descendants

To *Zina*, *Avlana*, and *Cherina*
for their understanding while I pursued
the fascinating history of our specialty

Contents

THE EARLY DAYS

X-ACTLY SO!

The Roentgen Rays, the Roentgen Rays,
What is this craze?
The town's ablaze
With the new phase
Of X-ray's ways.

I'm full of daze,
Shock and amaze;
For nowadays
I hear they'll gaze
Thro' cloak and gown—and even stays,
These naughty, naughty Roentgen Rays.

Wilhelma
Electrical Review, April 17, 1896

CHAPTER 1

Predecessors of Roentgen

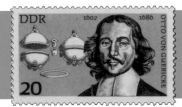 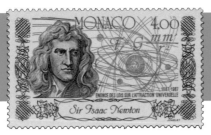 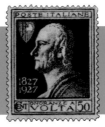 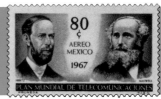

> In the history of Science, nothing is more true than that the discoverer, even the greatest discoverer, is but the descendant of his scientific fore-fathers; he is always essentially the product of the age in which he is born.
>
> SYLVANUS P. THOMPSON, 1897

The dramatic discovery of x-rays by Roentgen in 1895 was the culmination of centuries of observation and experimentation in electricity and magnetism. This discovery also required a series of mechanical and technical advances permitting the production of a strong vacuum in glass tubes.

More than 2,500 years ago, the Greeks observed that amber, when rubbed briskly, would attract or repel light objects such as feathers and small bits of paper. A semiprecious stone, although not especially rare, amber is a fossil resin that is primarily found on the shores of the Baltic Sea. It was a major article of trade for several thousand years before the scientific investigation of its properties began. Another curious material known in early times was lodestone, a naturally magnetic iron ore that is widely distributed in the Mediterranean islands and adjacent lands. Although masses of this ore were discovered to be especially magnetic and were highly valued, its strange properties could not be investigated until iron was discovered and worked. About 400 years ago, the analogy of the effect of friction causing amber to attract light objects and that of lodestone to attract iron led to the first true scientific study of the phenomenon.

William Gilbert, physician to Elizabeth I of England, was an enthusiastic convert to the Copernican hypothesis that the earth and other heavenly bodies were huge magnets held in their orbits by the same attraction as that exhibited by lodestone. Anticipating Sir Isaac Newton's theory of gravitation, Gilbert explained that ships and people do not fall off the planet because of the attraction of all bodies by the great mass of the earth. Gilbert's famous work, *De Magnete*, published in 1600, formed

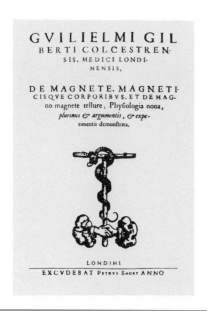

Title page of Gilbert's *De Magnete* (1600).

the scientific foundation for subsequent investigations of electricity and magnetism. One of the first scientists to become dissatisfied with the lack of logic and system in the "experiments" of the alchemists, Gilbert emphasized the importance of accurate and detailed observations and information. As he wrote, "There are many books about hidden, abstruse and occult causes and wonders . . . words alone, without experimental proof. All of my own experiments were repeated again and again under my own eyes."

Gilbert studied the lines of force, or "effluvia" as he termed them, around a small magnetic needle balanced on a pivot. In performing these experiments, he discovered magnetic induction and magnetic conductivity. By noting that the ordinary magnetic compass needle points toward the north because the earth is a great magnet and not because the needle is "attracted by the stars," Gilbert discovered terrestrial magnetism. But his most valuable accomplishment was the rediscovery of frictional electricity and the "electrical" properties of amber. Indeed, it was Gilbert

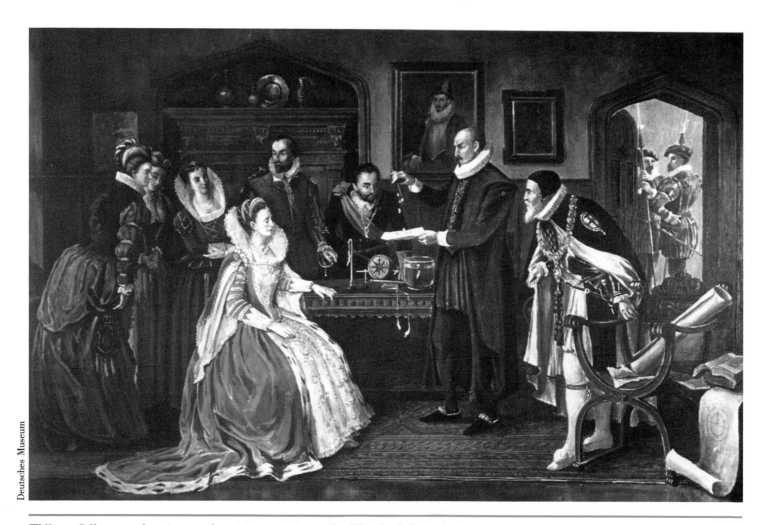

William Gilbert performing an electricity experiment for Elizabeth I in 1600.

who first used the term "electrical," from the Greek word for amber, to apply to properties of attraction arising from friction. He also found a series of other materials such as sulfur, glass, resin, sealing wax, and many crystals, which when rubbed possessed similar "electrical" properties. To measure electrical attraction, Gilbert devised a kind of electroscope that he called a "versorium." It consisted of a thin metal needle suspended in a horizontal plane so that it "could be attracted like a compass needle."

Gilbert was the first experimenter to investigate the effects of minute quantities of high tension electricity, the form of electricity capable of exciting a vacuum to eventually produce x-rays. This "static" electricity was the only form known until the discoveries of Galvani and the construction of the battery by Volta at the end of the eighteenth century. Indeed, static electricity continued to be the only usable form of high tension electricity until some 40 years later, when the co-discovery by Faraday and Henry of electromagnetic induction led to the invention of the coil, the dynamo, and the transformer.

In addition to electricity and magnetism, the third major physical principle involved in the production of x-rays is the vacuum and the evacuated glass tube. The first attempts to create an "empty space" by removing air from an air-tight vessel were made independently by the Italian, Evangelista Torricelli, and the German, Otto von Guericke. Torricelli, who was the secretary and companion to the blind Galileo in his old age in Florence, thought out an explanation of one of Galileo's unfinished problems—why a pump cannot draw water higher than about 33 feet. He reasoned that if the weight of the air forced up the column of water with each lift of the piston, then the atmosphere could sustain a column of mercury only $\frac{1}{14}$ as high, because mercury is 14 times heavier than water. He proposed to fill a glass tube with mercury so that it would stand upright, with the open end immersed in a cup of mercury. The mercury column sank to about 30 inches, leaving an empty space above. In this manner, in 1643, Torricelli invented one of the most important scientific instruments, the mercury barometer. Of major interest to the radiologist, however, was the empty space above the mercury that represented the first permanent vacuum. (The unit of measurement for the degree of vacuum, the "torr," is named for Torricelli.)

Otto von Guericke, the burgomaster of Magdeburg, was another ardent disciple of Copernicus. He reasoned that the earth, moon, and other heavenly bodies observed through the telescope of Galileo must be moving in empty space, for otherwise the resistance of air would long since have brought all to a standstill. Acting on this idea, in 1646, von Guericke made the first air pump for the distinct purpose of forming a vacuum with which to study celestial conditions close at hand. He later constructed an improved vacuum pump consisting of a vertical cylinder in which the piston could be moved up and down by means of a lever. An automatic leather valve replaced the stopcock that he had used on his initial apparatus. Von Guericke demonstrated that animals could not live in a vacuum and that all bodies, feathers and stones alike, fell with equal velocities within a vacuum.

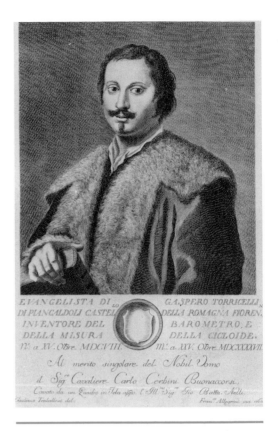

Evangelista Torricelli (1608-1647).

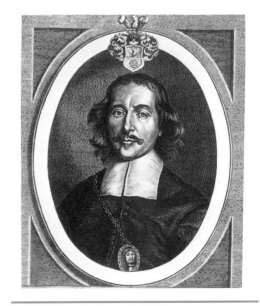

Otto von Guericke (1602-1686).

Demonstration of von Guericke's
Magdeburg hemispheres.[2]

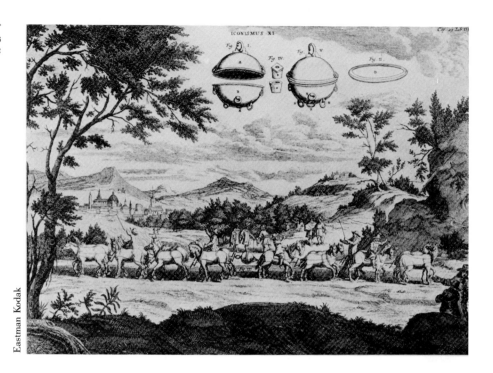

Demonstration of von Guericke's
Magdeburg hemispheres.[2]

Eastman Kodak

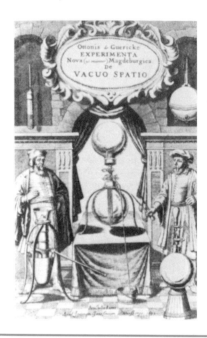

Air pumps on title page of von Guericke's
book.[2]

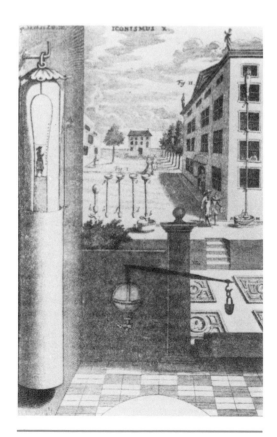

Von Guericke's barometer.[2]

Von Guericke's best known experiment was the celebrated Magdeburg
hemispheres, which he devised as a demonstration for his royal patron,
Emperor Ferdinand III. These were halves of a heavy metal sphere that
would fit together to be air-tight, with a stopcock permitting air to be
pumped out. Heavy rings on each hemisphere could be attached to
chains. A classic print shows eight horses hitched to each hemisphere
and attempting to pull in opposite directions without success. However,
as soon as von Guericke turned the stopcock and let in some air, the
hemispheres fell apart by themselves.

Without knowledge of Torricelli's work, von Guericke built a water
barometer 60 feet high outside his house. On the top of the column of
water in the barometer he placed a small wooden figure, the outstretched
hand of which pointed to a scale to indicate the barometric pressure. By
observing changes in barometric pressure, von Guericke was able to
make extraordinary weather predictions.

Von Guericke also invented the first electrical machine, a rotating
sulfur sphere made by pouring sulfur into a glass globe that was broken
away after the sulfur hardened. Rotation of the sulfur sphere with the dry
hand pressed against it yielded static electricity of a potential high
enough to produce phosphorescent light and brush discharges, or even
small sparks. Von Guericke found that the excited sulfur ball would
attract all sorts of light objects (paper, shavings, particles of gold and
silver leaf), which was a different and more universal attraction than
occurred with lodestone. This attraction could even be communicated
over a linen thread a yard in length. Although this was the first transmission of an electrical impulse over a conductor, von Guericke did not
perceive this to be either an impulse or a current. He did allow himself
some fanciful speculation, believing that the earth was a great electrical
machine "rotated by the hand of the Almighty and excited by the friction
of the solar rays."

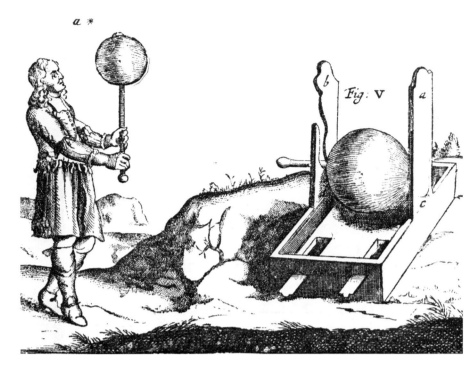

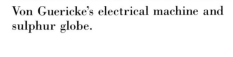

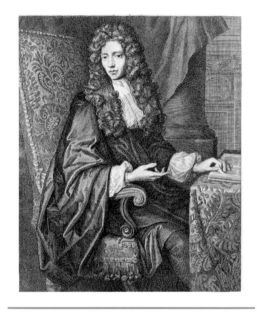

Robert Boyle (1627-1691).

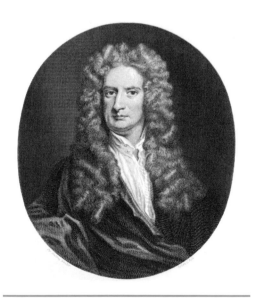

Sir Isaac Newton (1643-1727).

Over the next few years, several scientists made observations and apparatus that set the stage for major future advances. Robert Boyle, with his assistant, Robert Hooke, improved on von Guericke's air pump, or "pneumatic engine" as he called it, and added the pinion movement to it. With this machine, Boyle studied the behavior of gases when enclosed in glass tubes and formulated the gas law that bears his name. In 1676, he made the important observation that the electrostatic effects of rubbed amber and the effects of magnetism also occur in a vacuum.

Sir Isaac Newton (1675) built an electrical machine with a rotating glass sphere with which he made a large series of important experiments. One interesting observation was that it was possible to electrically charge one side of a glass plate by rubbing the other side with a cloth.

The production of a luminous glow within a vacuum chamber was first described in 1678 by Jean Picard, a French priest and astronomer, who supplied Newton with the calculations necessary to prove gravitation as a law of the universe. One evening, Picard was carrying his Torricelli barometer up some steps in his dark observatory when he noticed a glow in the vacuum of the instrument. He found that he could produce the glow at will by agitating the mercury. Twenty years later, the German professor of mathematics, Jakob Bernoulli, came across Picard's notes and performed experiments of his own by shaking mercury in tubes with and without a vacuum. He produced considerable light, which he called "mercurial phosphorus," and believed that he had invented a mechanical substitute for candles. The underlying mechanism for this phenomenon was demonstrated by Francis Hauksbee, the leading figure in the early history of electrical exploration.

Francis Hauksbee was the curator of experiments and instrument maker to the Royal Society of London. Instead of working with a miniature vacuum chamber in the end of a barometer, Hauksbee exhausted much larger tubes and bell jars by means of an air pump of his own

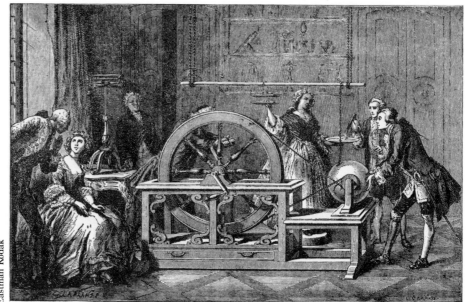

Hauksbee's electrical machine.

design. He finally demonstrated that the Picard glow or Bernoulli's "mercurial phosphorus" was due to the friction of mercury on glass, which produced electricity. Hauksbee designed an extensive set of experiments to investigate the phenomenon of electrical excitation in a vacuum. He built machines for the rapid rotation of vacuum bulbs 6 or 8 inches in diameter and found that the friction of his dry hand on the outside of these globes gave a purple glow of sufficient brilliance to permit reading of large type. The wall of the room, 10 feet away from the globe, also became visible. Later, he rubbed wool against glass and leather against amber to produce a striking luminescence. Hauksbee observed that as small amounts of air were permitted to enter the globe, the glow diminished. Encouraged by these experimental successes, he replaced the glass globe with a glass cylinder on which he performed an extensive series of experiments that revealed unusual properties of attraction and glow. He then ingeniously constructed dual-rotating equipment, whereby one glass cylinder was placed within another so that each could be exhausted of air separately and each could be rotated independently in the same or in opposite directions.

Experiment showing electrical attraction and repulsion using a Hauksbee machine (Watson, 1745).

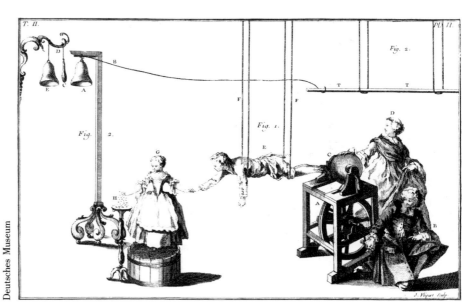

Hauksbee observed that a quiescent vacuum tube lying near one that was excited would glow without being touched. Finger tips held near the excited tubes would emit a brushlike radiance. Thus Hauksbee discovered *electrostatic induction*, although he offered no name or explanation for this phenomenon. For the first time, a vacuum tube, the ancestor of all x-ray tubes, was excited by an electrical machine.

In addition to luminescence and brush discharges, Hauksbee also obtained sparks larger than had ever been seen in a laboratory. As he wrote, "I have observed the light to break from the agitated glass like lightning, and if the hand is held near the fricated glass a light will be seen to dart from it with a noise like that of a green leaf in a fire, but not so loud." The artificial production of sparks demonstrated so beautifully by Hauksbee created a sensation throughout the world. Stephen Gray, a pensioner in the London Charterhouse, described "light and crackling noises" that could be produced by rubbing hair, silk, linen, wool, paper, leather, wood, and other materials from one body to another. Gray discovered that electricity is a current and will flow over conductors, as well as remain a charge on the surface of glass or sulfur. His source of electricity was a glass tube or ivory ball excited by friction. Gray showed that electricity resides on the surfaces of bodies thus electrified, that conductors must be insulated, that insulators are not conductors, and that a charge is induced in a conductor closely parallel to a line carrying a current. By using a fishing rod and insulating glass rods, he succeeded in carrying currents as far as 34 feet. With his friend, Granville Wheeler, Gray attempted to conduct the "electric virtue" through a hemp cord 800 feet long but was unsuccessful until Wheeler suspended the string on silk threads to thus insulate the conductor. In a spectacular experiment, Gray suspended boys of the Charterhouse by cords and electrified them.

Many of Gray's experiments were repeated by his French contemporary, Charles-François de Cisternay Du Fay, Director of the Royal Gardens in Paris. Du Fay's greatest contribution was the discovery that resinous bodies (silk or paper) and glass, when rubbed with wool and silk, respectively, yield two different types of electricity. He noted that the two electricities repelled themselves and attracted each other. These observations paved the way for Benjamin Franklin's single-fluid theory of positive and negative electricity. Later, Du Fay constructed an electroscope that was similar to the "versorium" described by Gilbert. When this instrument was charged with glass electricity and a rubbed resin rod was brought near, the deflection of the filaments of the electroscope was decreased and vice versa. Du Fay showed that all bodies, even metals, could be made "electric" by heating and then rubbing them; however, they must be suspended on insulating silk threads to stop the electrical charge from being dissipated.

During the next several years, stronger electrostatic machines, wire conductors, and insulators enabled experimenters to produce stunning effects at incredible distances.

Public interest became insatiable and electric demonstrations supplanted the theater. There was no end to displays of artificial electric sparks, glowing brush discharges from the human body in darkened rooms, the ignition of spirits by fire from a piece of ice or a jet of water, the explosion of gun powder at a distance, the electrocution of small animals, and innumerable other thrilling demonstrations.[3]

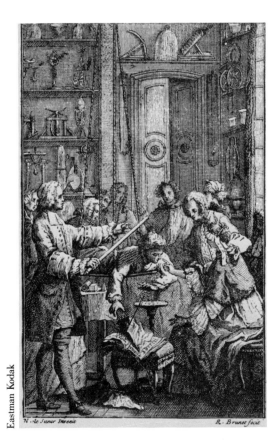

Eastman Kodak

Abbé Nollet exhibiting Gray's experiment on the electrified boy.

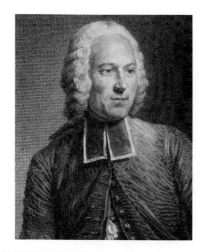

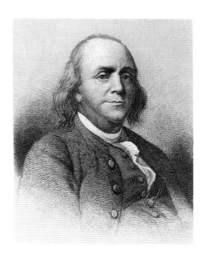

Jean Antoine (Abbé) Nollet (1700-1770).   Benjamin Franklin (1706-1790).

The next important advance in the knowledge of electricity was the work of the Frenchman, Jean Antoine (Abbé) Nollet. Unlike Hauksbee, who placed the source of high tension electricity within an evacuated tube, Nollet placed it outside and led the high tension to the glass vessel by means of iron chains sealed into the vessel wall. This "electrical egg," so-called because of its shape, contained the essentials for production of x-rays—a vacuum tube and an outside source of high tension electricity. A little higher vacuum and another wire sealed in the opposite end of the electrical egg could have led to the production of x-rays. However, even if x-rays had been produced at this time, no one would have known. The x-ray was invisible to the eye. The photographic plate, serving as an artificial retina, did not evolve until 90 years later. Also lacking was the fluorescent screen, which could transform the invisible short x-rays into longer waves that the eye could perceive.

Living in France at this time was the American, Benjamin Franklin. Franklin is well known for his experiments and theories relating to atmospheric electrical discharges during thunderstorms, especially his proof that lightning is an electrical discharge and his construction of the lightning rod. Franklin revolutionized the underlying concept of electricity. As late as 1747, electricity was defined as "that Property of Bodies by which when they are heated by attrition they attract and repel light bodies at sensible distances." The sparks resulting from friction were not regarded as electrical but as fire, which was believed to be inherent in all bodies. Franklin postulated the single-fluid theory of electricity, in which he coined the terms *positive* and *negative* and described electricity as composed of "particles infinitely subtile."

In 1745 and 1746, devices were designed to collect and store large amounts of static electricity. The spectacular shocks that could be generated from these Kleist or Leyden jars proved a popular spectacle. Nollet, in the presence of the King, killed small birds and animals by a discharge of the jar. He discharged a jar through 180 soldiers of the Royal Guard, as well as through a line of Carthusian monks 180 yards long, which made them all jump together. Many experimenters conceived the idea of using this newly found agent to cure certain diseases. The effects were tried on paralytics but without success. Sir William Watson in

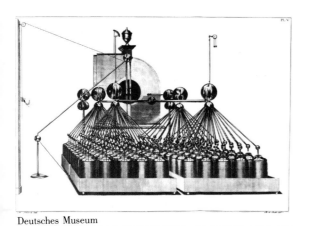

Leyden jar battery (1795).

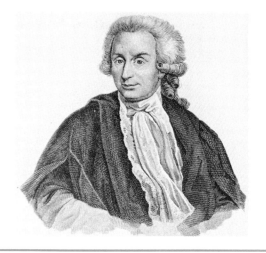

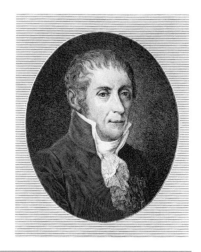

Luigi Galvani (1737-1798).   Alessandro Volta (1745-1827).

England tried to determine the longest distance through which the discharge from a Leyden tube could be transmitted through wires. In 1747, he made his famous experiment "to convey the electric shock across the river Thames, making use of the water of the river for one part of the chain of communication."

Until this time, all electrical phenomena observed came from frictional or atmospheric electricity. In the late eighteenth century, two Italians, Luigi Galvani and Alessandro Volta, discovered a new kind of electricity. Galvani demonstrated the twitching of a frog's legs suspended by a copper hook to an iron rail. He termed this phenomenon *animal electricity* and erroneously thought that the tissue itself was the source. Several years later, Volta determined that the source of the electrical current originated in the metals themselves and that it was created when two different conductors were placed in contact. His most important

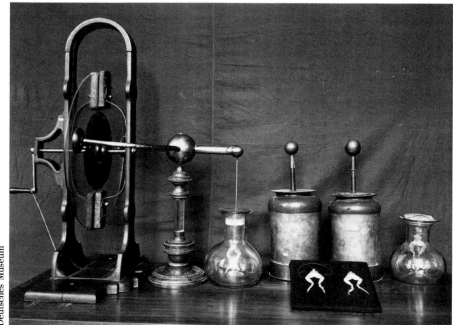

Apparatus for the classic frog legs experiment (Galvani, 1780).

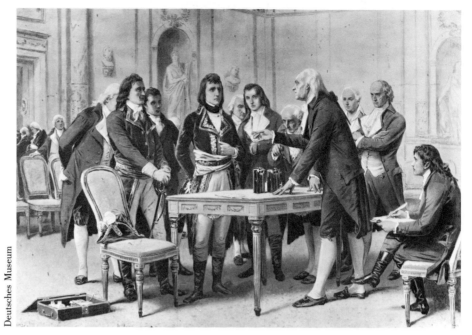

Volta demonstrating the principles of electricity for Napoleon Bonaparte in 1801.

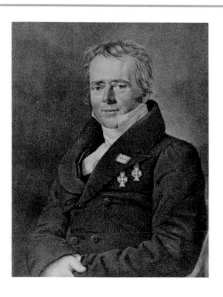

Classic experiment using plates of zinc and copper (*left*) and voltaic pile (Volta, 1800).

discovery was the "voltaic pile," a column of alternating plates of silver and zinc or copper and zinc soldered together on one end and separated by moist cardboard or leather, which could furnish a constant current of electricity. These initial experiments resulted in the construction of the voltaic cell, which revolutionized the science of physics and chemistry. The generation of electricity by means of the voltaic pile was so different from that produced by the classic static machines that there were serious doubts that both electricities were of the same nature.

The link between electricity and magnetism was first noted by the Danish professor, Hans Christian Oersted. In 1820, Oersted discovered the deviation of a magnetic needle by a conductor through which a current was flowing. Later that year, the French mathematician, André Marie

Hans Christian Oersted (1777-1851).   André Marie Ampère (1775-1836).   Georg Simon Ohm (1787-1854).

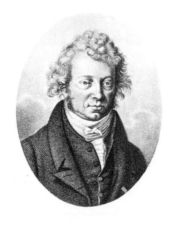

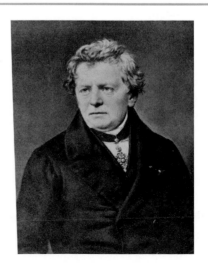

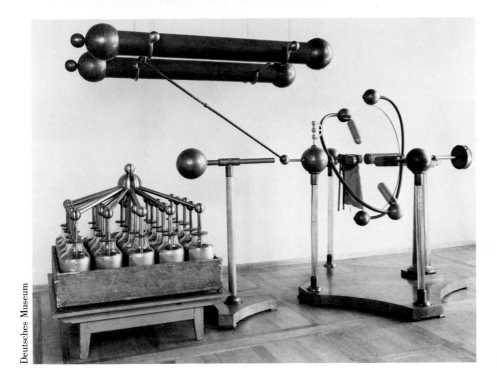

Electricity producing apparatus, including a battery composed of 25 Leyden jars (Ohm, 1840).

Ampère, developed the mathematical principles to determine the direction in which the electrical current deviated the needle. He observed that the connecting wire of a voltaic battery could magnetize iron. Ampère showed that electrical conductors have a dynamic effect on each other. He found that conductors in which current flows in the same direction repel each other, whereas those in which it flows in the opposite direction attract each other. Ampère made a sharp distinction between electrical current and electrical tension and laid the foundation for the study of electrodynamics. The mathematical formula stating the relationship of current, electromotive force, and resistance was the work of Georg Simon Ohm. Ohm's law states that in an electrical circuit, the current is in direct proportion to the electromotive force and inversely proportional to the resistance.

In 1831, the British scientist, Michael Faraday, repeated and extended the experiments of Oersted and Ampère to better understand the correlation between electrical and magnetic forces. He reasoned that since a magnet is influenced by an electrical current, a magnetic current must produce electrical forces in conducting wires. When moving a magnet inside a copper wire coil, Faraday discovered that an electrical current was flowing through the coil. This important principle of electricity, termed *electromagnetic induction,* eventually led to the construction of the induction coil and transformer that produced the strong electrical currents of high voltage used by Roentgen when he discovered x-rays. In addition to the discovery of electromagnetic induction, Faraday pointed out magnetic and electrical lines of force, described magnetic induction, and laid down the principles for the production of continuous induction currents from a coil rotating between magnetic poles.

The behavior of an electrical current flowing through a glass tube was shown to follow the pattern described by Faraday in his description of current flow through liquids. He considered solutions and chemical compounds carrying currents to contain electrically charged atoms. Such liquids he called "electrolytes." When a difference of electrical potential was applied to two points in an electrolyte, Faraday concluded that the negatively charged particles moved toward the positive terminal and the positively charged ones moved toward the negative terminal. Faraday

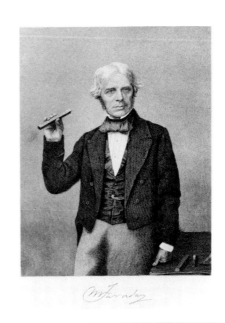

Michael Faraday (1791-1867).

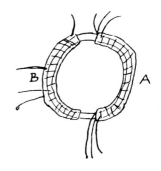

Faraday's induction ring. *A*, Primary and *B*, secondary windings (copy of Faraday's original drawing).[4]

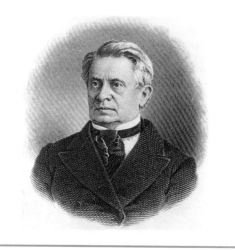

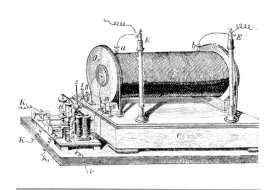

Ruhmkorff induction coil.[5]

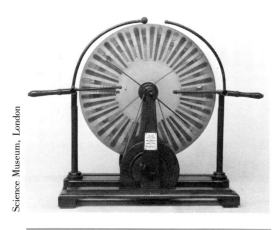

First Wimshurst electrostatic machine.

designated these charged particles as *ions* ("travelers" in Greek), or carriers of electricity. He also coined the words *anode* and *cathode*. Faraday's exquisite precision in measuring the amount of electricity required to deposit a certain quantity of silver in the process of electroplating first demonstrated that electricity existed in quanta or multiples of a unit of either energy or matter.

Faraday studied the peculiar discharges in glass tubes that contained small amounts of rare earth. His name became associated with the dark space surrounding the negative electrode, the size of which depended on many factors such as vacuum and the potential differences at the electrodes. At the time, three states of matter (solid, liquid, and gaseous) were recognized. Faraday suggested that the luminosity of highly rarefied gaseous material in a vacuum tube when excited by electricity was a property of matter in a fourth state. Faraday termed this *radiant matter*.

A contemporary of Faraday who made important experiments along the same lines was Joseph Henry, an American. He made an electromagnet capable of sustaining 50 times its own weight and developed the principle of the first electromagnetic telegraph and the dynamo.

The earliest coils based on Faraday's electroinduction principles were built in the 1830s. The best induction coils of that time were constructed by the Parisian mechanic, Heinrich Daniel Ruhmkorff, and most of the coils constructed afterward (including Roentgen's) carried his name.

Substantial improvements also were being made in electrostatic machines, often called "influence machines." The most famous of these were produced by Wilhelm T. B. Holtz and James Wimshurst. Wimshurst used glass plates with tinfoil, while Holtz changed to hard rubber plates (see Chapter 7).

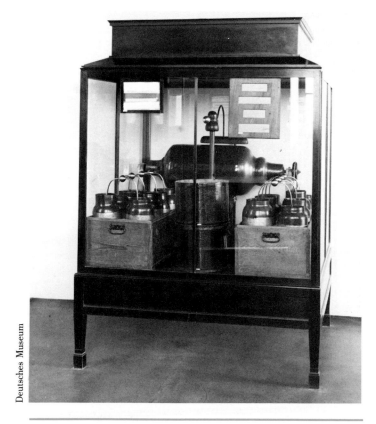

Early electrical machine using an induction coil and two batteries, each of which consisted of 8 Leyden jars (Feddersen, 1858).

The construction of instruments to measure potential and current also underwent considerable improvement. Rudolf Kohlrausch, a German physicist, used a swinging wire suspended on a thin glass thread and studied electrostatic deflections with this instrument. William Thomson, a British mathematician and physicist, who later became Lord Kelvin, designed the quadrant electrometer to provide more accurate measurements.

Faraday's experiments awakened a renewed interest in the study of electrical discharges from evacuated tubes. Limiting factors were the quality of the glass tubes and the inefficient methods of producing high vacuums. In the 1850s, glass tubes of many shapes and sizes were produced by Johann Heinrich Geissler of Bonn. Geissler, a skilled glass blower, was called on to form complex glass shapes for physics and chemistry experiments. His skill in the construction of scientific apparatus also produced a second major improvement, an advanced form of the mercury air pump invented by Hermann Sprengel in 1865. With this new pump, enough air could be extracted from glass tubes to produce a relatively high vacuum (to 0.01 Å). Platinum wire electrode terminals were fused into both ends of the tubes (Hauksbee's tube had no wires and Nollet's had one). By applying high voltage currents from a Ruhmkorff coil and admitting small quantities of various gases into these tubes, Geissler produced luminous color effects of extraordinary brilliance and beauty.

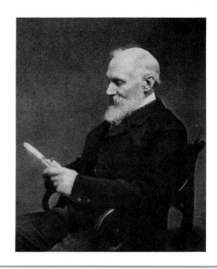

Lord Kelvin (William Thomson) (1824-1907).

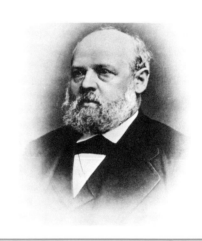

Johann Heinrich Geissler (1815-1879).

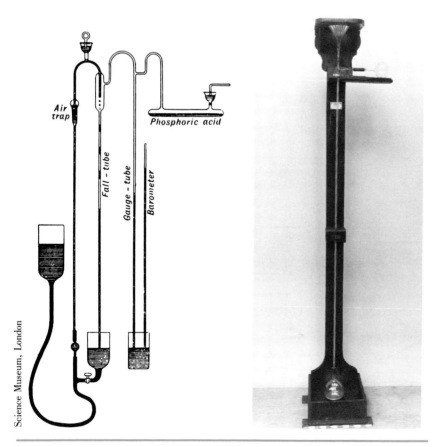

Sprengel air evacuation pump (1865). *Left*, Diagram[5] and *right*, actual instrument. A mercury rather than a piston type of air pump was developed to achieve the higher vacuums required in cathode ray and x-ray experiments.

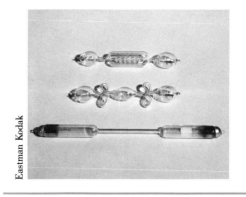

Geissler tubes.

15

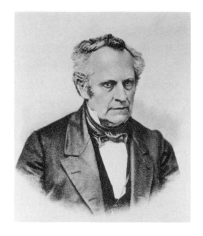

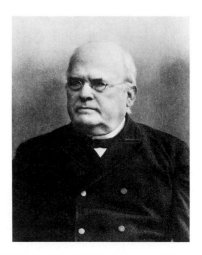

Julius Plücker (1801-1868).   Johann Wilhelm Hittorf (1824-1914).

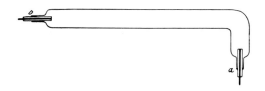

Hittorf's L-shaped tube used to demonstrate the cathode as the source of electrical discharges.[7]

The discharges in Geissler tubes were also investigated by the German physicist, Julius Plücker. Plücker was the first to observe glass fluorescence (green in glass of British manufacture and blue in German glass) in the tubes opposite one of the electrodes. With his student, Johann Wilhelm Hittorf, Plücker discovered that the diffuse light emanating from the cathode could be concentrated with the use of a magnet.

Hittorf made tubes with a much higher vacuum to identify the source of Faraday's "radiant matter." By designing an L-shaped tube and noting that the electrical discharge always occurred in the arm with the negative electrode, Hittorf identified the cathode as the source of the phenomenon. By placing a screen in the path of the ray and observing the resulting shadow on the phosphorescent spot, Hittorf concluded that the light from the cathode of a vacuum tube moved in straight lines. He also showed that the rays produced heat and caused fluorescence at the point where they impinged on the glass of the tube. A few years later, Eugen Goldstein, a German physicist, used the term *cathode ray* to describe the colored stream visible between the terminals of electrically excited vacuum tubes.

Sir William Crookes, who discovered the element thallium, was fascinated by Faraday's hypothesis and designed a wide variety of vacuum tubes containing various terminals and interior devices for demonstrating the properties of "radiant matter." He succeeded in developing tubes of high vacuum and employed an induction coil to supply a controllable current. Crookes showed that as soon as matter entered into the fourth or "ultra-gaseous state," entirely new phenomena were produced. In contrast to Hittorf, who published his results with great modesty in somewhat inaccessible journals and whose books were very technical and dry, Crookes was a brilliant writer, demonstrator, and lecturer. He was successful in conveying his information about the cathode rays to a great many scientists and thus is generally given credit for some observations that had really been made years before by Hittorf. Consequently, high vacuum tubes became known as "Crookes tubes."

The research work done by Crookes on the cathode ray established a

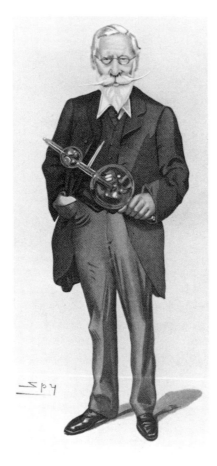

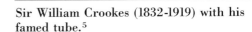

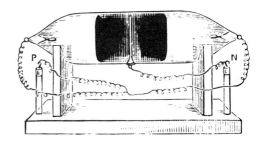

Crookes tube demonstrating the "Faraday dark space."[7]

number of its properties. Although in ordinary air it required a potential difference of nearly a million volts to penetrate an air gap a foot in length, the voltage needed to penetrate an equivalent length of partially exhausted space in a long vacuum tube was considerably reduced. Watching the continued process of exhaustion from such a tube, Crookes observed the beginning of a pale white light established between the electrodes within the tube ends. On further exhaustion, a purple quivering beam of light became visible, which with higher vacuum broadened into a misty crimson glow that ultimately filled the entire tube. Further evacuation, on the order of a millimeter of mercury or less, strengthened the light closer to the anode and somewhat away from the cathode, leaving a recognizably dark space first observed by Faraday and thus known as the "Faraday dark space." A bright violet-bluish glow clung to the cathode, which also developed the narrow dark space named after Crookes. Still further exhaustion caused the beam to break up into a number of striations and quivering disks of light. Beyond this state of vacuum, further withdrawal of gas increased the electrical resistance and diminished the glow and the gas particles to support it. Finally, all visible manifestations ceased.

A controversy had arisen regarding the true nature of the cathode rays. Crookes and his supporters, mostly English, maintained that they were emanations of particles. Most German experimenters were convinced that they were disturbances in the ether and that their character was similar to ultraviolet rays. In 1897, Sir Joseph John Thomson of Cambridge confirmed that cathode rays consisted of negatively charged particles (electrons), thereby confirming Crookes' position.

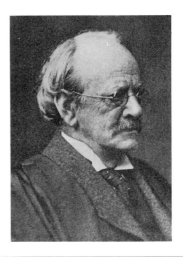

Joseph John Thomson (1856-1940).

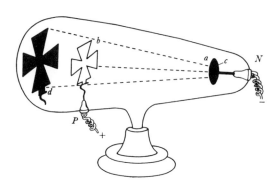

Demonstration by Crookes that cathode rays travel in straight lines. *a*, Cathode; *b*, aluminum cross and anode; *d*, dark shadow; *c*, phosphorescent image.[5]

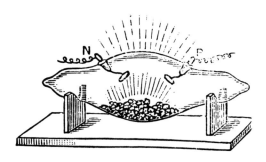

Crookes phosphorescent ruby pebble tube.[7]

When the negative terminal of the tube was attached to only one of two adjacent electrodes, the beam travelled parallel to the axis of the tube. When the negative terminal was connected to both electrodes, however, two parallel streams of radiant matter were energized and were seen to diverge, indicating that they represented two streams of electrified molecules rather than streams similar to wires carrying a current.

Crookes demonstrated that the light emanating perpendicularly from the cathode surface moved in straight lines regardless of the position of the anode. In tubes having a relatively low vacuum, the glowing bands would turn corners and enter side tubes to reach the anode. The phosphorescent or fluorescent glow was shown to result from impact with solid material in the ray's path. This impediment might be the wall of the tube itself or some other solid placed between the cathode and anode. In a classic experiment, Crookes placed a Maltese cross of mica in the ray's path. He energized the tube and showed, on the opposite side, the clear black shadow of the cross in the otherwise phosphorescent glow. Various chemical compounds and gems such as diamonds or rubies placed in the path of the rays glowed with distinct and vivid colors. The particulate nature of the rays was demonstrated in another experiment in which Crookes placed a delicate paddle wheel with vanes of transparent mica in a spherical tube. When current was applied across electrodes fastened to the outside of the tube, the wheel revolved; when the current was reversed, the wheel rotated in the reverse direction. The speed of revolution was in proportion to the intensity of the incident rays. That the rays generated heat was shown by concentrating them by means of a concave cathode on pieces of metal. Even refractory metals such as platinum were melted and fused by the intense heat. Finally, Crookes confirmed that the stream of cathode rays could be deflected by bringing a magnet close to their path.

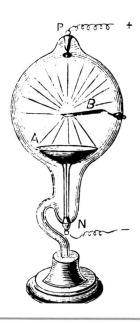

Demonstration by Crookes that cathode rays yield heat. The concave cathode (*A*) focuses the rays on a piece of metal (*B*), which heats to fluorescence.[7]

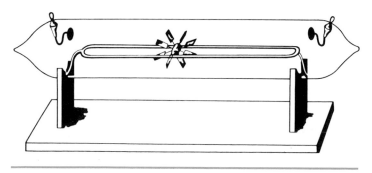

Crookes paddle wheel experiment.[7]

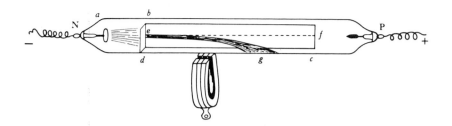

Demonstration by Crookes of the bending of cathode rays by a permanent magnet. *a*, Cathode; *b* to *d*, ray-defining aperture; *e* to *f*, path of undeflected beam; *e* to *g*, path of deflected beam.[7]

Crookes emphasized that the metallic electrodes in his series of experiments were all fastened to the outside of the glass tube and did not penetrate it. Other scientists had questioned whether the glass itself was not energized and particles torn from the glass sides and projected across the tube space. To counter this suggestion, Crookes painted a coat of yttria on the inside of the tube over the area covered by the silver negative electrode fastened to the outside of the tube. When energized, the tube demonstrated the characteristic dull blue of the lead glass but not the golden yellow of yttria. This proved that the glow was the radiant matter of the residual gaseous molecules and did not represent particles torn off from the negative electrode.

When using tubes with a vacuum raised to a millionth of an atmosphere, Crookes unknowingly was generating x-rays in more than sufficient quantity and penetration for practical diagnostic work. As he stated in his first lecture, "On Radiant Matter":

> This bulb is furnished with a negative pole in the form of a cup. The rays will, therefore, be projected to a focus on a piece of yttrial-platinum supported in the center of the tube.
>
> I first turn on the induction coil slightly so as not to bring out its full power. The focus is now playing on the metal, raising it to white heat . . . I increase the intensity of the spark. The yttrial-platinum glows with an almost insupportable brilliancy and at last melts.

This description perfectly depicts an x-ray tube in full action, pushed to the point of destruction as experienced by many early radiologists. Crookes also found photographic plates in unopened boxes that were strangely fogged and often blackened. When he complained to Ilford, the leading manufacturer of photographic plates, he was promptly sent replacements. After repeated fogging of each fresh supply, Ilford implied that the damage had occurred at the physicist's institute, since no other complaints had been received. Although Crookes could not appreciate the reason, it is now clear that these photographic effects were due to x-rays passing through the pasteboard boxes.

Yet Crookes was not the first to unknowingly produce x-rays. This distinction probably belongs to an Englishman, William Morgan, who in 1785 experimented to find if electricity would pass through a perfect vacuum. After forming such a vacuum by boiling the mercury of a Torricellian barometer to expel all the gases, Morgan demonstrated that electricity could not be forced through this vacuum. But in the course of one of his experiments, the glass tube cracked and began to admit air slowly. Morgan then observed a continuing succession of beautiful colors, beginning with yellowish-green and passing through blue and purple to red. He suggested that it might be possible to estimate the degree of a vacuum by determining the resultant color of the electrical discharge. After Roentgen's discovery, the identification of the yellow-green shade with x-rays made it clear that Morgan was the first to produce them.

James Clerk Maxwell (1831-1879).   Hermann von Helmholtz (1821-1894).   Heinrich Rudolf Hertz (1857-1894).

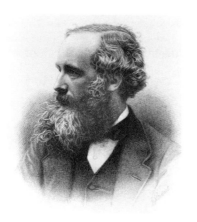 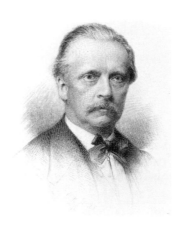 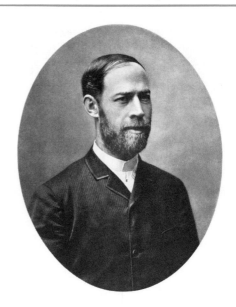

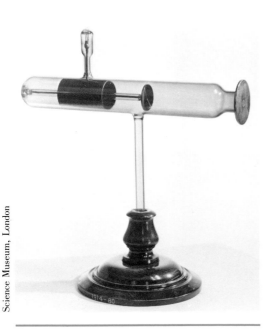

Lenard tube (1894). The tube has a perforated end piece over which gold leaf or aluminum foil could be fitted before the tube was evacuated.

At the same time that Crookes was discovering the properties of cathode rays and designing the tubes that would be used by Roentgen, a theoretical prediction of the existence of x-rays was being developed. James Clerk Maxwell, a Scottish physicist, interpreted Faraday's work in terms of higher mathematics to form the profound electromagnetic theory of light. Maxwell contended that any change of an electrical field results in an electric current with which magnetic effects are associated. In addition, he deduced that regular oscillations of electricity travel from any source of rapid and regular changes of electrical discharge with the velocity of light and with the same frequency. Maxwell's theoretical equations were experimentally substantiated 20 years later by Heinrich Rudolf Hertz, a German physicist, who constructed a receiving resonator with which he was able to detect oscillations from a specially constructed spark gap through the air anywhere in his laboratory. He observed that the receiving oscillator had the same frequency as that of the sender.

Maxwell's theories had strong influence on Hermann von Helmholtz, the mathematical discoverer of x-rays before their physical discovery by Roentgen. In his "dispersion theory of the spectrum," von Helmholtz allowed for x-rays and for radio waves, specifying their properties (including their power to pass through opaque material) years before either was known or named. This theory of von Helmholtz led two English physicists, Sir Oliver Lodge and Sir Joseph John Thomson, to conclude only 8 months after Roentgen's discovery (but 15 years before it was experimentally proven) that x-rays belonged to the short-wave end of the light spectrum.

Hertz was assigned by his teacher, von Helmholtz, the task of producing some of these unknown electromagnetic waves in his laboratory. In 1888, he discovered the wireless or radio waves. Hertz then turned to investigations of the electric discharge from evacuated tubes and made the important observation that the cathode rays could pass through a thin layer of aluminum placed within the tube. Hertz's pupil, Philipp Lenard, exploited his teacher's discoveries by constructing a vacuum tube with a thin (0.00265 cm) aluminum window sealed in the glass wall of the bulb at a point where the cathode rays were focused. Using a few particles of fluorescent potassium phosphate, Lenard could see that the cathode rays

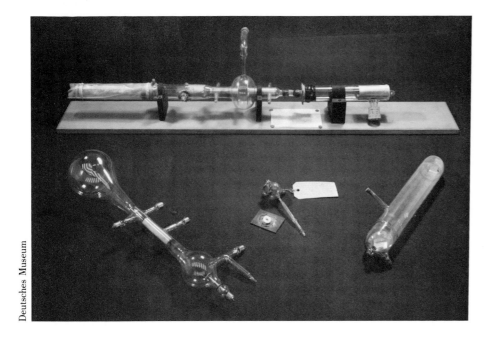

Deutsches Museum

Early cathode ray tubes. *Back*, Evacuated tube of Lenard for the first quantitative measurement of cathode rays (1893-1898). *Right*, Evacuated tube of Hertz for investigating the ability of cathode rays to pass through thin metal foils (1892). *Middle*, First tube of Lenard (1892). *Left*, Evacuated tube of Thomson for estimating the emission of cathode rays (1897).

not only penetrated through the window but also travelled several inches in the free air. Although the cathode rays were invisible, their effects could be studied with fluorescing substances such as phosphates and ketones. In addition, the cathode radiation could darken a photographic plate securely protected by a lightproof holder.

Lenard observed that the rays, which were propagated in straight lines within the tube, scattered in all directions like a diffuse fan once outside the window. From this he reasoned that molecules of air scattered the rays, which therefore must be extremely fine. Comparing the absorption of the cathode rays by different solids and gases, Lenard showed that the densest substances were the most absorbent, while the lightest substances were the most transparent. Lenard also developed an aluminum "ladder," which contained one to nine layers of aluminum foil (0.0014 mm thick), to analyze the penetration of various cathode ray beams. Such metal ladders were frequently employed for absorption measurements of x-rays after Roentgen's discovery.

Lenard did not realize that the cathode rays, after passing through the aluminum window, were mixed with an abundance of another kind of ray. He was unaware that he was making "x-ray pictures." Indeed, years later Lenard became embroiled in a bitter controversy as to whether he, rather than Roentgen, should be honored as the discoverer of x-rays (see Chapter 2).

All portraits in this chapter courtesy Eastman Kodak.

Bibliography

Crane AW: The research trail of the x-ray. Radiology 23:131-148, 1934.

References

1. Glasser O: Scientific forefathers of Röntgen. AJR 54:545-546, 1945.
2. Glasser O: The genealogy of the roentgen rays. I. AJR 30:180-200, 1933.
3. Crane AW: The research trail of the x-ray. Radiology 23:131-148, 1934.
4. Glasser O: The genealogy of the roentgen rays. II. AJR 30:349-367, 1934.
5. Dibner B: The new rays of Professor Röntgen. Norwalk, Conn, Burndy Library, 1963.
6. Pusey WA and Caldwell EW: The practical application of roentgen rays in therapeutics and diagnosis. Philadelphia, WB Saunders, 1904.
7. Lerch IA: The early history of radiological physics: A fourth state of matter. Med Phys 6:255-266, 1979.
8. Lenard P and Becker A: Handbuch der Experimental Physik. Leipzig, Akademische Verlagsgesellschaft MBH, 1927.
9. Brecher R and Brecher E: The rays: A history of radiology in the United States and Canada. Baltimore, Williams & Wilkins, 1969.

CHAPTER 2

Roentgen and the Discovery of X-Rays

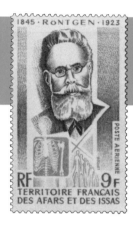

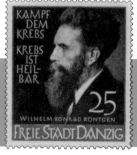

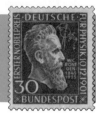

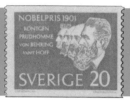

THE DISCOVERY

It was late afternoon on Friday, November 8, 1895. As was his custom and preference, Wilhelm Conrad Roentgen was working alone in his laboratory. He had recently repeated Lenard's experiments in which invisible cathode rays escaping from the thin aluminum window of an evacuated glass tube produced luminescent effects on certain fluoroscopic salts and darkened a photographic plate. It had occurred to Roentgen that if similar experiments were made with heavier-walled Hittorf-Crookes tubes without aluminum windows, the cathode rays might penetrate the glass directly and excite a cardboard screen painted with fluorescent barium platinocyanide. However, this effect might possibly be obscured by the strong luminescence of the tube itself. Taking a pear-shaped tube from the rack, Roentgen carefully covered it with pieces of black cardboard and then hooked the tube onto the electrodes of a Ruhmkorff coil. After darkening the room to test the opacity of the black paper cover, Roentgen started the induction coil and passed a high tension discharge through the tube. To his satisfaction, no light penetrated the cardboard cover.

As Roentgen was preparing to interrupt the current to set up the fluorescent screen for the crucial experiment, he suddenly noted a faint flickering glow shimmering on a small bench he knew was located nearby. It was as though a ray of light or a faint spark from the induction coil had been reflected by a mirror. Not believing this possible, Roentgen passed another series of charges through the tube and again the same fluorescence appeared, this time looking like faint green clouds moving in unison with the fluctuating discharges of the coil. Excitedly, Roentgen lit a match and to his great surprise discovered that the source of the mysterious light was the barium platinocyanide screen lying on the bench several feet away. He repeated the experiment again and again, continually moving the little screen further away from the tube. But each time the

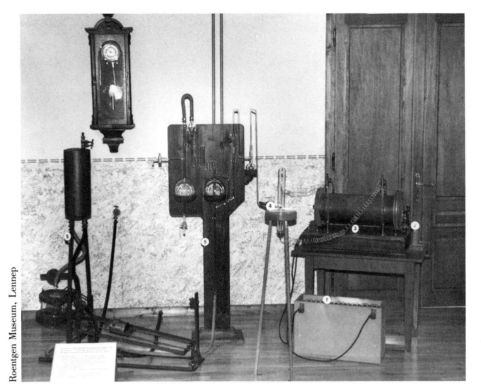

Roentgen Museum, Lennep

Reconstruction of the apparatus with which Roentgen discovered x-rays. *1*, Lead battery; *2*, mechanical interrupter (15 to 20 interruptions per second); *3*, Ruhmkorff spark inductor (200,000 windings, 40 to 60 kV); *4*, simple discharge tube; *5*, vacuum pump (evacuation time several hours to one day).

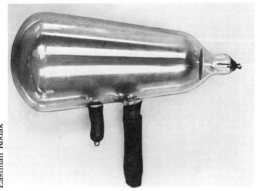

Eastman Kodak

Pear-shaped Hittorf-Crookes tube without aluminum windows used in Roentgen's initial experiments.

result was the same, and the glow persisted even when the painted surface of the fluorescent screen was turned in the opposite direction. After a careful search and eliminating all possibilities, there seemed to be only one explanation for the phenomenon. Something was emanating from the evacuated tube that produced an effect on the fluorescent screen at a much greater distance than he had ever observed in his cathode ray experiments, even when using Lenard tubes with their thin aluminum windows.

If this curious emanation could escape the lightproof cardboard box, perhaps it could penetrate other substances. To test the truth of this conjecture, Roentgen held a variety of objects between the tube and the screen and closed the switch to the inductor. Most showed little or no reduction in the intensity of the glowing screen. Only lead and platinum seemed to obstruct the rays completely. As he held the various materials between the tube and the fluorescent screen, Roentgen was amazed to visualize the ghostly shadow of the bones and soft tissues of his own fingers. The flesh was transparent, and the bones were fairly opaque.

How could he document these evanescent images wondrously appearing on the fluorescent screen? Fortunately, Roentgen remembered that cathode rays darkened a photographic emulsion. Therefore he replaced the fluorescent screen with a photographic plate and succeeded in producing an image using the vacuum tube as a light source. When he placed a piece of platinum on the plate before the exposure, a light area appeared on the developed plate where the platinum had absorbed the rays. It became clear to Roentgen that this was a new form of light, which was invisible to the eye and had never been observed or recorded. Thus x-rays were discovered and Radiology was born.

For the next 7 weeks, Roentgen remained secluded in his laboratory, concentrating entirely on a large number of carefully planned experi-

Deutsches Museum

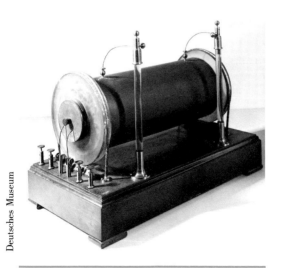

Ruhmkorff induction coil used in Roentgen's initial experiments.

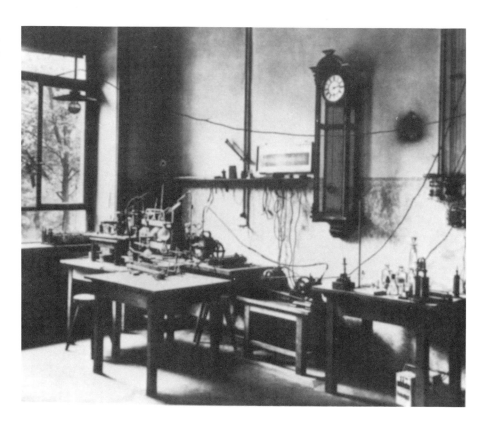

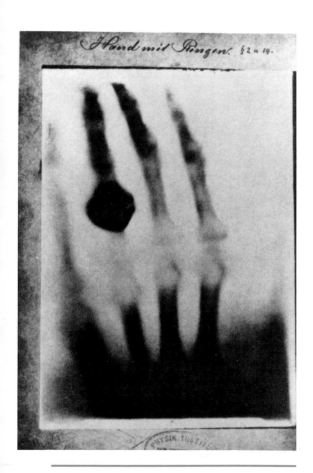

First Roentgen photograph of Mrs.
Roentgen's hand.[2]

ments. He was determined to continue his work in secret until he was certain of the validity of his observations and was confident enough to hand the results over to other scientists for confirmation or refutation. As his wife reported, Roentgen had his meals served in the laboratory and even had his bed moved there so that he could remain undisturbed and ready day or night to try out any new ideas that might come to him. Only once did he mention to one of his few good friends, Theodor Boveri, "I have discovered something interesting but I do not know whether or not my observations are correct."

Roentgen constructed a sheet metal cabinet about 7 feet high and 4 feet square at the base to have a permanent darkroom instead of draping his laboratory with ineffective blinds and curtains. Into one side of the zinc-walled chamber he inserted a circular aluminum sheet 1 mm thick and about 18 inches in diameter through which the new rays would pass. A zinc door on the side of the booth opposite the aluminum disk permitted his entry and exit. The vacuum tube was placed outside and focused on the disk's center. A lead plate was added to the zinc wall between the tube and himself. In this way, Roentgen effectively protected himself from the yet unknown harmful effects of radiation.

One evening, Roentgen persuaded his wife to be the subject for an experiment. He placed her hand on a cassette loaded with a photographic plate and made an exposure of 15 minutes. On the developed plate, the bones of her hand appeared light within the darker shadow of the surrounding flesh. Two rings on her finger had almost completely stopped the rays and were clearly visible. When he showed the picture to her, she could hardly believe that this bony hand was her own and shuddered at the thought that she was seeing her skeleton. To Mrs. Roentgen, as to many others later, this experience gave a vague premonition of death.

Roentgen's first communication. *Left*, First page of the hand-written manuscript (1895). *Middle*, First page of the published article on a new type of ray. *Right*, Front cover of reprint of the initial paper.

THE FIRST COMMUNICATION

After extensive experimentation, Roentgen was convinced that he was dealing with an entirely new kind of ray different from all others. Knowing that the announcement of such a discovery could not be long delayed, Roentgen prepared a short manuscript entitled "On a New Kind of Rays, a Preliminary Communication," which he handed to the secretary of the Würzburg Physical Medical Society on December 28, 1895. Since no meetings or lectures were to be given during the long Christmas vacation, Roentgen made the unusual request that the paper be published in the annals of the Society even before it had been presented at one of the meetings.

In this epochal announcement, which appeared in the last 10 pages of the 1895 volume, Roentgen reviewed his wealth of experimentation establishing the existence of these new "x-rays" (to distinguish them from other rays already known), as well as a perceptive description of their properties. He first described the generation of x-rays and stressed that the black envelope around the tube, which was opaque to visible light or to ultraviolet rays from the sun or from an electric arc, did not filter or reduce the effect of the rays on a fluorescent screen. Roentgen demonstrated that almost all materials were transparent to the x-ray, although in widely differing degrees. As he wrote, "Paper is very transparent: I observed that the fluorescent screen still glowed brightly behind a bound book of about 1,000 pages; the printer's ink had no noticeable effect. Likewise, fluorescence appeared behind a double pack of Whist cards; the eye can hardly detect a single card held between the apparatus and the screen." Similarly, a single sheet of tinfoil was hardly observable, and only the addition of several layers began to show a distinct shadow on the

Experiment using Roentgen's laboratory door. *Left,* Photograph of the laboratory door. *Right,* Corresponding radiograph shows the various thicknesses of stiles and panels, as well as streaks representing areas on which lead-based paint had been brushed.

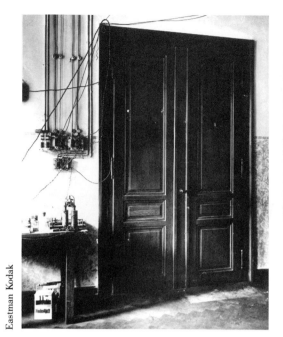

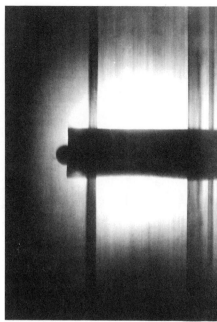

Eastman Kodak

Roentgen's request to tube makers in Erlangen to buy x-ray tubes at a lower price.

screen. Pine boards 3-cm thick remained partially transparent to the rays. The behavior of glass remained a special phenomenon because, although generally transparent to visible light, the amount of lead contained in the glass showed up markedly on the screen. Most dramatically, Roentgen described the stark image produced by the shadow of a hand with its relatively transparent fleshy parts and darker shadows of the bones.

Various substances—gases, liquids, or solids—were shown to be as transparent as air. Sheets of copper, silver, lead, gold, and platinum showed transparency of different degrees. Roentgen concluded that "the transparency of various substances assumed to be of equal thickness depends primarily upon their density" (that is, inversely as the molecular weight of the substance). Platinum and lead were the most opaque substances. Noting that 1.5-mm thick lead was practically opaque, Roentgen used this substance in his experimental work to show its contrast effect on photographic plates. For example, a stick of wood having a 20-mm square cross-section that had one side painted white with lead paint acted differently depending on how it was held between the glass tube and the screen. Although it had practically no effect when the direction of the x-rays was parallel to the surface, the stick showed as a dark streak on the plate when the painted face was turned across the beam.

Roentgen showed that barium platinocyanide was not the only substance that fluoresced when exposed to x-rays. He also listed calcium compounds, uranium glass, ordinary glass, calcite, and rock salt. He considered it fortunate that photographic dry plates were sensitive to x-rays, since "one is able to make a permanent record of many phenomena whereby deceptions are more easily avoided." Simply wrapping the photographic plate in heavy black paper or a routine holder enabled Roentgen to perform his experiments in daylight. However, it was no longer possible to leave wrapped photographic plates lying around the laboratory lest they be exposed to incidental x-rays that would spoil them.

Roentgen showed that the new rays were propagated in straight lines and that they were neither reflected nor refracted. He proved that the x-ray intensities followed the inverse square law relative to the distances between the screen and discharge apparatus.

A critical issue was to differentiate the new rays from the cathode rays described by Lenard. Roentgen showed that air (and most other substances) absorbed a much smaller portion of transmitted x-rays than cathode rays. The fluorescent glow from x-rays could be produced as far as 6 feet from the discharge tube, compared with only several inches for cathode rays. Unlike cathode rays, x-rays could not be deflected by a magnet, even in strong magnetic fields. Roentgen showed that the area on the wall of the discharge apparatus that showed the strongest fluorescence had to be considered the main point of emission of x-rays, which radiated in all directions. Thus the x-rays were arising from the area where previous investigators had determined the cathode rays impinged on the glass wall. If he deflected the cathode rays within the discharge apparatus by means of a magnet, he observed that the x-rays were now emitted from another area, namely from the new terminating point of the cathode rays. Therefore Roentgen concluded that "x-rays are not identical with cathode rays, but they are produced by the cathode rays in the glass wall of the discharge apparatus."

Roentgen also showed that the new rays were not ultraviolet rays, since they were not refracted in passing from air into various substances nor were they polarized. Because they formed shadows, fluoresced, and exerted chemical effects, Roentgen postulated that the new rays might be related to light and speculated that they might represent "longitudinal vibrations in the ether."

Roentgen then reviewed the various photographs taken with his apparatus to demonstrate the true "ray" character of the emanations. The most dramatic were photographs of the hand showing the bony structures and one made through his laboratory door that not only showed the varying thickness of stiles and panels but also several streaks representing areas on which lead-based paint had been brushed. Other radiographs showed a set of weights in a covered wooden box, the shadow of a wire wrapped around a wooden spool, and needle and degree markings of a compass in its enclosed metal case.

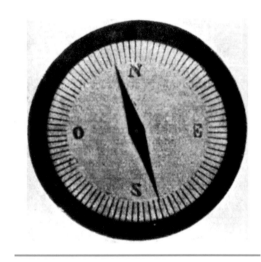

Early radiograph of a compass in which the magnetic needle is entirely enclosed by metal (Roentgen, 1895).[2]

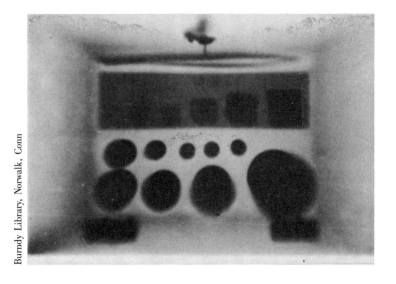

Early Roentgen radiograph. One of the first x-ray photographs sent by Roentgen to his colleagues to demonstrate the new ray was part of a set of metal weights contained in a closed wooden box. It bears the stamp of the Physical Institute of the University of Würzburg where the discovery was made.

To speed critical reading and evaluation of his work, even before news of the discovery was published, Roentgen sent copies of the article and examples of prints of the x-ray pictures he had taken to a number of well-known physicists, many of whom he knew as friends. Probably sensing that his days of peaceful relative obscurity were coming to an end, he exclaimed "Now the devil will be to pay!" to his wife after dropping the reprints in the mail.

NEWS OF THE DISCOVERY SPREADS

Professor Franz Šerafin Exner of Vienna, a friend of Roentgen's since their college days in Zurich, received one of the New Year's packets and showed the pictures to a small gathering of fellow scientists. One of those in attendance, Professor Ernst Lecher of Prague, asked Exner to lend him the prints until the next morning. Lecher, in turn, showed them at once to his father, Z. K. Lecher, who was then the editor of the Vienna *Presse*. Realizing the enormous news value in the story of the new rays, Lecher immediately prepared an elaborate article on the revolutionary discovery by the "Würzburg Professor" for the next morning edition. During the rush to meet his deadline, the editor misspelled Roentgen's name, and the discovery of "Routgen" echoed throughout the world. However, Lecher perceptively appreciated that "biologists and physicians, especially surgeons, will become interested in the Ray as it might open new trails for diagnostic purposes."[1]

The news was quickly copied by other European papers, and on the evening of January 6 it was cabled from London to all of the civilized countries of the world in the following words:

> The noise of war's alarm should not distract attention from the marvelous triumph of science which is reported from Vienna. It is announced that Prof. Routgen of the Würzburg University has discovered a light which for the purpose of photography will penetrate wood, flesh, cloth, and most other organic substances. The Professor has succeeded in photographing metal weights which were in a closed wooden case, also a man's hand which showed only the bones, the flesh being invisible.

Ironically, Roentgen's hometown paper first reported news of the sensational discovery on January 9. Compounding delay with inaccuracy, the Würzburg newspaper assumed that scientific societies met during the Christmas holidays and stated that Roentgen had first presented his discovery in a lecture.

The most astounding confusion concerning Roentgen's discovery was created by Thomas Smith Middleton, who in 1895 was a student at Würzburg University. When returning home to Chicago, he came up with this widely circulated fable:

> On the afternoon of April 29, 1895, Roentgen was suddenly called to the telephone while observing the fluorescence of a tube connected with a Ruhmkorff coil. Without disconnecting anything, he placed the loaded tube on a book which contained a key as page marker. A photographic cassette happened to lie underneath the book. On his return from the telephone, Roentgen disconnected the tube and spent the rest of the afternoon outdoors, photographing flowers. The following morning, while developing the plate, he noticed the radiograph of the key.

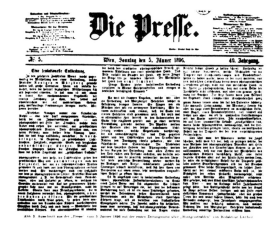

Photographic reproduction of the front page of "Die Presse" of January 5, 1896, reporting the discovery of x-ray by Professor Routgen.[1]

Thus April 30, 1895 was marked as the anniversary of the great discovery in Chicago and elsewhere where the imaginative public believed in the myth of the book and the key.

An appreciation of the potential medical use of the new rays could be found in the morning edition of the Frankfurter *Zeitung* on January 7:

> At the present time, we wish only to call attention to the importance this discovery would have in the diagnosis of diseases and injuries of bones, provided that the process can be developed technically so that not only the human hand can be photographed but that details of other bones may be shown without the flesh. The surgeon then could determine the extent of a complicated bone fracture without the manual examination which is so painful to the patient; he could find the position of a foreign body, such as a bullet or piece of shell, much more easily than has been possible heretofore and without any painful examinations with a probe. Such photographs also would be extremely valuable in diagnosing bone diseases which do not originate from an injury and would help to guide the way in therapy.

Almost overnight, Roentgen was

no longer a middle-aged Professor of Physics at the University of Würzburg but the focus of international praise, condemnation, and curiosity. From all over the world came letters of congratulation and incredulity as well as reports of duplication of the original experiments and a few of failures. To the Würzburg Institute were sent tubes of various construction and other equipment for the production of the rays. Through its modest doors passed scientists, reporters, the sympathetic, and the curious. The location of the Roentgen residence in the Institute left no escape from the heterogeneous horde that descended upon it. "Our domestic peace is gone," complained Mrs. Roentgen to a friend, and Roentgen was forced to adjust from the satisfying freedoms of a quiet private life to a tacit acceptance of public demands. Some visitors went so far as to filch x-ray photographs from the laboratory, and postcards with Roentgen's signature failed to reach their destination.[1]

"The light that never was." Report of Roentgen's discovery that appeared in the *St. Louis Post-Dispatch* on January 7, 1896.

Report of Roentgen's discovery hinting at its possible medical usage.

The response of scientists and laymen seemed completely out of proportion to the simple, unpretentious, rather dry style of the published communication. Unquestionably, if not for the many pictures of hands made quickly after the communication was published, which demonstrated the importance of the new rays in the study of anatomical structures and pathological changes, the discovery might have been consigned for some time to the relative oblivion of the physical laboratory.

Roentgen received 1,000 pieces of mail during the first week alone. Among these were several suggesting that there might be monetary gains in the proper exploitation of the new rays. Sometime later, Max Levy, an engineer in the German electric firm A.E.G., who had done some excellent work with x-rays, approached Roentgen regarding the firm's interest in the development of the rays. Roentgen answered him without hesitation: "According to the good tradition of the German university professors, I am of the opinion that their discoveries and inventions belong to humanity and that they should not in any way be hampered by patents, licenses, contracts, nor should they be controlled by any one group." The opposite point of view was taken by Thomas A. Edison, who freely admitted to the commercial exploitation of science for personal gain. He was quoted by an American newspaper as saying, "Professor Roentgen probably does not draw one dollar profit from his discovery. He belongs to those pure scientists who study for pleasure and love to delve into the secrets of nature. After they have discovered something wonderful, someone else must come to look at it from the commercial point of view. This will also be the case with Roentgen's discovery. One must see how to use it and how to profit by it financially."

Roentgen's communication was immediately translated into several languages. The newspaper speculations on the medical use of x-ray photographs, although seemingly unwarranted at first, led to innumerable experiments that offered unequivocal proof of the value of the new rays. Within 2 months, virtually all the major medical and nonmedical scientific journals printed x-ray illustrations and articles on the value of x-rays in medicine. In all of 1896, more than 1,000 papers relating to x-rays were published.

Roentgen detested the excessive publicity and complained that "on January 1st I sent out the offprints and then all hell broke loose!" He declared that "they blew the trumpet out of proportion." Roentgen especially disliked the sensationalization of radiography, which he considered only as a means to document his astounding fluoroscopic observations.

FIRST PUBLIC DEMONSTRATION

The first public demonstration of x-rays before a scientific body occurred on the evening of January 23, when Roentgen addressed the Würzburg Physical Medical Society before a large and crowded audience. Every seat in the auditorium was filled long before the meeting began, and Roentgen's appearance was greeted with a veritable storm of applause that was repeated several times during the presentation. With genuine modesty, Roentgen first gave credit to his predecessors in the investigation of cathode rays, mentioning Hertz, Lenard, and Crookes in particular. After a discussion of his experimental protocol and results and a demonstration of several radiographs, Roentgen invited a University colleague, the famed anatomist Albert von Kölliker, to have his hand photographed by the new rays. Von Kölliker eagerly complied, and a little later an excellent x-ray picture of his hand was shown to the audience amid tremendous

Letter written to Professor Röntgen informing him of his election to honorary membership in the Röntgen Society of Great Britain (1897).

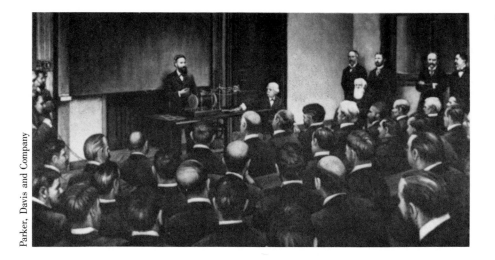

Parker, Davis and Company

Roentgen's first public demonstration of x-rays painted by Robert Alan Thom. In the painting, Roentgen speaks to the audience while Kölliker's hand is exposed to the rays.

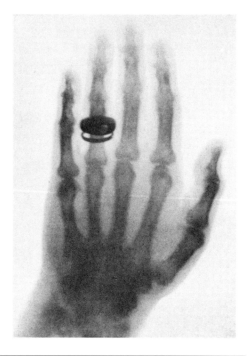

First x-ray made in public. The picture of the hand of the famed anatomist, von Kölliker, was made during Roentgen's initial lecture before the Würzburg Physical Medical Society on January 23, 1896.[2]

applause. The anatomist then noted that in his 48 years as a member of the Society, he had never attended a meeting with a presentation of greater significance, neither in the field of natural science nor in medicine. After leading the audience in three cheers for the discoverer, von Kölliker proposed that the new rays should henceforth be designated as "Röntgen's rays," and this proposal was approved by unanimous and enthusiastic applause. Although Roentgen lived 27 years longer, this was the only formal lecture he gave on the subject of the discovery of x-rays.

SECOND AND THIRD COMMUNICATIONS

Ten weeks after his initial paper, Roentgen issued his second "communication" (March 9, 1896). Roentgen observed that positively or negatively electrified bodies in air were discharged by x-rays. Replacing air by hydrogen or reducing the air pressure caused a corresponding reduction in the rate of discharge. He reported a scale for measuring the intensity of the rays by observing the degree of fluorescence on a screen or the intensity of blackening of a photographic plate. He recommended the insertion of a Tesla apparatus (condenser and transformer) between the vacuum tube and the induction coil. This arrangement generated less heat and maintained the vacuum for a longer period, produced a more intense penetrating beam, and could compensate for vacuum tubes that had been too much or too little exhausted.

Roentgen showed that glass and aluminum were not the only generating sources for x-rays. Any solid body could produce x-rays when cathode rays were directed on it. He noted that the amount of x-rays produced depended on the type and thickness of the material on which the cathode rays fell. The most intense x-rays were produced from a tube in which the cathode was an aluminum concave mirror and the anode a platinum sheet placed in the focus of the mirror but inclined at a 45-degree angle. Although x-rays emanated from the anode in this case, it made little difference in the intensity of the ray whether the emanations were from the anode or from another point.

The third and final communication by Roentgen, "Further Observations on the Property of the X-ray," appeared in May 1897. It was submitted to the Prussian Academy of Sciences in Berlin rather than the Würzburg Physical Medical Society to which the first two communications had been sent. In this work, Roentgen discussed x-ray diffraction and proceeded to an analysis of the eight variables that produced differ-

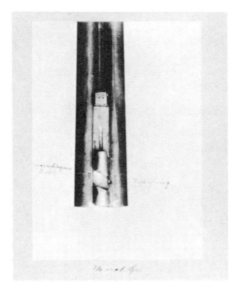 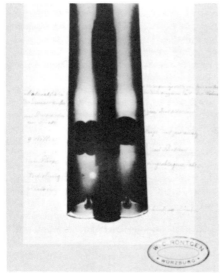

Roentgen's favorite gun. *Left*, X-ray picture of the double-barrel shotgun with marginal notes and the Institute's seal sent to some of Roentgen's friends. Note the shells with lead pellets and shot, primer, wadding, and powder in place. *Right*, Photographic picture shows the stamped bore and indent markings.[2]

ing intensities of x-ray brightness on a fluorescent screen. He noted that some tubes were more penetrating ("hard"), while others were weaker ("soft"). Roentgen explained how he selected among these various tubes the one best suited to the object to be photographed. For example, the bone structure of the hand was best imaged using a harder tube, whereas a soft tube was preferred for the fleshy parts. Roentgen observed the tendency of tubes to become harder with continued use, thereby indicating a continued self-exhaustion of the remaining gas particles. Using such a hard tube, Roentgen took a remarkable x-ray photograph of his favorite double-barreled hunting gun with cartridges in place. Not only were the internal parts of the cartridges visible, but even the construction and embossing details of the barrels could be seen. As the eminent British physicist, Silvanus P. Thompson, complained in a book written that year, "Roentgen had so thoroughly explored the new properties of the new rays by the time his discovery was announced, that there remained little for others to do beyond elaborating his work."

BIOGRAPHY

After the news of Roentgen's discovery had been published, the general public wanted to know more about the man himself. The first newspaper accounts were meager and inaccurate. Because news of the discovery came from Vienna, it was erroneously reported that Roentgen was an Austrian professor. Soon, however, enterprising reporters were able to find out more about his personal affairs and were able to present their readers with good biographies of the great scientist.

Wilhelm Conrad Roentgen was born on March 27, 1845, in Lennep, a small town on the Lower Rhine in the heart of the industrial Ruhr Valley of Germany. He was the only child of Friederich Conrad Roentgen, a manufacturer and textile merchant, and Charlotte Constance Frowein, his father's first cousin who came from a Dutch family well known in industrial and shipping circles. When Wilhelm was 3 years old, the Roentgens moved to Apeldoorn in Holland, about 100 miles to the northwest, where Charlotte's parents made their home. As the only child of a conservative and well-to-do merchant, Wilhelm had a pleasant childhood and was certainly indulged if not spoiled. His initial schooling was erratic, and at

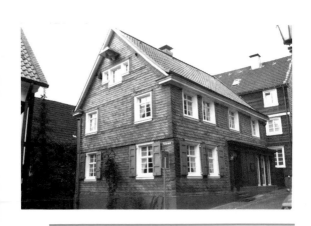

Roentgen's birthplace in Lennep.[2]

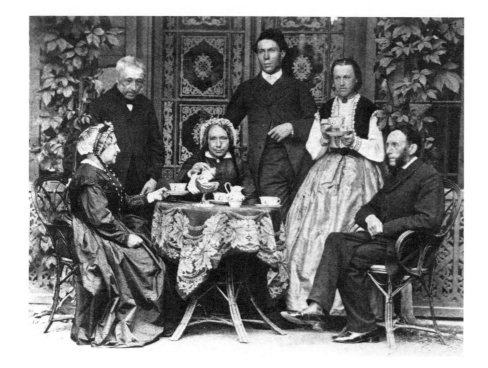

Roentgen with his parents and other relatives.[2]

age 17 he began his studies at the Utrecht Technical School. This institution prepared its students in 2 years for entrance into a technical high school but did not fill the prerequisites for matriculation to a university. Although only an average student, Roentgen was progressing satisfactorily until a harmless student prank got him into trouble. Unwilling to divulge the name of a fellow student who drew a caricature of an unpopular teacher, Wilhelm took the blame and was expelled from the school.

When the unfortunate incident in the Utrecht school promised to be serious enough to interrupt Wilhelm's education, his father attempted to obtain permission for a private examination that would give his son credentials to enter a college. After many months, this permission was finally granted, and for almost a year Wilhelm prepared for the examination. Unfortunately, on the day before the examination the examiner, who was sympathetic toward Wilhelm, became ill and was replaced by a teacher who had taken part in the former suspension proceedings. With this handicap, Wilhelm failed the examination. Again, his path to a university had been blocked.

Wilhelm and his parents had almost become resigned to his seeming inability to adjust to the requirements of the Dutch educational system and to obtain the credentials necessary to become a regular university student. Luckily, a Swiss friend living in Utrecht informed them that the Polytechnical School in Zurich would accept students lacking the usual credentials if they could pass a stiff entrance examination. Thus Wilhelm began classes in Zurich in November, 1865, and received his diploma as a mechanical engineer 2½ years later. Ironically, Roentgen had only a single course in physics, given by Rudolf Clausius, the father of thermodynamics.

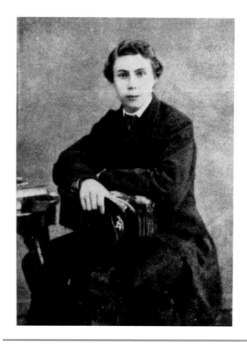

Roentgen as a young student.[2]

Of all the professors who helped shape Roentgen's mind during these formative years, the one who proved to be of greatest influence was August Kundt, a brilliant experimental physicist who succeeded Clausius in the Chair of Physics at the Polytechnical School. Roentgen remained in Kundt's laboratory after graduation and began physical experiments on various properties of gases. After 1 year he submitted his thesis to the University of Zurich, housed in the same building as the Polytechnical School, and on June 22, 1869, Roentgen obtained his doctorate in philosophy from that University.

Roentgen (*right*) and college friends.[2]

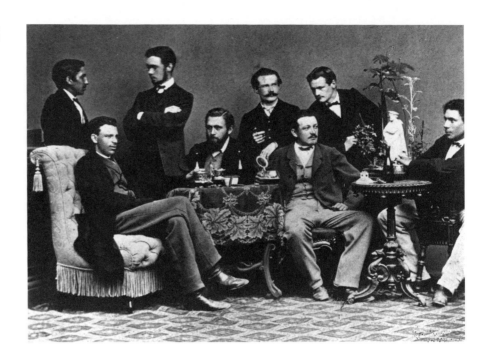

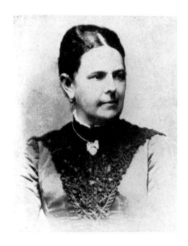

Anna Bertha Ludwig Roentgen
(1839-1919).[2]

While living in Zurich, Roentgen often visited a popular student cafe run by Johann Gottfried Ludwig, a former student at the University of Jena who had fled from Germany in the 1830s during a revolutionary uprising. He fell in love with Ludwig's daughter, Anna Bertha, who was 6 years older and "a tall slender girl of extraordinary charm." Although his parents, who were anxious to see him married to the daughter of some prominent and wealthy family, expressed some disappointment, Wilhelm and Bertha married on July 7, 1872.

When Kundt moved to the University of Würzburg in Germany, he invited Roentgen to become his assistant. However, once again Roentgen was held back by his inadequate formal education. Before he could be appointed to a salaried position on the faculty, it was necessary that Roentgen climb the first step of the academic ladder and be appointed a "privat-dozent," or unpaid lecturer recognized by the University. Lacking the high school matriculation degree, as well as satisfactory training in the classical languages, Roentgen was prevented by the strict traditions of the old institution from getting this initial academic title. Fortunately, this disappointment was short lived, for 2 years later both Kundt and Roentgen accepted appointments to the faculty of the newly established University of Strasbourg. After 2 years of hard work, Roentgen was appointed a privat-dozent and the stage was now set for an unimpeded academic career.

During the 7 years that he spent at Strasbourg, Roentgen investigated a wide variety of problems in physics. These included the determination of specific heats, electrical discharges, the sun's radiation, telephonic improvements, electromagnetic rotation, and the properties of crystals.

Roentgen's work began to appear in publications and to attract interest in the rapidly expanding field of physics. In 1879, he was invited to become Professor of Physics at the University of Giessen in Hesse, an important post that he accepted when only 34 years old. While at Giessen, Roentgen intensified his research on electromagnetic and gas phenomena, on pyroelectrical and piezoelectrical properties of crystals, and on surface phenomena of liquids. He also undertook an extensive investi-

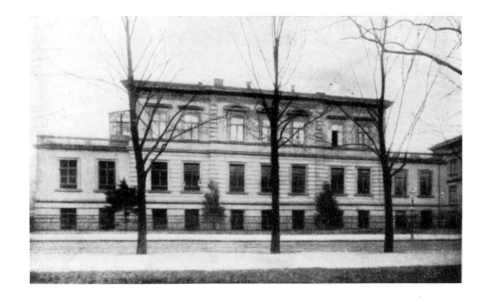

gation of the "Rowland effect," named for the American, Henry Rowland, who had shown that a charged body in motion produced a magnetic field similar to that generated by an electric current in a conductor. Roentgen proved that when a dielectric is moved between two electrically charged condenser plates, magnetic effects result. He later considered this demonstration of the "Roentgen current" as having an importance equal to that of his discovery of x-rays.

On October 1, 1888, Roentgen was offered the prestigious post as Professor of Physics and Director of the new Physical Institute of the University of Würzburg. Unlike his old, meagerly equipped laboratory at the University where he had begun work 16 years before as a newlywed, the new Physical Institute on the broad, tree-lined Pleicher Ring had two spacious floors, a basement, and a lecture room. The second floor comprised the private residential quarters of the Director of the Institute and had ample room for a conservatory, much to Mrs. Roentgen's delight. One can only imagine Roentgen's feeling of triumph on assuming the Chair of Physics at the same university that had previously refused to give him an academic title.

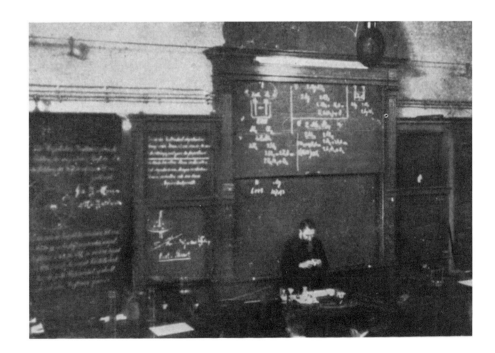

Roentgen lecturing in Würzburg.[2]

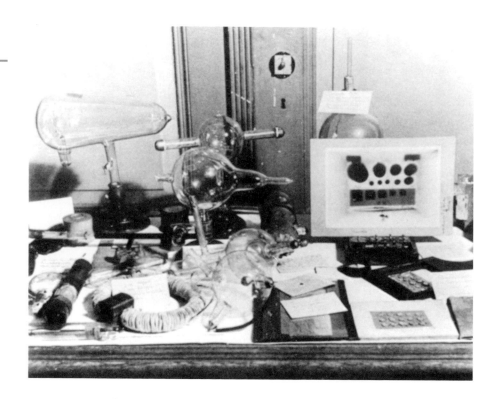

Roentgen's laboratory apparatus. Crookes tube (*left background*), several Hittorf tubes (*center*), and a glass jar for ionization of air with the classic print of a box of weights standing against it. There are prisms along the right edge with masks of lead and aluminum in the *right foreground*. In the *left foreground* at the edge is an "absolutely evacuated" tube (Roentgen used many of these) with an electromagnet beside it.[5]

At Würzburg, Roentgen obtained important results in studies on the influence of pressure on various physical properties of solids and liquids. He investigated the compressibility of many liquids, notably ether and alcohol, and continued studies of the effect of pressure on the dielectric constants of water and ethyl alcohol. He examined the refractive indexes of these liquids and the conductivity of various electrolytes.

In 1894, Roentgen became Rector of the University of Würzburg. In his inaugural address, he repeated the words of Professor Athanasius Kircher, one of his predecessors in the Chair of Physics and Philosophy, who had stated more than 2 centuries before, "Nature often reveals the most astonishing phenomena by the simplest means, but these phenomena can only be recognized by persons who have sharp judgment and the investigative spirit, and who have learned to obtain information from experience, the teacher of all things." Little did Roentgen realize that in less than a year these words would apply to him.

By October, 1895, Roentgen found his entire attention captivated by the work of Hittorf, Crookes, Hertz, and Lenard on cathode rays. He had already repeated some of Lenard's original experiments, notably his observations on the effects produced by cathode rays in free air and hydrogen. Although at first he used Lenard's aluminum-window tube, Roentgen found that he could obtain the same results with ordinary tubes, which he preferred since flaws in the thin aluminum window tended to weaken the vacuum in the Lenard tube. By now totally absorbed by this field that challenged the most competent experimental talent, Roentgen decided to drop further studies on the influence of pressure on dielectric constants of various liquids and to devote himself exclusively to research on cathode rays.

Following Roentgen's discovery of x-rays, numerous decorations and special honors poured in from all over the world. Among the most outstanding ones were the gold Rumford medal from the Royal Society in London, the Elliot-Cresson medal of the Franklin Institute in Philadelphia, and the Barnard medal awarded by Columbia University at the recommendation of the American Academy of Sciences. In 1901, Roent-

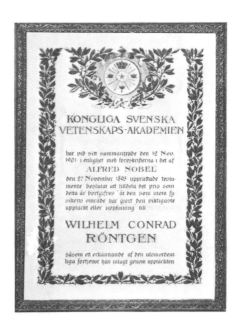

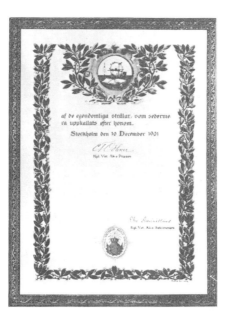

First Nobel Prize for Physics, presented to Roentgen in 1901.[2]

gen became the first recipient of the Nobel Prize for Physics. Contrary to his usual rule of not personally attending the awarding of an honor, Roentgen travelled to Stockholm to receive the diploma, gold medal, and prize from the hands of the Swedish Crown Prince in a ceremony at the Music Academy. He declined to give an official Nobel lecture, but at the impressive supper after the ceremony he spoke a few words of appreciation for the honor and said that this recognition would stimulate him to continue scientific research that might prove of benefit to humanity. Roentgen gave the prize money (50,000 kroner) to support scientific research at the University of Würzburg, the site of his immortal discovery.

Roentgen was summoned by the German Emperor to demonstrate the new ray at the imperial palace. The Prince Regent awarded him the Royal Order of Merit of the Bavarian Crown, which carried with it not only the honor and decoration but also personal nobility. Roentgen accepted the

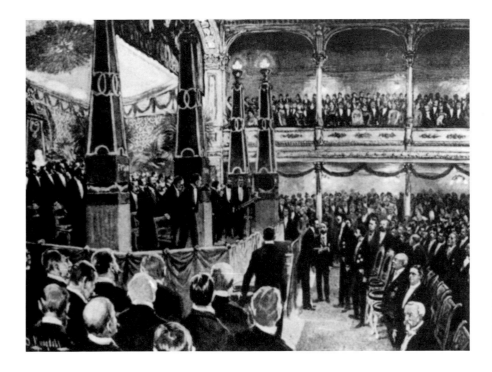

Nobel ceremony in the Great Hall of the Academy of Music, Stockholm, on December 10, 1901. Roentgen is receiving his prize from the hands of the Swedish Crown Prince.[6]

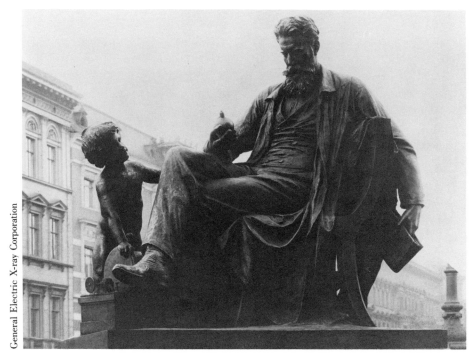

General Electric X-ray Corporation

Burndy Library, Norwalk. Conn

Photograph of Roentgen taken in 1906
while he was director of the Institute of
Physics at the University of Munich.

decoration but declined the status of nobility. He also declined to use the coveted "von," a symbol of status in a most status-conscious nation. Busts and monuments were erected in Roentgen's honor, and even a statue on the Potsdam Bridge in Berlin. Roentgen's portrait could be found on special stamps in various lands and on German currency.

In 1900, at the special request of the Bavarian government, Roentgen agreed to become Professor of Physics at the University of Munich and Director of the new Physics Institute. He resumed his research on the physical properties of crystals, their electrical conductivity, and radiation influences on them. The outbreak of World War I and the ultimate defeat of Germany affected Roentgen deeply. Strong national feelings convinced Roentgen to turn in his gold decorations (including the Rumford medal) when the call for gold was made to continue the war effort. Roentgen even was persuaded by some patriotic colleagues to sign a proclamation of 93 intellectuals in an "appeal to the civilized world" not to believe the reports of German excesses during the war. Later, in his older and calmer years, he regretted both of these actions.

In October, 1919, Roentgen's beloved wife Bertha died after a prolonged illness. The memory of their wonderful companionship for almost 50 years intensified Roentgen's loss, and in his loneliness he would read important news items to her picture and pretend that she still shared his thoughts.

Roentgen retired from his post as Professor of Physics early in 1920, but two laboratory rooms were set aside for his continued use. Three years later, at age 78, Roentgen was still able to walk to the laboratory to eagerly complete some experimental investigations that he had begun some months earlier. However, he complained that walking was becoming more difficult and that his sight and hearing were proving inadequate for the observations required. On February 10, 1923, the discoverer of x-rays died in Munich.

The funeral cortege assembled prominent scientists from all parts of Germany and neighboring countries, who came to pay their respects to a great fellow researcher and benefactor of mankind. Then, in accordance with his will, his body was cremated and his papers and personal correspondence also given to the flames.

Among the many eulogies was one by Rudolph Grashey, a pioneer radiologist, who stated[3]:

An angel from heaven presented the wonderful new ray to the scientists. Medicine has received the lion's share of his discovery. Nature manifests itself in such a way only to those who, through restless exploring, have developed an instinct for its intricacies and laws . . .
Nobody could have been more dignified, predestined to receive this present from nature. Life has given him much, but more than he has received he has given us. A spark of his mind has kindled a light which illuminated dark trails of science. Immortal is his work, immortal his name.

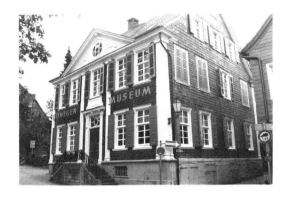

Roentgen Museum in Lennep.

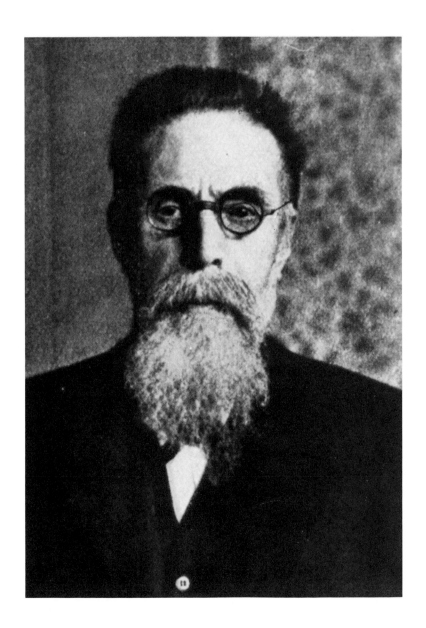

Roentgen a few weeks before he died.[2]

39

PRIORITY CLAIMS

Was Roentgen the first to produce x-rays? As with all major discoveries, a number of often vociferous scientists came forward to claim priority in having observed the penetrating rays.

The first x-ray picture was actually produced almost 6 years before Roentgen's discovery. After an experimental session testing electrical sparks and brush discharges as photographic light sources, Professor Arthur W. Goodspeed began demonstrating the properties of a Crookes cathode ray tube to William Jennings, a photographer. Next to the tube, Jennings had stacked several unexposed photographic plates, on top of which were two coins, reportedly his fare for the Woodland Avenue trolley. When Jennings later developed the plates, some were mysteriously fogged and one contained two dark round disks, as well as the usual tracing of the electrical sparks on the negative. This curious shadowgraph could not be explained, and so the plates were filed away and forgotten for nearly 6 years. Only after Roentgen's discovery did the men recreate the setting of that February night and grasp the magnitude of the observation that they had failed to make. Although he claimed "no credit for the interesting accident," Goodspeed maintained that "without doubt, the first Roentgen picture was produced on February 22, 1890 . . . (at) the University of Pennsylvania."[7]

In 1890, Ludwig Zehnder, Roentgen's assistant at Würzburg, was using black cloth to cover a vacuum tube and thus eliminate the disturbing light emanating from the cathode. In this way, he hoped to detect fluorescence of the screen, not only nearby but also at some distance from the tube. When Zehnder turned the current on, he noticed a momentary flash where the remote screen was lying, but the tube was immediately punctured. Zehnder felt terribly upset and was willing to replace the tube at his own expense. Roentgen, however, consoled his friend with the prophetic remark that "many more tubes will have to be punctured before all their mysteries are solved." After the discovery of x-rays, Zehnder recalled the incident and that he had noticed the instantaneous glow from the nearby fluorescent screen. However, Zehnder never made a priority claim and remained a loyal friend of Roentgen for the rest of his life.[8]

First x-ray shadow picture. Taken by accident by Arthur W. Goodspeed at the University of Pennsylvania on February 22, 1890.

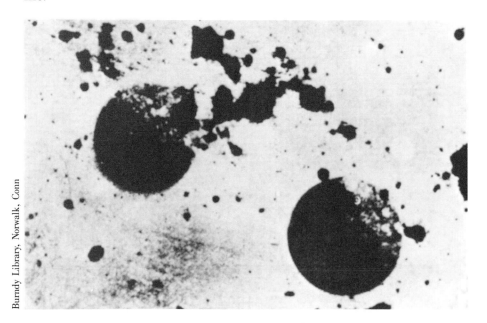

A number of scientists working with electrical discharges through evacuated glass tubes had in all likelihood produced x-rays. Crookes (see Chapter 1), Jackson, Hittorf, Goldstein, and Lenard had observed the fluorescent glow in materials located near their tubes. However, none had properly recognized or identified the nature or source of the fluorescence, let alone reproduced the phenomenon with full awareness and command. As one of the earliest investigators of x-rays, Max Levy of Berlin, reminisced later, "I have no doubt that x-rays were seen in laboratories even before Roentgen's time, but they were not recognized as such by the investigators. The credit due Roentgen is not decreased but is considerably increased by this fact because his genius discovered the significance of a thing which others had seen but did not recognize."

The most bitter contender for the credit given Roentgen was Philipp Lenard. Lenard initially respected and admired Roentgen and sent him a letter congratulating Roentgen on "your great discovery."[9] In turn, Roentgen acknowledged the work of Lenard and his teacher Hertz in his Würzburg lecture. Roentgen and Lenard even shared two prestigious prizes, in Vienna in 1896 and in Paris a year later.

Lenard's unquenchable animosity began when Roentgen alone was awarded the first Nobel Prize in Physics in 1901. Lenard felt not only disappointed but actually betrayed, for he was certain that he would share the prize. Consequently, Lenard proclaimed himself the true discoverer of the x-ray.

The real story of the Nobel decision was kept secret for almost 70 years, until the transcripts of the many meetings were made available to the public. A Board of Members of the Swedish Academy of Sciences was empowered to make the selection. A special Advisory Committee of five leading Swedish physicists (headed by Svante Arrhenius and Anders Ångström) was also appointed. Physicists in different parts of the world were invited to submit names for the prize. Among these physicists was Roentgen himself, who suggested Lord Kelvin of Edinburgh.

When the time for nominations had expired, 29 proposals had been submitted. Of these, 12 suggested Roentgen, one Lenard, and five recommended a division of the Prize between these two scientists. The Advisory Committee recommended that the Prize be divided equally between Roentgen and Lenard. Nevertheless, the Academy in full session disregarded the recommendation of the Advisory Committee. They decided against sharing the Prize, since the late Nobel had specified that it be given only to the most distinguished scientist of the year. The decision was unanimous in favor of Roentgen.[10]

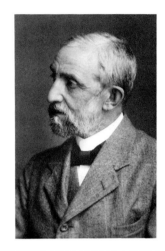

Philipp Lenard (1862-1947).[9]

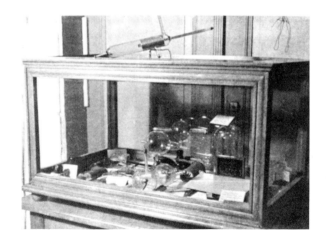

The cabinet in Roentgen's library in the Physical Institute of the University of Würzburg, containing the historical collection. The original and only Lenard tube with which he experimented is shown outside the case, so placed by the Physics Faculty as symbolic of the fact that it was not essential in Roentgen's discovery.[9]

Even after being awarded his own Nobel Prize in 1905, Lenard's animosity continued unabated. Among his statements downgrading Roentgen's efforts while glorifying his own are the following[9]:

A comparison can best make clear to the neutral observer Roentgen's role in the discovery. I shall make this striking comparison here because it may throw a light on the even now widespread historical confusion and untruth! Roentgen was the midwife at the birth of the discovery. This helper had the good fortune to be able to present the child first. She can only be confused with the mother by the uninformed who knows as little about the procedure of the discovery and the preceding facts as children of the stork.

I am the mother of the x-rays. Just as a midwife is not responsible for the mechanism of birth, so is Roentgen not responsible for the discovery of x-rays, which merely fell into his lap. All Roentgen had to do was push a button, since all the groundwork had been prepared by me.

In effect, Lenard claimed that anybody could have discovered x-rays after *his* (Lenard's) work on cathode rays. However, Lenard never gave a satisfactory explanation as to why he himself had not accomplished this task. Also, he never mentioned that the so-called Lenard tube was actually based on Hertz's work.

Roentgen took all these insinuations philosophically and contended it was beneath his dignity to react publicly. To his friend, Zehnder, he wrote: "Well, dear heaven, the envious are never lacking when something occurs as with me. That is always the case."[8]

Lenard's unbridled hatred of Roentgen climaxed during the time of his lofty and commanding position in the Nazi hierarchy of scientists. In his four-volume work on German physics, there is no mention of Roentgen (or Einstein) in the text, but the foreword is a lengthy diatribe against the Jews. The implication, drawn by many persons in Germany, was that Roentgen was a Jew. In answer to a direct query from the American radiologist, Lewis E. Etter, "Was Roentgen a Jew?," Lenard replied, "No, but he was friend of Jews and acted like one."[9]

It is interesting to note that at the time of the fiftieth anniversary of Roentgen's discovery, the Physical Medical Society of Würzburg applied to the Nazi Minister of Post and Telegraph to have a memorial stamp made for Roentgen similar to the ones issued for Robert Koch and other scientists. But it so happened that the minister (Ohensorg) had been a physicist and student of Lenard's at Heidelberg. He rejected the request saying the proposal was not in order, since such an honor was reserved "only for the illustrious."[9]

Bibliography

Dibner B: The new rays of Professor Röntgen. Norwalk, Conn, Burndy Library, 1963.

Glasser O: Wilhelm Conrad Röntgen and the early history of the roentgen rays. Springfield, Ill, Charles C Thomas, 1933.

Glasser O: Dr. W. C. Röntgen. Springfield, Ill, Charles C Thomas, 1958.

References

1. Kraft E and Finby N: Beginning of radiology in 1896: First newspaper report of discovery of x-ray. NY State J Med 81:805-806, 1981.

2. Glasser O: Wilhelm Conrad Röntgen and the early history of the roentgen rays. Springfield, Ill, Charles C Thomas, 1933.

3. Kaye GWC: Roentgenology: Its early history. New York, Hoeber, 1928.

4. Kraft E and Finby N: Wilhelm Conrad Röntgen (1845-1923): Discoverer of x-ray. NY State J Med 74:2066-2070, 1974.

5. Etter LE: Post-war visit to Röntgen's laboratory. AJR 54:547-552, 1945.

6. Knutsson F: Röntgen and the Nobel Prize. Acta Radiol 8:449-460, 1969.

7. Brecher R and Brecher E: The rays: A history of radiology in the United States and Canada. Baltimore, Williams & Wilkins, 1969.

8. Kraft E: W. C. Roentgen: His friendship with Ludwig Zehnder. NY State J Med 73:1002-1008, 1973.

9. Etter LE: Some historical data relating to the discovery of the roentgen rays. AJR 56:220-231, 1946.

10. Knutsson F: Röntgen and the Nobel prize: The discussion at the Royal Swedish Academy of Sciences in Stockholm in 1901. Acta Radiol (Diagn) 15:465-473, 1974.

CHAPTER 3

Marie and Pierre Curie and the Discovery of Radium

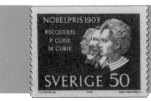
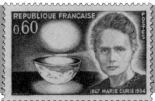
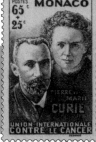
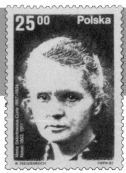

Soon after Roentgen's discovery of x-rays, several scientists observed that the multicolored fluorescence of the glass walls of vacuum tubes caused by the impact of the cathode rays indicated the spot where the energy of the cathode rays was transformed into x-rays. The French scientist, Jules-Henri Poincaré, suggested that since the fluorescence of the glass apparently was a necessary condition for the formation of x-rays, it might be worthwhile to investigate whether rays similar to x-rays could also be produced by ordinary fluorescent or phosphorescent substances. Antoine-Henri Becquerel, professor of physics at the Polytechnical School in Paris, followed Poincaré's suggestion and began to experiment with uranium salts, especially the double sulfates of uranium and potassium that were known to be highly fluorescent. Employing a method similar to that used to detect x-rays, Becquerel put the uranium compounds into small metal trays of aluminum or copper and then placed the trays on a photographic plate that was protected from any direct light by several wrappings of black paper. After he exposed the uranium compounds to sunlight for several hours to produce strong and prolonged phosphorescence, the photographic plate was developed. Dark spots seen on the plate correlated with the position of the uranium salts. At first, Becquerel concluded that the radiation that had passed through the paper wrapping and affected the photographic plate was due to the phosphorescence produced by solar energy. However, a few days later a spell of inclement weather led Becquerel to the correct interpretation. In late February, 1896, Becquerel prepared to repeat and expand his experiments. However, the sky had become cloudy and dark. Unable to expose the photographic plates and trays with the uranium salts to sunlight, Becquerel instead placed them in a drawer for safekeeping. For several more days the sun failed to shine. Tired of waiting, on March 1 Becquerel decided to develop the plates before exposing them to sunlight. Knowing that the phosphorescent light from the uranium salts persisted for no more

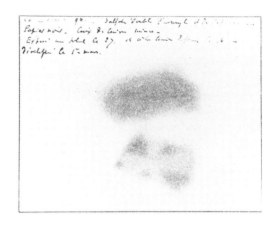

First autoradiograph indicating the discovery of radioactivity (March 1, 1896). Clear outline of a cross made of thin sheet-copper that had been placed on a photographic plate under a layer of uranium salt and kept in a dark drawer.[2]

than $\frac{1}{100}$ of a second after termination of exposure to light, Becquerel expected to find only weak darkening of the plates. However, he was amazed to find that the results were identical to his previous experiments. The dark spots representing the silhouetted images of the uranium salts on the photographic plates clearly indicated that the plates had been subjected to intense radiation that had been in progress while they were lying in the box. Becquerel concluded that neither sunlight, fluorescence, nor phosphorescence was necessary to produce this effect, which apparently came from the substance itself and was able to penetrate the bottom of the metal tray and darken the photographic plate. By repeating and extending his experiments, Becquerel discovered that these penetrating and invisible rays were emitted spontaneously and persistently from all uranium compounds, whether fluorescent or not, and even from metallic uranium itself. Like x-rays, the radiation emanating from uranium could not be reflected by mirrors nor refracted by prisms and could discharge an electroscope by ionizing the surrounding air even when it was placed a considerable distance from the radiant source. Unlike x-rays, this new radiation was a specific property of the atom itself and actually represented an entirely new and unexpected property of matter.

Becquerel presented his discovery the following evening at the weekly Monday meeting of the French Academy of Sciences and published his findings 10 days later in a paper entitled "On visible radiations emitted by phosphorescent bodies."

Becquerel's discovery excited the curiosity of many scientists. One was Marie Sklodowska, who was born in Warsaw, Poland, on November 7, 1867. The youngest daughter of two teachers, Marie demonstrated an early aptitude for mathematics. Unfortunately, Marie had to discontinue her studies as a teenager and take a position as a governess for 6 years so that her father could afford to send her eldest sister to the Sorbonne for medical training. Finally, in 1891, Marie joined her sister at the Sorbonne to study mathematics and physics. Although poverty stricken and in poor health, Marie received her master's degree in physics 2 years later, graduating first in her class; 1 year later, she graduated second with a master's degree in mathematics.

The major turning point in Marie's life came in 1894 when she met Pierre Curie, a physicist working at the Sorbonne. Born on May 15, 1859, Pierre was the son of a Paris physician. With his brother Jacques, Pierre

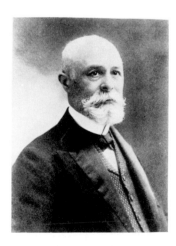

Antoine-Henri Becquerel (1852-1908).[1]

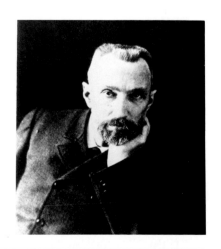

Marie Curie (1867-1934).[3]

Pierre Curie (1859-1906).[1]

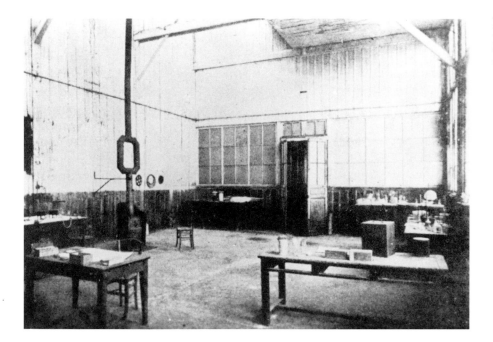

Interior of drafty and leaky shed at the School of Physics where radium was discovered.[1]

discovered piezoelectricity, a phenomenon in which certain types of crystals when compressed produce electrical charges on their surfaces. When voltage is applied to these crystals, they also change shape slightly. Pierre and Jacques constructed an electrometer that later was given the Curie name. After Jacques left for Montpelier, Pierre became an instructor at the School of Physics on the Rue Lhomond, where he organized the physics laboratory and instructed numerous pupils. Although he possessed no private laboratory and only meager equipment, Pierre achieved valuable scientific results, especially in studying the magnetic properties of crystals under various temperatures.

Pierre became acquainted with Marie when she requested permission to do some research in his laboratory. He quickly became attached to the young foreigner, who like himself was dedicated to science. On July 26, 1895, Marie and Pierre were married.

Three years after their marriage, Marie selected the topic of Becquerel's "spontaneous radioactivity" for her doctoral research. A major obstacle was to locate a place that would be suitable for Marie to carry out her experiments. After numerous unsuccessful attempts to acquire space at local laboratories, Marie was offered a small room in the basement of the municipal school where Pierre was now professor of physics. This drafty, leaky, floorless shack filled with old machinery was to be her second home for more than 4 years and the birthplace of immeasurably valuable discoveries.

Marie Curie's first task was to develop a method to accurately measure the intensity of the new rays. Because the photographic method was too imprecise, Marie decided to use the power of uranium rays to make air a conductor of electricity so as to discharge an electroscope. For this purpose, Marie used an ionization chamber and two devices invented by Pierre—a Curie electrometer and a piezoelectric quartz. Her initial experiments demonstrated that the intensity of the radiation was proportional to the amount of uranium, independent of the chemical structure in which the uranium was found and independent of outside conditions such as temperature and pressure.

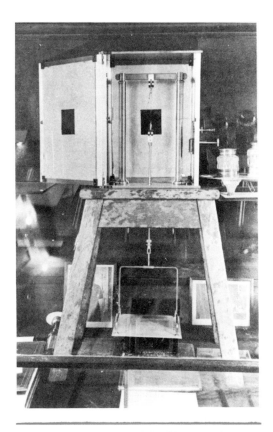

Piezoelectrometer used by Marie and Pierre Curie in their early work on radioactivity.[3]

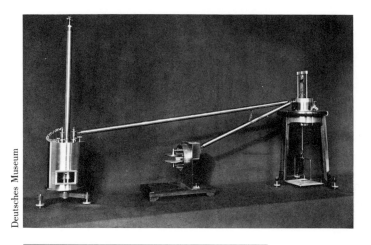

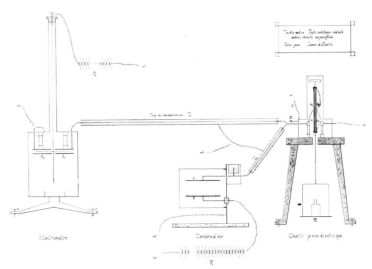

Complete apparatus for measuring radioactivity (Pierre and Marie Curie).
Left, Photograph and *right*, diagram of
(left to right) electrometer, condenser, and
quartz piezoelectric device.

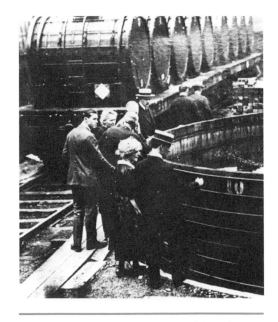

Separation of radium from pitchblende in
the early 1900s. Marie Curie is on the left.[5]

Marie's next step was to determine whether other substances emitted similar radiation. By studying virtually every element or compound of elements known at that time, she found that only thorium compounds had properties similar to those of uranium. As with uranium, the intensity of radiation emitted from thorium compounds was independent of their chemical form. Marie called the new form of energy seen in uranium and thorium *radioactivity.*

The radioactivity from a pure uranium compound was roughly proportional to its uranium content; that is, it was an atomic, not chemical, property. The one notable exception was a crude form of uranium oxide called *pitchblende*, which was far more radioactive than the pure oxide of uranium that could be extracted from it. Marie logically concluded that pitchblende must contain small quantities of some other substance that was much more radioactive than either uranium or thorium and that this substance could not be one of the known chemical elements (all of which she had already examined with her electrometer). According to the Curies' most pessimistic calculations, they thought that the new element should represent about 1% of pitchblende ore. In reality, the radioactive element they sought accounted for only one part in a million.

Joined by her husband, Marie carried out a systematic chemical analysis of pitchblende using such well-known chemical reactions and procedures as pulverization, precipitation, and fractional crystallization. Each separated portion of the ore was carefully examined for radioactivity using the electrometer. Large quantities of pitchblende had to be treated to obtain small traces of the radioactive material. The process of chemical analysis was tedious and complicated, since for each pound of pitchblende that was treated, they needed 5 pounds of chemicals and 25 liters of water. Eventually, a strong radioactive substance was found in association with the bismuth extract of the ore. Marie and Pierre Curie announced the discovery of this substance on July 18, 1898, in the *Proceedings of the Academy of Science:* "We believe the substance we have extracted from pitchblende contains a metal not yet observed, related to bismuth by its analytical properties. If the existence of this new metal is confirmed we propose to call it *polonium*, from the name of the original country of one of us."

Proceeding further with the chemical separation of the impurities in pitchblende, the Curies recognized a second substance that was strongly radioactive and entirely different from the first in its chemical properties. This highly radioactive substance, which emitted 2 million times as much radiation as uranium, was called *radium* and its discovery was announced in December, 1898.

Although the Curies did not doubt for a moment that they had discovered two new elements, polonium and radium, the French chemists were critical. Before these elements could be given official status, they would have to be separated into their pure forms and their atomic weights determined. Considering that 1 part of radium is found in about 4 million parts of pitchblende (25 pounds of ore to extract ⅟₁₀₀₀ of a gram of radium), it was clear that isolation of the element required huge quantities of the crude ore. The Curies were faced with three agonizing problems—lack of sufficient amounts of suitable ore, lack of adequate working space, and lack of funds to continue their work.

The only uranium mine at that time was Austrian state property and located in Joachimstal, Bohemia, now part of Czechoslovakia. Uranium, used mainly to produce glass with a beautiful green color, was of little value. Through the efforts of an influential Austrian geologist, Eduard Suess, the Austrian government generously offered the Curies a ton of pitchblende residues for which the Curies had to pay only the transportation charges. Since Marie had no income, the costs were covered by Pierre's modest salary. Only gradually, after the publication of their first results, did they obtain financial support from the Academy of Sciences and an anonymous donor.

The Curies' search for a suitable workroom was unsuccessful. After vain attempts to find space in one of the numerous buildings attached to the Sorbonne, Marie and Pierre returned to the School of Physics (where Pierre taught) to the little room in which Marie had performed her first experiments. The room opened onto a courtyard, and on the other side of the yard there was a wooden shack, an abandoned shed with a skylight roof in such bad condition that the rain seeped through. The Faculty of Medicine had formerly used the place as a dissecting room, but it had long been considered unfit to cover even the cadavers. Lacking a floor, the room was finished with some worn kitchen tables, a blackboard, and an old cast-iron stove with a rusty pipe.

In summer, because of its skylights, the shed was as stifling as a hothouse. During the rainy season, the water dripped with a soft, nerve-wracking noise onto the ground or the worktables, places that the Curies had to mark to avoid putting delicate apparatus there. Because the shed possessed no chimney to carry off noxious gases, most of their treatment of pitchblende had to be made in the open air of the courtyard. When a shower came, the physicists hastily moved their apparatus inside; to keep working without suffocating, they set up draughts between the opened door and windows. In such horrendous conditions, Marie and Pierre Curie worked for 4 years from 1898 to 1902. They decided that it was most practical to separate their efforts. Pierre Curie devoted most of his time to a study of the properties of the newly discovered elements, while Marie Curie continued the exhausting chemical treatments that would permit her to obtain salts of pure radium.

As Marie wrote, "I came to treat as many as 20 kilograms of matter at a time, which had the effect of filling the shed with great jars full of precipitates and liquids. It was killing work to carry the receivers, to pour off the liquids and to stir, for hours at a stretch, the boiling matter in a smelting basin."

In the face of an increasing workload, the Curies sought collaborators

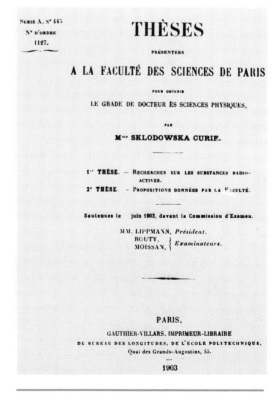

SÉRIE A, N° 443
N° D'ORDRE
1127.

THÈSES

PRÉSENTÉES

A LA FACULTÉ DES SCIENCES DE PARIS

POUR OBTENIR

LE GRADE DE DOCTEUR ÈS SCIENCES PHYSIQUES,

PAR

Mᵐᵉ SKLODOWSKA CURIE.

1ʳᵉ THÈSE. — RECHERCHES SUR LES SUBSTANCES RADIO-ACTIVES.

2ᵉ THÈSE. – PROPOSITIONS DONNÉES PAR LA FACULTÉ.

Soutenues le   juin 1903, devant la Commission d'Examen.

MM. LIPPMANN, *Président.*
BOUTY, } *Examinateurs.*
MOISSAN, }

PARIS,

GAUTHIER-VILLARS. IMPRIMEUR-LIBRAIRE
DU BUREAU DES LONGITUDES, DE L'ÉCOLE POLYTECHNIQUE,
Quai des Grands-Augustins, 55.

1903

Cover page of Marie Curie's doctoral thesis (1903).[3]

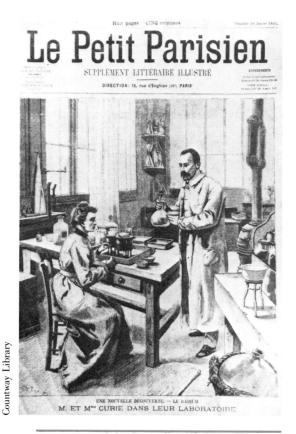

Le Petit Parisien
SUPPLÉMENT LITTÉRAIRE ILLUSTRÉ
DIRECTION: 18, rue d'Enghien (10º), PARIS

UNE NOUVELLE DÉCOUVERTE — LE RADIUM
M. ET Mᵐᵉ CURIE DANS LEUR LABORATOIRE

The Curies in their laboratory.
Cover *Le Petit Parisien*, 1904.

to share in their efforts. One of the scientists whom they enlisted, André-Louis Debierne, conducted research that led to the discovery of a third new radioactive element (*actinium*) in their pitchblende residues. At last in 1902, 45 months after announcing the probable existence of radium, Marie finally succeeded in preparing a decigram of pure radium chloride with a calculated atomic weight of 225.

Despite the success of their research and the accolades of the scientific world, Marie and Pierre were treated badly by the French academic community. To improve their financial status, Pierre, on the advice of associates, attempted three times unsuccessfully to gain a professorship at the Sorbonne. He was forced to accept a professorship at the School of Physics in Paris, while Marie took a position at a girls' school. Marie developed tuberculosis, while Pierre was agonized by rheumatism.

Nevertheless, the Curies continued to study the effects and properties of the new radioactive substances. They determined that radium emitted three different kinds of rays, described a gas that was produced by radium (*radon*), and noted that radium spontaneously gave off heat and light. Marie Curie postulated that the radioelements were in a state of spontaneous evolution, such that the more rapid the rate of transformation the more powerful their "activity." Her predictions proved true in 1903 when two English scientists, Sir William Ramsay and Frederick Soddy, demonstrated that radium was continually releasing helium gas.

Marie Curie also noted the "contagious" nature of radium. Objects, persons, plants, and minerals exposed to radium would develop "activities" of their own that would interfere with the precise measurements she attempted. As she wrote in her notebook, "When one studies strongly radioactive substances, special precautions must be taken if one wishes to be able to continue taking delicate measurements. The various objects used in a chemical laboratory, and those which serve for experiments in physics, all become radioactive in a short time and act upon photographic plates through black paper. Dust, the air of the room, and one's clothes, all become radioactive." Indeed, to this day the working notebooks of the Curies continue to emit radioactivity.

With Becquerel, the Curies began to study the physiological effects of radium rays. In 1900, two German scientists (Friedrich Oskar Giesel and

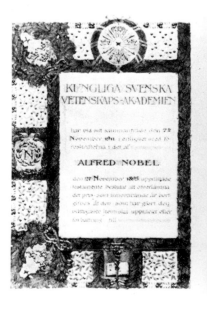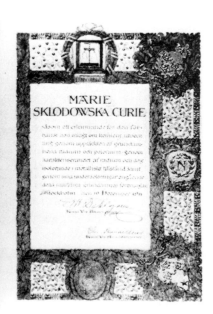

Marie Curie's second Nobel Prize (1911).[1]

48

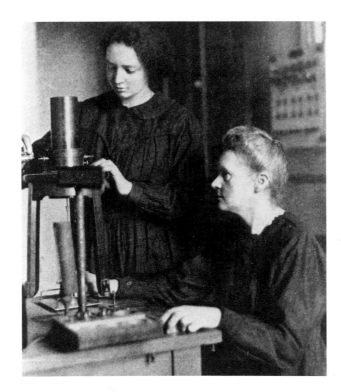

Friedrich Otto Walkhoff) reported that the rays emitted by radium had a destructive action on the skin. Intrigued by these results, Pierre intentionally placed a radium sample on his arm for 10 hours, producing a skin reaction that was similar to sunburn and took several months to heal, although not without leaving a mark behind. Becquerel, who had borrowed some radium from the Curies, also suffered a radiation burn after carrying the sample in his vest pocket. The reddened patch that appeared on his abdomen soon became a necrotic, suppurating wound that took some time to heal. After these experiences, Pierre and Marie Curie started numerous animal experiments that led to the treatment of patients with what was to become known as Curie therapy.

In 1903, the Curies and Becquerel shared the Nobel Prize in physics for their work on radioactivity. Earlier in the year, Marie had been awarded her doctoral degree, 5 years after she had begun her research project. In 1905, Pierre was belatedly presented a professorship at the Sorbonne and was elected to the Academy of Science (to which Marie was admitted in 1911). In 1911, Marie Curie obtained the chemistry prize alone, thus being the only person to ever be awarded two Nobel Prizes. In 1935, her daughter, Irene, and son-in-law, Frédéric Joliot, were given the prize for their fundamental discovery of artificial radioactivity. The Curie family thus possessed five Nobel medals.

The Curies could have become quite wealthy by securing a patent for the process of producing radium. However, like Roentgen, the Curies published detailed accounts of their complete experimental protocols so that anyone interested in them could make use of their work.

Tragedy struck the Curie household in 1906 when Pierre absentmindedly darted into the path of a heavy horse-drawn wagon on a rain-swept street and was killed instantly. Marie, deeply devoted to her brilliant husband, was crushed and withdrew from all human contact for months. Eventually, she returned to work and managed to isolate radium in its pure metallic form. Next came the development of a method for measuring

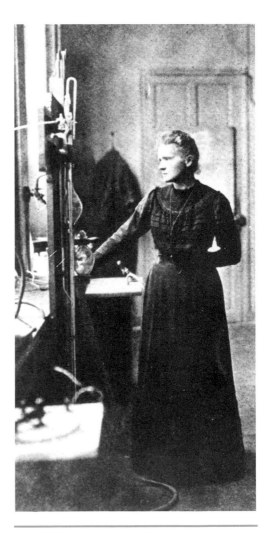

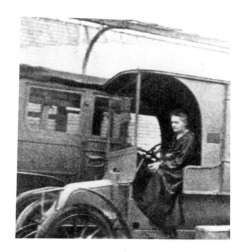

Marie Curie at the wheel of an ambulance in World War I.[1]

radium and the preparation of the first international standard—22 mg of pure radium chloride, which was presented to the Office of Weights and Measures at Sevres, near Paris. Marie Curie was offered and accepted her husband's Chair of Physics at the Sorbonne. At her instigation, in 1912 the Radium Institute was organized. However, the opening of the institute was delayed by the outbreak of World War I. Marie immediately offered her services to develop France's medical x-ray facilities. With funds provided by the Union of the Women of France, Marie equipped the first radiological car, a mobile unit containing radiographic apparatus with a dynamo to supply electricity. As the war raged, citizens donated cars to the energetic woman scientist, who then equipped them with x-ray equipment and dispatched the affectionately named "little Curies" where they were most needed. Disdaining dependence on others, Marie taught herself the skills of radiography, driving, and even auto mechanics so that she could operate her radiological car unaided. She traveled from hospital to hospital, where she spent long hours beside surgeons, radiographically examining the wounded.

In 1920, during the course of a conversation with Mrs. Meloney, a New York editor, Marie admitted that she wished she had a gram of radium to work with since hers was tied up treating patients at the Radium Institute. On returning home, Mrs. Meloney initiated a nationwide campaign to raise the necessary $100,000. The gift was given to Marie in Washington by President Harding, and she was most warmly welcomed by numerous institutions during her stay in the United States.

Sadly, Marie Curie eventually fell victim to the ravages of the element she had discovered. Although she possessed intimate knowledge of radiation, she never adequately protected herself in all her years of contact with the powerful agent, even though she insisted that safety precautions be taken by her colleagues and students. Constant direct handling of radium produced severe burns on her hands, and she died on July 4, 1934 of aplastic anemia.

The story of the discovery of radioactivity would not be complete without noting the grimly prophetic remarks of Pierre Curie in his Nobel lecture of 1904. "One may also imagine that in criminal hands radium might become very dangerous, and here we may ask ourselves if humanity has anything to gain by learning the secrets of nature, if it is ripe enough to profit by them, or if this knowledge is not harmful." Within 40 years of these words, the "secrets of nature" learned by humanity had grown to include nuclear fission and fusion, culminating in the development and detonation of the atom bomb.

Bibliography

Curie E: Madame Curie. New York, Doubleday, 1949.

Curie M: Pierre Curie. New York, MacMillan, 1923.

Foley JJ: Marie Curie: The birth of a science. Radiol Technol 47:134-140, 1975.

Glasser O: Pierre and Marie Curie and the discovery of radium. In Glasser O (ed): The science of radiology. Springfield, Ill, Charles C Thomas, 1933.

Hevesy GC: Marie Curie and her contemporaries: The Becquerel-Curie memorial lecture. J Nucl Med 25:118-131, 1961.

Klickstein HS: Marie Sklodowska Curie. St. Louis, Mallinckrodt Classics of Radiology, 1966.

Knutsson F: Becquerel and the discovery of radioactivity. Acta Radiol (Diagn) 16:113-116, 1975.

Leucutia T: Heuristic gems from the American Radium Society. AJR 121:653-660, 1974.

Mould RF: A history of x-rays and radium. 1980.

Nobel Lectures: Physics 1901-1921. Amsterdam, Elsevier, 1967.

References

1. Curie E: Madame Curie. New York, Doubleday, 1949.

2. Nobel Lectures: Physics 1901-1921. Amsterdam, Elsevier, 1967.

3. Klickstein HS: Marie Sklodowska Curie. St. Louis, Mallinckrodt Classics of Radiology, 1966.

4. Glasser O: Pierre and Marie Curie and the discovery of radium. In Glasser O (ed): The science of radiology. Springfield, Ill, Charles C Thomas, 1933.

5. Mould RF: A history of x-rays and radium. 1980.

CHAPTER 4

Early Radiology

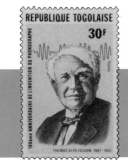
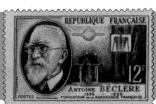
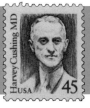
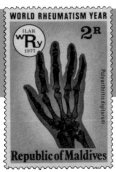

FLUOROSCOPY VERSUS RADIOGRAPHY

The first important improvement on the original roentgen apparatus was a device to permit direct observation of an object, such as a hand, rather than image it on a photographic plate. This instrument, first described by the Italian physicist, Enrico Salvioni, in February, 1896, also permitted examination in a lighted room rather than a completely darkened chamber. His "cryptoscope" consisted of a tube with a fluorescent screen at one end and an opening for the eyes at the other. If x-rays were present, the screen would glow with characteristic fluorescence, "resembling somewhat a ground glass window pane as seen at night with a light at some little distance away and behind it." An opaque substance placed between the evacuated tube and the fluorescent screen would produce a dark shadow. Of course, there was no permanent shadow left on the screen. As soon as the generation of x-rays ceased, the crystals stopped fluorescing and the screen became dark.[1]

Other forms of hooded fluoroscopic screens were soon reported. William Francis Magie produced a tubular "skiascope," while Edward Pruden Thompson[2] used a truncated cone rather than a cylinder for his "kinetoskotoscope." John MacIntyre and Thomas A. Edison used truncated pyramids, the form that prevailed in the later construction of the hooded fluoroscopic screen "through the romantic and tragical days of its rise, decline and fall."

Edison's intense interest in scientific advances compelled him to plunge into the new field of radiology with tremendous energy and enthusiasm. He had read Roentgen's original paper and noted that Roentgen had used only barium platinocyanide and a few other fluorescent materials to detect the presence of x-rays. He wondered if it might be possible to find other chemicals that would fluoresce even more brightly when excited by the new rays. Just as they had tested thousands of substances to determine the best material for use as filaments in incandescent light bulbs, by late March, four men in Edison's laboratory had tried over 1,800

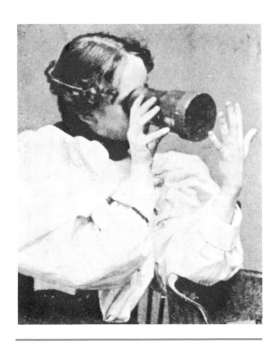

Early fluoroscope (1896). A quick way to test the x-rays being produced was to place the hand between a vacuum tube and fluorescent screen.[2]

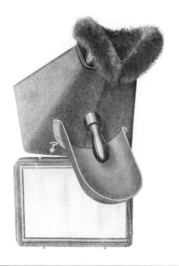

Early fluoroscope (1896).[3]

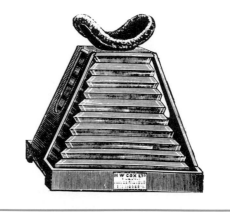

Cryptoscope (1902).[4]

different salts and found that 72 fluoresced. Eight months later, some 8,000 substances had been tested, and the best was found to be calcium tungstate. Having produced this substance in finely divided form, Edison coated a plain support and covered this fluorescent screen (through which x-rays could easily penetrate) with a hood in the shape of a truncated pyramid to exclude daylight. He placed an aperture formed for the eyes at the line of truncation and a supporting handle on one of the sides of the pyramid. Initially termed the *vitascope*, the device was later called a *fluoroscope*.

Edison jubilantly cabled the news to England on March 17, 1896:

> Please inform Lord Kelvin that have just found calcium tungstate properly crystalized gives splendid fluorescence with Roentgen ray far exceeding platinocyanide rendering photographs unnecessary.

Subsequent events, however, proved the fallacy of this hasty assumption.

In his usual dramatic fashion, Edison arranged a demonstration of his new fluoroscope in conjunction with the annual display of the National Electrical Exposition in New York (May, 1896). Preparations were made for a substantial number of people to examine their hands with a portable fluoroscope or walk in single file before an open fluoroscopic screen.

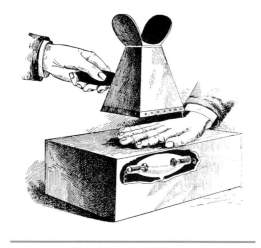

Edison's "Vitascope" (1896).[6]

Edison's demonstration at the National Electrical Exposition (1896). Huge crowds lined up to see their own hands through the new fluoroscopic equipment.

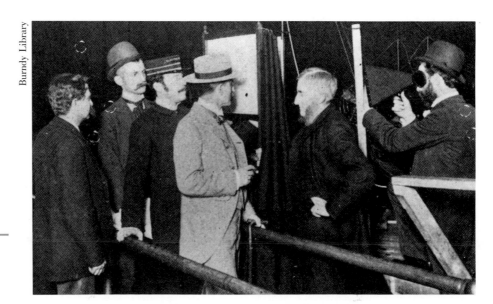

Many more people than were expected turned out for the demonstration, and Edison's assistants had to cope with shock, incredulity, and mirth as the crowd moved through darkened chambers hung with somber black cloths to improve their visual sensitivity. The visitors were guided through heavy iron railings, and signs along the way instructed them to slip a key or coin into a gloved hand so as better to see the bones of their hand and the object in the glove.

Among the team of highly trained men that conducted the demonstration was Clarence M. Dally. Dally was in charge of controlling the output of the induction coil and often held his hand over the x-ray tube to make small adjustments. Lengthy exposure to the virulent rays resulted in burns of the face, degenerative skin changes in the hands, and early loss of hair on the anterior scalp, eyebrows, eyelashes, and backs of the fingers and hands. As with most right-handed individuals, who tested the strength of the x-rays with their opposite hand, Dally's *left* hand was the first to be affected. Once the safety-conscious Edison realized what was happening, he immediately discontinued experimenting with x-rays. However, Dally's fate was already sealed. He died in 1904, one of the earliest x-ray martyrs.

Nevertheless, in 1896, Edison and almost all other x-ray workers were enthusiastic supporters of the fluoroscope. As Edison wrote in April, "there is no occasion to take photographs, shadowgraphs or radiographs. I stopped that long ago. You can see for yourself, the fluoroscope does the work in a moment." The demand on the early radiologists for the "quick" use of the fluoroscope (still largely a hooded screen) in emergency surgery or in the more gross pathology of the thorax was one of several factors responsible for the high incidence of radiation dermatitis during the early years (see Chapter 11).

A somewhat offbeat adaptation of the fluoroscope was the "seehear" of William Rollins. This extraordinary instrument combined a fluorescent screen and a stethoscope so that the sounds of the heart and lungs could be heard while the image of the heart and lungs was seen. Among Rollins' more practical contributions (see p. 69) were the interposition of a screen of heavy lead between the fluorescent screen and the physician's eyes to prevent the blindness he had produced in animals with what he termed *x-light*. He also insisted that the fluoroscope be made of a nonradiable material to prevent diffuse light from entering. Since the fluoroscope was often used in patients having contagious diseases, Rollins recommended that it be made of metal that could be easily sterilized by heat, rather than cloth-covered pasteboard or wood that would fall to pieces if heat sterilized.

Edison changed the configuration of the fluoroscope to the shape of the familiar stereoscope, so that both eyes could be comfortably focused on the image simultaneously. He turned his fluoroscope over to an associated company, Aylsworth & Jackson, to manufacture and sell at a low price. Thus before the end of March the fluoroscope was no longer merely a device to read about in scientific publications, but one that could be easily purchased on the open market.

Many early users of the fluoroscope used one hand to hold the screen and held the other hand between it and the tube to gauge the strength of the x-ray emanation. The long time required for the eyes to adjust to the subdued light became a hazard to the hand, and this all too often led to a disastrous chain of burns, lesions, amputations, and ultimate death.

Even with its more brilliant visual image, Edison's new fluorescent screen of calcium tungstate still had many disadvantages relative to the

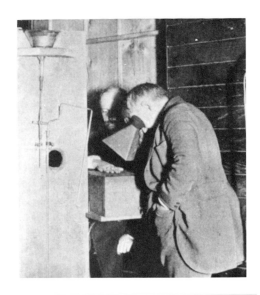

Edison examining a hand through a fluoroscope (1896). His unfortunate assistant, Clarence M. Dally, is seen holding his hand over the box containing the x-ray tube. Edison is looking through a fluoroscope of his own design.[2]

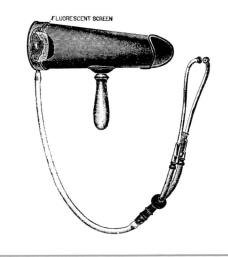

Seehear of Rollins (1904). The device combined a fluorescent screen and a stethoscope.[7]

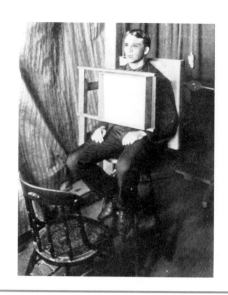

Use of an open fluoroscopic screen (1901).[10]

photographic plate. In the examination of the thicker parts of the body, the image was difficult to decipher because of its grain and the presence of secondary radiation fog. Detail, even in the thinner parts, was almost impossible to appreciate. The photographic plate provided a permanent record that was clearer and had greater definition and detail. In addition, the effect of the x-rays on the sensitive plate was cumulative, so that an image only faintly perceptible on the fluoroscopic screen could be shown on a plate by merely prolonging the exposure. For example, a radiograph of an adult pelvis could be made, whereas a detailed image could not be observed directly on the fluoroscopic screen.[9]

The first radiologist to consistently use the *open* fluoroscopic screen was probably Francis Williams of Boston. As a practicing internist for many years, Williams was attracted by the possibilities of the fluoroscope to assist in the diagnosis of diseases of the lungs and heart. His preference for the open screen also was due to his practice of making tracings on glass, celluloid, or the patient's skin of his observations covering the entire thorax. At least one free hand (often two) was needed for this procedure, since the foot-control of current supply was unknown at that time.

Another advocate of fluoroscopy in thoracic diagnosis was Augustus W. Crane. In 1900, Crane wrote an article correlating radiographic findings with the physical signs of chest pathology and exclaimed,[11] "I trust that in this paper may be shown the superiority of the fluoroscope over the dry plate (the radiograph) in the examination of the lungs." As an aside, in the same paper Crane described his "skiameter," which was a manual instrument for measuring shadow-densities by means of a gauging scale, at first of metallic wires of varying cross-section and later of layers of tinfoil arranged in various thicknesses. The depth of a given shadow beneath the screen surface could be determined from its intensity by an ingenious, if somewhat complex, application of mathematics.[11]

In a presentation to the first meeting of the Roentgen Society of the United States (1900), Mihran Kassabian summarized the relative advantages and disadvantages of fluoroscopy and skiagraphy (radiography)[15]:

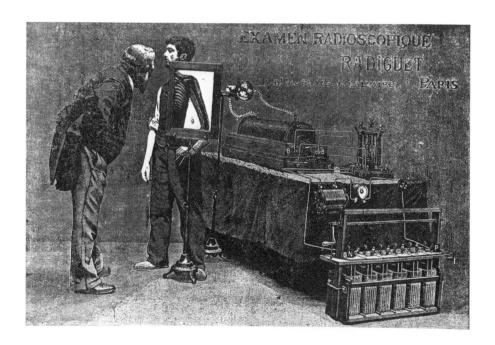

Fluoroscopic examination (1900).[16]

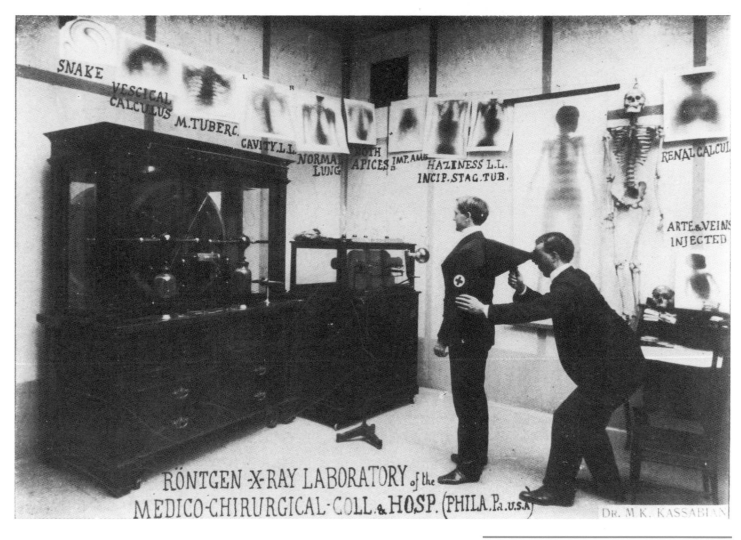

SNAKE
VESCICAL CALCULUS
M.TUBERC.
CAVITY.L.L.
NORMAL LUNG
BOTH APICES
IMP.AMB
HAZINESS L.L.
INCIP.STAG.TUB.
RENAL CALCUL.
ARTE&VEINS INJECTED
RÖNTGEN-X-RAY LABORATORY of the
MEDICO-CHIRURGICAL-COLL.&HOSP.(PHILA.Pa.U.S.A)
DR. M.K. KASSABIAN

Kassabian's clinic (1901).[15]

The fluoroscopic examination is merely temporary, while the view is limited to a few individuals. On the other hand, the skiagraph is a permanent record, visible to everybody, and moreover, capable of use in legal cases, the lecture room, clinics, etc. Fluoroscopy, however, is easy, quick, and affords ready facilities for comparison with the normal corresponding part. In these respects it has an advantage over the skiagraph, which requires considerable time to effect, and is more tedious. Fluoroscopy also has an advantage when the heart, joints and respiratory movement are concerned; as it offers better opportunities for studying them, and from different directions, when necessary. The skiagraph shows a blurred effect in the case of moving organs. Fluoroscopy is at a disadvantage when the pelvis, kidney, spine and deeper tissues are to be examined; but the skiagraph shows them plainly.

Kassabian[15] concluded that "both are important and useful, yes, necessary since they confirm each other."

In the early 1900s, there was a definite decline in the use of fluoroscopy. One major reason was the increasing realization, especially among practical users of x-rays, that the fluorescent screen could be the source of real danger to the operator. George Pfahler (1905) admitted that he had discontinued the use of fluoroscopy in examining the chest "because of its

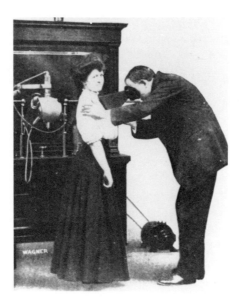
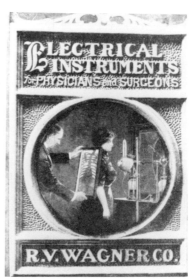

Fluoroscopic examinations. *Left,* Hand-held fluoroscopy and *right,* open-screen fluoroscopy from the cover of the 1907 catalogue of Chicago x-ray manufacturer Rome Wagner, who died of the results of radiation exposure 1 year later.

inaccuracy and of the dangers attending its use." The other reason for the decline of fluoroscopy was the steady improvement in radiographic methods resulting from the production of more powerful generators and the development of intensifying screens of better quality (less granularity and phosphorescence).

A resurgence of interest in fluoroscopy occurred during the next decade, because of the development of gastrointestinal radiology (see Chapter 15) and the x-ray needs of the military in World War I (see Chapter 22). Unfortunately, the apparatus constructed for military purposes was simply constructed and woefully inadequate as far as protection of the operator was concerned. Soon after the end of the war, possible results of overexposure to x-rays in the Army were suggested by the occurrence of aplastic anemia and other blood dyscrasias. Wide publicity led to an even greater reaction than had been the case 15 years before. With the onset of the "second fluoroscopic depression," many radiologists completely abandoned the use of the screen. Various national and international committees established protection standards (see Chapter 11). Nevertheless, as Percy Brown warned (1935)[17]:

> In spite of these organized precautionary measures, to which the registered American radiologist must subscribe and comply, and thus may practice his profession with absolute safety to his patient and relative safety to himself, the untoward potentiality of uncontrolled fluoroscopic practice is still with us. There yet endures the unprincipled charlatan who, within the mystifying aura of the

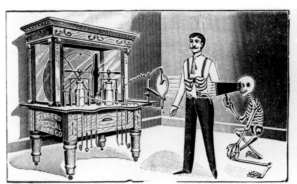

Great Reduction
IN PRICE OF
HIGH GRADE
X RAY and STATIC MACHINES,
GALVANIC, Portable, Dry Cell,
FARADIC COMBINATION Batteries,
Cabinets, Wall and Table Plates, Switchboards, Cautery and Illumination Batteries, Rheostats, Meters and Electrodes.
Our new Catalogue No. 8 will be sent free on application.
Electro-Medical Mfg. Co.
350 Dearborn St., CHICAGO, ILL.

Fanciful advertisement (1902) for an x-ray unit featuring a skeletal fluoroscopist.[14]

roentgenoscope, seeks to hoodwink his trusting victim as he shamelessly lies into credulous ears as to what the luminous screen reveals. We still have the manufacturer who is so far unmindful of the respect of the qualified radiologist that he continues to persuade the internist or the general practitioner of the advantage in the possession of the fluoroscope as a bit of decorative office furniture, which it is ultimately to become after producing its yield of disappointment. Also, there is the less serious matter of the commercially wolfish shoe dealer garbed in the sheep's clothing of science, as he asks us to enjoy, with him, by fluoroscope, the sublime vision of our hallux valgus which he proposes to fit, plus or minus, into the tight leather of vanity. Roentgenoscopy, with all our modern devices for protection of the operator, is still, in unpracticed hands, a procedure potentially serious, to use no stronger an adjective.

CINERADIOLOGY

Radiographic plates and film could capture the appearance of a structure at a given moment in time; the fluoroscopic screen could show the motion of a structure over time. However, there was no mechanism to provide a permanent record of the movement of the fluorescent screen image to use for future reference and study or to enable the observer to study a rapidly occurring event in slow motion.[8] The solution to this problem was the development of cineradiography. The earliest procedure was *indirect* cineradiography, which consisted of photographing the shadows on a fluorescent screen by means of an ordinary camera. In June, 1896, the fluoroscopic image was first photographed by Julius Mount Bleyer, a laryngologist who used this device "in shadowing out tumors, growths, foreign bodies, and various diseased conditions of the larynx and bones of the face and their accessory cavities and the lungs with their many complicated ailments"[19] (see Chapter 12). In Angelo Battelli and Giorgio Garbasso's first attempts with this method, only the image of the metallic holder of the photographic lens was seen on the camera plate. The x-rays penetrated the fluorescent screen and the plate holder of the photographic camera and darkened the plate before the weak light from the fluorescent screen could make any impression. This problem was solved by placing a heavy lead diaphragm with a hole the size of the lens in front of the camera. This apparatus visualized the shadows of the fluorescent screen and a photographic record could be made at the same time.[20] In Scotland, John MacIntyre initially used the indirect method of cineradiography but found the procedure too slow. Consequently, he developed the technique of *direct* cineradiography in which the movements of a hind limb of a frog were recorded serially on film passing behind the aperture of a motion-picture camera encased in a lead box. When MacIntyre first demonstrated his results in late 1896, the *Archives of Skiagraphy* reported[21]:

> Doctor MacIntyre has for some time been experimenting on the best methods of obtaining rapid exposures with a view to recording the movements of organs within the body. Two methods have been adopted, one in which the shadow of the object, as seen upon the potassium platino-cyanide fluorescent screen, was photographed by means of the ordinary camera. This, however, was found to be too slow for the purpose. The other method was to allow the sensitive film to pass underneath the aperture in the case of thick lead covering the cinematograph. This opening corresponded to the size of the picture, and was covered with a piece of black paper, upon which the limb of an animal, say a frog, could be photographed. As yet, the move-

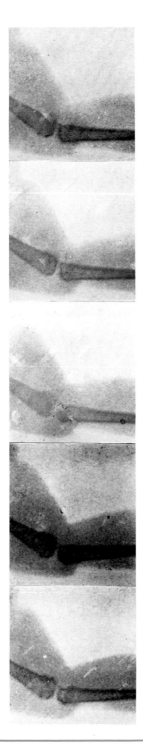

First moving picture made with roentgen rays (1897).[21] Five views of the motion of a frog's leg.

ments must be slow, and consequently carried out by an artificial or slow anaesthesia. In the present state of our knowledge the former gives the more satisfactory results. Some months ago, Doctor MacIntyre showed, by means of the mercury interruptor, that he could obtain instantaneous photographs of the bones of his fingers by a single flash of the tube, due to one vibration of the contact breaker. At a meeting of the Glasgow Philosophical Society recently, he was able to pass a film forty feet in length through the cinematograph; the movements of the leg of a frog could clearly be seen when demonstrated on a magic lantern screen by means of the cinematograph.

EARLY RADIOLOGISTS

Radiography was initially considered a new specialty in the field of photography. Most of the workers who were actively engaged in making radiographs were photographers or physicians who practiced photography as a hobby. Others were professors in university physics laboratories who were intrigued by the phenomena of the x-rays as an addition to pure science. Still others were from the rank and file of amateur experimenters and inventors.

Following the discovery of x-rays,[9]

many men attracted by the unknown, men not well trained, but of an inquisitive mind or mechanical bent procured the necessary apparatus to produce these new rays. Their tribulations with equipment were many. Much of the apparatus had to be built by the experimenters. Tubes were the poorest. Exposures were long, and the results were disheartening. But when the basic principle of the rays (the ability to penetrate objects and cast shadows in proportion to their density) was brought to the attention of medical men, they recognized the advantage their use would produce in the localization of foreign bodies and in the diagnosis of fractures. This demand for its use soon became general. As many of the very early experimenters had no medical and little scientific training, it was to these untrained investigators that medical men most often had to turn, for its use demanded that it be obtained wherever possible. In many parts of the country these men were the first to produce roentgenograms.

Who was best equipped to use x-rays for medical purposes? As Percy Brown[22] described at the 1908 meeting of the American Roentgen Ray Society (ARRS):

(Medical radiography) was a piebald proceeding, a sort of Joseph's coat of many colors, which fitted no one. The attendant wires and sparks suggested an electrician's work, surely; . . . but there were the plates, darkroom and chemicals, considered usually the accessories of the photographer. Neither of these artisans, on the other hand, could be expected to intrude themselves so far into the realms of medicine as to offer a diagnostic verdict . . .

The electrician, after dallying in the darkroom with the chemicals, produced photographic results of no higher quality than might be expected of an electrician; the photographer, after producing a generous display of pyrotechnics in the immediate vicinity of the patient, finally met with a practical electrical problem quite beyond his depth; while the surgeon, albeit well-versed in all heretofore employed methods of diagnosis, skillfully cut for renal stone in an endeavor to find what was, in reality, the elusive suspender button . . ."

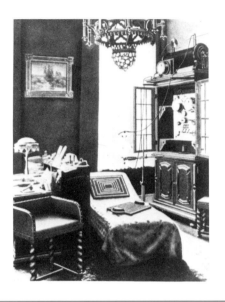

Diagnostic corner of Alban Kohler's office (1900).

The *Electrician* of January, 1896 considered x-rays to be the province of traumatic and orthopedic surgery when its editorial stated, "so long as individuals of the human race continue to professionally inject bullets into one another, it is well to be provided with easy means for inspecting the position of the injected lead, and to that extent aiding the skilled operators whose business and joy it is to extract it."

The difficulty in operating and procuring suitable x-ray apparatus in 1896 caused many physicians to rely on independent operators for radiography of their patients. As a consequence, "Roentgen studios" sprang up in America and Europe, advertising the fact that they were conducting a business in "Roentgen photography" and that appointments could be made for "x-ray sittings." These studios extensively solicited physicians so that the majority of their work was essentially medical or surgical in character. Occasionally, curious persons requested radiographs of various opaque objects such as pieces of sculpture, jewelry, pearls, diamonds, metal castings, mummies, and other objects of similar nature—foreshadowing modern industrial radiography.[9]

The *Electrical Engineer* reported on June 3, 1896, of the opening of an x-ray studio in New York "where pictures of the interior human structure, etc., will be taken. The consultation hours are from 1 to 2 and 5 to 6. A lady assistant is in attendance." Another curiosity was *free* x-ray service offered as a "public service" by Colonel Charles F. Lacombe in Denver. The laboratory "was besieged by persons who were certain that their physicians were wrong, and wanted x-ray photographs to prove it." This prompted Colonel Lacombe to establish a rule that no patient would be x-rayed unless his physician was present.

Broadsheet (1896) advertising public demonstration of x-rays the Crystal Palace Exhibition in London.[24]

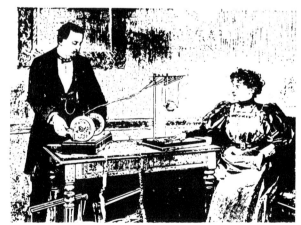
Advertisement for x-ray studio.

Many of the initial x-ray applications required little or no medical knowledge. However, once equipment was available to demonstrate more detailed anatomy and subtle pathological changes, it became apparent that mere technical proficiency was insufficient and actual medical knowledge was required. "Some of the pioneers, stimulated by the contact with medicine, acquired a large amount of medical knowledge and rendered good service. Some even took the necessary work to acquire a medical degree."[25] However, there were no set standards of training and few places where a budding x-ray worker could gain even a meager knowledge of the work. The field looked lucrative from the outside and appeared to offer a higher professional standing. Thus many physicians, some failures in general practice and with little special knowledge, entered the field. These men often possessed poor technical ability, so that in addition to the technician without medical knowledge there was now the poorly trained physician, who was actually more dangerous to radiology than the nonmedical technician because nothing distinguished him from his well-trained medical colleagues. Because of a lack of knowledge on the part of the profession and of the laity, reports of the charlatan and the misinformed were given the same credence as were the scientific opinions of qualified men. As Murphy[25] wrote in 1933,

> lay technicians, who render medical reports, have almost passed. However, because of past history, a heritage still remains in the minds of many persons connected with medicine and hospitals; it is the idea that roentgenologists require no elaborate medical training. Many still feel that production of films of sufficient excellence is enough and that anyone can interpret them. This is much in evidence among surgeons and internists, men who would be the first to denounce the roentgenologist for removing an appendix or treating a case of nephritis, but who at the same time do not hesitate to diagnose a gastric ulcer from a set of roentgenograms made by a technician, even though in the present day system of medical training the roentgenologist is far better trained in surgery and medicine than the surgeon or the internist is in roentgenology.

In another lecture at the 1908 meeting of the ARRS, a prominent New York surgeon, Reginald H. Sayre,[26] explained why many physicians who had formerly used x-rays themselves had now abandoned them and were referring their patients to specialists like Dr. Brown. He indicated that he had begun to experiment back in 1896 and had continued to use x-rays in his practice for several years thereafter. But after a lapse of a few years, he found that if he were to do x-ray work on a par with that performed by the specialists, he would have no time to practice surgery: "The demands of my surgical practice were too exacting to permit me to do justice to the x-ray work." Rather than dropping his specialty and become a radiologist, Dr. Sayre concluded that he would stop taking x-ray photographs and refer his patients to someone who "had become more competent than I."

One of the most vigorous proponents of medical radiology as a specialty was Russell D. Carman of St. Louis. As he wrote in 1910,[27]

> the evolution and progress of medical science and art necessitate division and subdivision of labor—specialization. In medicine, as in everything else, the fewer things a man does, the better he can and ought to do them . . . The right of a specialty to existence has only this test—that it employ the specialist's entire time and attention with increased benefit to himself, to the profession and to the public. Judged by this test, Roentgenology is and of right ought to be, a legitimate specialty.

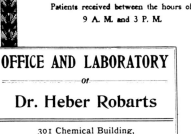
Advertisement for x-ray office and laboratory for Dr. Heber Robarts.[23]

Carman complained that "the only valid adverse criticism of the Roentgen Ray is based upon the fact that during its brief existence an abundance of poor work has been done with it by incompetent or inexperienced men, in many instances working with crude apparatus." He described one flagrant example reported by the well-known radiologist, Eugene W. Caldwell, who also favored specialization and said,

> When this point of view has become more prevalent, the pictorially excellent skiagraph of a hand or a foot made by some enthusiastic amateur will no longer excite wonder, and the photographers, electricians and janitors who now make the so-called x-ray photographs in many hospitals, will have their activities transferred to other fields, where they will be less a menace to the public health.

Successful employment of the x-rays, Dr. Carman continued, "demands an intimate knowledge of a highly complex apparatus, practical acquaintance with the essentials of a good radiogram, ability to interpret a radiograph properly, detailed instruction in the art of localizing foreign bodies, familiarity with the therapeutic use of the rays, and appreciation of the dangers which may attend their careless or unskilled application." These requirements were so difficult that he was forced to come to the following conclusion: ". . . there are in the United States to-day barely a dozen Roentgenologists who are capable of performing really expert service."

How did the early radiologists learn the x-ray manifestations of various disorders? In the absence of textbooks and experience, they availed themselves of what later came to be known as "retrospectoscopy." A radiologist made his plates, examined them, and failed to reach a sound diagnosis. The patient either was operated on or died and was examined at autopsy. The radiologist attended the operation or the autopsy and learned the true diagnosis. Then, in retrospect, he reexamined his plates and searched, often with intense embarrassment, for the clues that he had missed before. The rewards of retrospectoscopy came later, when an examination of another patient revealed similar findings and the radiologist could now make the diagnosis with confidence.

Who were the pioneer radiologists? Dr. Brown sent a survey to all members of the ARRS in 1910 and received replies from about half. The great majority of those responding had received their medical degree during the years 1896-1903. Thus the specialty in 1910 was staffed primarily with younger men, most of whom were still in undergraduate or medical school when Roentgen's discovery was announced. Among those receiving their degrees between 1900 and 1903, a considerable number had begun working with x-rays in 1896 or 1897 as physicists, engineers, electricians, photographers, or in other technical capacities. Brown concluded that these individuals, including several leaders of the profession such as Kassabian of Philadelphia, Caldwell of New York, and Dodd of Boston, had returned to school and earned their medical degrees specifically for the purpose of qualifying as radiologists.

Brown's survey indicated that only 20% of ARRS members in 1910 were limiting their practice to radiology. The remainder were about equally divided between general practice and some other specialty. Almost all the respondents agreed that the demand for their x-ray services was increasing.

Even at this early date, a considerable split had developed between diagnostic and therapeutic radiology. Only 30% of the ARRS members responding stated that they were engaged in both x-ray diagnosis and therapy. About half worked only in diagnosis, and a significant minority (19%) specialized solely in therapy.

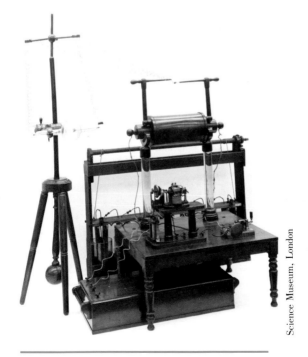

X-ray apparatus of John and Russell Reynolds in England (1896-1897). The x-ray tube is a "Watson Penetrator" focus tube.

Choosing a Name

What should this new field of medicine be called? In his first public presentation in Würzburg in January, 1896, Roentgen modestly suggested the term, *x-ray*, as a designation for his discovery. At that same meeting, the famed anatomist, von Kölliker, whose hand served as the experimental object, suggested that the discovery be called *Roentgen's rays*, a recommendation enthusiastically supported by the entire audience.[28]

Using the Greek suffix "gram" (the written message) or "graph" (to write), a German orthopedic surgeon, Carl Thiem, proposed calling the new procedure *Röntgographie*. Arthur W. Goodspeed, a Professor of Physics at the University of Pennsylvania, offered the term *radiography*. For years, the eponym and the prefix "radio-" competed bitterly for etymological supremacy. In France, Antoine Béclère coined the term, *radiologie*. Further support for use of the prefix "radio-" came with the Curies' discovery of "activité radiante," which soon was changed to "radio-activité." At this time, the prefix has virtually supplanted the eponym throughout the English speaking world, except for the title of one of the two major American journals.[23]

Various other names were suggested for the new medical procedure. An anonymous article in the *Archives of the Roentgen Ray* (1897) suggested the terms *skiagraphy* (Greek *skia-*, meaning shadow) or *pyknography* (Greek *pyknos*, meaning dense or obscure).[29] According to Grigg,[23] Apollodorus Skiagraphos was a fifth century BC Athenian shadow painter said to have originated the art of silhouette drawing. In 1801, the Swiss illustrator, Johann Heinrich Füssli, defined skiagrams (silhouette pictures) as outlines of shades without any other addition of character or feature but what the profile of the object thus delineated could afford. Many early x-ray plates were underexposed and underpenetrated, with additional loss of detail occurring during printing or when transferred to a slide for projection. Because the final result seldom showed more detail than the bare outlines of the bones, a name derived from the Greek word for shadow seemed appropriate. Indeed, the term *skiagraphy* was used for the first regular journal, *The Archives of Clinical Skiagraphy*, although this was changed 1 year later to the *Archives of the Roentgen Ray*.

Other terms suggested by early x-ray workers included actinography (Greek *actino-*, meaning ray), diagraphy (Greek *dia-*, meaning through or penetrating), and scotography (Greek *scoto-*, meaning dark). The term *fluoroscopy* was suggested by Thomas A. Edison, while Max Levy, an early German engineer and writer, preferred kryptoscopy from the Greek *krypto-*, meaning hidden.[23]

A curious term that appeared only once in the literature (*London Globe*, July 16, 1897) described radiology as the new "Ithuriel." This referred to the angel Ithuriel, who appears near the end of the fourth book of Milton's *Paradise Lost*. Satan, disguised as a toad, seduces Eve while she sleeps. The angel Ithuriel, who has been sent to protect the two mortals, discovers the treachery and with his spear touches the toad near Eve's ear. Immediately, the toad is revealed in his true nature and appears as Satan. Thus Ithuriel is the force that reveals the true nature of things, an apt description of radiology.[30]

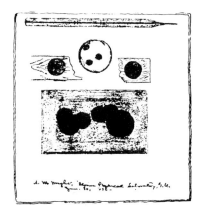 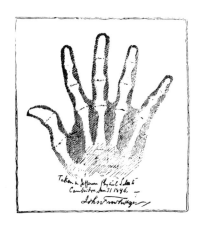

Left, First published American radiograph by Arthur W. Wright, Yale University, February 1, 1896. *Right*, Second published American radiograph by John Trowbridge, Harvard University, February 2, 1896.

HISTORIC FIRSTS

As described previously (see Chapter 2), the first American radiograph had been made inadvertently by Arthur W. Goodspeed almost 6 years before Roentgen's discovery of x-rays. The first intentional American radiograph was made on January 27, 1896 by Arthur W. Wright, Director of Yale's Sloane Physical Laboratory. On cardboard-covered bromide photographic paper, Wright placed several small objects: a lead pencil, a pair of scissors, and a 25-cent piece. Using an exposure time of 15 minutes, he obtained "a very clear representation of the objects employed." The historic event was published 4 days later in the *Engineering and Mining Journal* (February 1, 1896). Meanwhile, John Trowbridge, Director of Harvard's Jefferson Physical Laboratory, was making similar experiments. His article in the *New York Journal*, which included a photograph of the bones of the human hand, appeared on February 2, 1896, just 1 day after Wright's report.

The first clinical radiograph in the United States was made by Edwin Brant Frost, a Professor of Astronomy at Dartmouth. Frost was asked by his physician brother to radiograph the fractured forearm of one of his patients. After a 20-minute exposure, the plate of a Colles' fracture of Eddie McCarthy's left arm became immortalized as the first clinical radiograph obtained in America (February 3, 1896).

First clinical application of x-rays in the United States by Edwin B. Frost, Dartmouth College, February 3, 1896. *Left*, Professor Edwin Frost is sitting, watch in hand. The patient is seated to the right of the table, while Dr. Gilmon Frost is standing to the extreme right as his wife observes. *Right*, First American radiograph of a pathological condition, fractures of the distal radius and ulna.[31]

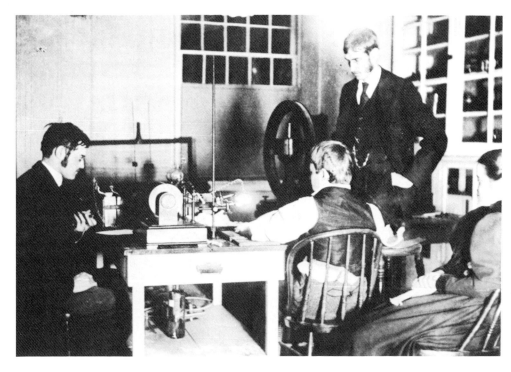 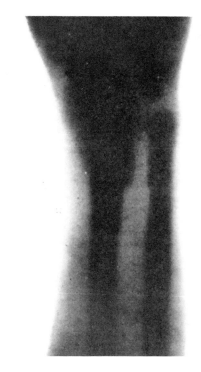

First clinical application of x-rays in Canada by John Cox in the Physics Lecture Theatre of McGill University in Montreal in 1896.[33]

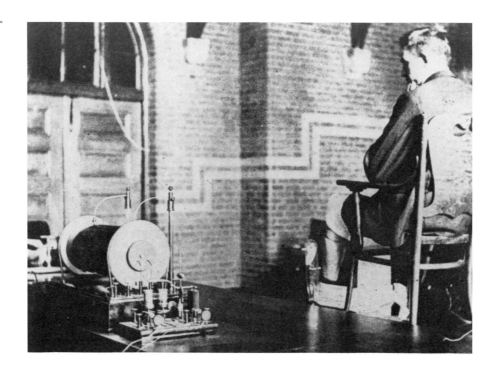

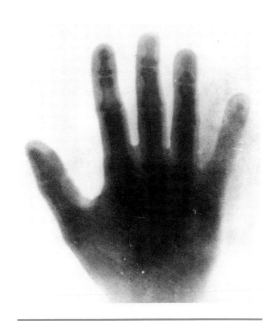

First radiograph made in Great Britain (Campbell-Swinton, January 13, 1896).

In Canada, John Cox, Professor of Physics at McGill University in Montreal, was the first in North America to use x-rays successfully as an adjunct to surgery when he localized a bullet in the leg of a gunshot victim (February 3, 1896). As the *Montreal Medical Journal* noted 4 days later[33]:

> The experiment was made this morning in one of the laboratories of McGill's Physics Building. A table was procured, a chair placed upon it, the left leg of the young man was stripped, and when he had taken his seat, a camera holder containing a sensitized Stanley plate was placed against a heavy block of wood at one side of the leg, the latter being held in a steady position by means of bandages and towels.
>
> When all was in readiness, the electric current was turned on. The light immediately began to flare and flicker, but after a short interval became quite steady. At the end of 45 minutes, the current was cut off, the bandages loosened, and the plates taken to the dark room for developing.
>
> After the lapse of 15 minutes, Professor Cox reappeared. One could detect at once, from the beaming countenance, the success of the experiment.

As Cox was quoted as saying as he entered the room, "The bones in the calf of the leg are plainly discernible in the plate, and in addition there is a solid substance there which I am convinced is the bullet." The bullet was successfully removed, and the patient recovered rapidly.

But there was more to the story. The patient later brought suit against the man who had shot him, and Cox's x-ray plate was entered into evidence.

The earliest intentional radiograph made in Great Britain (and possibly, after Roentgen, in the entire world) was by the Scottish engineer, Alan Archibald Campbell-Swinton. On January 7, 1896, Campbell-Swinton made what he called a "poor roentgenogram," but this was followed the next day by a series of more satisfactory radiographs of coins, keys, and similar objects. These plates were first reproduced in *Nature* on January 23, 1896. Soon afterward, on the advice of several eminent physicians and surgeons, Campbell-Swinton established what was probably the earliest x-ray laboratory in the country to which medical men could send patients for radiography.[34] On one occasion in this laboratory he made a radiograph of the head that successfully located the position of a bullet. However, the skin dose was so high that the patient's hair fell out, and Campbell-Swinton was threatened with legal proceedings. Fortunately, nothing came of this for the hair began to grow again. Many distinguished people visited the laboratory, among whom were Lord Salisbury, the Prime Minister, and Lord Kelvin, the famous scientist.

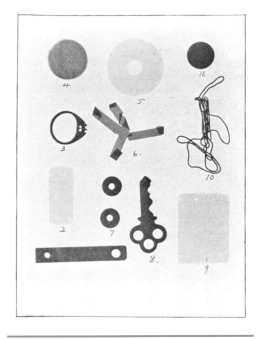

"Shadow pictures" from Trevert's book (1896) showing relative opacification of eleven items using a 30-second exposure. *1*, Sheet brass; *2*, aluminum; *3*, diamond ring; *4*, eye glass; *5*, mica; *6*, tin foil; *7*, copper; *8*, steel key; *9*, hard rubber; *10*, fine wire; *11*, silver 10-cent piece.

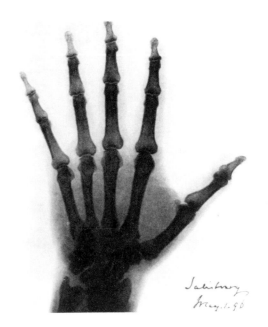

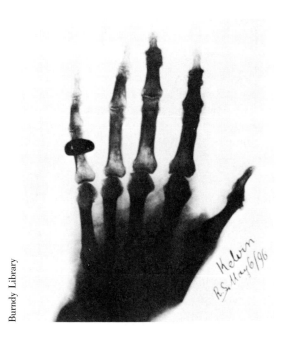

Burndy Library

Radiographs made by Campbell-Swinton in 1896 of the hands of British Prime Minister, Lord Salisbury (*left*), and Lord Kelvin (*right*). Their approvals are indicated by their signatures.[34]

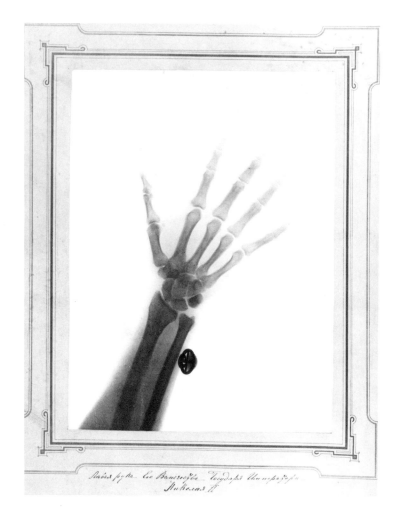

Radiographs of the hands of the Tsar (*top*)
and Tsarina (*bottom*) of Russia (c. 1896).

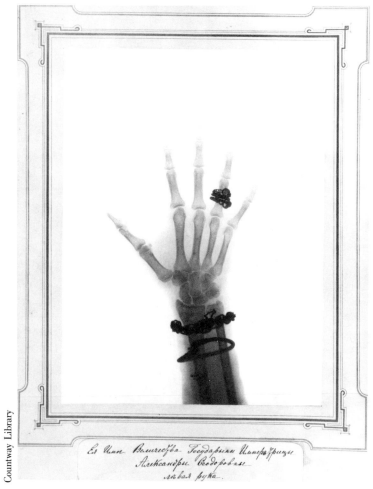

66

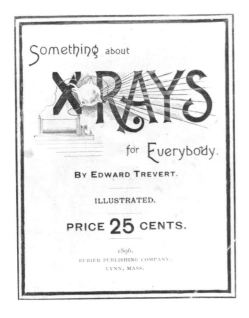

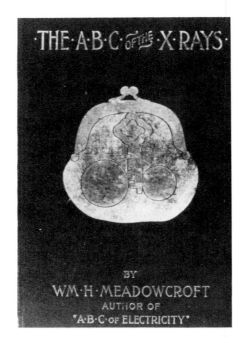

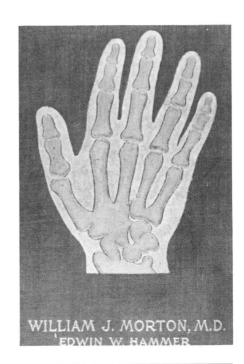

Front cover of Trevert's *Something about X-rays for Everybody* (1896).[3]

Front cover of Meadowcroft's *The ABC of the X-rays* (1896).[1]

Front cover of Morton and Hammer's *The X-ray* (1896).[8]

The first English language books on radiology were written by Edward Trevert (*Something About X-rays for Everybody*, June, 1896),[3] Edward P. Thompson[2] (*Roentgen Rays and Phenomena of the Anode and Cathode*, August, 1896), and William H. Meadowcroft (*The ABC of the X-rays*).[1] The first book published by a physician was *The X-ray* by William J. Morton (and Edwin Hammer), whose preface bears the date of September 1, 1896.[8]

In Britain, the first x-ray monograph was *Practical Radiography* by Henry Snowden Ward. Perhaps due to "unfamiliarity of human anatomy in the light of x-rays,"[35] one of MacIntyre's chest skiagrams over the title "The Human Heart, in situ" was printed upside down on the frontispiece of the book!

EARLY HOSPITAL RADIOLOGY

Hospitals considered x-rays as low priority, assigning limited resources to this curious new form of photography. George E. Pfahler[36] reminisced that:

> the meager space and equipment which were available in 1899 is illustrated by my own experience at the Philadelphia General Hospital, but the importance of the subject can best be gauged by the fact that a special ground floor room was built of concrete 12 by 15 feet—180 square feet of floor space; three feet were separated for a photographic developing room, leaving a total space of 12 by 12 feet for the equipment and furnishings, consisting of a Ruhmkorff coil and a small adjustable tube stand and roentgen-ray tube. A ward carriage was used as a table.

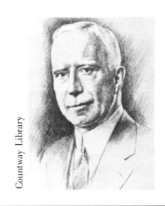

Countway Library

George E. Pfahler (1874-1957).

First x-ray unit at the Massachusetts General Hospital.

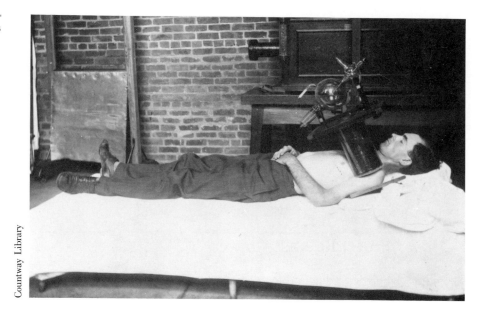

Countway Library

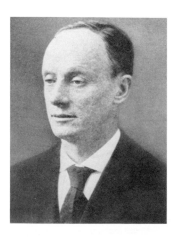

Walter J. Dodd (1869-1916).[38]

In Boston, the first Crookes tube arrived at the Massachusetts General Hospital in early 1896. As Harvey Cushing,[37] then an intern and later a famous neurosurgeon, remembered, "Dr. John Collins Warren had just brought back from Roentgen's laboratory a small tube about the size of a goose's egg and with it (Ernest A.) Codman and I ground out on the old static machine the first faint x-ray picture of the hand ever taken (at the Massachusetts General Hospital)." During the remaining 6 months of his stay in Boston, Cushing became extremely interested in x-rays and actually put up the money to purchase "an x-ray machine," confidently expecting that when the medical staff had learned to appreciate its usefulness he would be reimbursed. As he wrote to his mother in May, "It is great sport—very useful in the Out Patient to locate needles, etc. We looked through the chest readily this morning—count the ribs, see the heart beat, the edge of the liver. It is positively uncanny." However, the person most deeply involved with radiology at the Massachusetts General Hospital was Walter J. Dodd,[38] who had begun his scientific career as a janitor in a chemical laboratory at Harvard. In 1892, Dodd was listed among the employees as an assistant apothecary, but his interest and skill in photography led him to also become the hospital's official photographer. He kept his equipment, developed his negatives, and made his prints in a small building on the hospital grounds. Because x-rays were initially viewed as a new photographic discovery, it was only natural that responsibility for this area become Dodd's (especially once Cushing, who was not reimbursed, left for Baltimore in October, 1896, taking his x-ray tube with him). The first true x-ray room was then set up in "one of the vaulted, dungeon-like small rooms under the front steps of the Bulfinch Building." Meanwhile, Cushing developed the x-ray department at Johns Hopkins Hospital, exposing the photographic plates with the aid of a medical student who had to turn the crank of a static machine for 45 minutes to generate sufficient current.[37]

Children's Hospital in Boston established a Department of Roentgenology in 1903 under Percy Brown[39]: "The first X-ray Department at the Children's Hospital was limited in its function by reason of the fact that the hospital was not equipped with electric current, and was obliged to obtain its power from the Opera House nearby. A wire was run from the

Opera House to the Hospital, but when there was no music there was no current. No opera, no x-rays!" At the Peter Bent Brigham Hospital, a letter written as late as 1911 saw no need for the services of a roentgenologist, specifying[37]: "in regard to a roentgenologist we have put down no salary figure. This Department will probably involve the employment of one or more technical assistants not graduates in medicine, with the probable supervision of a resident or visiting graduate in medicine."

One reason for the generally low opinion of radiologists among other medical specialists was the fact that in the early days radiologists were not willing to delegate the operation of their machines. Thus they were perceived as something lower than physicians, more like technicians.[41]

William Herbert Rollins

The major American advocate for radiation protection was William Herbert Rollins. A New England dentist practicing in the Boston area, Rollins subsequently earned a medical degree but soon settled down to practicing dentistry exclusively. Rollins loved work that required manual dexterity, since it put him closer to his true desire to be a machinist—a goal he could not realize because he was allergic to the irritating metal dust then associated with that trade.[42]

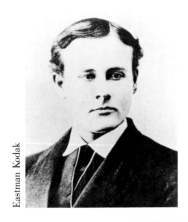

William Herbert Rollins (1852-1929).

Soon after the news of Roentgen's discovery reached the United States, Rollins began to investigate the properties of x-rays. He was a tireless inventor, endlessly designing x-ray tubes and related apparatus for his brother-in-law, Francis H. Williams of Boston City Hospital, who the Brecher's labelled "America's first radiologist." In his own field of dentistry, Rollins described a fluoroscope through which a dentist could observe portions of the oral cavity (see Chapter 21). Much of his work was directed toward methods of improving the radiographic image and creating better x-ray generating apparatus. Accordingly, he pointed out that scattered radiation was of no value for radiography and suggested the use of collimating diaphragms and leaded tube housings.

In January, 1898, while exposing his hand to a highly evacuated tube subjected to a high potential, Rollins suffered a severe burn. This experience probably initiated his intense interest in radiation protection.

Instead of seeking to determine how large a dose could be safely administered, Rollins almost from the beginning urged radiologists to use, especially in diagnostic work, the smallest exposure that would accomplish the purpose. His experiments with guinea pigs showed that the adverse radiation effects were a result of the x-rays themselves and prompted Rollins to offer three precautionary maxims to medical x-ray users (see Chapter 11). But Rollins' suggestions were generally neglected, either because of expense, inconvenience, or simple apathy.

Rollins recommended painting the inside of the tube-enclosing box with several coats of nonradiable paint, white lead in japan. He proposed a quantitative standard that such a tube should meet: "The test . . . is to expose a photographic plate in contact with the outside of the case. If the plate is not fogged in 7 minutes, the coating is sufficient." Misinterpretation of this simple test has credited Rollins with establishing what amounts to the first "tolerance dose" or maximum permissible exposure. However, this was certainly not Rollins' intent, and when it is recalled that at the time and for years thereafter many radiologists were exposing themselves and their patients to the stray radiation from tubes with no

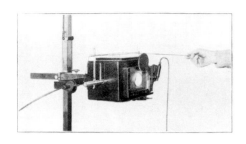

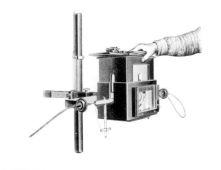

Nonradiable box for an x-light tube (1904). *Top,* Intact unit. *Bottom,* Top being removed to allow the tube to be taken out.[7]

shielding at all, Rollins' 7-minute standard (measured at the face of the tube enclosure, not at the radiologist's position) represented an enormous initial stride toward the minimization of exposure.

Rollins' observations of x-ray hazards were not limited to the effects of the rays themselves. He recognized those effects associated with the production of ozone and oxides of nitrogen by x-ray generating apparatus and suggested that a fan inside the case be used to exhaust these fumes through a chimney.[43] Rollins advised shielding for workers who were constructing and testing x-ray tubes, pointing out that it was unsafe to be near excited tubes for long periods.[44]

Early radiologists often placed their tubes quite close to the patient. Rollins soon recognized that it was safer, as well as optically better, to station the tube farther away. He even built an apparatus containing a protruding rod that made it necessary to keep the tube at least 1 m away from the photographic plate.

Rollins decried the common practice of "warming up" the tube with the patient in its beam. Using this method, the radiologist waited until the fluorescence emitted by the tube indicated that conditions were right before exposing his plate. As an alternative, Rollins designed an instantaneous shutter that worked so that "by pressing and releasing a bulb the shutter is opened, the plate exposed to the most suitable radiation and the shutter closed." Of course, the shutter "should be lined with white lead in japan until nonradiable" and it should overlap the tube-case opening by about 15 mm "to prevent the escape of x-light" through the cracks.

Rollins was the first to suggest the use of two fluorescent screens to decrease the amount of radiation exposure required. As a result of the coarse grain and lack of uniformity of early intensifying screens, Rollins noted that "a single screen makes the developed image blotchy." Accordingly, he recommended the use of more than one intensifying screen, "because the time of exposure is shorter and the blotches are less apparent, for the bright places on one screen usually correspond to darker places on the other."

Importance of relative position of tube and screen or plate (1901). "*Left,* Photograph of the experimental procedure showing the relative positions of a cork containing multiple pins placed at various distances from the vacuum tube and plate. *Right,* Resulting radiograph. The figures in black give the distance of the plate from the tubes; those in white the distance of the pins from the plate (in inches). Clearly, the sharpest images are produced the farther the pin is from the tube and the closer it is to the plate."[10]

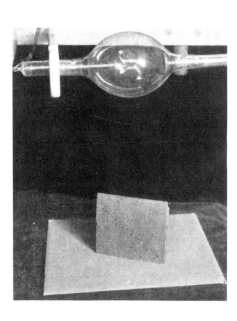

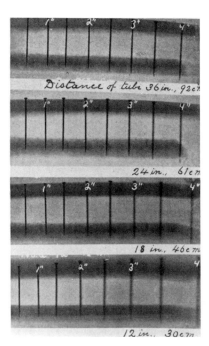

Rollins developed the concept of rectangular collimation. As he stated, "If we use a round opening, the section of the cone of x-light escaping from the tube box is a circle . . . While the patient will be illuminated by the whole cone, it is evident that the only part of the illumination which will be useful will be that included in the rectangular area." As was frequently the case, Rollins' idea was years before its time; the modern "rectangular collimator" was not introduced into general use until the 1950s.

Rollins also designed an arrangement of handles making it possible to control the size of the collimator opening by remote control, so that the radiologist could enlarge or reduce the size of the opening (i.e., the area of the patient's body being radiated) while watching the effects through the fluoroscope. He also described a centering device that would aid in aiming the collimator.

Rollins realized that fluoroscopy produced a much greater exposure both to the radiologist and to the patient than the making of an x-ray plate. Consequently, he made numerous proposals for reducing the degree of fluoroscopic exposure. The fluoroscope

> must have a plate of heavy lead glass to absorb the x-light which has passed unchanged through the fluorescent screen, to prevent injury to the observer's eyes. The walls of the cryptoscope must be made of nonradiable material. The patient should be covered during the photographic exposures with a non-radiable sheet, exposing only the necessary area. An experimenter who works much with x-light should use a non-radiable face mask, the eye holes of which are glazed with thick plates of heavy lead glass.

To reduce patient exposure during fluoroscopy, Rollins recommended that a pulsating rather than a steady current should be fed into the x-ray tube. Since the image on the fluorescent screen persists for a brief interval after the rays cease to excite it, and since the human eye also exhibits a brief persistence of vision, it was possible to take advantage of these two types of persistence "to reduce the total amount of x-light required to make the diagnosis. The best way to do this is (by) sending the electric current in surges, each of very short duration, producing pulses of x-light, that persist as fluorescent light on the screen and in the eyes, allowing intervals between the surges during which, though the light appears continuous to the eye, no (x-)light is shining on the tissues."

Rollins also was probably the first to suggest the use of selective filtration of the x-ray beam,[45] which apparently went unnoticed until emphasized several years later by George Pfahler.

Why was Rollins' work so neglected? According to Kathren,[42]

> It is not difficult to understand why Rollins' efforts have scarcely been recognized, for he was a reserved and highly unpretentious person. He did not make use of his academic degrees, even though this was dictated by the protocol of that era. Although deeply interested in the study of x-rays, he seldom if ever attended meetings of the various societies dedicated to the study of this phenomenon. His name was not carried on the rolls of these organizations, even at the time when he was most actively engaged in his experiments. Even when finally awarded honorary membership in the American Roentgen Ray Society, he had to be persuaded to accept the accolade. The citation, however, made no mention of Rollins' x-ray protection efforts.

Rollins' writing style tended to be sketchy and superficial. His work appeared in only two journals, one of which was a local medical journal of limited circulation. Most of his articles were published in an engineering journal and thus escaped medical attention. Even his book, *Notes on X-Light* (1904), a compilation of his writings on x-rays from 1896 through 1903, was privately printed and had a limited distribution.

As Rollins ruefully wrote in 1903, "Most of these precautions are neglected even at the present time, as may be seen by examining the illustrations in the catalogues of the makers of apparatus and in the papers and books of those who are writing on the subject, where open tubes are almost invariably figured. If masks are used to protect patients during the therapeutic application of x-light, they are in many cases made of rubber cloth or other radiable material."

How many radiation injuries might have been prevented if Rollins had embarked on a career as a commercial manufacturer of x-ray equipment? As Percy Brown observed,[17]

> If, by some turn of the wheel of destiny, William Rollins and others of his type had lent their genius to the commercial production of apparatus embodying their foresight and caution, the picture of American pioneer roentgenology might have been limned in brighter pigments.

Francis Henry Williams

Often labeled America's first radiologist, Francis Henry Williams of Boston was particularly suited by both training and experience to pioneer in the use of x-rays for medical diagnosis. Having graduated from the Massachusetts Institute of Technology before taking his medical degree, Williams had a better understanding than most physicians of the technical problems involved in radiology. A member of the medical staff of Boston City Hospital, Williams used patients in that hospital for his early studies. He worked closely with two staff members at MIT, Charles L.

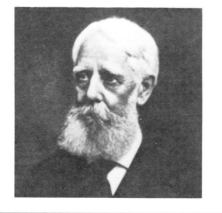

Francis Henry Williams (1852-1936).

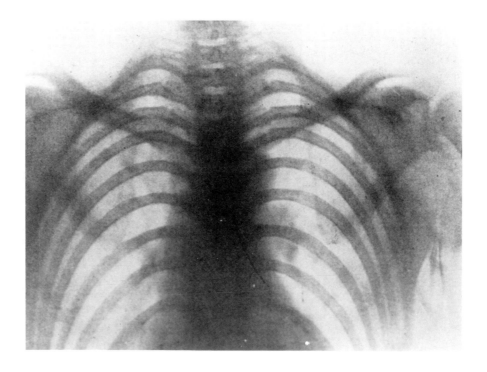

Radiograph taken at the Massachusetts Institute of Technology in early 1896 using an exposure of 45 minutes.[10]

Norton and Ralph R. Lawrence, who designed more powerful x-ray equipment that permitted the taking of sharper radiographs with shorter exposures (as little as ⅕ second by May, 1896).

The first x-ray picture published by Williams appeared in the *Boston Medical and Surgical Journal* (now the *New England Journal of Medicine*) on February 20, 1896. Two months later, Williams gave a demonstration at MIT showing the value of x-rays in diagnosis of diseases of the thorax. As the editor of the Journal reported on April 30, 1896, in addition to the usual demonstrations of the hand and wrist,[46]

> what was more wonderful than what was actually shown to the audience was Doctor Williams' account of what had been accomplished with the fluoroscope in the diagnosis of diseases of the thorax. Doctor Williams and Messrs. Norton and Lawrence had found the thorax much more transparent to the x-rays than the abdomen. The lungs were particularly transparent, the rays passing clearly through them, and the outline of the ribs being plainly seen. The liver was comparatively opaque to the rays, and they were able to mark out accurately the position of the upper border of the liver in extreme inspiration and expiration, and there was found to be a difference of three inches in these levels.

The climax of the meeting came when Williams brought in a patient from the City Hospital who had a greatly enlarged heart. The outline of the heart, as determined by percussion, had been drawn on the skin of the man's chest, but this outline could not be seen through the shirt he was wearing. With the shirt still on, Williams drew on it the outline of the

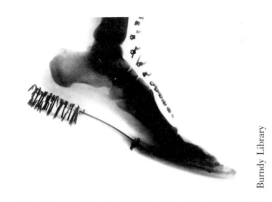

Foot with shoe (Williams, 1896). Time of exposure, 20 minutes.[28]

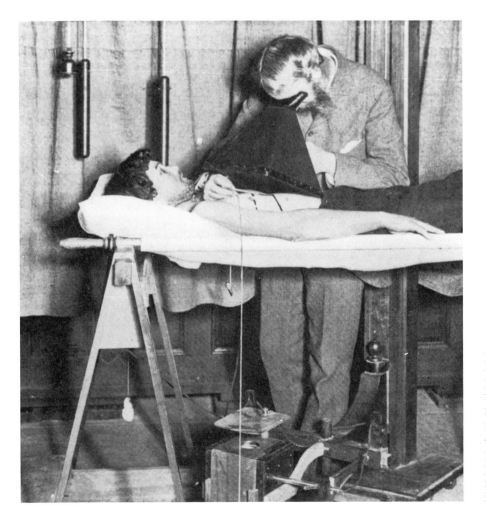

Method of drawing the outlines on the patient's skin while looking through the fluoroscope (1901). "The fluoroscope is held farther away from the patient than is necessary in practice in order that the pencil which is under it may be shown in the picture. The observer usually stands on the patient's right, but in order to show the method of examination better, he is standing on the patient's left."[10]

heart as it appeared on the screen of the fluoroscope. When the shirt was removed, the outline that Williams had drawn on it "everywhere corresponded very closely with the area previously drawn on the skin by percussion." As the Journal concluded,[46] "Dr. Williams was warmly applauded at the close of his most interesting and successful demonstration."

When the extremely impressed editor of the Journal asked for further details of his experiments, Williams wrote him a letter that also appeared in the publication. As Williams stated,

> During the past few weeks . . . I have tested the application of the rays to medical practice in various ways . . . Our aim has been to make the rays pass through the body; and recently (April 22) this was attained, when Mr. Norton saw in a dark room by means of the fluoroscope the ribs and backbone of an adult. On the same evening, I examined Mr. Norton from behind, and saw, besides his ribs and backbone, that the lighter portion of the area of the right lung was limited below by a darker outline at about the height of the 4th rib, and that this outline moved up and down with expiration and inspiration. Evidently this was the upper border of the liver . . . It seemed to me desirable to examine some of my patients by the x-rays. The first case was that of a man with an enlarged heart (7 inches in transverse diameter). I found that the outline of the heart as seen from the front of the body through the fluoroscope, corresponded in a general way to the outline drawn on the skin with percussion as a guide. Messrs. Norton and Lawrence confirmed my observation. It was interesting to note that the heart could be made out through the man's waistcoat and two shirts. The next case was that of a man with an enlarged spleen who had leukemia. The outline of this spleen could be followed in part; but it was so obvious by palpation that the latter was a readier way of tracing it. One of the most interesting cases was that of a patient suffering from tuberculosis of the right lung, who was under the care of one of my colleagues . . . After looking at him from behind for a moment the difference in the amount of rays which passed through the two sides of the chest was very striking, as seen through the fluoroscope. The diseased lung, as I had predicted, being darker throughout than the normal lung. The ribs on the left side were much more distinct than those on the right, and the heart of this patient could be seen more clearly than usual.

In early 1897, Williams summarized his broad medical experience with x-rays in a classic 57-page paper published in the *Medical and Surgical Reports* of the Boston City Hospital.[47] In this work, Williams accurately described the radiographic features of a wide variety of thoracic abnormalities, including tuberculosis, pneumonia, emphysema, pleural effusion, pulmonary edema, cardiac hypertrophy, pericardial effusion, and intrathoracic aneurysm (see Chapters 12 and 13). In addition to long sections describing the radiographic findings in a broad spectrum of thoracic abnormalities, there were chapters on surgical conditions containing numerous superb illustrations of fractures, dislocations, foreign bodies, and bone diseases that compared favorably with radiographs obtained many years later. In the section on gastrointestinal disease, it was clear that Williams had been one of the first to use bismuth meals in examinations on humans. The section on therapeutic uses of x-rays detailed surprisingly good results in the treatment of superficial conditions, even at a time before filtration or methods of measurement were known.

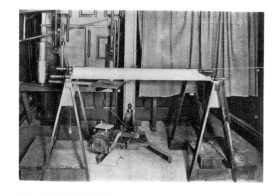

X-ray apparatus at Boston City Hospital (1901). "The poles of the stretchers used in the hospital are kept apart by steel rods, at the head and foot, which have an opening in each end through which the ends of the stretcher poles pass. Fastened to the wooden horses at either end, there is a step on which the orderlies stand when they lift the stretcher with the patient lying upon it onto the horses; the horses would be too high to reach without this aid. Under the stretcher is seen a tube holder, with a very thin aluminum screen (which is grounded) above it."[10]

Williams stressed the use of a diaphragm to produce a sharper image and even to protect the patient. He recommended "a piece of sheet metal (e.g., brass) six inches wide by twelve inches long, and thick enough to prevent the passage of the x-rays, toward one end of which is cut a rectangular opening—this is preferable to a circular one—about two by three inches being a convenient size. After taking a general survey with the fluoroscope, the part of the body that is to be carefully examined is selected, and the metal plate held . . . in such a position that the x-rays coming from the Crookes tube fall directly through the opening, while the surrounding area is shielded by the metal. The fingers should be protected from the rays while holding the plate, and to accomplish this object leather straps are fastened onto the plate, so that the fingers may be inserted under them on the upper side; the plate may be moved about and any special part examined." To study a large field, Williams moved the brass plate closer to the tube; for a smaller field, he moved it closer to the patient. Another handy device introduced by Williams was a pencil "made of metal, with a crayon point suitable for marking the skin." Alternatively, a strip of lead wire could be fastened with adhesive plaster to an ordinary crayon and its movement followed through the fluoroscope.

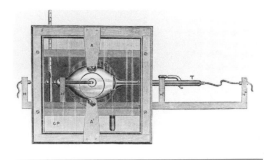

Nonradiable x-light tube box with centering diaphragm plate.[7]

In this article, Williams included an introductory lesson in the physics of radiation, a discussion of the relative merits of fluoroscopy vs x-ray photography, and a brief review of radiation geometry. This was illustrated by a discussion of the detection of stones in the kidney and bladder: "Before attempting to detect any form of calculi in the body, I first placed several different kinds over a photographic plate, which was enclosed in dark paper to shield it from the light, and exposed them for a few minutes to the x-rays. The rays penetrated the calculi made up of uric acid, of cholesterine, and biliary salts very readily, but were obstructed by calculi containing oxalate of calcium in considerable proportion, phosphate of calcium, or other inorganic constituents." Williams therefore concluded "that any attempt to detect in the body calculi made up of organic compounds would, so far as our knowledge now goes, be futile, whereas those of inorganic origin might be detected."

This need for physical experimentation before clinical trials became a standard procedure for Williams. For example, he compared the effect of x-rays through clear water with x-rays through "the various fluids formed in the body in health or disease, such as the blood, ascitic and pleuritic fluid, the urine, pus, fluid from hydrocele, etc.," and reported that all were "found to offer about the same resistance to the passage of the rays."

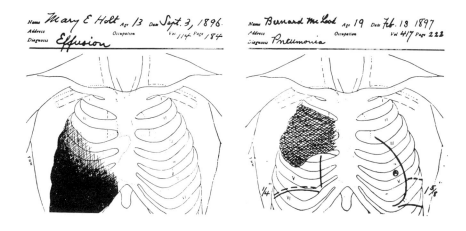

Examples of Williams' short medical x-ray reports.

Williams predicted that the best approach to medical diagnosis with x-rays depended on the differential opacity of *air* as opposed to water or organic tissue. As he wrote, "It is readily seen of how much importance is this difference in permeability of air and water by the rays, on account of the great contrast which is thereby afforded in health between the lungs and their adjacent tissues or organs." This probably was one of the considerations that led Williams to initially concentrate his efforts on radiology of the chest.

In collaboration with his physicist co-workers, Lawrence and Norton, Williams appreciated that the higher the voltage the greater the penetrating power of the resulting x-rays. "It is sometimes of service to be able to vary the length of the spark (in modern terminology, the voltage applied to the tube while observing it with the fluoroscope), and the character of the picture changes with the character of the light. For instance, with a long spark (high voltage) the medullary canal of the long bones is distinctly visible while with a short one this disappears and the bones become darker."

Williams' understanding of the fundamentals of radiologic geometry was evidenced by his clinical suggestions for using the fluoroscope:

> It is important to bear in mind the relative position of this instrument (the fluoroscope), the Crookes tube, and the organ which is under observation. For example, in examining the heart a good position for the tube is about on a level with the heart in front of the patient and a little to the right of his median line; the patient should not face the tube squarely, but should be placed with his right side turned a little toward it; the observer, standing behind the patient and holding the fluoroscope to the left back of the latter, thus sees a shadow of the apex projected on the screen of the fluoroscope far to the left, even touching the left posterior axillary line, thus bringing a large part of the heart into view.

With his brother-in-law, Rollins, Williams recognized early the potential dangers of fluoroscopy and stressed the need for performing it under stringent precautions. Therefore unlike many of the other early x-ray workers, Williams never suffered any serious radiation injury.

Williams' 1901 book, *The Roentgen Rays in Medicine and Surgery,* was the first major textbook in American radiographic literature. In the opening pages, Williams produced a half-tone illustration that graphically showed the comparative densities as revealed by x-rays of many of the substances constituting human tissues. Originally produced 4 years previously, it was republished with the following paragraph:

> This experiment suggests how we may recognize some changes in chemical composition made in the body by pathological processes. The ability to do this without beaker or re-agents or without disturbing the vital processes is a step in the application of chemistry and physics and practical medicine, which hints that which the future may have in store for us.

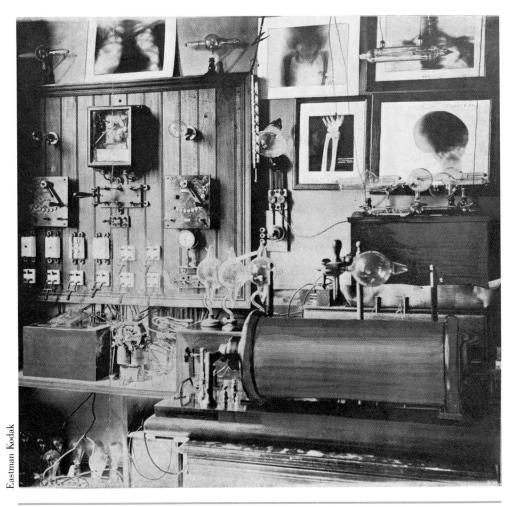

X-ray laboratory of William Fuchs.

As an editorial[48] entitled "A Pioneer in Roentgenology" noted in 1925,

> The directions given by Dr. Williams nearly a quarter century ago for the examination of the chest are delightfully precise, differing from many later works where too much is taken for granted. I quote the following: 'In making examinations the three following stages should be kept distinctly and separately in mind; first, attention should be given to observing carefully the appearances which present themselves; second, a very careful record should be made of these appearances in some simple and direct way which will be a record of facts, not of opinions; third, the observations made should be well considered by themselves and in connection with information furnished from other sources. The evidence from each source should be given just, but not exclusive consideration for making a diagnosis.' It would be hard to find three more useful rules for the examination of patients.

Bibliography

Brecher R and Brecher E: The rays: A history of radiology in the United States and Canada. Baltimore, Williams & Wilkins, 1969.

Evans WA: American pioneers in radiology. In Glasser O (ed): The science of radiology. Springfield, Ill, Charles C Thomas, 1933.

Glasser O: Wilhelm Conrad Roentgen and the early history of the Roentgen Rays. Springfield, Ill, Charles C Thomas, 1934.

Rollins W: Notes on x-light. Boston, Privately published, 1904.

Williams FH: The roentgen rays in medicine and surgery. New York, Macmillan, 1901.

References

1. Meadowcroft WH: The ABC of the x-rays. New York, Excelsior Publishing House, 1896.
2. Thompson EP: Roentgen rays. New York, 1896.
3. Trevert E: Something about x-rays for everybody. Lynn, Mass, Bubier, 1896.
4. Walsh D: The Röntgen rays in medical work. New York, Wood, 1902.
5. Henshaw GB: The roentgen rays: Their production and use. Boston, American Roentgen Ray Company, 1897.
6. Electrical World 27:360, 1896.
7. Rollins W: Notes on x-light. Boston, Privately published, 1904.
8. Morton WJ and Hammer EW: The x-ray. New York, American Technical Book Co, 1896.
9. Fuchs W: Historical notes on x-ray plates and films. In Bruwer AJ (ed): Classic descriptions in diagnostic roentgenology. Springfield, Ill, Charles C Thomas, 1964.
10. Williams FH: The roentgen rays in medicine and surgery. New York, MacMillan, 1901.
11. Crane AW: Skiascopy of the respiratory organs. Phila Med J 1:154-170, 1899.
12. Londe A: Technique et applications médicales. Paris, Gauthier-Villars, 1898.
13. Martin JM: Practical electro-therapeutics and x-ray. St. Louis, The CV Mosby Co, 1912.
14. American X-ray Journal 9:111, 1902.
15. Kassabian MK: Technique of x-ray work. Amer X-Ray J 8:867-876, 1901.
16. Brunel G: Manuel de radioscopie et de radiographie. Paris, Tignol, 1900.
17. Brown P: American martyrs to science through the roentgen rays. Springfield, Ill, Charles C Thomas, 1936.
18. Lusted LB and Miller ER: Progress in indirect cineroentgenography. AJR 75:56-62, 1956.
19. Bleyer JM: On the Bleyer photo-fluoroscope. Elect Engin 22:10-11, 1896.
20. Battelli A and Garbasso A: Concerning the rays of Roentgen. Il Nuovo Cimento 4:40-61, 1896.
21. MacIntyre J: X-ray records for the cinematograph. Arch Skiag 1:37, 1897.
22. Brown P: Trans Amer Roentgen Ray Soc 232-237, 1908.
23. Grigg ERN: The trail of the invisible light. Springfield, Ill, Charles C Thomas, 1964.
24. Burrows EH: Pioneers and early years: A history of British radiology. Channel Islands, England, Colophon, 1986.
25. Murphy JT: Influences affecting the future of roentgenology. AJR 30:718-722, 1933.
26. Sayre RH: Trans Amer Roentgen Ray Soc 238-239, 1908.
27. Carman RD: Medical roentgenology as a specialty. J Missouri State Med Assoc 7:121-123, 1910.
28. Glasser O: Wilhelm Conrad Röntgen and the discovery of the roentgen rays. In Glasser O (ed): The science of radiology. Springfield, Ill, Charles C Thomas, 1933.
29. Arch Roentgen Ray 2:36, 1897.
30. Lang EF: From earlier pages. AJR 130:586-587, 1978.
31. Cipollaro AC: The earliest roentgen demonstration of a pathological lesion in America. Radiology 45:555-558, 1945.
32. Western Electrician 18: February 15, 1896.
33. Montreal Med J 24:661-665, 1896.
34. Ramsey LJ: Some notable early contributors to radiography: Thompson, Jackson and Campbell-Swinton. Radiography 46:289-297, 1980.
35. Posner E: The early years of chest radiology in Britain. Thorax 26:233-239, 1971.
36. Pfahler GE: The early history of roentgenology in Philadelphia. AJR 75:14-22, 1956.
37. Fulton JF: Harvey Cushing. Springfield, Ill, Charles C Thomas, 1946.
38. Macy J: Walter James Dodd. Boston, Houghton Mifflin, 1918.
39. Sosman MC: Roentgenology at Harvard. Harvard Medical Alumni Bulletin, 1947.
40. Mould RF: A history of x-rays and radium. 1980.
41. Feldman A: A sketch of the technical history of radiology from 1896 to 1920. RadioGraphics 9:1113-1128, 1989.
42. Kathren RL: William H. Rollins (1852-1929): X-ray protection pioneer. J Hist Med 19:287-294, 1964.
43. Rollins W: Removing the irritating gases produced by x-light generators. Boston Med Surg J 144:403, 1901.
44. Rollins W: Pumping x-light tubes. Elect Rev 40:538, 1902.
45. Rollins WA: A grouping of some of the axioms mentioned. Elect Rev 43:849, 1903.
46. Boston Med Surg J 134:447-448, 1896.
47. Williams FH: The Röntgen rays in thoracic diseases. J Am Med Sci 114:665-687, 1897.
48. Hickey PM: A pioneer in roentgenology. AJR 13:484-486, 1925.

CHAPTER 5

Stereoscopic Radiology

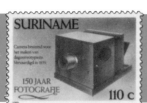

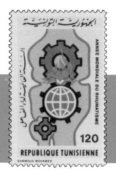

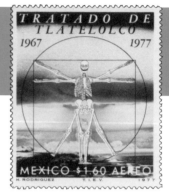

Stereoscopy is a method for producing a pair of two-dimensional pictures that can be perceived as a single three-dimensional image. At the time of the discovery of x-rays, the technique of making stereoscopic photographs had been well known for decades. Modern stereoscopy was born with the final development of the theory of binocular vision and the invention of the stereoscope by Sir Charles Wheatstone in 1838.[1] Five years later (1843), Sir David Brewster invented the lenticular, or refracting, stereoscope.[2] The Brewster hand stereoscope was later used extensively in viewing stereoscopic photographs of radiographs.[3]

To make a stereoscopic photograph, the photographer simply took a picture, moved his camera 1 inch or so to the side, and took a second picture. When the two pictures were viewed in a stereoscopic viewer, so that one eye saw only one picture and the other eye only the other, the illusion of depth and solidity was readily achieved. It was easy to judge the relative position of objects in the foreground, middle ground, and background.[6]

The first publication suggesting the application of stereoscopy to radiography was written by Elihu Thomson and appeared on March 11, 1896.[7] As Thomson[7] wrote,

> while experimenting with the making of shadow pictures, it occurred to the writer that it would be desirable to secure some indication of the position in space of various embedded solid objects, or, in other words, to obtain a pair of pictures which, when placed in a stereoscope would show solidity. This would manifestly be useful in surgical examinations, as the true relations in space of the parts of a bone, or of a foreign body and the bone would become evident. The ordinary Röntgen pictures are simple shadows on a plane surface. It is impossible to tell from such a shadow whether one object or part of an object is front or back of another. There is, however, no difficulty in determining the real positions when resort is had to the production of stereoscopic shadow pictures.

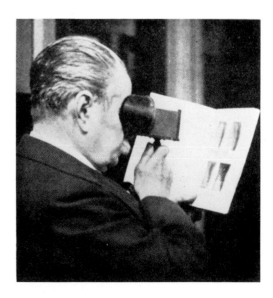

Brewster hand stereoscope, modified for stereoscopic viewing of photographic reproductions of radiographs.[3]

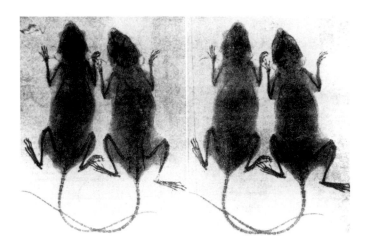

First published stereoscopic radiographs depicting two mice.[8]

As with plain photography, Thomson exposed two plates with a Crookes tube in slightly different positions. He then made paper prints from the negatives and mounted them for use in an ordinary stereoscopic viewer. With justifiable pride, Thomson reported the complete success of his first trial:

> The effect is very curious. A cork or block of wood having nails or screws driven into it in various directions is clearly shown and the screws or nails in their proper positions. When two heavily insulated wires twisted together constitute the object, the metal wires alone are seen, but standing apart in space, one around the other. The bones of two superimposed figures are to be seen in their correct positions.

Stereoscope for examining binocular radiographs (1902). "A set of four pairs of prints can be tacked on the square pillars and examined in succession by turning the pillars round on their pivoted base. These pillars slide on a sledge to any focal distance from the pair of small mirrors set at right angles on the central post and marked MM. This post slides backward and forward to any focus. For inspection, level the two prints with their lines running in the same directions as shown by the two knives in the plate. *Bottom,* Then place the stereoscope so that the light will equally fall on the right and left side of the view, sit in front of the reflecting mirrors with the bridge of the nose engaging the angle of meeting, and each eye looks squarely into one mirror. Then with each hand draw up or slide back the pillars until they are equally in focus with the eyes and both pictures appear as one. Complete the exact adjustment by sliding the post with the mirrors until the landmarks of the two pictures exactly cover each other. The view is then correct. To view the hands cutting a pear, the pillars must be given a quarter turn to bring them into a position facing each other and the mirrors."[5]

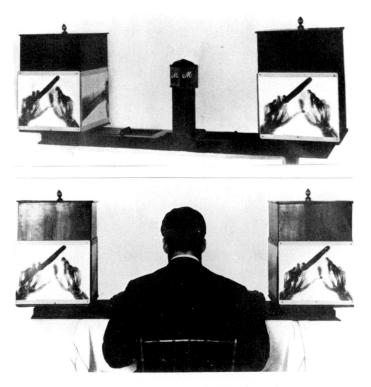

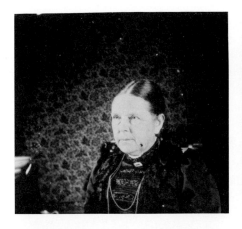
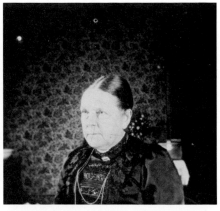
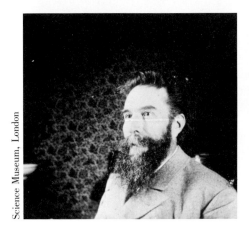
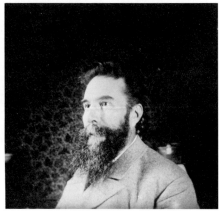

Stereopair photographs taken by Roentgen. *Top*, Mrs. Roentgen. *Bottom*, Roentgen himself.

Thomson also suggested the use of stereoscopic fluoroscopy, which never enjoyed the popularity of stereoradiography, probably because of the complexity of the equipment required.

Within 2 weeks of Thomson's article, an independent report by Armand Imbert and Henri Bertin-Sans was published in the French literature.[8] Among the many European investigators who applied stereoscopy to radiography was Sir James McKenzie Davidson, who stressed the value of this technique for foreign body localization.[9] Davidson also described a method for viewing stereoscopically without a stereoscope by crossing the visual axes (i.e., looking at the two images cross-eyed).

Stereoscopy was employed in many areas of radiology. The skull, including the facial bones and sinuses, could be beautifully demonstrated stereoscopically. However, pneumoencephalography could be better interpreted using right-angle views. Stereoradiographs of the cerebrovascular system after the injection of opaque contrast yielded superb results. In the thorax, stereoscopy was useful for studies of the lungs, spine, and ribs; the heart and gastrointestinal tract were poorly imaged because they appeared as disks rather than three dimensional and their movements resulted in undesirable parallax. Accurate measurements of the pelvis could be made on stereoradiographs, and the bladder, rectum, and uterus filled with opaque contrast could be demonstrated to good advantage. Certain areas of the skeleton, such as the shoulder, were better viewed stereoscopically than with right-angle views.[3]

The development of modern cross-sectional imaging effectively marked the end of the stereoscopic era in diagnostic radiology.

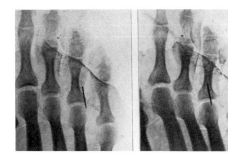

Stereoscopic radiograph of a piece of needle in the sole of the foot (1904). The skin of the sole was rubbed with powdered bismuth subnitrate.[10]

Four physicians using hand stereoscopes to view a pair of stereoscopic chest radiographs.

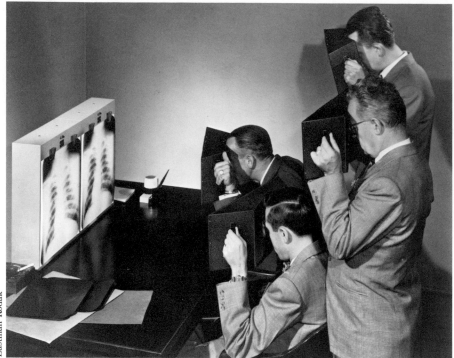

Eastman Kodak

References

1. Wheatstone C: Contributions of the physiology of vision: Part the first. On some remarkable, and hitherto unobserved, phenomena of binocular vision. Philosoph Trans Royal Soc London. Part I. 371-394, 1838.
2. Brewster D: Stereoscopy: Its history, theory and construction. John Murray Publishers, London, 1856.
3. Keats TE: Origin of stereoscopy in diagnostic roentgenology. In Bruwer AJ (ed): Classic descriptions in diagnostic roentgenology. Springfield, Ill, Charles C Thomas, 1964.
4. Davidson JM: Localization by x-rays and stereoscopy. London, Lewis, 1916.
5. Monell SH: A system of instruction in x-ray methods and medical uses of light, hot-air, vibration and high-frequency currents. New York, Pelton, 1902.
6. Brecher R and Brecher E: The rays: A history of radiology in the United States and Canada. Baltimore, Williams & Wilkins, 1969.
7. Thomson E: Stereoscopic roentgen pictures. Electrical Engineer 21:256, 1896.
8. Imbert A and Bertin-Sans H: Stereoscopic photographs obtained by means of x-rays. CR Acad Soc (Paris), p 786, March 30, 1896.
9. Davidson JM: Remarks on the value of stereoscopic photography and skiagraphy: Records of clinical and pathologic appearances. Brit Med J 2:1668-1671, 1898.
10. Pusey WA and Caldwell EW: The practical application of roentgen rays in therapeutics and diagnosis. Philadelphia, WB Saunders, 1904.

TECHNOLOGY OF RADIOLOGY

"X-RAY"

My father is a Doctor Man,
And he does the queerest things;
Finds hooks and eyes and safety pins,
Down little babies' long red lanes.
The "Grown-ups" all have aches and pains,
And sometimes have the queerest names.
He takes them in a room that's dark,
And pulls a switch that makes a spark.
He says, "Now steady, hold your breath!"
The spark goes "buz-z-z-z," and he says, "All right!"
And last he asks them "Name and Age,"
And "When they've had a fall."
But now I'll tell you,
'Tis very strange to say,
That all this rigmarole is simply called—
                    X-RAY!

Helen Ashbury, age 12
AJR 7:484, 1920

CHAPTER 6

X-ray Plates, Film, and Screens

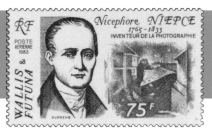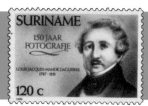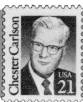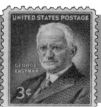

Radiology is actually a form of photography, since it is a process whereby images are obtained on sensitized surfaces by the action of light or other radiant energy. Like photography, radiography may use visible light as emitted from fluorescent screens, or it may use invisible light (x-rays) that differs from visible light only in wavelength. Since radiography uses photographic emulsions as recording media, this aspect of its history reaches back to the beginning of photography in the eighteenth century when it was observed that some silver compounds blackened when exposed to light.

THE BEGINNINGS OF PHOTOGRAPHY

The prototype of the modern camera was developed in the sixteenth century by Giovanni Battista della Porta, who illustrated and described (1553) the "camera obscura." It consisted of a box with a small aperture through which an observer could view a distant scene and copy it on paper. Danielo Barbaro (1568) fitted the camera obscura with a simple lens and a movable diaphragm to sharpen the image.

In 1727, a German chemist, Johann H. Schultz, discovered that a paste of silver carbonate or silver chloride mixed with chalk became dark when the glass tube it was in was exposed to light. After stencils of letters were placed on the tube and the material was exposed to sunlight, black-lettered images were seen when the stencils were removed. However, these images were only transient. Since no way was known to make them permanent, the areas originally protected from light eventually darkened.[2] A few years later, a Swedish chemist, Carl Wilhelm Scheele, coated a paper with silver chloride and, by using a prism to refract the sun's rays, produced an image of the solar spectrum on the paper.

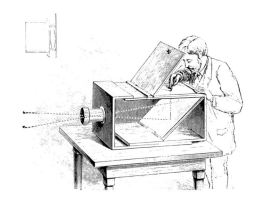

Camera obscura. This first camera was constructed by making a small hole in a large box. An image formed by a lens and reflected by a mirror onto a ground glass was then traced.[1]

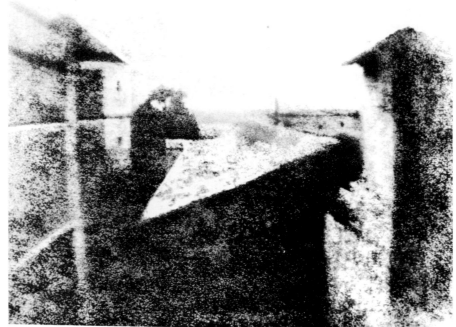

First known photograph taken by Niepce in 1826. Crude photograph of his house in St. Loup-de Varenness using a camera obscura and an exposure time of 8 hours.[1]

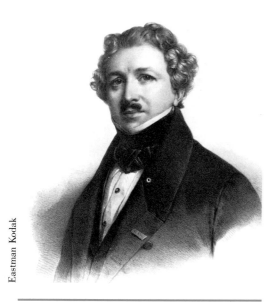

Louis J. Daguerre (1789-1851).

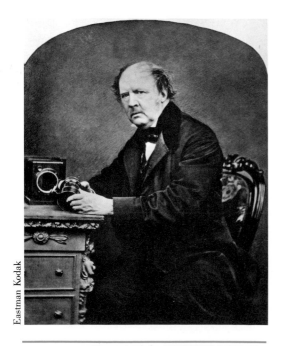

William Henry Fox Talbot (1800-1877).

Thomas Wedgewood and Sir Humphrey Davy (1802) recorded silhouettes on glass by contact printing on paper coated with silver chloride. Fourteen years later (1816), Joseph-Nicéphore Niepce obtained negative images from a crude camera consisting of a jewel box in which a lens from a microscope was inserted. Unfortunately, none of the images could be made permanent, although in 1826 Niepce did apply an engraving process to fix the image and is thus credited with making the first permanent photograph. In 1819, the great astronomer, Sir John Herschel (who discovered the planet Uranus in 1781), found that "hypo" (sodium thiosulfate) would dissolve away residual silver chloride. However, the Reverend J. B. Reade was the first (1839) to use hypo to dissolve the unexposed silver salts remaining in the photograph. This treatment prevented the image from darkening on further exposure to light.

A French painter and inventor, Louis-Jacques-Mandé Daguerre, recorded images (1839) on plates covered with a silver salt that had been fused with iodine to form a layer of silver iodide. Long exposures of these plates in a camera produced faint, unsatisfactory visual images. One day, Daguerre placed one of the exposed plates in his cupboard. When he removed the plate later, he found that there was a well-defined positive image on it. Some mercury had been spilled in the cabinet, and its fumes had "developed" the image completely. The unexposed silver iodide was removed by a solution of sodium chloride. In this way, Daguerre established the basis for chemical *development* of a photosensitive material.

In the same year, William Henry Fox Talbot, an English physicist, exposed silver chloride paper in a camera obscura to secure a visible image that was made permanent by washing the paper with a solution containing weak reducing agents (silver nitrate and gallic acid). Of much greater value was the discovery that it was not necessary to expose the paper in the camera until a clear image appeared. An image that was barely visible could be developed further by applying an additional amount of the reducing agent. An exposure of more than an hour was no longer necessary; a picture could be taken in half a minute. This process of developing a latent image to a negative form from which any number of positive prints could be made (negative-positive method) was the ancestor of modern photography. It is interesting to note that Herschel, who discovered hypo, in a letter to Talbot dated February 28, 1839 coined the word *photography* (drawing with light) in referring to Talbot's work. Herschel also was the first to use the terms *negative* and *positive* to describe the photographic images.[2]

Paper negatives were used up to this time, but the objectionable grain of the paper was reproduced on the prints. To overcome this condition, Claude-Félix-Abel Niepce de Saint-Victor (1847) coated glass with an albumin emulsion containing silver iodide to produce a plate that could be used in cameras. Gallic acid was used for development and resulted in a good quality image of fine grain.

In 1851, Frederick Scott Archer of England published the details of a process for using wet collodion (a sticky substance) as a binder for coating silver salts on glass plates. The glass plate had to be prepared immediately and exposed while still wet; development also had to be performed immediately before the collodion dried. Although this method soon supplanted all other processes, it was laborious and inconvenient and various attempts were made to find a system for coating a plate that could be dried and stored until used.

Richard L. Maddox of England (1871) invented the *dry* plate, using an emulsion of silver bromide in gelatin (rather than collodion), which served as the basis for modern photography. The plate was slow and the salts often crystallized in the emulsion, since Maddox did not realize the necessity for washing away the excess of silver salts. The speed and stability of the plate was improved by J. Burgess, who in 1873 manufactured the first practical dry plate with a *washed* emulsion. In that same year, H. W. Vogel discovered that such plates, normally sensitive only to blue and violet light, could be made sensitive to all colors by the addition of certain dyes.

Dry plates were found to be several times faster than wet plates and were soon manufactured in several countries. Although at first coated by hand, a plate-coating machine for mass production was invented in 1879 by George Eastman. Another important accomplishment of Eastman (1885) was the introduction of a stripping film (*American Film*), which used paper as a temporary support for the emulsion. The paper was coated with two layers of gelatin, one soluble and the other insoluble but light sensitive. After processing, hot water was used to dissolve the soluble gelatin. The gelatin bearing the image could then be transferred to a clear sheet of gelatin, which was dried flat on glass and stripped from it, leaving a thin transparent "film" from which prints could be made. Eastman also began the manufacture of paper sensitized with an emulsion for use in cameras (*Negative Paper*). After exposure and development, the paper was made transparent for printing by chemical treatment. Four years later (1889), Eastman's company was the first to introduce roll film consisting of a flexible transparent base of cellulose nitrate coated with a sensitive silver halide emulsion.

The trademark *Kodak* was introduced in 1888. Eastman wanted a short and easily spelled word that could be readily pronounced in any language. The letter "K" was one of his favorites, and after experimenting with many combinations starting and ending with the letter "K," Eastman decided on the word *Kodak*.[2]

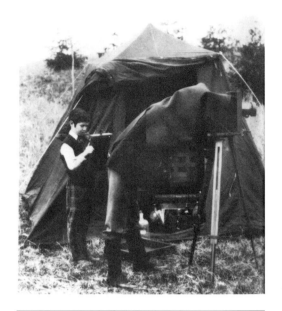

Photographer in operation in the field in the early 1870s. Note the amount of equipment and the size of the camera required to make a photograph of the landscape. It is also interesting to note that the photographer needed an assistant—in this case, a young boy. Today, the boy would take the picture with a simple hand-held camera.[2]

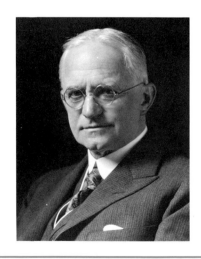

George Eastman (1845-1932).

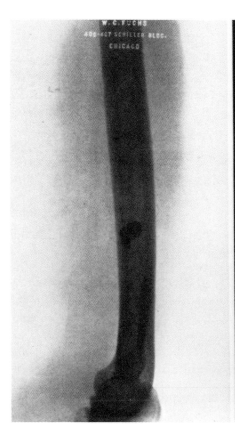

Photograph of a compass card and needle completely enclosed in a metal case (originally published in *Roentgen's First Communication* in *Nature* 53:274-276, January 23, 1896).[3]

EARLY RADIOGRAPHY

Roentgen's original paper[3] indicated the importance of the photographic plate as a means of *recording* the radiographic image and contained illustrative examples of Mrs. Roentgen's hand and a compass box:

> Of special interest in many ways is the fact that photographic dry plates show themselves susceptible to x-rays. We are thus in a position to corroborate many phenomena in which mistakes are easy, and I have, whenever possible, controlled each important ocular observation in fluorescence by means of photography.

In 1896, it was difficult to produce a satisfactory radiograph because the photographic plate then available and designed for exposure to light was affected by only a small proportion of the x-ray energy that fell on it. Nevertheless, superb images can be seen in the reproductions of photographs obtained by some early radiologists, who possessed no more elaborate equipment than a low-power induction coil, a temperamental gas tube, and a photographic dry plate. Of course, many of these early radiographs required an exposure of one or more hours to make a simple image of the hand. If it were possible to compare an early radiograph with a modern one, it would be obvious that the image in the former lacked density and contrast. Regardless of the length of the x-ray exposure, after-treatment of the radiographs often was necessary to make satisfactory prints from them. Since the early radiographer followed the procedure practiced by the professional photographer, positive prints of radiographs were usually made on a sensitive photographic paper that possessed considerable contrast. Moreover, the density and contrast in the print could be increased, thereby enhancing details that were only faintly visible in the plate. The prints were often gold-toned to produce a pleasing sepia positive.[4]

Comparison of early and "modern" radiographs. An unusual historical item showing an early radiograph and "follow-up" made 35 years later. The patient was a girl who had been shot by a rifle bullet in 1897. The radiographic examination was made in the laboratory of Wolfram C. Fuchs in Chicago. After the examination, gold-toned contact prints were made from the *original glass plate*. One was sent to her physician; another was given to the patient and is reproduced on the left. The patient was reexamined in 1932 with "modern" x-ray film (*right*), and the bullet may still be seen in its original position.[6]

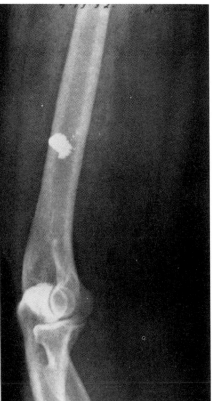

A major controversy at that time was the nature of the effect of x-rays on the photographic plate. Did x-rays act directly on the sensitive emulsion or indirectly by inducing "phosphorescence" or some unknown action at the back of the dry plate? Some investigators recommended the use of Celluloid (trade name for a colorless product composed of pyroxylin and camphor used for photographic film) instead of glass because it was more fluorescent and thus would produce a denser image. This entire concept was disproved by workers who obtained radiographs by exposing emulsion stripped from the glass or celluloid backing. According to one theory, the exposure action of x-rays was thought to be due almost entirely to fluorescence within the emulsion aided by the fluorescence of the glass support. Some even stated that x-rays exerted no *direct* action on the sensitive plate! This speculation was disproved by the ability to make radiographs on bromide paper, a substance that does not fluoresce.

Eventually, it was shown that the action of x-rays was similar to that of light. Radiation reaching the emulsion was primarily responsible for exposure of the silver halide emulsion. Any fluorescence of the emulsion or support was slight and did not produce a significant image. Of course, this applied only to direct x-ray exposure. When intensifying screens were used, it was the fluorescent light from the screen that exposed the film.

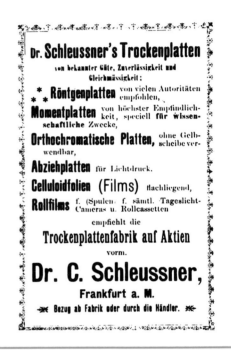

Schleussner advertisement (1899) listing roentgen plates and celluloid films.[6]

PHOTOGRAPHIC PLATES

The earliest plate made strictly for radiographic purposes was probably produced by Carl Schleussner, a German photographic plate manufacturer, who at the request of Roentgen made some plates with a heavier-than-average silver bromide emulsion. These plates allowed for greater photographic density and became popular in the United States and Europe. The first American plate strictly for x-ray purposes (February, 1896) was made by John Carbutt in cooperation with Arthur W. Goodspeed of Philadelphia. This product, called the *Roentgen X-Ray Plate*, had a thicker and heavier silver emulsion than the usual photographic plate and permitted a dramatic reduction in the time of exposure (20 minutes vs an hour or more for an examination of the fingers). Within 2 months, further improvements in apparatus and x-ray plates permitted exposures to range from a few seconds for a hand to 30 to 60 seconds for heavy parts of the body. Projections of the trunk, however, were still a problem because exposures were on the order of minutes rather than seconds.

The early photographic dry plates were slow to x-rays, prompting a real need for more sensitive emulsions. The proper characteristics of an x-ray emulsion, as stated by Carbutt,[5] were that "it should be of medium sensitiveness, have a good body of emulsion, be capable of absorbing the x-rays, thereby giving more detail and perspective to the bones." Multiple experimenters tried every conceivable method for increasing the emulsion speeds. Dry plates were immersed before exposure in solutions of iron chloride or uranium nitrate but no better images were produced. Heating the plates or soaking them in solutions of fluorescent salts only resulted in a loss of sensitivity and the production of extreme fog, which made the plates worthless. In England, Alan Archibald Campbell-Swinton mixed the silver emulsion with powdered fluorspar and calcium tungstate, but this produced excessive granularity of the image without any substantial increase in sensitivity.

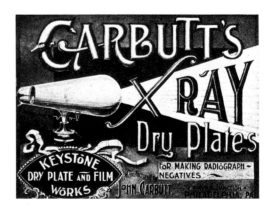

Advertisement of John Carbutt, first manufacturer of plates in America specifically designed for x-ray work (1896).[6]

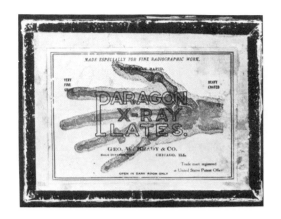

Paragon x-ray plates (c. 1914). This was a popular American brand of roentgen plate used before the advent of x-ray film.[6]

X-ray workers in 1896 were faced with a bewildering array of plates with each manufacturer claiming that his emulsion was the most sensitive. Some claimed that a plate slow-to-light was fast to x-rays and vice versa, although the majority felt that a plate fast-to-light was correspondingly fast to x-rays. The prevailing types of emulsions recommended or used in early x-ray work were the orthochromatic, useful because of its sensitivity to the yellow-green fluorescence of the barium platinocyanide screen; the collodion, or wet emulsion, which was but slightly affected by x-rays; mixtures of silver bromide gelatin emulsions, with small quantities of silver iodide or chloride, which were quite satisfactory; and pure silver chloride emulsions that were virtually useless. The common agreement was reached that the emulsions, regardless of their color sensitivity, should be much thicker than those for pictorial photography and should contain more silver. The recommendation advanced by most of the best workers was simply to use a plate with which the x-ray operator was familiar. This recommendation was so widely accepted that it tended to delay whatever efforts manufacturers were willing to make in producing a special x-ray emulsion. As long as the consumer was content with the photographic plate, it was apparently advisable to leave well enough alone.

A major problem in processing the exposed plate or film was to obtain adequate density. Radiographs at that time tended to be thin and lacking in contrast. To overcome this difficulty and to shorten the exposure time (which was essential if this "new photography" was to be of any practical value), multi-emulsion coated plates and gelatin or celluloid films were made. It was claimed that this technique provided greater detail and contrast than with a single-coated plate or film. Special plates and film also were coated on both sides of the support. The rays passed through the support and, in the case of film, affected the emulsion on both sides to the same degree so that the image on one side reinforced that of the other. This method doubled the density of the image and greatly improved the diagnostic value of the radiograph. However, with plates, the absorption of the rays by the glass produced less density on one side as compared with the greater density on the tube side of the plate.

Glass plates were popular in spite of several serious deficiencies. They were so fragile that shipment was extremely difficult. Glass plates also were heavy—a 14-inch × 17-inch glass plate weighed about 2 pounds, compared with a modern x-ray film of similar size that weighs only about 1.5 ounces (a factor of 20:1). Glass plates also were expensive. In 1906, a 14-inch × 17-inch plate cost about $1 (about $100 in today's dollars), but in that same year a good suit of clothes cost $7, a pair of shoes cost $3, and steak was 15¢ a pound.

Manufacturing defects in plates were a critical problem because the artifacts they produced interfered with diagnosis. In a discussion at the 1902 meeting of the American Roentgen Ray Society dealing with the diagnosis of calculi, Wolfram C. Fuchs of Chicago noted that:[7]

> I have not found a plate maker yet whose product does not have some defect. After the negative has been developed we find spots all over it. The hardest stones to locate are the small stones. The large ones you can see at a distance. Take a very small stone, as for instance, in this radiograph. You can distinctly see the outline of the kidney and the darker shadow in the center, with many darker spots all over.

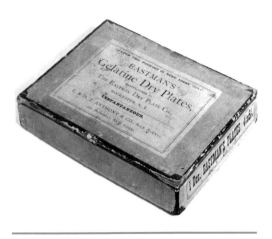

Eastman's gelatine dry plates (1884).[6]

They are even visible to the patient and that is not good. I usually take two plates, one on top of the other, and expose them at the same time with the envelope around them. In this way, while the spots (artifacts) will still show on a plate, yet the spots are not in the same place on both plates. In that way you can overcome the difficulty of the plate defects. I have spoken to the expert plate makers about this and they recognize this; they try to remedy it, but have not, as yet, succeeded in doing so.

Photographic plates for radiology initially were inserted in lightproof wrappers and sealed. However, it was found that the plates deteriorated through interaction between the chemicals in the paper and the emulsion. This led to the development of separate double envelopes with the operator "loading" the x-ray plate as needed, first in a black envelope and then in an orange- or ruby-colored envelope for protection.

In reality, the diagnostic quality of most of these radiographs was largely confined to the depiction of gross appearances. The presence of secondary radiation fog and the granularity of the image when screens were used tended to discourage the photographic recording of x-ray images. This resulted in increased acceptance of fluoroscopy and did much to delay the production of better photographic-sensitive materials. Even by 1901, when over 3 million plates were used for radiography, the production of "special" x-ray plates was still limited and more than 75% of the plates exposed were those that had been made for the photography trade![9]

As the volume of radiographic work continued to dramatically increase, the demand for specific x-ray plates increased. Major products included the Paragon, Ilford, Cramer, Wratten, and Seed x-ray plates. In 1912, Kodak introduced the Wratten x-ray plate, which was coated with a heavy silver halide emulsion impregnated with a high-atomic-weight bismuth salt, the purpose of which was to absorb the roentgen rays and increase the effect on the silver halide crystals in the emulsion. As late as 1923, Schleussner introduced a plate with fluorescent salts incorporated in the emulsion. However, the plate was expensive and difficult to handle and its commercial life was short, for by that time the photographic plate era was coming to an end.

EARLY METHODS FOR DEVELOPING AND PRINTING

In the early days, the radiographer developed radiographs and prints by means of the old "four bottle" photographic method. In succession, the photosensitive material was covered with solutions containing the developing agent, preservative, accelerator, and then the bromide. As development proceeded, the radiographer used his experience to add a little more of the solution from one or another of the bottles until development was completed. In this way, the radiographer hoped to bring out the desired anatomical detail. The most prevalent method of increasing the density of the image was through after-treatment (intensification) of the negatives, and many of the leading x-ray workers of that time resorted to this practice.[4]

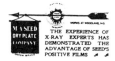
Advertisement for the Seed Dry Plate Company (1899).[6]

Advertisement (1914) for the Wratten x-ray plate, a unique type that contained a heavy metal salt in the emulsion.[6]

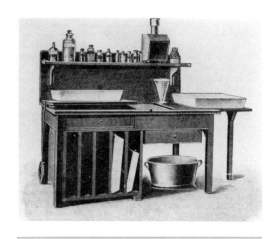

Accessories for developing plates.[8]

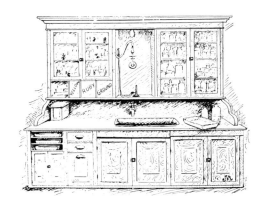

Illustration of an early bench used to process x-ray plates (c. 1899). Note the chemical bottles and trays.[9]

Because many pioneer radiographers were photographers or physicians who practiced photography as a hobby, they were used to the complicated and nonstandardized photographic methods of those days. Thus they accepted these inconveniences with little thought that the procedure could be simplified. All types of developers, no two alike, were employed in the days of the glass plate. Every plate manufacturer printed developing formulas to be used with his product. The types and quantities of chemicals employed in the various formulas were not standardized, and thus development was entirely empirical with each x-ray worker. The more successful developers contained pyrogallic acid, metol, or hydroquinone as reducing agents. Various quantities of alkali, sodium sulfite, and potassium bromide were employed to accelerate or retard developer activity.[4]

The density of the radiograph was influenced by the relative proportions of the different parts of the developer used. Excellent results could be obtained when the operator understood the function of each component in the developer and fixer. Indeed, a thorough knowledge of existing photographic chemistry was mandatory if good radiographic results were to be obtained. However, of major importance was the need for greater amounts of reducing agents. These all-important chemicals were included in only small amounts in most of the developing formulas.

The development process was influenced by the type of exposure equipment and the type of emulsion. Radiographs made with a small coil, having a low electric output, and a "soft" tube were said to present little difficulty in development. Such radiographs were made of small body parts and with low voltage, resulting in a short scale of contrast but relatively high density. Radiographs made with a "hard" tube and a powerful apparatus produced images of generally low density and a long scale of contrast. In developing these images, the radiographer had to carefully increase the degree of contrast.

Soft emulsions swelled rapidly when placed in the developer, and quickly became saturated with the solution. Conversely, a hard emulsion was difficult to saturate, since the gelatin was slow in swelling. Therefore the developer only acted on the surface of a hard emulsion and yielded a thin image.

Multilayered emulsions were difficult to process because the developers did not penetrate quickly. Because the type and quantity of alkali were seldom adequate, the procedure was time-consuming and the images were often mottled because of unequal development.

Before 1900, plates were largely hand processed in trays. Since each plate required special treatment in development (because of the erratic exposures received by the emulsion), close inspection of the developing image was required. Once the speed of plates became somewhat standardized (and the radiation quality and quantity could be better controlled with the advent of the Coolidge hot-cathode tube), it became possible to more accurately time the period of development, which varied from about 10 to 25 minutes.

During development, the plate had to be constantly agitated so that uniform development of the entire image could be accomplished. This was a tedious job until the development of a mechanical rocker (titubator), which was operated by a motor or a foot pedal attached to suitable cams that would produce a gentle rocking motion of the tray. This time-saving device also precluded the need for prolonged exposure of the radiographer's hands to the developer solutions.

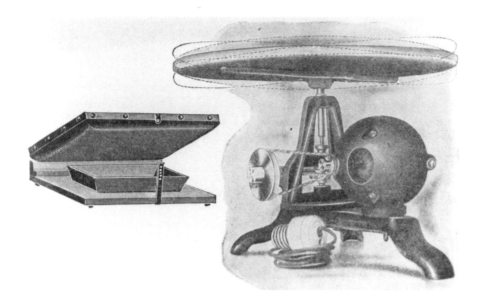

As the amount of x-ray work grew, it was necessary to invent more efficient and speedier processing methods. This often was difficult to accomplish since hospitals were hesitant to provide additional funds to secure proper equipment. By 1906, wooden tanks were made with slotted sides so that plates could be easily inserted in the slots and the development period accurately timed. Compartments in the tanks were set apart for the various size plates then in use. A slotted plate developing hanger became available in 1910. It had a crossbar at the top that made it possible to suspend the plate in the solutions. The hangers could be readily removed for transfer to other sections of the tank so that separate compartments for plates of various sizes could be abolished.

David Bowen (1912) modified the tanks to provide for a developing compartment, a rinse area, a fixer compartment, and a large washing area. At first, these tanks were made of wood or wood lined with lead sheeting; later they were constructed with soapstone. These tanks permitted greater uniformity of results than could be achieved with tray development and substantially reduced the space required for processing the plates.[11]

As radiographic film replaced glass plates, a system of standardized tank development was developed in 1929 by Frederick C. Martin and co-workers at the Eastman Kodak Company. They recommended the establishment of a constant time of development for a given temperature based on the rate of exhaustion of the developer. This "exhaustion system" assured uniformity of results and was a valuable aid in checking exposure time.[12]

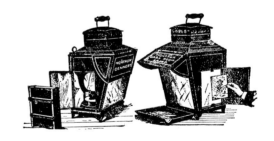

Darkroom lantern.[10]

In 1947, Crabtree and Henn of Kodak described the "replenisher system" of development. This technique was designed to maintain the activity of the developer by the addition of developer replenisher solution at a constant rate. This method made possible the use of a constant time of development for a given temperature for the life of the solution.[13]

In the 1940s, medical x-ray films still had to be hand processed. The exposed radiographic film was immersed successively in individual containers of developer, stop bath, and fixer solution, and it was then washed in running water. The washed radiographs were hung up to drip and air

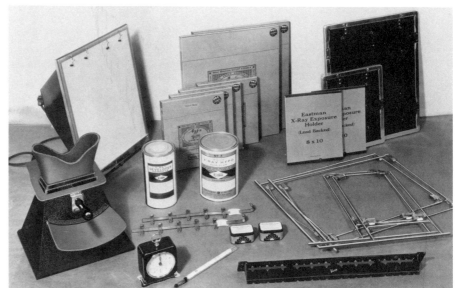

General Electric

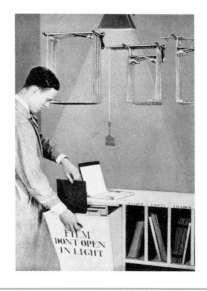

Darkroom in the 1940s containing a film
bin, loading bench, cassettes, exposure
holders, and hangers for manual development of x-ray film.[1]

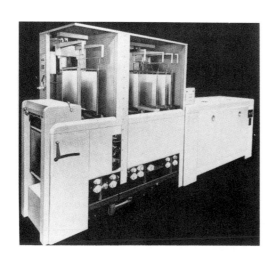

Pako automatic film processor.

dry. Image quality, reproducibility of results, and patient exposure were
dependent on the user's control of processing time, solution temperatures,
solution freshness, agitation, and general housekeeping. Frequently, exposure was increased to permit shortened development time for early
inspection of the radiograph. This procedure tended to reduce contrast
and to increase patient exposure.

The increased volume of x-ray examinations led to the introduction in
1942 of the Pako automatic film processor. The first commercial model
(1945) used conventional x-ray films with square-cut corners, which were
unloaded in the darkroom and impaled by a stamper on the sharp retainer
claws of specially designed hangers. Although the sharp corners and the
much sharper tags left by the claw perforations were eventually trimmed
from the dry film with a corner cutter, bandages and antiseptics were
routine accessories in the film-handling area. The Pako system could
process 120 films per hour by successively dipping the films in developer,
washer, and hypo before taking them into a drying tunnel. The total cycle
time for one film was about 40 minutes.[14]

The hanger-type processor was superseded in 1956 by the Kodak
X-Omat processor (1956), the first roller transport processor for medical
radiographs.[15] The initial X-Omat processor was about 10-feet long,
weighed nearly three fourths of a ton, and sold for approximately $33,000
($150,000 based on today's dollars). Film fed into a loading slot at one
end moved along nylon rollers and could be taken out dry and ready for
interpretation in 6 minutes without the need for hangers and conventional
processing tanks. About 600 films of mixed sizes could be processed
each hour using this technique. In 1965, 90-second rapid processing was
introduced, using a device only 36-inches long, 30-inches wide, and 42-
inches high.

Automatic processing eliminated the variability in results caused by
the human element. It enabled radiologists and radiographers to further
standardize techniques, so that fewer retakes were needed. By reducing
the time before radiographs were available, automatic processing decreased the time that a patient had to spend in the radiology department,
thus improving efficiency and work flow and increasing the number of
examinations that could be performed in a day.

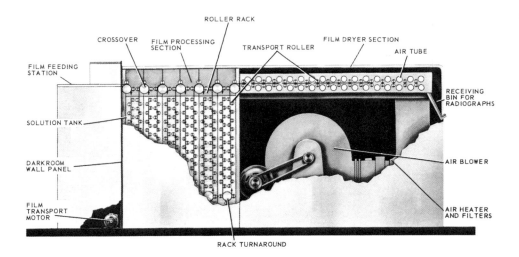

ROLLER RACK

CROSSOVER   FILM PROCESSING SECTION   TRANSPORT ROLLER   FILM DRYER SECTION   AIR TUBE

FILM FEEDING STATION

SOLUTION TANK

DARKROOM WALL PANEL

FILM TRANSPORT MOTOR

RECEIVING BIN FOR RADIOGRAPHS

AIR BLOWER

AIR HEATER AND FILTERS

RACK TURNAROUND

Cutaway of first X-Omat processor.[2]

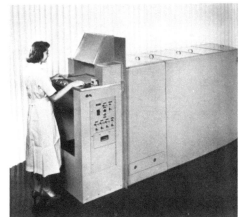

First Kodak X-Omat automatic roller transport processor.[2]

INTENSIFYING SCREENS

Although the principle of the intensifying screen was first proposed by Angelo Battelli and Giorgio Garbasso of Italy and by A. A. Campbell-Swinton of England in January, 1896, Michael Pupin of Columbia University was the first to use fluorescence to reinforce the exposure of a medical radiograph. A surgeon had sent Pupin a well-known lawyer who had sustained a shotgun wound to the hand. Pupin was asked to make a radiograph so that the shotgun pellets could be located and extracted. The first attempts were unsuccessful because the patient was in severe pain and too weak and nervous to stand "a photographic exposure of nearly an hour." Having recently been sent a calcium tungstate fluoroscopic screen by his friend Thomas Edison, Pupin decided to attempt an exposure by placing the fluorescent screen on the photographic plate and the patient's hand on the screen. With an exposure of a few seconds, he obtained a beautiful image of the 77 pellets in his patient's hand.[16] As Pupin wrote, the photographic plate showed the numerous shot as if "they had been drawn with pen and ink." The shot were removed by the surgeon, and the appreciative patient offered to establish a fellowship at a certain club that would entitle Pupin to two toddies a day for the rest of his life.[17]

Early x-ray workers coated their own intensifying screens. Typically, a card or other support material would be covered with an adhesive-like fish-glue or a varnish-type binder made from collodion and castor oil. The powdered phosphor would be sprinkled on the wet surface and allowed to dry before use. Barium platinocyanide was the most effective material, although it was extremely expensive. It also tended to become unstable on exposure to heat, dry atmospheric conditions, and continued use. To inhibit the loss of moisture, these screens were often treated with wax, and manufacturers recommended that they be stored in humidors when not in use. Another drawback was that the spectral emission of barium platinocyanide was mainly in the yellow-green range, which made it useful for fluoroscopy but of limited value as an intensifying screen with the predominantly blue-sensitive plates. Potassium platinocyanate, which

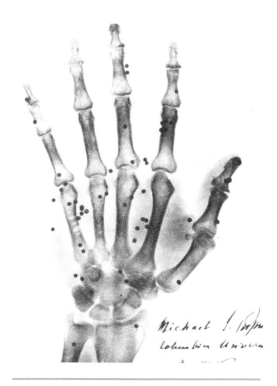

First screen-film radiograph (Pupin, February, 1896).[6]

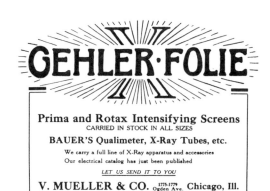

Advertisement for Gehler-Folie intensifying screens (American Quarterly of Radiology, 1911).

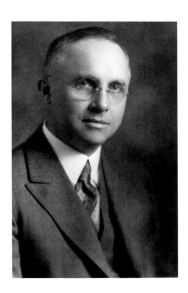

Carl V. S. Patterson.

fluoresced with a pale blue color, was a closer match for the radiographic plates than the barium salt. Unfortunately, it not only had a lower emission intensity but had to be kept moist by spraying it with water from time to time. Several zinc salts were tried, but they suffered from problems of intense afterglow.[18]

Edison had determined that calcium tungstate was the most suitable material for making fluorescent screens. Adopting this idea, the German, Gehler, soon began manufacturing intensifying screens using calcium tungstate. Under the name "Gehler-Folie," large quantities were exported to radiologists throughout Europe and the United States. At first, these screens were crude and, when washed, the water dissolved the binder and the screen was ruined. Another problem was that at that time, calcium tungstate crystals varied greatly in their fluorescence. The relative degree of brilliance of any screen depended on the quantity, as well as the quality, of the salt used in its preparation. Because rapid screens capable of producing good radiographs required a large quantity of this high–specific gravity material, good calcium tungstate screens were heavy.

Since glass plates were coated with emulsion on one surface only, the screen could be placed either on the front or the back of the plate as long as it was in contact with the emulsion side of the plate. Depending on the choice, considerable inconsistency of results arose. The lack of uniformity of coating thickness led to image variations that were most marked when a front screen was used. When a back screen was used, however, the image density was reduced due to x-ray absorption by the glass of the plate.

Although intensification screens were introduced early in the history of radiology, they dropped out of use for many years. The major reason was that the old screens had an extreme amount of fluorescent lag and excessive grain as a result of the use of large fluorescent crystals. Their surfaces became easily marred, making it necessary to cover them with some form of transparent cellulose. Unfortunately, these coverings invariably produced an abundance of static electricity that affected the x-ray film.[18]

The manufacturer most responsible for the development of high-quality intensifying screens was Carl V. S. Patterson. He determined that the two vital research problems to consider in producing a successful screen were the development of a satisfactory fluorescent chemical and exact methods of manufacture, since fluorescent chemicals were greatly influenced by minute additions of other substances. Patterson demonstrated the importance of maintaining uniformity in production, so that all screens in an x-ray laboratory would have as nearly as possible the same intensification factor. He stressed that the ideal screen should be made of a pure, fine-grain, fluorescent chemical with brilliant and uniform fluorescence and minimal afterglow. In 1916, Patterson produced a screen of synthetic calcium tungstate that fluoresced brightly, was coated with improved uniformity, had minimal afterglow, and overcame difficulties associated with impurities in the natural mineral. Patterson later introduced a cassette containing two intensifying screens, which was appropriate for the new double-coated films. This cassette consisted of a "thin" front screen and a "thick" back screen, both to avoid excessive absorption of x-rays and to shorten the exposure time.[18]

In 1922, the Eastman Kodak Company introduced its first intensifying screen. It incorporated calcium tungstate crystals in a cellulose binder that was coated on a cellulose sheet for support. Although this screen was durable and entirely waterproof, some undesirable characteristics led to it being discontinued in favor of a cardboard-supported coating of crystals having great speed.

Early intensifying screens had the disadvantage of being easily marred and required care in handling. They were difficult to clean, since particles of dirt and grit worked into the screen surface and could not be removed. Although several types of protective surface coatings were developed, they were generally unsuccessful. The coating materials lacked toughness and adhered poorly, leading to the development of wrinkles and blisters. Discoloration and lack of clarity inhibited the transmission of luminescence from the chemical, and the thickness of the coating contributed to radiographic unsharpness. In 1921, Patterson introduced a cleanable fluorescent intensifying screen that contained a thin protective covering over the phosphor. Cleaning could be readily accomplished using mild soap and water on a soft wool cloth or tuft of cotton. The impact of this cleanable screen was dramatic, since with reasonable care and periodic cleaning a pair of screens might perform well for years, whereas previously replacements had been frequent and costly.[19]

To produce excellent radiographs using intensifying screens, it was essential that there be precise contact between the screen and the photographic plate or film. To accomplish this, cassettes were developed to provide a light-tight container in which to hold the screen and plate in close contact during exposure. Early cassettes were made of wood and beautifully constructed; later they were made of metal.

In 1948, intensifying screens composed of a barium lead sulfate phosphor were introduced. These were the first commercially successful radiographic screens not made of calcium tungstate and provided greater speed in the 70 to 100 kVp range.

Research in several laboratories with rare earth phosphors for color television tubes and image-intensifier tubes culminated in work by Buchanan, Finkelstein, and Wichersheim in the early 1970s that suggested the use of rare earth screens for medical radiography.[20] First available commercially in 1974, these new rare earth screens used a high-absorption, green-emitting gadolinium oxysulfide phosphor and were coupled with orthochromatic films, sensitive to green as well as to blue light. Other manufacturers marketed screens composed of such phosphors as lanthanum oxybromide, yttrium oxysulfide, and barium fluorochloride. Because of their absorption characteristics and increased efficiency in converting x-ray energy to light, rare earth phosphors made possible the production of faster screen-film combinations than were previously available.

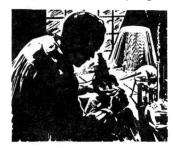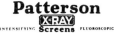
Advertisement for Patterson screens.

PHOTOGRAPHIC PAPER

The search for a more sensitive material than glass plates for radiography led many workers to experiment with bromide paper as used in general photography. In America, the first paper radiograph was made by A. W. Wright at Yale University on January 27, 1896. The first sensitized paper prepared especially for radiographic purposes was marketed by Kodak in 1901. The title of the announcement, "Eastman's x-ray bromide paper takes the place of plates in radiographic work," indicated the high hopes that were held for paper as a recording medium. The *stated* advantages of paper over plates included the following: it was nonbreakable; it could be bent to conform to the shape of the body and thereby secure better contact; its latitude was greater; it was cheaper and simpler to handle; there was no need to make a negative before a print; unlike glass plates, there was no useful limit to their size; the time required to produce a finished radiograph was only 5 minutes; and since each sheet of this paper was packed in special envelopes, the trouble of "loading" them was eliminated. In addition, any number of "prints" could be made with one exposure, since the paper was "transparent" to x-rays. Unfortunately, the sensitivity of x-ray paper was much less than that of traditional glass plates.

X-ray paper continued to be used sporadically until the 1940s, especially during World War I when the severe economic conditions in Europe made it necessary to use the cheapest radiographic recording medium available if examinations were to be done at all. However, photographic paper has never played a major role in radiology, primarily because of its inability to show detail and contrast as clearly as the glass plate or x-ray film. This characteristic is inherent in the use of a reflecting surface rather than a transparent base for the support of the sensitive emulsion. The blackest "black" that can be produced on paper reflects an appreciable portion of the incident light, whereas the image on a light-transmitting base can readily be made so dense that no light is visible through it when using a standard x-ray illuminator. This means that the range of densities that can be rendered on paper is much less than that which can

Advertisement for Carbutt plates and films (American Journal of Photography, October, 1896).[6]

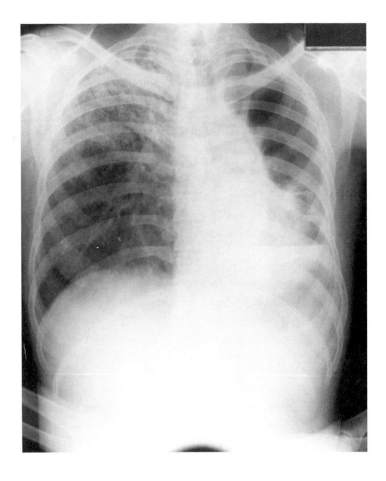

be recorded on film. The limitation of the useful density range of x-ray film is the amount of illumination that it is practical to use in viewing the film; the limitation in the useful density range of paper, however, is confined to the narrow range of reflecting powers possible in the paper surface, which cannot be extended regardless of the amount of illumination.

RADIOGRAPHIC FILM

Although Roentgen's original paper had indicated that either plates or films could be employed to record the x-ray image, the use of photographic film was initially limited. In 1896, Eastman Transparent Film-New Formula with a cellulose base was still being manufactured and occasionally used in radiography. Films used for x-ray purposes in England were the Austin-Edwards' snapshot film and the Cristoid made by the Sandell Plate Company. These films were essentially gelatin-based rather than cellulose-based. They were made of two emulsions, one rapid and one regular speed, that were coated on glass and then stripped off. The films were supplied packed in dark envelopes, difficult to develop, and much slower than fast plates.

Neither gelatin nor celluloid films were desirable because of their tendency to curl or crack, but they had the advantage of being thin and could be used with one or two intensifying screens with a consequent reduction in exposure. Also, they were not subject to breakage as were the glass plates.

In Germany, x-ray film was produced by the Schleussner Company in

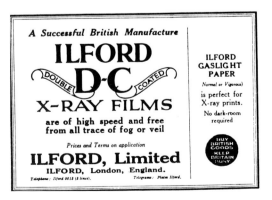

Advertisement for Ilford x-ray films and paper.

Early Kodak advertisement (April, 1914) of the first single-coated x-ray film.[6]

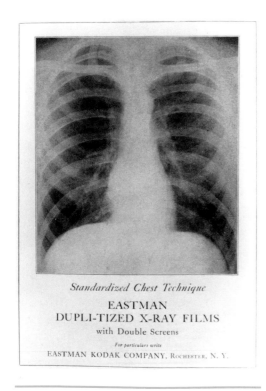

Standardized Chest Technique

EASTMAN
DUPLI-TIZED X-RAY FILMS
with Double Screens

For particulars write
EASTMAN KODAK COMPANY, ROCHESTER, N. Y.

Early Kodak advertisement describing "Dupli-Tized X-Ray Films" (AJR, 1919).

1896. The film had a double emulsion on each side, making four coats in all. This company also made radiographic plates and was probably the only firm in those days making an emulsion that approached the density, contrast, and speed suitable for x-ray work. Results with this film were good, but the high cost and considerable manufacturing difficulties led to its limited use and reduced production.

Before World War I, the glass used for photographic plates was obtained from Belgium. The German warfare on Allied shipping and the invasion of Belgium soon curtailed this source, and the procuring of glass for photographic purposes became a serious problem. The demand for radiographic plates in Army hospitals became so great that it was almost impossible to satisfy them. Even when glass plates were available in large quantities, their bulk and fragility made them exceedingly difficult to transport without breakage. These problems finally made it imperative to provide some support other than glass for the emulsion.

Radiography made special demands on a film support for the emulsion. Sensitive surfaces of a large area were required. The base had to support the coated emulsion without buckling and be glass-clear and flexible. The only solution at the time was to adapt the cellulose nitrate base used in the manufacture of photographic film. Consequently, in 1914, Kodak introduced a single-coated x-ray film with an emulsion of greater sensitivity than that of any x-ray plate (or film) on the market. However, even this film was not ideal since it curled excessively and was therefore difficult to develop in trays.

The use of portable x-ray equipment in the field during World War I demanded greater efficiency and speed in x-ray films. This need accelerated the extensive research work then being conducted on a film coated on both sides of a transparent base that made possible a double-screen technique. Finally, in 1918, Kodak's "Dupli-Tized" (double-coated) x-ray film was made available. The double-screen technique using double emulsion film produced an enormous increase in speed and made practical the use of the Potter-Bucky diaphragm for the control of scattered radiation. The improved diagnostic quality of the resulting radiographs was a significant factor in the growth of radiology in this period.

X-ray film coated on both sides of a transparent support made all other forms of radiographic recording media obsolete overnight. Nevertheless, the introduction of film was no easy task, for there were years of prejudice to overcome. Radiographers had so accustomed themselves to glass plates that it took time to convince them that film offered any significant advantages. New cassettes and other types of film holders had to be invented. The then current practice of tray development was a deterrent to the rapid adoption of double-coated films. A few laboratories used deep tanks for processing plates vertically and were able to change over rapidly when a suitable film hanger soon became available.

In 1923, a still faster x-ray film became available. It permitted a radical shortening of exposure time or a lowering of the kilovoltage with consequently less wear and tear on tubes and apparatus. The base of this film, like that of its predecessors, was cellulose nitrate.

Cellulose nitrate as a film base had always presented a fire hazard, which hospitals and laboratories were forced to recognize because of several fires caused by careless handling and storage of such film. Despite intensive efforts, the search for less flammable material was unsuccessful until 1906, when it was found that cellulose acetate could serve as the base for a "safety film," especially for motion picture use. The value of making x-ray film from this substance was not seriously considered at that time, because glass plates were then in universal use.

The actual production of a useful cellulose acetate base required many years of research and development. Problems that had to be solved included elimination of impurities, reduction in brittleness, improved clarity, and greater strength. Great strides also were made in the recovery process of by-products of the chemical reactions in cellulose acetate manufacture, which permitted the price to be kept down. In addition, World War I provided great impetus for the production of cellulose acetate for other than photographic purposes. This huge consumption made it possible to greatly increase the knowledge regarding the efficient manufacture of cellulose acetate. Finally, an x-ray film on a safety base of cellulose acetate was produced and marketed by Kodak in 1924. However, because this new film still tended to wrinkle and grow moldy and was somewhat more expensive, flammable film continued in general use and accumulated in huge quantities in radiological offices and hospital radiology departments. In 1929, disaster struck. A film fire at the Cleveland Clinic claimed 124 lives. Thereafter, an improved cellulose acetate film became available and the use of the nitrate base was soon discontinued.

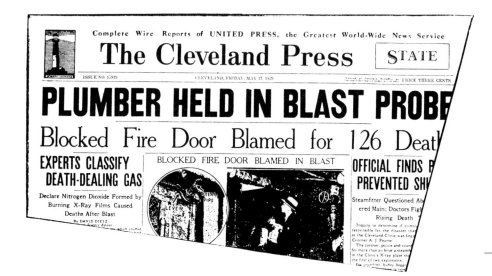

Cleveland Clinic fire.

The early 1930s saw the introduction of Diaphax film, which consisted of a translucent base with a faster emulsion that permitted viewing of the radiograph before any light source, such as a window. Up to this time, all x-ray film was colorless. In 1933, the DuPont Film Manufacturing Company added a blue tint to their base, which enhanced the diagnostic quality of their film. This practice has since been adopted universally by all manufacturers of x-ray film.

The first film for direct x-ray exposure (*Non-Screen*) was marketed in 1936 by Ansco (later purchased by Agfa). Intended for x-ray exposure without fluorescent screens, this film had higher speed, contrast, and definition than screen-type films and was used primarily for examinations of the extremities. Four years later, Kodak introduced the *Blue Brand* x-ray film, which was coated with a new type of emulsion that gave greater speed and contrast and could be used for either direct exposure or screen radiography.

To meet the demand for decreased x-ray exposure to patients, increases in film sensitivity continued to be made together with improvements in contrast and keeping qualities and reduction in the basic fog level. Kodak's high-speed film (*Royal Blue*), introduced in 1958, provided good contrast despite its adaptability to higher kilovoltage and lower milliamperage technique and the use of finer focus x-ray tubes.

In 1960, 10 years after its introduction in general photography, polyethylene terephthalate was introduced by DuPont as a new support for medical x-ray films. Compared to cellulose esters, this new material had greater stiffness, greater dimensional stability, lower water absorption, and greater resistance to tearing. The stiffness of polyethylene terephthalate improved transport reliability in automatic roller processors, and the lower water absorption simplified the drying of the radiographs. Since the early 1960s, polyester bases have replaced cellulose-based film for all conventional (noncinefluorographic) radiography.

In the 1970s, DuPont introduced a Daylight film loading and processing system that could be used without the usual darkroom. It consisted of shielded film magazines that could be placed in radiographic rooms and from which special cassettes could be loaded under daylight conditions. Included in the package were special film processors into which the film could be transferred from the cassette under daylight conditions. These systems, which have become relatively popular, have decreased dark-

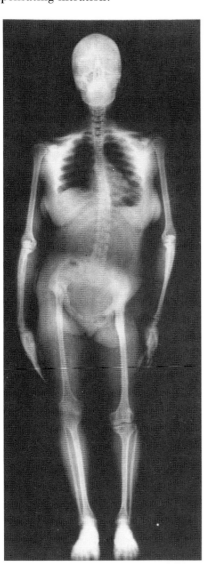

Largest x-ray film (32 × 72 inches) used for entire body radiography of a 33-year-old woman who exhibited hip pathology. The radiograph was made with a one-second exposure, 75 kVp, 150 ma, 12-foot film distance, fast screens, and tissue compensating filtration.[6]

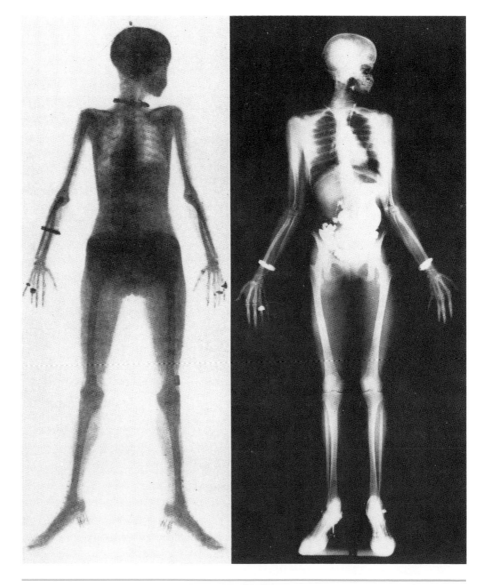

Entire body radiographs. *Left*, Film made by William J. Morton (1897) on a single sheet of photographic film with an exposure of 30 minutes. *Right*, Radiograph made by Arthur W. Fuchs (1934) on a single sheet of x-ray film using compensating filtration and an exposure of 1 second.[9]

room costs, increased departmental efficiency, and reduced the number of cassettes required for an installation or department. Daylight loading systems also eliminated many problems of screen damage and maintenance, since the screens are always within the protective interior of the special cassette and thus never exposed to damage in the darkroom.[21]

The size of radiographic film has varied widely to satisfy its many medical applications. The smallest film, used for examining children's teeth and the lacrimal duct, is $\frac{7}{8} \times 1\frac{3}{8}$ inches. The largest film, 32×72 inches, can make a radiograph of the entire body.

The first entire body radiograph of a living person was made in 1897 by William J. Morton of New York City.[22] It is interesting to compare that radiograph, requiring an exposure of 30 minutes, with one reported by Arthur W. Fuchs in 1934, using a filter to compensate for various tissue opacities and an exposure of only 1 second.

XERORADIOGRAPHY[23]

Unlike conventional film, xeroradiography uses no solution and thereby derives its name from the Greek word *xeros* meaning dry. It is photoelectric rather than photochemical. Xeroradiography is an outgrowth of an electrostatic photographic process in which a metallic plate coated with a thin layer of selenium (a semiconductor) is given a homogeneous electrostatic charge and is then exposed to x-rays in the same manner and with the same equipment one would use if ordinary x-ray film were employed. The x-rays that pass through the subject and strike the plate selectively dissipate the electric charge on the selenium; the rate of loss of charge is a direct function of the intensity of x-ray exposure. This process results in the production of a latent electrostatic image, which can be made visible by dusting the surface of the selenium with finely divided powder granules. The powder is attracted to the charged portions of the plate and adheres to these areas tenaciously. The irradiated portions of the plate, being discharged, are unable to retain the powder and it rolls off. A permanent record of this image is made by electrostatic or adhesive transfer of the powder to paper or other sheet material. After the plate is cleaned by brushing, it is ready for reuse. The development process is rapid and it is easily possible to have a completed xeroradiograph ready for interpretation within 30 seconds after the x-ray exposure is completed.

The dry development and absence of need for a darkroom facilitate the use of the process in many work locations. There are no problems of film or chemical storage nor danger of fogging in areas where radiation may be present. Since a plate can be reused for hundreds of exposures, the process is more economical than film.

The forerunner of xerography and xeroradiography was an electrostatic recording method called *electrography*, developed by Paul Selenyi of Hungary (1935).[24] In Selenyi's apparatus, a beam of negative ions was driven by an electric field through a hole in a control electrode onto an insulating covering on a metal drum, which was rotated and advanced screw-fashion so that the beam deposited a spiral line of charge on the drum. The intensity of the beam was controlled by an input signal produced by scanning a photograph or drawing at the sending station to cause variations in density of charge deposited and thereby reproduce the pattern of the original image. Dusting the drum covering with powder made the image visible.

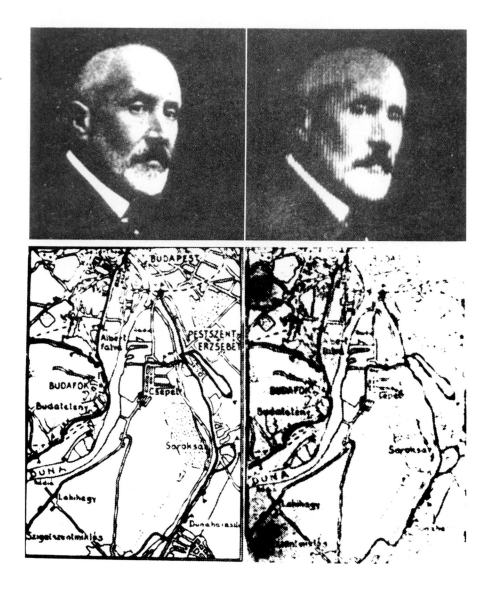

Electrography. *Top*, Transmission of a photograph. *Bottom*, Transmission of an India ink drawing. *Bottom left* is the original.[24]

At the same time, Chester Carlson, a New York patent attorney who was also a graduate physicist, was interested in devising a simple duplicating method that could be used in offices to produce quick copies of documents and drawings. After seeing a brief account of Selenyi's work and realizing the value and convenience of the powder development method, Carlson set out to find a new photoconductive coating that would also be a good insulator in the dark and hold an electrostatic charge which might be developed with powder. Among the photoconductive insulating materials with the desired characteristics, Carlson chose pure elemental sulfur. After the first successful test of the process in 1938, Carlson tried unsuccessfully to interest several companies in taking over further development of the process. In 1944, Battelle Memorial Institute, a nonprofit research organization in Columbus, Ohio, entered into an agreement with Carlson under which Battelle would support further development in return for a share of the invention. One of their most significant advances was the discovery of the photoconductivity of selenium, the material that has proven to be the most useful photosensitive coating for xerographic plates. During this period, Schaffert, McMaster, and Bixby conducted experiments showing that the selenium-coated plates displayed relatively high sensitivity to x-ray exposures and thus developed the process of xeroradiography.

In 1946, the Haloid Company (now known as Xerox Corporation), a photographic manufacturer in Rochester, New York, acquired a license under the xerography patents and eventually marketed the first commercial xerographic copying equipment in 1951. The first xeroradiographic

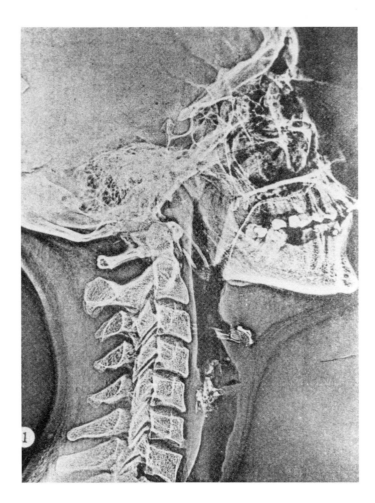

equipment was marketed by General Electric X-ray Company under arrangement with Haloid-Xerox in 1956.

Although some excellent results were obtained in many radiologic studies, especially those of peripheral soft tissues and the larynx,[25] the need for higher radiation doses in thicker body parts significantly limited the widespread medical use of this technique. In the 1960s, John N. Wolfe championed the use of xeroradiography for breast imaging (see Chapter 20). For more than 2 decades, xeromammography was extremely popular, especially in high volume centers; however, most mammography is now performed using the film-screen technique.

MEDICAL IMAGING MANAGEMENT SYSTEMS

Medical imaging management systems (MIMS), also referred to as picture archiving and communication systems (PACS), are being designed to replace film and file rooms with digital storage and retrieval.[27] These systems acquire and format, transmit, display and manipulate, and archive digitally formatted data. In the present systems, a patient's digital image data is displayed on the video monitor of an interactive display station. Appropriate window and level values are selected by the operator to best demonstrate the regions of interest. Converting the digital data to an analog film image by using a multiformat camera interfaced to the display station video monitor permits referring physicians to receive analog hard copies of selected images supporting the consultation report.[28]

The traditional film jacket gives physicians access to all of a patient's conventional and digitally formatted examinations. Viewboxes are a widely available and inexpensive means of viewing these films. However, as the number of digitally formatted examinations increases, a more efficient means of managing and viewing digital image data will be required. Currently, access to a patient's film jacket is limited to a single user or single display site. Transfer of the film jacket from user to user takes significant time. Because of the diversity of modern imaging techniques and the geographic separation of imaging areas, offices, and consultation rooms, the most recent examinations or consultation reports may not have been incorporated into the patient's film jacket when they are most needed by the radiologist or referring physicians. Digital networks have the potential for rapid access, transmission, and simultaneous multisite display. However, there is need to develop a low cost, long-term archiving system capable of managing a huge amount of image data. As this technique becomes cost effective and the digitization of plain radiographic studies (chest, skeletal, and abdomen) meets spatial- and contrast-resolution requirements, medical image management systems will play an increasingly important role in radiologic practice settings.[28]

Another application of computers in radiology is teleradiology, the transmission of radiographic images from one location to another. Images can be transmitted from clinics or other medical facilities with no full-time radiologist to large medical centers where they are viewed on television monitors and interpreted by specialists in diagnostic radiology.

Bibliography

Fuchs AW: Evolution of roentgen film. AJR 75: 30-48, 1956.

Fuchs AW: Historical notes on x-ray plates and films. In Bruwer AJ (ed): Classic descriptions in diagnostic roentgenology. Springfield, Ill, Charles C Thomas, 1964.

Haus AG and Cullinan JE: Screen film processing systems for medical radiography: A historical review. RadioGraphics 9:1203-1224, 1989.

References

1. Haus AG and Cullinan JE: Screen film processing systems for medical radiography: A historical review. RadioGraphics 9:1203-1224, 1989.
2. Kodak and radiography. Med Radiogr Photog 46:79-106, 1970.
3. Roentgen WC: On a new kind of ray. Sitzungsberichte der Würzburger Phys-Med Ges 1895, 1896.
4. Martin FC and Fuchs AW: The historical evolution of roentgen-ray plates and films. AJR 26:540-548, 1931.
5. Carbutt J: The new photography. Photographic Times, June 1897, pp 280-283.
6. Fuchs AW: Evolution of roentgen film. AJR 75:30-48, 1956.
7. Fuchs WC: Discussion. Trans Amer Roentgen Ray Soc, 1902, pp 172-175.
8. Monell SH: A system of instruction in x-ray methods and medical uses of light, hot-air, vibration and high-frequency currents. New York, Pelton, 1902.
9. Fuchs AW: Historical notes on x-ray plates and films. In Bruwer AJ (ed): Classic descriptions in diagnostic roentgenology. Springfield, Ill, Charles C Thomas, 1964.
10. Martin JM: Practical electro-therapeutics and x-ray therapy. St. Louis, CV Mosby Co, 1912.
11. Bowen DR: System of development for roentgen laboratories. AJR 18:308-314, 1914.
12. Martin FC, Smith EE, and Hodgson MB: A new system of standardized tank development. X-ray Bulletin 5:6-10, 1929.
13. Crabtree JI and Henn RW: Developer solutions for x-ray films. Med Radiogr Photog 23:1-12, 38-46, 1947.
14. Angus WM: A commentary on the development of diagnostic imaging technology. RadioGraphics 9:1225-1244, 1989.
15. Russell HD: Rapid processing of x-ray film. Photogr Sci Eng 3:32-34, 1959.
16. Ramsey LJ: Luminescence and intensifying screens in the early days of radiography. Radiography 42:245-253, 1976.
17. Pupin M: From immigrant to inventor. New York, Scribner's, 1923.
18. Fuchs AW: Radiographic recording media and screens. In Glasser O (ed): The science of radiology. Springfield, Ill, Charles C Thomas, 1933.
19. Turner WH: History of x-ray screens and cassettes. Unpublished material.
20. Buchanan RA, Finkelstein SI, and Wickersheim KA: X-ray exposure reduction using rare earth oxysulfide intensifying screens. Radiology 118:183-188, 1976.
21. Krohmer JS: Radiography and fluoroscopy, 1920 to the present. RadioGraphics 9:1129-1153, 1989.
22. Morton WJ: X-ray picture of an adult by one exposure. Electrical Engineer 23:522, 1897.
23. Beeler JW: Xeroradiography. In Bruwer AJ (ed): Classic descriptions in diagnostic roentgenology. Springfield, Ill, Charles C Thomas, 1964.
24. Selenyi P: Electrography: A new electrostatic recording procedure and its uses. Elektrotech Z 56:961-963, 1935.
25. Roach JF and Hilleboe HE: Xeroradiography. Arch Surg 69:594-596, 1954.
26. Gold RH, Bassett LW, and Widoff BE: Highlights from the history of mammography. RadioGraphics 10:1111-1131, 1990.
27. Arenson RL, Seshadri SB, Kundel HL et al: Clinical evaluation of a medical image management system for chest images. AJR 150:55-59, 1988.
28. Cox GG, Templeton AW, and Dwyer SJ: Digital image management: Networking, display, and archiving. Radiol Clin North Am 24:37-54, 1986.

CHAPTER 7

Power Generation

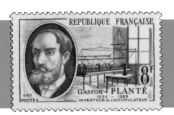
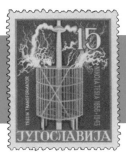
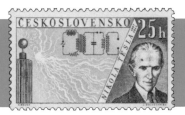
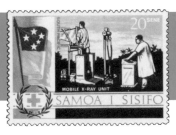

At the time of Roentgen's discovery of x-rays, the three common sources of power were static machines, induction coils, and the Tesla (high-frequency) apparatus.

Static machines were the earliest electrical generators. Already in common use before 1896 for the treatment of various diseases (electrotherapeutics) and for laboratory demonstration of electrical phenomena, several hundred had been reportedly sold to lightning-rod dealers to demonstrate the effectiveness of their wares in the protection of buildings. The electrostatic induction machine was invented in 1865 by the German physicist, Wilhelm T. B. Holtz. An improved, widely used version was developed by the English engineer, James Wimshurst.

Static machines were essentially devices for producing a high-voltage electrical potential by means of friction between sets of revolving and stationary disks. The disks were made of glass, hard rubber, or mica, with the last two being less fragile and permitting the use of greater speed. Some of the static machines were of gigantic proportions, with glass plates as large as 6 feet in diameter and complex units containing as many as 50 revolving glass plates.

One problem with static machines was the difficulty in precisely timing exposures. The current produced by the machine increased gradually and did not attain its maximum until the plates were turning rapidly. Similarly, when the revolving plates were slowing down, the current died out by degrees rather than a sudden cut off. Therefore radiographic exposures could not be limited to an exact number of seconds of maximum radiance when starting and stopping the static machine in the usual way. One ingenious solution offered by Monell was a metal "short-circuit stick" with a nonconducting handle. Placing the stick across the poles of the static machine shunted the current from the x-ray tube. Once the plates were revolving at full speed, the operator lifted the stick from the poles to excite the tube for the required exposure time.[4]

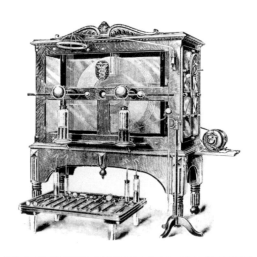

Holtz static machine (1904).[1]

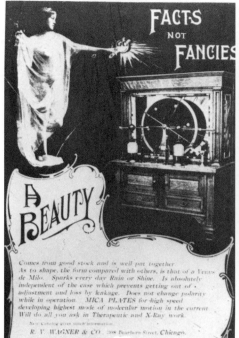
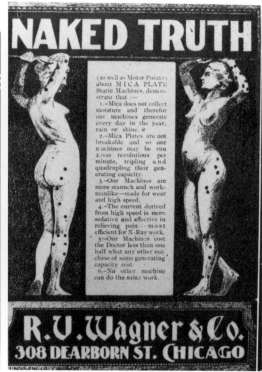
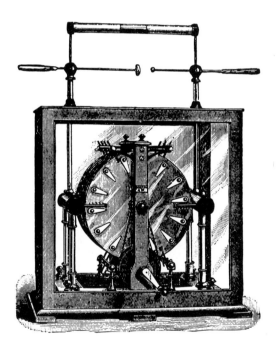

Wimshurst influence machine (1904).[2]

Large static machine of Francis Williams (1901). There were 4 revolving plates 6 feet in diameter and 4 fixed plates 6 feet 4 inches in diameter. The front of the case has been removed.[3]

Static machines were initially operated by hand power, but larger units required water power or electrical motors. The average static machine produced high voltages (up to 100 kV), but only little current (about 1 mA). The larger static machines designed to increase amperage were noisy and tended to work poorly on humid days. A large bowl of calcium chloride or a kerosene lamp placed in the same cabinet helped to absorb the moisture. Although their unidirectional current was ideal for diagnostic tubes, the low current output necessitated long exposure times and for this reason they were used primarily for therapy.

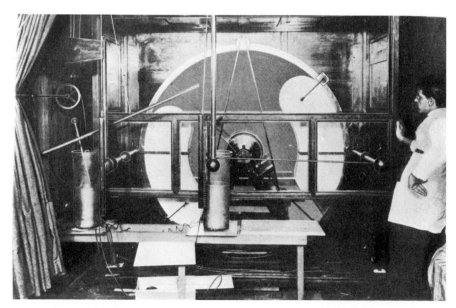

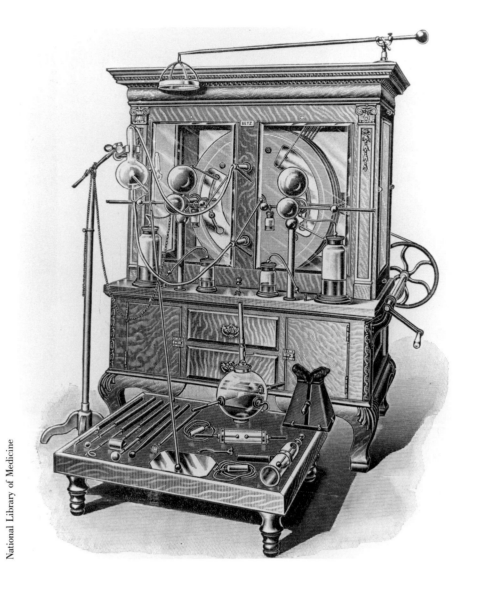

Static machine for general diagnostic and therapeutic x-ray work (1903). Note the hand crank at the right.

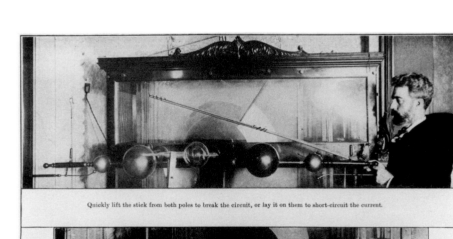

Quickly lift the stick from both poles to break the circuit, or lay it on them to short-circuit the current.

Short-circuit stick (Monell, 1902). In the *lower* figure, the stick is laid on the poles and shunts current from the tube. In the *upper* figure, the operator is seen lifting it from the poles to let the current excite the tube for the required exposure time.

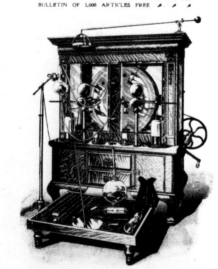

It Is the BE·T·Z 1903
The Finest Machine Made in the World. Send for booklet.
800 BETZ STATIC AND X-RAY OUTFITS NOW IN USE
BULLETIN OF 5,000 ARTICLES FREE

Frank S. Betz & Co.
37 Randolph St.   CHICAGO, ILL.

Advertisement for Betz static machine (1903).

109

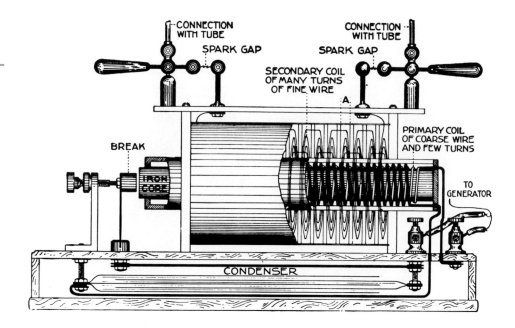

Induction coils consisted of two coils of wire, a primary and a secondary, both wound around an iron core. The primary winding was composed of a few turns of heavy wire; the secondary contained many turns of fine wire. The most popular model was known as the Ruhmkorff coil, the one used by Roentgen in his experiments (see Chapters 1 and 2). Induction coils acted as voltage multipliers and amperage reducers. When current of low voltage and high amperage was fed into the primary coils, current of high voltage but low amperage emerged from the secondary. After overcoming the problem of breakdowns of the insulation between the primary and secondary, commercially available induction coils produced almost 200 kV and currents up to 20 mA, energies that far exceeded the capacities of x-ray tubes in those days.

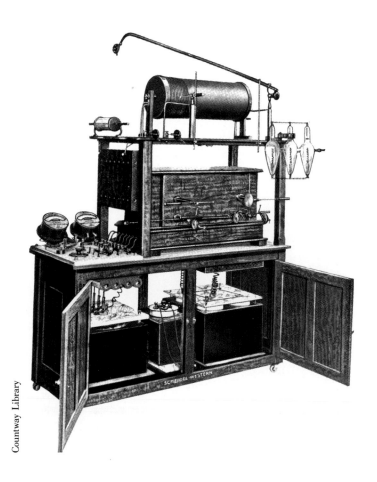

Induction coil unit for general diagnostic and therapeutic x-ray studies (Scheidel-Western, 1909).

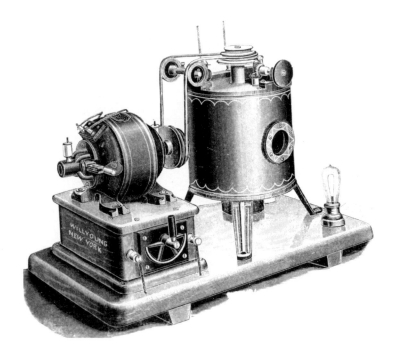

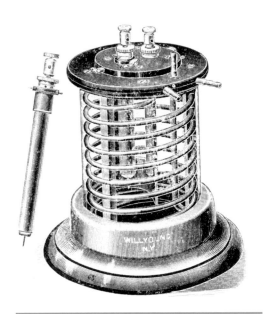

Interrupters. *Left*, Mercury-jet type. *Right*, Wehnelt electrolytic interrupter (1904).[5]

The major drawback of induction coils was that they would not work on steady direct current. An induction coil required either alternating current (often not easily available) or a pulsating current turned off and on many times a second by an "interrupter." Mechanical or electromagnetic interrupters initially were used, but they were noisy and their contact points were quickly pitted and burned with consequent changes in regularity of the energy output of the coil. Mercury interrupters were an improvement over the mechanical type because they operated quietly and permitted a higher current input. In this device, a motor-driven turbine wheel was used to make and break a mercury contact. However, arcing and consequent oxidation of the mercury surface necessitated frequent cleaning of the unit.[6]

Around 1905, the Wehnelt electrolytic interrupter came into more general practical use. It consisted of a plate and a conducting point, both of which were immersed in a conducting dilute acid bath. When the x-ray switch was closed, current flowed between the plate and the point. Hydrolysis at the point quickly produced a nonconducting hydrogen bubble that broke the circuit. Conduction was immediately reestablished by collapse or movement of the bubble, and the cycle was rapidly repeated. The Wehnelt interrupter improved regularity of the current and permitted a higher current input. However, with prolonged use the electrolytic interrupter became heated and emitted intolerable acid fumes. It also leaked on carpets, and floors were ruined. Thus it could not be used for fluoroscopy or therapy.

Induction coils cost substantially more than static machines and were much more expensive to maintain. Although they produced a materially increased energy output, were more rugged and reliable, and were less affected by atmospheric conditions, induction coils still left much to be desired in control and quantity of the energy output. Their gradual disappearance from the x-ray field began in 1907, following the introduction of the so-called "interrupterless transformer."

The third type of x-ray power supply was the *Tesla apparatus*, named for Nikola Tesla, who had developed it several years before. The Tesla apparatus was a series of coils designed to step up the voltage to high potentials and simultaneously to increase the frequency of current alternation to millions of cycles per second by passing the current through

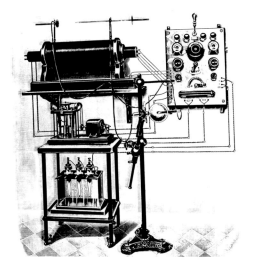

Induction coil unit designed for use with an electrolytic or mercury-jet interrupter (Reiniger, Gebbert, and Schall, 1906).

111

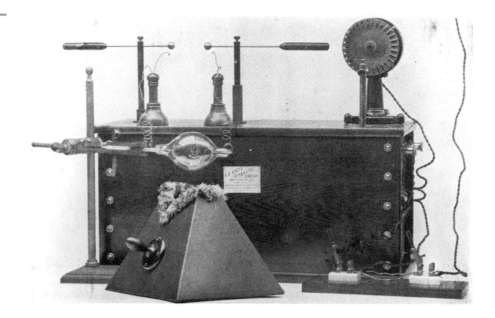

condensers and spark gaps. Although the Tesla apparatus permitted much shorter exposures, it delivered alternating instead of direct current and frequently blew out tubes.

Whether the x-ray worker used static machines, induction coils, or the Tesla apparatus, the high-voltage currents fluctuated widely and reproduction of output from day to day was difficult to obtain. No precise measurement of the output of these various kinds of power supply was possible at that time. Voltage could only be measured by a rough rule of thumb. While the tube was being operated, the spark gap was gradually closed until a spark jumped. The number of inches of spark, multiplied by 10,000, plus 10,000, gave a rough estimate of the voltage. Thus a potential that produced a spark across a 4-inch gap was deemed to be 50,000 volts. Amperage was judged on the basis of the "fatness" of the spark; the fatter it was, the higher the presumed amperage. With such primitive measuring techniques, it was obviously difficult to know just what current was being fed into a tube or to duplicate in one laboratory the findings reported by another.

Method for determining tension of static current (Monell, 1902). "Sit on insulated platform and ground either pole. Let out strands till they fall to floor. Note degree of strain. Then let them fly from hand. A large current will hold out six feet of light cotton cord and drive it ten feet or more when released. This far surpasses the usual spark test. A current not equal to this illustration is too small for fine x-ray or therapeutic work. The author's machine is at the right of the patient and omitted from the cut."[4]

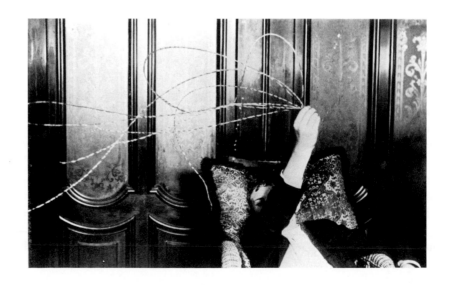

Because the degree of vacuum varied from tube to tube and from minute to minute with a single tube, the voltage fed into the tube had to be matched to the vacuum if one wanted to generate x-rays in abundance. The higher the vacuum within the tube, the higher the voltage required. Experimenters gradually learned to gauge the characteristics and power requirements for their tubes by the tint and brightness of the fluorescence observed. They could raise or lower the input voltage to keep the tube fluorescing. However, it was difficult to repeat an experiment precisely and impossible to convey the conditions of an experiment in repeatable form to workers operating different tubes in other laboratories.

Another problem plaguing early workers was the nonhomogeneous quality of x-rays, which cover a considerable range in the spectrum and vary in wave length much as light varies in color. Most x-ray workers did not realize that an activated Crookes tube emitted a beam composed of x-rays having varying degrees of penetrance. Some rays in the beam were "soft" and barely able to pass through the skin. Others were so "hard" that they easily passed through the thickest bones. In general, the higher the voltage fed into the tube, the "harder" the x-rays emitted. However, some soft rays accompanied the hard rays even at maximum voltages. Although Fred S. Jones of the University of Minnesota had shown that x-ray penetration varied with the input voltage, his report in the *Western Electrician* (March 21, 1896) was either not read, not believed, or forgotten. Most experimenters were at the mercy of whatever rays might emerge from their tubes at the voltage they happened to be using. Therefore they were in much the same position as photographers using a light that varied in color from minute to minute—but able neither to see the light nor to determine its color in other ways.

By 1904, the induction coil combined with an interrupter was by far the most frequent source of power for x-ray work. However, even the best interrupter had a major defect. For a Crookes tube to function at its best, the current through it must always flow in one direction—from the cathode to the target. When an interrupter was used in the power supply, an "inverse current" flowing in the wrong direction through the tube during a part of each cycle reduced efficiency and impaired operating life of the tube. A Swiss-born inventor employed by General Electric, Hermann Lemp, patented an "alternating current selector" (later known as a rotating rectifier switch) that came close to solving the problem.[8] Although invented in 1897, this device was never the subject of a published paper and only patented in 1904. Lemp's device was a switch that was rotated by a synchronous motor so that it completed exactly one revolution (or an exact multiple of one revolution) during each alternating current cycle. When one terminal of the induction coil secondary was strongly negative, the switch connected it to the cathode. Thus the Crookes tube theoretically received a high-voltage pulsating direct current from an induction coil that was operating on an alternating current. During low-voltage portions of the cycle, no voltage was fed to the tube. This reduced the quantity of heat generated in the tube without reducing the x-ray output.

Lemp's rectifier was not immediately put to wide use in radiology because of two major disadvantages. The alternating current supplies available at that time were poorly regulated, so that the switch frequently fell "out of sync" with the current. In addition, the commonly used induction coils were inefficient when powered with alternating current. Therefore most radiologists continue to use direct current and the often problematic interrupters.

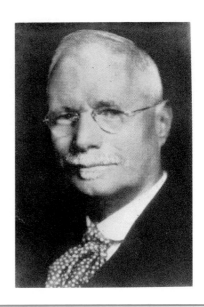

Hermann Lemp (1862-1954).[7]

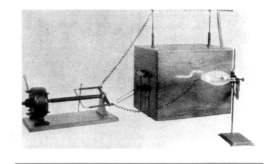

Lemp's mechanical rectifier.[7]

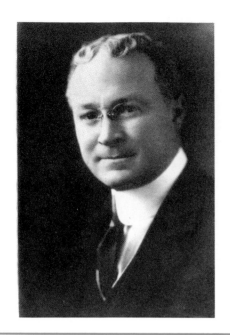

Homer Clyde Snook (1878-1942).[7]

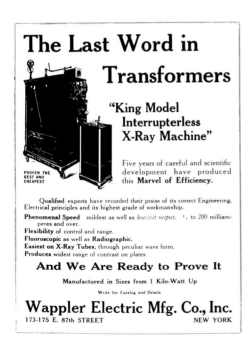

Advertisement for interrupterless transformer (AJR, 1913).

Snook "interrupterless transformer" (1910).

The solution to the problem of induction coils and interrupters was provided by Homer Clyde Snook, a Philadelphia physicist and x-ray equipment manufacturer, who was one of the few nonmedical members admitted to the American Roentgen Ray Society.[9,10] In June 1907, Snook installed his first "interrupterless transformer" in Jefferson Hospital in Philadelphia. It was an immediate success and apparently amazingly sturdy, for a photograph taken 10 years later showed that the machine was still the major unit in use in the Hospital.

Snook understood that the existing supplies of alternating current were too unstable to keep in step with Lemp's switch. Therefore he used a direct current motor and applied a rotary converter to change it to alternating current. The rectifying switch was then mounted on the converter shaft. This locked the switch to the alternating current cycle and ensured that only the negative phase of the current would be fed to the cathode of the Crookes tube.

For locations where no direct current was available, Snook used the alternating current supply to run a motor that drove a dynamo. The dynamo generated alternating current with a cycle independent of that of the dynamo. The rest of the circuit was the same as for direct current installations.

The Snook system resulted in high voltage being applied to the x-ray tube near the peaks of the voltage cycle and only in the correct polarity. Thus while current flowed in the tube, the average voltage was near the peak, a situation that yielded efficient production of x-rays and used both halves of the voltage wave form.[11]

In addition to his rotary converter, Snook replaced the conventional induction coil with a much more efficient closed-magnetic-circuit transformer that had minimal magnetic leakage and was sealed in an oil-filled tank. He added a rheostat for varying the current continuously from a fraction of a milliampere to the full output of the transformer, and a switch

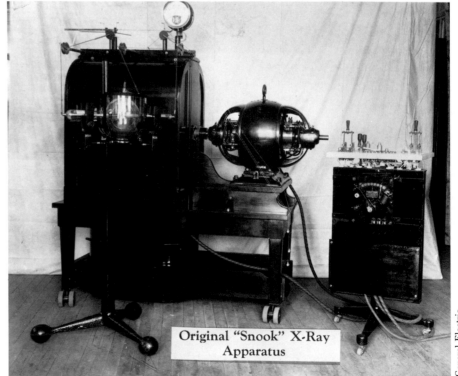

Original "Snook" X-Ray Apparatus

General Electric

for varying the voltage in steps from 70,000 to 120,000 volts. Thus the voltage and amperage fed to the tube and the quantity and hardness of the x-rays generated could be independently controlled. Because the energy output (more than 100 kV at 100 mA) of the Snook machine was far beyond that of the available gas x-ray tubes, the power supply was no longer the limiting factor in radiological procedures. The high voltage source was now dependable and could be adjusted by means of a rheostat or autotransformer in the primary leads to the high voltage transformer. A milliammeter in the secondary circuit could be used to read the tube current. Now all that was needed was an x-ray tube with predictable operating characteristics and capable of operation at higher power—the Coolidge "hot cathode" tube (see Chapter 8).

The remaining problem with the Snook apparatus was that it contained a vacuum-tube rectifier (the Fleming valve) that permitted current to flow from its cathode to its anode but not in the reverse direction. However, the Fleming valve (like the Crookes tube) contained residual gas and was therefore inherently unstable. The combination of two or four unstable gas rectifiers with the erratic operation of a gas tube produced a situation that many physicians could not tolerate.

This problem was solved in 1914 by the development of a new rectifier tube (kenotron) by Saul Dushman, an associate of Langmuir and Coolidge at General Electric.[12] The kenotron, or valve tube, was basically a hot-cathode Fleming valve from which almost all the gas had been evacuated. Initially, kenotrons were primarily used in radiotransmitters, which required continuous operation at a fixed voltage. The initial units were poorly designed for x-ray application, which called for operation for short periods of voltage and current that varied with the technique being used. A variable drop across the kenotron from exposure to exposure resulted in poor duplication of radiographic results. Nevertheless, when tube currents in excess of the 100 mA capability of the mechanical rectifier became desirable in the early 1930s, Dushman and his associates succeeded in designing a kenotron that met all x-ray requirements and became generally used.

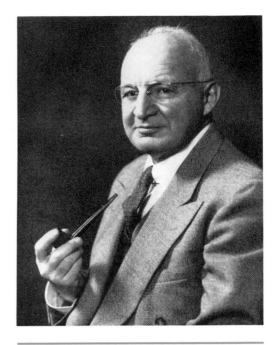

Saul Dushman (1883-1954).[7]

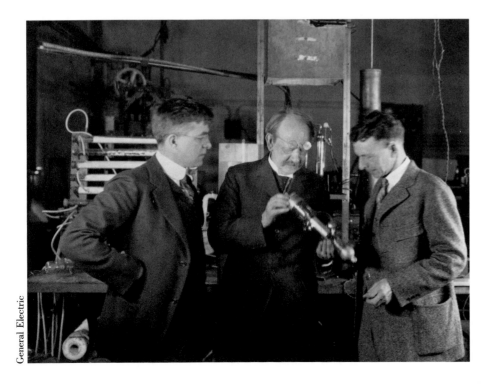

General Electric

Hot cathode kenotron. Irving Langmuir (*left*) and William Coolidge (*right*) watch intently as Sir Joseph John Thomson inspects the new valve tube.

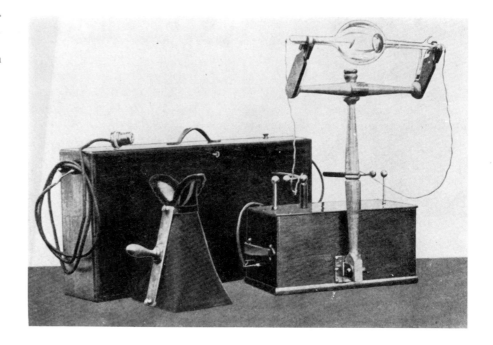

Portable apparatus (1901). The smaller box contains the coil; the larger, the interrupted electrolytic interrupter, two vacuum tubes, and the tube-holder. The tube-holder is shown fastened to the smaller box.[3]

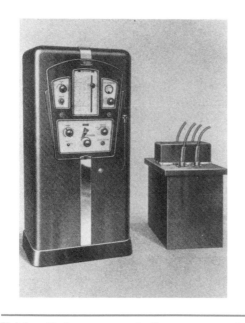

Keleket Techron anatomically programmed generator.[14]

Coolidge developed models of the hot-cathode tube that were capable of operating directly from a transformer without an auxiliary rectifying device.[13] This "self-rectifying" tube could be enclosed in the same metal container with the transformer (simplifying the equipment and facilitating protection from high voltage and from stray radiation) and made possible the construction of a portable x-ray unit with a capacity of 85 kV and 10 mA. However, for applications in which light weight and simplicity were not too important, it was still desirable to have rectified current. If the x-ray tube was not required to act as a rectifier, the focal spot could be made appreciably smaller. In addition, x-ray tubes could, by abuse, be brought into such a condition that they would not operate satisfactorily on unrectified current but could work well with a rectifier. Four kenotrons, placed in the same tank with the high-voltage transformer, could provide the full-wave cycle rectification required.

Line voltage fluctuations altering the temperature of the cathode filament could rapidly change the milliamperage in a high vacuum x-ray tube. To solve this problem, William K. Kearsley developed a milliamperage stabilizer (1920). This unit automatically guarded against the effects of line voltage change and a consequent alteration in the electron emission and production of x-rays.[13]

An important technical development in the late 1920s was the Keleket Techron generator, which was the forerunner of all of the anatomically programmed x-ray units that were developed later. To use the Techron generator, it was necessary to measure the centimeter thickness of the part to be radiographed. This measurement was set on the "Techron" dial, which essentially set the kilovoltage so that the kilovolt peak (kVp) equaled 2 × Techrons + 23. The vertical slide pointer was then set at the appropriate anatomical part, the desired density was selected, and the exposure was made. The heart of the operation of the Techron generator was essentially a built-in technique chart that was entered and checked at the time of installation and checked again at later service calls.[14]

THREE-PHASE GENERATORS

The voltage in early radiological equipment was produced by single-phase electric power. This resulted in a pulsating x-ray beam, caused by the alternate swing in voltage from zero to maximum potential that occurred many times per second. The x-rays produced when the single-phase voltage wave form had a value near zero were of little diagnostic value because of their low penetrability. To overcome this deficiency, some sophisticated electrical engineering principles were utilized to generate three simultaneous voltage wave forms out of step with one another. Using this "three-phase power," multiple voltage wave forms were superimposed on one another to result in an effective wave form that maintained a nearly constant high voltage that never dropped to zero during the exposure. Three-phase generators also permitted a much higher tube rating for extremely short x-ray exposures, since near-maximum loading was applied to the tube throughout the exposure with the electron beam spread across a sizable area of the rotating anode. Three-phase generators made it possible to produce radiographs with extremely short exposure times and high repetition rates, as in angiography.

The first three-phase unit, produced by Siemens in 1928, could be operated at a then amazing 2000 mA at 80 kVp. Five years later (1933), Picker introduced the first three-phase unit to be built in the United States.

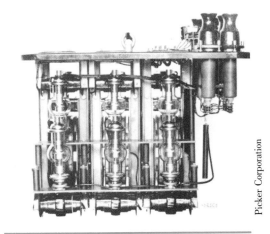

Picker Corporation

Internal design of the Picker three-phase generator.

PORTABLE RADIOGRAPHY

Portable x-ray units were developed to permit examinations to be made outside the traditional hospital or office setting. An early use of portable apparatus was in a military environment (see Chapter 22). In civilian life, Francis Williams (1901) described a portable unit that "weighs 40 pounds and can be easily carried by a man, one box in each hand. In places where no 110-volt circuit is available, I have used an electric cab or carriage by running insulated wires from the storage batteries in the cab to the patient's room, and connecting them with an x-ray apparatus."[3] A more unusual approach to providing energy for portable units was horse power, and exotic transportation techniques included x-ray tricycles and airplanes.

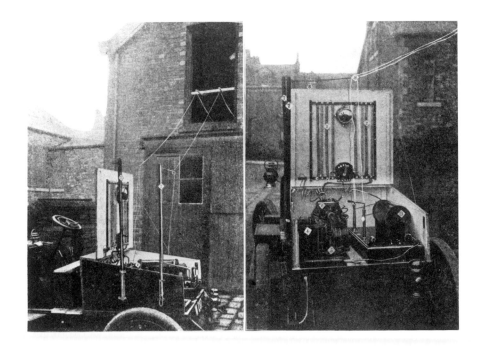

X-ray automobile (1913). "*1*, Dynamo driven by a pulley from a countershaft, the latter being driven by a silent chain from the engine shaft. The winding of the dynamo is compound. At 1,710 revolutions per minute the output is 65 volts and 20 amperes. *2*, Variable resistance with the ampere meter and switch. *3*, 12-inch spark coil; *4*, motor mercury interrupter; *5*, main switch. A small resistance to control the speed of the motor is shown just below this; *7*, two removable poles fitted into sockets at the side of the car. A piece of strong elastic rubber is attached to the top of each pole. At the end of the rubber is an eyepiece (*8*), through which passed the high-tension leads from the secondaries of the coil. These leads next passed to two ebonite rods, which are clamped to the bottom of the window-sash, as shown on *left*, and thus to the focus-tube at the bedside of the patient."[15]

X-ray aeroplane (1918). This proposal to the French Ministry of Inventions consisted of a single-engined, three-seater biplane that carried a pilot, radiologist, and surgeon. The aeroplane engine was designed to provide power for the x-ray apparatus and the equipment for emergency surgery.[16]

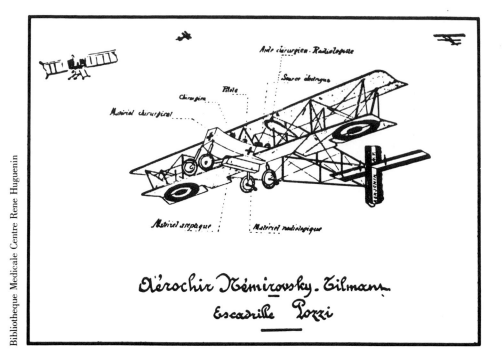

A variety of portable radiographic units were developed by major x-ray equipment companies. They typically operated at 30 to 50 mA and up to 80 or possibly 95 kVp. As late as 1933, some mobile units were still of the nonshockproof variety with cables exposed.

In 1958, Picker introduced a high-powered mobile unit that could produce 300 mA at 125 kVp. Other manufacturers followed, but because of the high cost of providing electrical outlets for these units, they have disappeared from the market and been replaced in recent years (with a sacrifice in power) by rechargeable, battery-operated and capacitor discharge mobile units that can be plugged into existing 115-volt outlets for charging or operation.

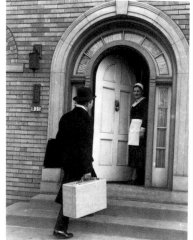

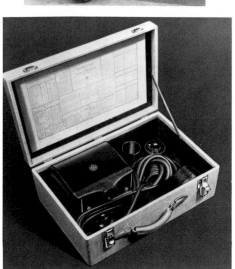

Later portable x-ray unit. *Top,* Doctor entering a home carrying the shock proof portable device. *Bottom left,* Portable diagnostic unit in its carrying case. *Bottom right,* Using the portable device to obtain an AP chest film on a woman patient at home in bed.

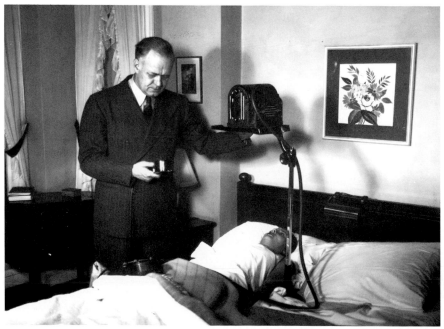

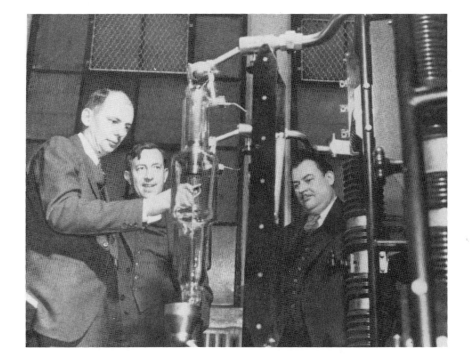

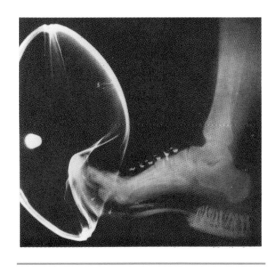

Charles Slack and the Micronex cold-cathode field emission tube.[14]

Micronex radiograph of a football kick using a 1-msec exposure.[14]

LATER TECHNICAL DEVELOPMENTS

In 1939, Charles Slack of Westinghouse X-Ray Company developed the "Micronex" field emission tube for microsecond exposures. During World War II, the Field Emission Corporation combined the field emission tube with a capacitor discharge unit to produce a 90-pound apparatus for the Armed Forces. In 1960, a commercial mobile version of this device (Fexitron) was introduced. Although it permitted exposures as short as 1/100 second, the Fexitron never became popular.

During the 1950s, the output of x-ray generators was increased to provide tube voltages up to 150 kVp and tube currents up to and exceeding 1000 mA, substantial increases from the 100 kVp at 500 mA that had been available at the start of the decade. In an effort to improve chest radiography, William Tuddenham (1954) reported on using a GE Maxitron 2000, 2-million volt x-ray generator for "supervoltage" chest radiography. Chest images obtained with this equipment had minimal bone masking and thus provided better information about the mediastinum and apices of the lungs. However, problems such as cost, excessive patient exposure, excessive focal spot size, and relatively low output caused this procedure to be abandoned, although this technique is still performed as "port filming" in radiation oncology departments.

In the next decade, Hewlett Packard, which had acquired the Field Emission Corporation, used the cold cathode field emission tube to produce a 350 kVp chest radiographic unit that could produce millisecond images. These images were somewhat comparable to the "supervoltage" images of the 1950s with little bone masking, but they could be made with much less expensive and more compact equipment and with better spatial resolution. Although these units never achieved great popularity, some are still in operation.

A major improvement (especially for technologists) was the development of programmed radiographic devices that reduced exposure variable selection to the depression of a single push button. Exposure factors and other variables, such as tube focus, auxiliary device (Bucky, spot-film,

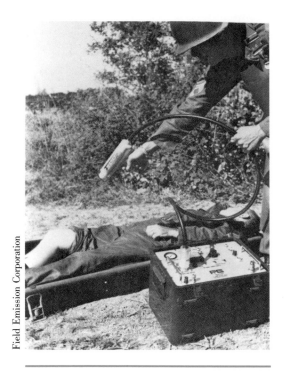

Field Emission Corporation

Fexitron. Prototype field model of suitcase size and weighing a total of 80 pounds. It used a 5-pound tube head and could take l-msec exposures at 70 to 120 kVp and 2500 mA.

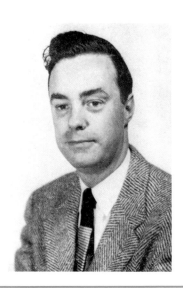

Russell H. Morgan.

etc.), automatic exposure control sensitivity, and measuring fields, were grouped on selector panels by body area and examination type. Pressing one button did away with a lot of busy work and left technologists free to attend to those tasks that a machine cannot perform.[17]

PHOTOTIMERS

The production of diagnostically excellent radiographs required correct x-ray exposure. However, the choice of a proper duration of exposure depended on several independent variables, such as the speed of the film, the kilovoltage applied to the tube, the milliamperage, the ray-absorbing characteristics of the grid, the thickness and opacity of the part being x-rayed, and the fatness or leanness of the patient. Although charts had been prepared to guide radiologists with respect to kilovoltage, milliamperage, film speed, and grid, each exposure required the exercise of judgment with respect to the other factors. Therefore it was not surprising many films emerged from the developer either underexposed or overexposed, especially when taken by a radiologist or technician with limited experience. As the volume of examinations increased yearly, it became increasingly urgent to design a simpler way by which technicians could consistently achieve proper exposure.

In 1942, Russell H. Morgan described an "exposure meter" based on photoelectric principles.[18] He mounted a fluorescent screen behind the film so that x-rays from the tube, after traversing the patient being radiographed and the film, caused the screen to fluoresce. Near the screen was a phototube, which emitted a slight electric current when light fell on its face. After amplification, this current was led to a condenser. When a specified amount of electricity was stored in the condenser, it discharged, tripping a relay that terminated the x-ray exposure. In this way, the radiologist or technician no longer had to guess how long an exposure would be required to secure a film of the desired density (blackness), since the phototimer automatically timed the exposure to achieve (at least in theory) the proper results.

During the next few years, Morgan and an associate, Paul C. Hodges, made many improvements on the initial phototimer model.[19] For a phototimer to work properly, it was essential that its detector "see" the object or area of interest. However, in many examinations it was extremely difficult to properly position the patient relative to the measuring aperture. Initially, a 2-inch × 2-inch fluorescent screen was used to sample the quantity of x-rays passing through the film. This proved too large for some purposes and too small for others. In both situations, the light striking the x-ray film and tube might be turned off too soon or too late. To remedy this difficulty, Morgan and Hodges introduced a series of "stops" instead of a single fluorescent screen. Stop 1, for example, allowed the x-rays to fall on the screen through a circular aperture 2 inches in diameter located at the center of the field. This proved satisfactory for sampling the x-rays during exposure of the skull, gallbladder, and certain other organs. Stop 2 allowed x-rays to reach the fluorescing screen through 16 apertures, each 1 inch in diameter, located four in each corner. This stop permitted sampling of a wide area and was used for filming the chest, abdomen, and pelvis. Stop 3 was similarly designed for filming the spine, while Stop 4 was used for the hand, wrist, fingers, and toes. By selecting the appropriate stop, the technician operating the apparatus could be assured that the exposure would be terminated at precisely the right time.

Some radiologists preferred their films a little darker or lighter than usual; at times, relatively light or dark films were required for special diagnostic purposes. To permit these variations from average or usual density, Hodges and Morgan designed a highly complex electronic circuit that added an adjusting device to the phototimer.

Although the Morgan-Hodges phototimer became standard equipment in radiographic apparatus, as well as in many automatic-exposure cameras, for a long time it was primarily used in chest radiography and spot filming. Acceptance of the technique in general radiography began some years later with the introduction of multifield ionization chamber detectors.

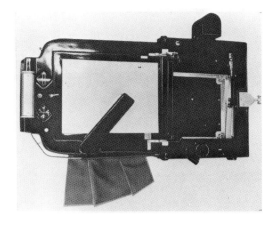

Westinghouse phototimer on a spot film device (1948). Using Morgan's principle, the sensing unit is contained in the movable arm, which also activates the cassette carrier.

Bibliography

Brecher R and Brecher E: The rays: A history of radiology in the United States and Canada. Baltimore, Williams & Wilkins, 1969.

Jerman EC: Roentgen-ray apparatus. In Glasser O (ed): The science of radiology, Springfield, Ill, Charles C Thomas, 1933.

Krohmer JS: Radiography and fluoroscopy, 1920 to the present. RadioGraphics 9:1129-1153, 1989.

Trout ED: Tubes and generators. In Bruwer AJ (ed): Classic descriptions in diagnostic roentgenology. Springfield, Ill, Charles C Thomas, 1964.

References

1. Beck C: Roentgen-ray diagnosis and therapy. New York, Appleton, 1904.
2. Pusey WA and Caldwell EW: The practical application of roentgen rays in therapeutics and diagnosis. Philadelphia, WB Saunders, 1904.
3. Williams FH: The roentgen rays in medicine and surgery. New York, MacMillan, 1901.
4. Monell SH: A system of instruction in x-ray methods and medical uses of light, hot-air, vibration and high-frequency currents. New York, Pelton, 1902.
5. Allen CW: Radiotherapy and phototherapy including radium and high-frequency currents. New York, Lea Brothers, 1904.
6. Trout ED: History of radiation sources for cancer therapy. In Buschke F (ed): Progress in radiation therapy. New York, Grune & Stratton, 1958.
7. Trout ED: Tubes and generators. In Bruwer AJ (ed): Classic descriptions in diagnostic roentgenology. Springfield, Ill, Charles C Thomas, 1964.
8. Lemp H: Alternating current selector. US Patent 774,090, issued November 1, 1904.
9. Snook HC: X-ray system. US Patent 954,056, issued April 5, 1910.
10. Snook HC: A new roentgen generator. Arch Roentgen Ray 13:186-188, 1908.
11. Feldman A: A sketch of the technical history of radiology from 1896 to 1920. RadioGraphics 9:1113-1128, 1989.
12. Dushman S: Electrical discharge device. US Patent 1,287,265, issued December 10, 1918.
13. Coolidge WD: The development of modern roentgen-ray generating apparatus. AJR 24:605-620, 1930.
14. Krohmer JS: Radiography and fluoroscopy, 1920 to the present. RadioGraphics 9:1129-1153, 1989.
15. Hazleton EB: An x-ray automobile. Arch Roentgen Ray 305-312, 1913.
16. Mould RF: A history of x-rays and radium. 1980.
17. Angus WM: A commentary on the development of diagnostic imaging technology. RadioGraphics 9:1225-1244, 1989.
18. Morgan RH: An exposure meter for roentgenography. AJR 47:777-784, 1942.
19. Hodges PC and Morgan RH: Photoelectric timing in general roentgenography. AJR 53:474-482, 1945.

CHAPTER 8

X-Ray Tubes

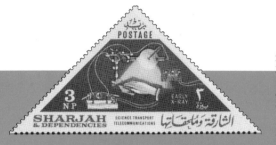

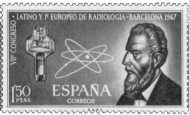

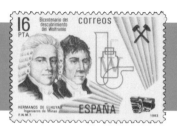

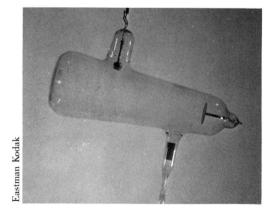

Eastman Kodak

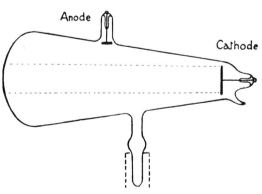

Top, Photograph and *bottom*, diagram of the original type of x-ray tube.[1] The cathode stream produced x-rays by impinging on the large area of the glass wall of the tube.

The basic method of producing x-rays today is essentially the same as that initially used by Roentgen. Electrons freed from a metal cathode are accelerated to a high velocity and then suddenly stopped by striking a dense target. However, since 1896 there have been many changes in the x-ray tube and in the means of accelerating its electrons.

GAS-TUBE ERA

The first x-ray tube was the type used by Crookes in his early experiments on electrical discharges through highly rarified gases. A high voltage current was applied between two metal electrodes sealed in the glass wall of the tube, either at opposite ends or (as in Roentgen's tube) with the anode off to one side. The electrons liberated by positive ion bombardment of the front surface of a flat aluminum cathode were emitted in a direction perpendicular to its surface and travelled in straight lines until they impinged on the glass wall of the tube, where the x-rays were generated.

The Crookes tube was substantially improved by Alan Archibald Campbell-Swinton, who placed a sheet of platinum in the path of the cathode rays to serve as the metal target instead of the glass wall of the tube. In most cases, the same metal surface that served as the target was connected to the positive terminal of the power supply, so that it also functioned as the anode. Using the anode as a metal target aligned with the axis of the tube was an important design change, since the metal had a much higher atomic number than glass and thus was more efficient in emitting x-rays. The surface of the anode was tilted so that the x-rays generated when the cathode rays struck it could emerge from the tube without being blocked by the cathode. Campbell-Swinton also designed a dual cathode x-ray tube for use when only an alternating current was available. As each disk alternately became the cathode, the cathode

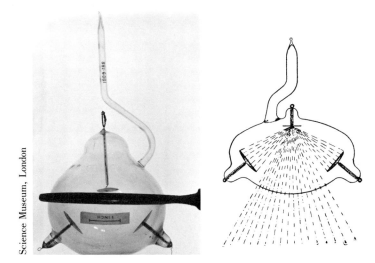

First dual cathode x-ray tube for use with alternating current (Campbell-Swinton, March 17, 1896). *Left*, Photograph and *right*, diagram.[2]

stream in both cases was directed at the target. A different approach to this problem was made by Thomas A. Edison, who developed a tube in which the two electrodes were inclined at an angle and opposite each other. Under the influence of oscillating discharges, each electrode alternately became anode and cathode, producing x-rays that could be observed at that part of the tube against which the cathode streams were directed.[3,4]

In 1894, Sir Herbert Jackson, utilizing an earlier discovery of Crookes, replaced the flat cathode with a concave one, thus focusing the cathode rays on a small area of the metal target. Because most of the x-rays in this "focus tube" emerged from a small region on the surface of the anode, they cast a much sharper shadow with less blurring. In addition, because the heat generated by cathode-ray bombardment was concentrated on the metal target rather than on the glass wall of the bulb, the glass was less likely to melt or crack and the useful life of the tube tended to increase.

Another early change in tube design was the inclusion of a separate anode connected electrically with the original anode facing the cathode. Although the function of this auxiliary anode was difficult to explain, it seemed to make the x-ray tube operate more steadily and became a standard feature in tubes produced after 1897.

The early x-ray tubes were small. As the power input was increased, better results could be obtained by greatly increasing the size of the glass bulb. This aided in reducing the pressure change that occurred during x-ray production and in decreasing the degree of local heating of the glass

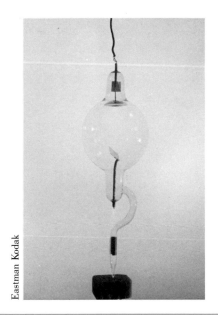

Early x-ray tube containing an angled metal target that also served as the anode.

Jackson "focus tube" (1896) diagram (*left*).[2] *K*, curved cathode; *A*, angled anode. *Right*, Photograph.

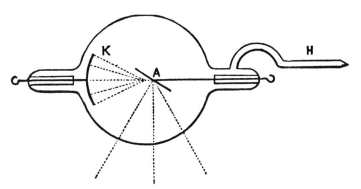

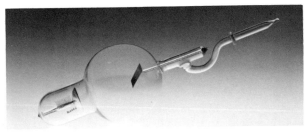

X-ray tubes with auxiliary anodes. *Left*, 1896 and *right*, 1900.

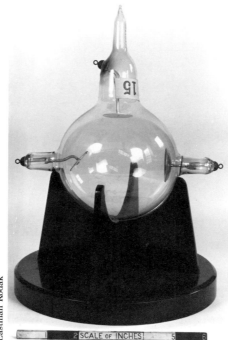

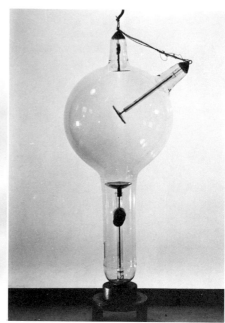

Eastman Kodak

resulting from its bombardment by electrons reflected from the focal spot.

The early aluminum cathodes were thin and thus easily melted by the positive ion bombardment to which they were subjected. Better results could be obtained by using relatively massive cathodes; for therapeutic work, cathodes were designed that were hollow and cooled by compressed air.

The thin metal target of the early tubes was soon replaced by a heavy mass of metal consisting essentially of two parts: a refractory metal face to take the cathode ray impact; and a heavy back plate consisting of a good heat-conducting metal that would serve to lead away and temporarily store the heat liberated at the focal spot. Platinum and copper came into general use for the refractory metal face and back plate, respectively. The platinum facing was made extremely thin (0.001 inch) and was welded to a disk of nickel, which in turn was soldered to a large mass of copper. The tube had a definite energy limitation, and, if this were exceeded even for an instant, the thin facing of platinum was ruined at the focal spot and the tube had outlived its usefulness.[6] Targets occasionally were made of osmium, iridium, tantalum, and other heavy metals with high melting points.

Early heavy anode tube (Campbell-Swinton, 1896). A thin piece of platinum was silver-soldered to a heavier disk of another metal, in this case a copper penny. This combination dissipated heat more effectively and permitted the use of larger currents that produced more x-rays.

Science Museum, London

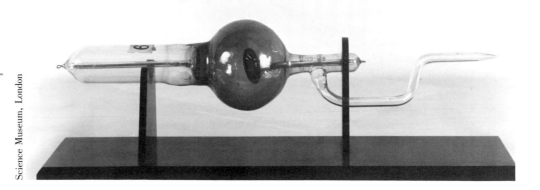

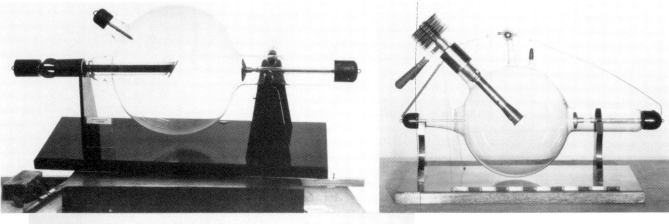

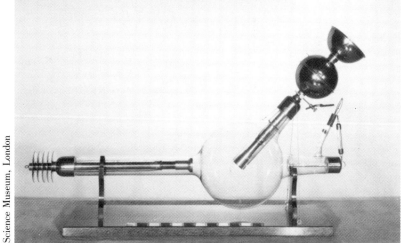

Science Museum, London

Top left, Heavy current tube with air-cooled anode (Gundelach, 1908). The rear of the anode was soldered to a heavy metal rod that projected outward from the bulb to a finned radiator that balanced the heat generated at about 200° C and prevented the anode from becoming incandescent. *Top right*, Tube cooled by means of removable metal tongs (Müller, 1912). When hot, the tongs could be exchanged for a cool pair so that the tube could be run almost continuously. *Bottom left*, Boiling water tube for intensive therapeutic work (Müller, 1918). In this ingenious tube, the hollow anode was connected to a water reservoir. When in use, the water boiled away so that the anode remained at a constant temperature.

X-ray tubes used for radiation therapy required the application of high currents for long periods and thus produced large amounts of heat that had to be dissipated. Among the ingenious devices developed were cooling fins (extension of the heat-conducting metal back plate outside the bulb to a finned radiator), removable cooling tongs, which when hot could be changed for a cool pair, and the boiling water tube, in which the hollow back plate of the anode was connected to a reservoir containing water which, when the tube was in use, boiled away to keep the anode at a constant and acceptable temperature.

The major problem with early x-ray tubes was regulating the vacuum within them. Although often called "vacuum tubes" in the 1890s, an inherent characteristic of Crookes tubes was their need to have a little air or other gas left inside. The gas pressure within these "gas tubes" during the time of exposure determined their operating characteristics. If the gas pressure in the tube became low (presumably a result of adsorption of gas on the inner surfaces of the tube), the discharge current became lower, but those electrons that succeeded in striking the anode had suffered fewer collisions with gas molecules and thus the x-ray spectrum was shifted toward higher photon energies. The decreased discharge current generally required the application of a higher voltage to maintain the discharge. This resulted in a more penetrating, though less intense, beam ("hard" tube) that led to a reduction in subject contrast. As the tube became warm with use, gas was driven off its inner surfaces, discharge current increased, and the energies of the electrons striking the anode decreased, resulting in a less-penetrating beam and a "soft" tube.[7]

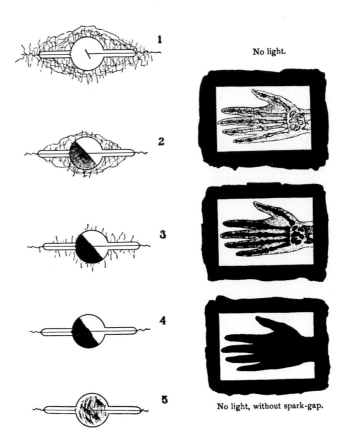

1

No light.

2

3

4

5

No light, without spark-gap.

Diagram showing the effect of the resistance of the tube on the x-ray picture thrown on the screen (1901). "The direction of the light is downwards and to the left. *1*, The current does not pass through this tube, since the resistance is high (a tube of such high resistance may be easily punctured). The amount of this resistance can be ascertained by measuring its equivalent of air resistance. *2*, The resistance of the tube is high; the picture of the hand on the screen is bright but without contrast. *3*, The resistance of this tube is not as high as in 2. The picture of the hand is good with well-marked contrast between the bones and flesh. *4*, Resistance of this tube is low; the picture of the hand on the screen is dark, and the contrast between the flesh and bones is not marked. *5*, The resistance of this tube is very low and no light is produced unless more of a multiple spark-gap is used. The light, which gives most penetration, is that obtained from 2, but the differentiation of the soft tissues is not as accomplished as with a tube of lower resistance. To increase the penetrating power of a tube with lower resistance, more energy must be passed through it."[5]

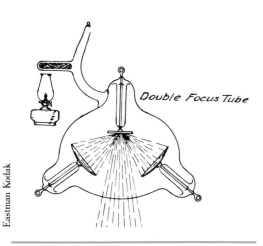

Eastman Kodak

Double Focus Tube

Chemical regulator (with heat source) attached to a double-focus tube developed by Elihu Thomson.

Unfortunately, it was virtually impossible to predict the characteristics of a tube at any time during its life, for they were constantly changing.

The finicky gas tubes played havoc with the practice of radiology. X-ray workers of the era kept a rack of tubes on hand, knew the history of each, and selected with care the right tube for each purpose. Tubes could last for several months or puncture after only a few hours. As Henry Hulst of Grand Rapids, Michigan, wrote[8]:

> Nature seems capricious to the savage mind; tubes do to the x-ray worker. He rests, pets, punishes, smashes tubes as the fetishist his idols. He learns to know them all by name, their temper and their capabilities. He has a number of them—the more the better. He has trained tubes, trick tubes, high-spirited, high-bred tubes as well as gentle steady tubes . . . A flashy tube is worse than a hysterical woman, it is incurably useless.

Many radiologists gave their tubes women's names; "I think I'll try Isobel this morning" was a typical remark of the gas-tube era.

The condition of each tube could be gauged by turning on the current and watching what happened. When a new tube was turned on for the first time, as Lewis Gregory Cole reported,[10]

> The anterior hemisphere lights up with a bright, yellowish-green fluorescence; this color gradually changes as the seasoning process advances into a purplish-yellow of less brilliancy (called) the "sunflower" light, because of its rich, mellow color. Eventually, in a very old tube there is scarcely any fluorescence whatever and Roentgen spoke of this as a dead tube . . .

Radiologists soon learned that the x-rays emitted by different tubes varied widely in their ability to penetrate human tissues. "Hard" tubes, which contained relatively little residual gas, required high voltages for their activation; the combination of high voltage and hard tube produced a more penetrating ray. Rays from a hard tube could produce an acceptable photographic plate with a shorter exposure, therefore making it less likely that the patient would move and spoil the image.

Excessive pressure within an x-ray tube could usually be reduced by operating the tube intermittently with small currents. When the pressure became too low, it could at first be raised by heating the bulb. After a time, however, this method would fail and the tube would have to be rebuilt.

To prolong the useful life of the tube, various methods were devised for the introduction of small amounts of gas whenever this was required. A common method consisted of attaching a side tube to the major x-ray generating bulb and placing within it a chemical such as potassium carbonate that emitted a gas when heated. If the vacuum rose too high, heat (initially by a flame, later by electrical means) was applied to the chemical in the "regulator." The gas that was released reduced the vacuum, and the tube began to function again. The Bauer valve was a successful regulator consisting of a small piece of unglazed porcelain sealed into the tube envelope. This porcelain was normally covered by liquid mercury, which could be displaced at will by squeezing a rubber bulb, thus allowing air from outside to diffuse through the pores of the porcelain into the tube. The osmosis regulator of Villard consisted of a tiny, thin-walled tube of platinum or palladium closed at one end and sealed at the other to the envelope of the x-ray tube. Heating the regulator with a Bunsen burner or other flame caused hydrogen to diffuse through the platinum or palladium into the x-ray tube.

Homer Clyde Snook developed a hydrogen x-ray tube with two osmosis regulators, one for raising and the other for lowering the hydrogen pressure. One osmosis tube was surrounded by a bulb containing pure hydrogen, which could be admitted to the x-ray tube by heating the regulator with a spark discharge. A second osmosis tube was exposed to the air and permitted the escape of hydrogen from the x-ray tube when electric heat was applied.

The most valuable vacuum regulator was introduced in 1897 by Henry Lyman Sayen, a designer of scientific equipment in the shop of Queen & Company in Philadelphia. Sayen devised a tube in which, whenever the vacuum rose too high, the current produced sparks between a second pair of electrodes. This *automatically* heated the potassium carbonate or other chemical lodged in the path of the sparks, released a little gas, and thus started the tube up again. Known as the Queen Self-Regulating X-Ray Tube, Sayen's tube became extremely popular.

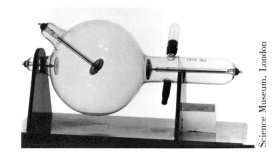

Osmosis regulator tube (Villard, 1898).

Advertisement for the Queen Self-Regulating X-Ray Tube with impressive testimonials.

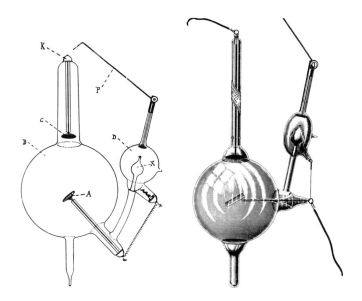

Queen Self-Regulating X-Ray Tube (Sayen, 1897). *Left,* "Diagram shows a small bulb (*X*) containing a chemical that gave off vapor when heated and reabsorbed it when it cooled, was directly connected to the main tube (*B*), and was surrounded by an auxiliary tube (*D*). The cathode of the auxiliary bulb was connected to an adjustable spark point (*P*), the end of which could be swung to any desired distance from the cathode (*K*) of the main tube. The anode of the small tube was directly connected to the anode (*A*) of the main tube."[9] *Right,* Drawing from 1901 catalogue of Queen & Company.

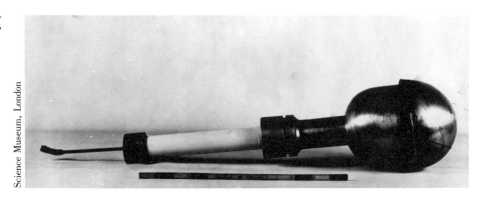

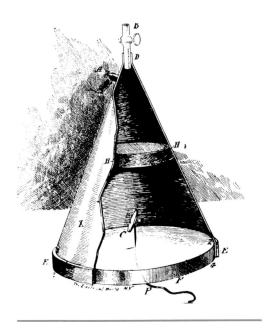

Woodward's metal x-ray tube (1896).[11]

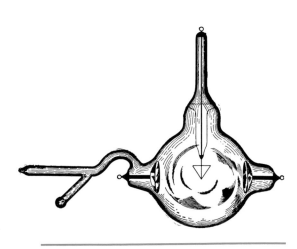

Thomson's double-focus x-ray tube (1896).[13]

Another approach to lowering the degree of vacuum was to "bake" the tube. It was thought that the glass, when heated, became sufficiently porous to permit the passage of air into the tube. More likely, the heating liberated gas trapped within or adjacent to the glass molecules themselves. If the tube was baked too long and the vacuum decreased excessively, the resulting soft (gassy) tube could then be used for superficial therapy until its vacuum was again raised (hardened) enough so that it could be returned to diagnostic tasks.

Numerous other variations on the Crookes design were introduced during the first year after Roentgen's discovery. Woodward at Harvard and Davies in London developed all-metal tubes[11] and John Trowbridge of Yale designed an oil-immersed tube to keep the glass cool and to eliminate the sparking that sometimes cracked or melted the glass of ordinary tubes.[12] Elihu Thomson of General Electric applied for a patent on a double-focus tube containing two cup-shaped cathodes (instead of only one) placed diametrically opposite to each other with a wedge-shaped platinum target electrode between them. When the tube was energized with direct current, the two focused cathode streams bombarded the platinum wedge to produce an abundance of x-rays. If alternating current were used, the electrodes rapidly took turns being anode and cathode.[13] Like many of these variations, even the dual-cathode design had been used by Crookes decades before and was described in a paper by Roentgen 5 months before Thomson's patent application.

The plethora of tube designs for the production of x-rays was best demonstrated in the January 28, 1897 issue of *Nature*, which illustrated 32 different types of tubes currently in use for the production of x-rays.[14] Slight modifications in the shape and form of the electrodes were made by various manufacturers, each one claiming some special advantage for his particular form of tube. The busy practitioner was confused as to which tube was the best to purchase. Consequently, John MacIntyre, the President of the Röntgen Society in London, decided to offer a gold medal to "the maker of the best practical x-ray tube for both photographic and screen work." A committee of experts was formed to act as judges, and some 28 tubes were sent in by manufacturers in England and abroad. Although the elaborate tests to which the tubes were subjected unfortunately were never published, six tubes were selected for a semifinal photographic test. Under identical conditions of electrification exposure, distance, and development, these tubes produced images that varied considerably in both density and sharpness. Two tubes were judged to be of virtually equivalent excellence, and the less expensive of the two was given the prize. Only later was it realized that both of these tubes were by the same maker, Carl H. F. Müller of Hamburg, Germany.[15]

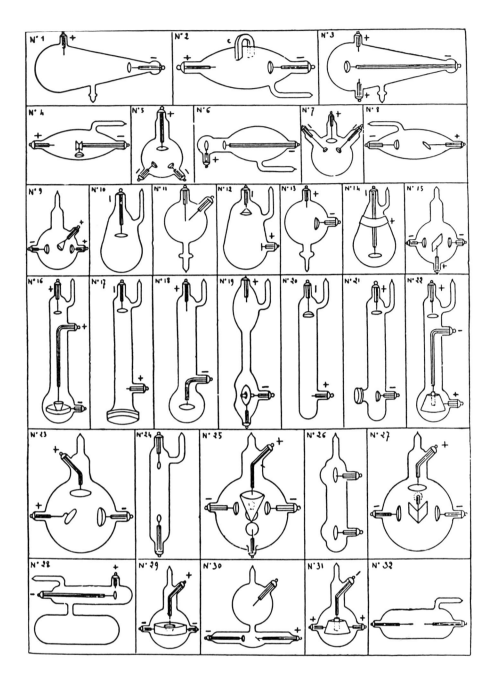

Forms of tube used for the production of cathode and x-rays. *1* and *2*, Crookes tube; *3*, Seguy tube; *4*, Wood tube; *5*, Seguy tube; *6*, Chabaud and Hurmuzescu tube; *7*, Seguy tube; *8*, "Focus" tube; *9*, Seguy tube; *10*, d'Arsonval tube; *11*, Seguy tube; *12*, Puluj tube; *13*, Seguy tube; *14*, d'Arsonval tube; *15*, Le Roux tube; *16*, *17*, and *18*, Seguy tubes; *19*, Rufz tube; *20*, Crookes tube; *21*, *22*, and *23*, Seguy tubes; *24*, Roentgen tube; *25*, Brunet-Seguy tube; *26* and *27*, Le Roux tubes; *28*, Colardeau tube; *29*, Seguy tube; *30*, Colardeau tube; *31*, Seguy tube; *32*, Roentgen tube.[14]

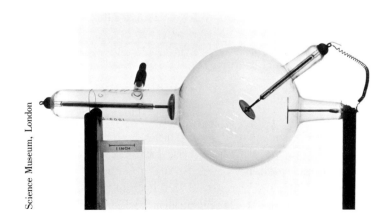

Science Museum, London

Müller "Gold-Medal" tube (1901). The tube contained an anode of nickel faced with platinum and had an auxiliary anode.

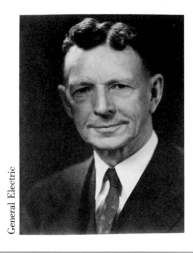

William David Coolidge (1873-1975).

COOLIDGE TUBE

In 1905, William David Coolidge moved from the Massachusetts Institute of Technology to the General Electric research laboratory in Schenectady, New York and was put to work on the problem of improving the filaments in electric light bulbs. Tungsten seemed to be the most promising metal for filaments, but it was a brittle metal that was difficult to handle. Coolidge (1910) discovered that ductile tungsten for filaments could be produced by working the metal at a lower temperature than usual.[18] Within 1 or 2 years, electric lamps with ductile tungsten filaments came into general use.

Having developed an important new metallurgical product, Coolidge searched to find additional uses for it. Soon his ductile tungsten replaced platinum for contact points on automobile ignition systems. Coolidge next turned to the possible use of tungsten instead of platinum for the targets in x-ray tubes.

Four principal properties were required for a metal to be suitable for use as a target in an x-ray tube: (1) high specific gravity (atomic number); (2) high melting point; (3) high heat conductivity; and (4) low vapor pressure at high temperatures. The denser the target, the more rapid the deceleration of electrons from the cathode and thus the greater the amplitude of the x-rays emitted (tungsten is only slightly less dense than platinum). A high melting point (3370° C for tungsten as against 1773° C for platinum) and high heat conductivity (to permit more rapid flow of heat from the focal spot to the surrounding metal) allowed sharp focusing of the cathode rays on the target even at higher voltages. Unlike tungsten, platinum vaporized freely when too hot, and the vapor thus released "condenses on the glass in finely divided form and absorbs relatively large amounts of gas, thus changing the vacuum. At high temperatures tungsten vaporizes least of all the metals."[19]

Although the tungsten target increased the power and the ruggedness of the gas tube, the results were still disappointing. When the focal spot of a tungsten target in a gas tube was overloaded, the tungsten vapor produced brought about a sudden and troublesome change in gas pressure. Tungsten vapor united with oxygen and nitrogen gases to form solid nitride and tungsten oxide, respectively, both of which deposited on the wall of the tube. In addition, when the tube was overloaded, the glass around the cathode became hot and frequently cracked. This was finally

Coolidge in laboratory scene from the movie "Exploring with X-rays."

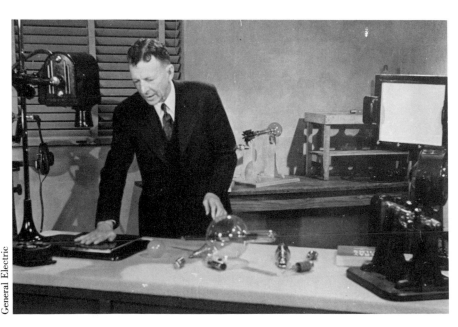

prevented by immersing the tubes completely in oil. Another difficulty then made its appearance—the aluminum cathode melted. To prevent this, a solid tungsten cathode was tried, but this made the tube exceedingly "cranky." No sooner would the tube be started than it would refuse to carry current until more gas had been introduced from the regulator.

"A consideration of the above-mentioned limitations," Coolidge reported, "showed that they were for the most part incident to the use of gas and that they could therefore be made to disappear if a tube could be operated with a very much higher vacuum."[20] However, in the ordinary Crookes tube activated with an electrical potential between the cathode and anode, the emission of electrons was triggered by positive ions of gas bombarding the cathode. A tube without enough gas to produce the initial ion bombardment of the cathode would not work at all. Therefore the problem of producing a stable tube by raising the vacuum seemed insoluble, unless electrons for bombardment of the target could be supplied in some other way.

A decade earlier, William Rollins had tried to solve this problem by using radium as a source of electrons but had not succeeded in obtaining the effect he sought. In 1912, Julius Edgar Lilienfeld incorporated an incandescent filament, which when heated, emitted electrons.[21] These electrons lowered the resistance of the tube and thus made possible x-ray production in a tube from which almost all the gas had been evacuated. Nevertheless, Lilienfeld's tube was still a gas tube and could not be operated if the pressure became too low.

The emission of electrons from a hot filament in a tube had been discovered years before by Thomas A. Edison in his work on the incandescent lamp. Early experimenters, however, had reported that this "Edison effect," like the emission of x-rays, depended on a residue of gas inside the tube. Could electric current flow through gas-free space between gas-free electrodes? Irving Langmuir of General Electric demonstrated that the electron emission from hot tungsten lamp filaments not only persisted in high vacuum but was actually favored by getting rid of the last traces of gas in the filaments and other parts of the tube.[22] Langmuir also developed a mercury vapor pump, which made possible the production of tubes with greatly reduced pressure. Encouraged by this work, Coolidge developed an x-ray tube with a tungsten target and a cathode consisting of a spiral-shaped wire that could be heated to incandescence when the tube was almost completely evacuated. On May 9,

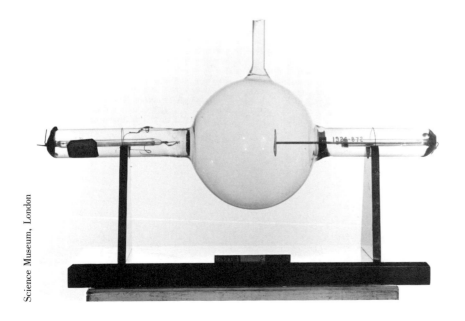

Experimental Coolidge tube. It consisted of a tungsten filament around which was a molybdenum ring, which helped to focus electrons on the small and light tungsten anode. The tube was not evacuated or sealed.

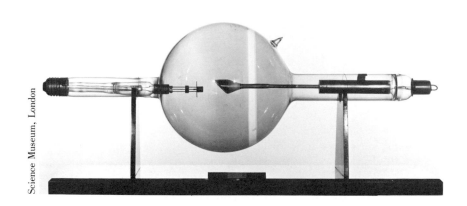

Science Museum, London

Commercial model of Coolidge tube (1913). The tungsten filament, in the form of a flat spiral, was hidden by the molybdenum focusing tube. The anode was a heavy piece of tungsten, which could become almost white hot when the tube was in use.

1913, Coolidge applied for a patent on his new "hot cathode" tube.[23] Unlike Lilienfeld's tube, which had a conventional cathode *plus* a hot filament to supply electrons, the cathode in Coolidge's tube was itself the electron-emitting tungsten filament. In addition, whereas Lilienfeld's patent application specified that the electrons from the hot filament were to be used to lower the resistance of the tube, Coolidge's patent application specified that the electrons from the filament-cathode were to bombard the target and thus directly produce the x-rays.

The new tube, containing gas at an extremely low pressure (about $\frac{1}{1000}$ of an ordinary tube), emitted far more x-rays than Coolidge had anticipated. Human skin could be burned in a few seconds. As Coolidge[24] recalled, "In our first experiments with this new type of x-ray tube, I temporarily and unintentionally sacrificed my own back hair. So I didn't like to practice on other living subjects. For further experiments I was, through the kindness of a medical friend, provided with a human leg which had outlived its usefulness."

After witnessing Coolidge demonstrating his tube, Preston M. Hickey (1913) wrote[25]:

> There was a decided warning given by the inventor as to the danger of the new tube in the hands of the inexperienced. Its apparent quiescence while producing the most tremendous quantity of high penetrating rays might easily lead to most disastrous over-dosage; the erythema dose has been given in a few seconds.
>
> It is hoped by Doctor Coolidge that owing to the extreme exhaustion, penetrating rays of the therapeutic value of the gamma rays of radium may be produced; this of course opens up the most wonderful new possibilities for treatment.

Coolidge then turned his tube over to a practicing radiologist for clinical trials on living patients. He wisely chose Lewis Gregory Cole of New York City, an eminent physician whose standards of quality were recognized as exceedingly high. In an article in the first issue of the *American Journal of Roentgenology*, Cole[26] reported seven advantages of the Coolidge tube over the old gas tubes:

1. Accuracy of adjustment
2. Stability
3. Exact duplication of results
4. Flexibility
5. Tremendous output
6. Long life of the tube
7. Absence of indirect rays

With gas tubes, any change in the electrical current might alter both the quantity of x-rays emitted and their hardness or penetrating power.

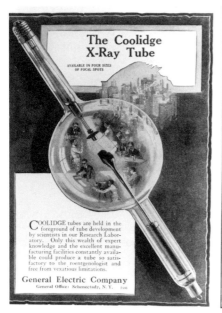
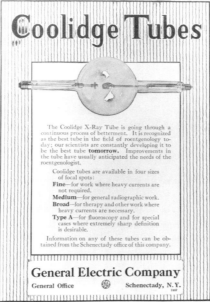
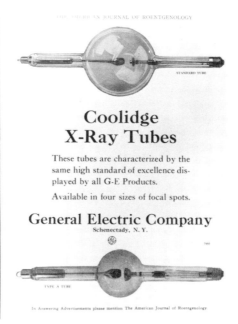

Advertisements for Coolidge x-ray tubes (AJR, 1918).

With the Coolidge tube, the quantity and hardness of the x-rays could be independently controlled. Increasing or decreasing the current to the hot cathode altered its temperature, thus controlling the amount of electron emission. Changing the voltage applied between the cathode and the target controlled the velocity of the electrons and thus the quality of the x-ray beam.

Unlike the gas tubes, where a "perfect" radiograph was difficult to achieve and almost impossible to duplicate, the Coolidge tube produced films of uniformly good quality[26]: "The apparatus can be set for a given penetration, and by using the same milliamperage through the tube, 100 roentgenograms can be made so nearly alike that it is impossible to tell them apart."

Cole noted that "the tube may be operated one instant at a penetration so slight as to show the anastomosis of the blood vessels of the extremities and the next instant, without leaving his seat in the operating booth, one may operate the tube at a penetration far exceeding anything possible with the ordinary (gas) tube." Because of the extreme vacuum, the Coolidge tube could produce high output that was "accurately adjustable and absolutely stable for an unlimited time." In addition, the tube could be operated directly from a transformer, making possible a simple x-ray outfit of relatively small size. Instead of wearing out, "the tube is more likely to meet its fate by being dropped or accidently broken in handling . . . It will not be punctured by any ordinary usage."

The high vacuum tube was also capable of operating directly from a transformer, without an auxiliary rectifying device. This made it possible to enclose it in the same metal container with the transformer, thus simplifying the equipment and facilitating protection from high voltage and stray radiation. In 1919, Waite and Bartlett developed a workable oil-immersed shockproof unit with a Coolidge tube. This led to the construction of a small, flexible, and safe unit for dental radiography. In addition to providing adequate electrical and x-ray protection, oil immersion also offered some favorable features in tube design. It permitted substantial reduction in the length of the anode arm of the tube and the anode stem, increasing the rate of heat removal from the anode and allowing increased x-ray output. It also eliminated the effects of altitude and humidity on tube performance.

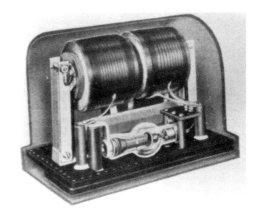

Interior view of CDX shock proof dental x-ray unit with all high-voltage elements in a single electrically grounded housing. At the bottom, note the small Coolidge tube immersed in oil along with the transformer.[27]

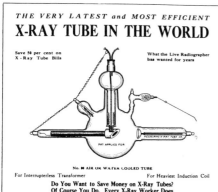

Advertisements for "the very latest and most efficient" x-ray gas tube in the world (AJR, 1913).

Even with Cole's glowing report, gas tubes were not altogether abandoned. Many radiologists had nostalgic moments remembering their beautiful, cantankerous, individualistic gas tubes, high-strung as a stable of thoroughbreds who had to be coaxed and cajoled and called by name before they would perform at their best. Cole continued to use them for certain diagnostic procedures as late as 1923, and "soft" rays from an old gas tube were still being used for some types of superficial therapy by Traian Leucutia at the Harper Hospital in Detroit at late as 1964.

LATER IMPROVEMENTS

Many improvements and variations on the Coolidge tube were introduced by General Electric and by other American and European tube manufacturers. The most significant changes were (1) reduced focal spot sizes for a given capacity, (2) reduction of leakage radiation to afford better protection to patient and operator, and (3) design of shockproof systems for protection from high-voltage shock.

The first step in reduction of focal spot size came with the development of the line-focus tube, in which the target was designed to allow a large area for heating while maintaining the small focal spot required to produce a sharp radiographic image. To accomplish this, the target was angled so that its effective area (effective focal spot size) was much smaller than the actual area of electron interaction. The lower the target angle, the smaller the effective focal spot size. Using the line-focus principle, it was possible to simultaneously produce the image sharpness of a small focal spot and the heat accommodation of a large focal spot. Initially explained and described by William Rollins in 1897, a United States patent for a line-focus tube was issued in 1916 to Elof Benson.[28] Most diagnostic x-ray tubes currently have two focal spot sizes, one large and the other small. The small focal spot is used when fine-detail images are required and for magnification studies. The large focal spot is used with techniques that produce large amounts of heat.

The major development in x-ray tube design permitting higher tube currents (and the virtually instantaneous exposures of rapid filming techniques) was the rotating anode. The rotating anode x-ray tube allowed the electron beam to interact with a much larger target area, so that the heating of the anode was not confined to one small spot as in a stationary-anode tube. The heating capacity increased with the speed of rotation of the anode (usually 3,400 revolutions per minute or more). However, if the

Line-focus tube (Müller, 1923).

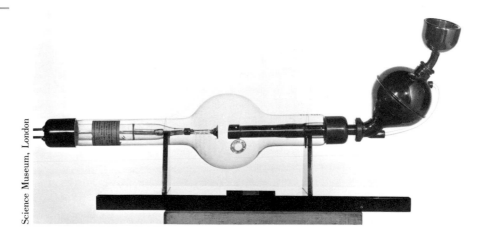

Science Museum, London

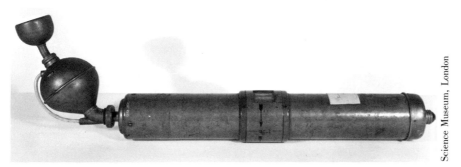

Science Museum, London

Müller protected x-ray tube.

rotor mechanism of a rotating-anode tube failed, the anode became overheated and pitted or cracked, resulting in tube failure. The first commercially available rotating anode tube (Rotalix, 1929) was designed by Albert Bouwers of Philips.[29] Although Rollins and Robert Wood had both proposed this principle for dissipating heat from gas tubes, they had suggested movement of the anode between (rather than during) exposures so that a new platinum target area could be moved into place should the one in use be melted. The development of powerful three-phase generators made it essential to have similar advances in rotating anode technology. To increase instantaneous loading of focal spots, stators with very specialized bearings and sophisticated electronic acceleration and braking circuits were designed that could bring a resting anode to 9,000 rpm in 0.8 seconds to minimize delay in making spot-film exposures. To accommodate the longer-term anode loads encountered in tomography and cinefluorography, anode thickness and diameter were increased. Heat exchangers were used to cool the oil in the tube shield. It was known that the x-ray output of a tube decreased steadily over its lifetime because

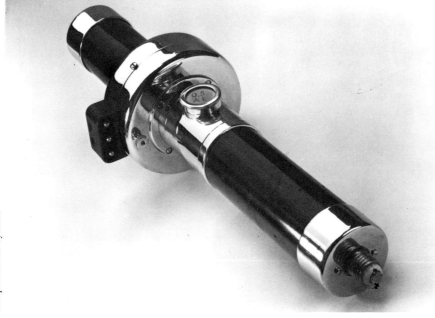

Philips Medical Systems

Rotalix tube (1929). First commercially available rotating anode tube.

Metalix tube (1927). The novel feature of this first self-protected tube was the use of a metal (chromium-iron alloy) for the center section of the tube. This was sealed to glass end sections, which insulated it from the electrodes. X-rays were emitted through a small window.

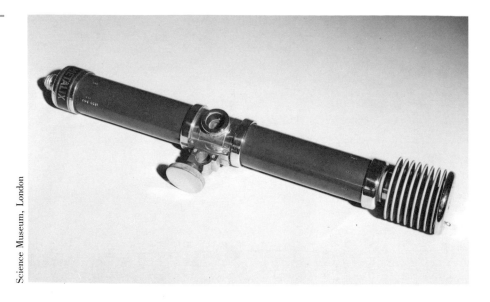

of anode micro-cracking and the deposition on the envelope (and consequently on the tube window) of evaporated tungsten. This was remedied by alloying tungsten and rhenium, which inhibited the deterioration of the anode and maintained over the useful life of the tube a favorable relationship of electrical input to x-ray output.[30]

Shielding from leakage radiation has long been a major goal in radiography. Various approaches to this problem have included tubes enclosed in lead boxes, open-top lead glass balls, and molded full-enclosing lead glass enclosures. The Philips Metalix tube (1927) was the first attempt to make the shielding an integral part of the tube. This was followed by many designs culminating in the present generally used format in which the tube is enclosed in a lead-lined, metallic cylinder filled with oil. These systems permit leakage radiation to be reduced to any level, the only limitation being the weight of the shielding that can be tolerated.[31]

Electrical hazards have long been a serious problem for radiologists. The first completely safe system, designed by Coolidge for use in dental machines (1921), placed the entire high-voltage system including the tube in an oil-filled, grounded metal tank.[32] The availability of shockproof cables in the 1930s made it possible to design tube systems providing protection from both radiation and high-voltage shock, since high-voltage cables could be combined with an oil-filled, lead-lined tube casing. By placing the high-voltage rectifiers in the tank with the high-voltage transformer, the entire system was shockproofed.

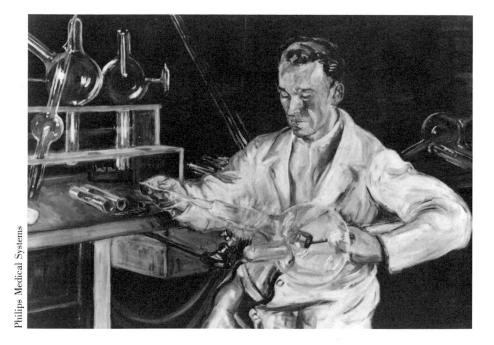

Philips Medical Systems

Craftsman glassblower in the Müller factory, c. 1925. Oil painting by Lore Alfter.

Bibliography

Brecher R and Brecher E: The rays: A history of radiology in the United States and Canada. Baltimore, Williams & Wilkins, 1969.

Coolidge WD and Charlton EE: Roentgen-ray tubes. In Glasser O (ed): The science of radiology. Springfield, Ill, Charles C Thomas, 1933.

Krohmer JS: Radiography and fluoroscopy, 1920 to the present. RadioGraphics 9:1129-1153, 1989.

Trout ED: Tubes and generators. In Bruwer AJ (ed): Classic descriptions in diagnostic roentgenology. Springfield, Ill, Charles C Thomas, 1964.

References

1. Ramsey LJ: Some notable early contributors to radiography: Thompson, Jackson and Campbell-Swinton. Radiography 46:289-297, 1980.
2. Electrical World 27:377, 1896.
3. Meadowcroft WH: The ABC of the x-rays. New York, Excelsior Publishing House, 1896.
4. Burrows EH: Pioneers and early years: A history of British radiology. Channel Islands, England, Colophon, 1986.
5. Williams FH: The roentgen rays in medicine and surgery. New York, MacMillan, 1901.
6. Coolidge WD: The development of modern roentgen-ray generating apparatus. AJR 24:605-620, 1930.
7. Feldman A: A sketch of the technical history of radiology from 1896 to 1920. RadioGraphics 9:1113-1128, 1989.
8. Hulst H: Joys and sorrows of an x-ray worker. Physician and Surgeon 24:492-498, 1902.
9. Pusey WA and Caldwell EW: The practical application of roentgen rays in therapeutics and diagnosis. Philadelphia, WB Saunders, 1904.
10. Cole LG: Amer Quart Roentgen 1:35-38, 1907.
11. Woodward EA: Electrical World 27:219-223, 1896.
12. Trowbridge J: Amer J Sci 1:245-246, 1896.
13. Thomson E: Inductorium and double-focus tube. Electrical Engineer 22:404, 1896.
14. Tubes for the production of Röntgen rays. Nature 55:296-297, 1897.
15. Gardiner JH: The origin, history and development of the x-ray tube. J Röntgen Soc 5:66-80, 1909.
16. Glasser O: William Conrad Röntgen and the early history of the roentgen rays. Springfield, Ill, Charles C Thomas, 1934.
17. Martin JM: Practical electro-therapeutics and x-ray therapy. St. Louis, The CV Mosby Co, 1912.
18. Coolidge WD: Ductile tungsten. Trans Amer Inst Elect Eng 29:961-965, 1910.
19. Coolidge WD: Trans Amer Inst Elect Eng 31:870-872, 1912.
20. Coolidge WD: A powerful roentgen ray tube with a pure electron discharge. Phys Rev 2 (2nd series):409-430, 1913.
21. Lilienfeld JE: US Patent 1,122,011, filed October 2, 1912.
22. Langmuir I: The effect of space charge and residual gases on thermionic currents in high vacuum. Phys Rev 2 (2nd series): 450-452, 1913.
23. Coolidge WD: Vacuum-tube. US Patent 1,203,495, issued October 31, 1916.
24. Coolidge WD: Speech on receiving I.R.E. medal at Columbia University, May 20, 1952.
25. Hickey PM: Editorial. AJR 1:91, 1913.
26. Cole LG: A preliminary report on the diagnostic and therapeutic application of the Coolidge tube. AJR 1:125-131, 1914.
27. Glenner RA: The dental office: A pictorial history. Missoula, Mont, Pictorial Histories, 1984.
28. Benson E: X-ray apparatus. US Patent 1,174,044, issued March 7, 1916.
29. Bouwers A: X-ray tube. US Patent 1,893,759, issued January 10, 1933.
30. Angus WM: A commentary on the development of diagnostic imaging technology. RadioGraphics 9:1225-1244, 1989.
31. Gross MJ: Roentgen ray and electrical protection with reference to roentgen tubes. AJR 39:278-283, 1938.
32. Bouwers A: Self-protecting tubes and their influence on the development of x-ray technique. Radiology 13:191-196, 1929.

CHAPTER 9

Diaphragms, Cones, Filters, and Grids

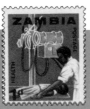 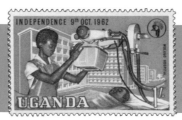 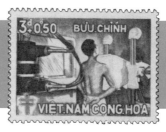

Scattered radiation has always been the bane of a radiologist's existence. The roentgen pioneers realized early that plates of thick parts of the body were clouded or fogged by some phenomenon, which they termed *extra-focal rays*, *glass-wall rays*, or *inverse currents*. To reduce this unwanted scatter, radiologists initially used a variety of diaphragms, cones, and filters between the x-ray tube and the patient and later added grids between the patient and the x-ray film.

APERTURE DIAPHRAGMS AND CONES

Aperture diaphragms and cones can reduce scatter in two ways. First, they limit the anatomical area irradiated and thus reduce the amount of secondary radiation generated by the body. In addition, diaphragms and cones screen out scattered radiation from the tube and surrounding objects. Both of these actions serve to limit the fogging of photographic plates that destroys image detail.

The initial x-ray tubes used by Roentgen employed an exceedingly broad "focal spot," 2 to 3 inches in diameter, which produced a wide x-ray beam and blurred, unsharp images. Because the entire tube was a source of x-rays, it was essential to concentrate the x-ray beam to decrease geometric unsharpness and thus produce a clearer image. This was accomplished by the development of a cup-shaped cathode (Sir William Crookes) and the placement of an angulated piece of platinum in the cathode stream at its approximate focus (Sir Herbert Jackson's "focus tube"). Other causes of image unsharpness were related to the low x-ray output produced by the small coils or static machines initially employed. This necessitated a long exposure time, permitting patient motion, and a short focus-film distance, which resulted in substantial geometric un-

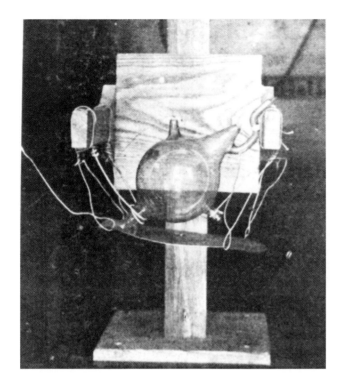

sharpness. These problems were solved with the development of more powerful generators with increasingly high x-ray output.

Paralleling the idea of a camera lens aperture, aperture diaphragms of various size began to be used to partially control image unsharpness. Unfortunately, to take full advantage of these favorable qualities, it was necessary to develop equipment capable of providing greater x-ray intensity, since longer exposures were needed with the use of aperture diaphragms.

The earliest type of aperture diaphragm employed in radiography was a piece of lead foil containing a central opening, which was placed immediately under the x-ray tube.[1] Because the placement of a diaphragm at the tube involved the use of some form of holder, it became easier to simply lay the foil directly on the part of the patient being examined and then to cut a hole in it large enough for the x-rays to pass through the area of interest (contact diaphragm).[2] This technique was soon supplanted by a number of often bizarre variations incorporating the aperture principle.

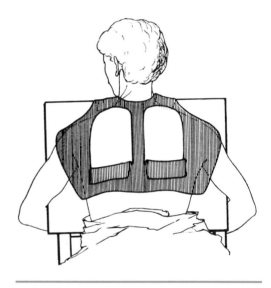

Drawing illustrating the use of a perforated lead foil attached to the body of the patient in radiography of the lungs (1905).[2]

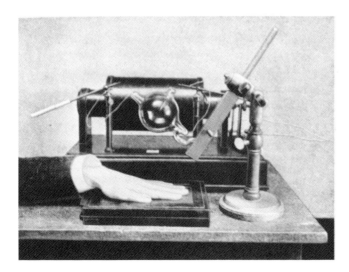

Unshielded tube with no aperture diaphragm for x-raying a hand (*McClure's Magazine*, May 1896).

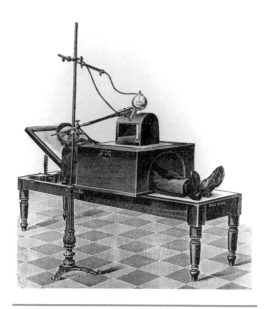

Lead covered box with cut out diaphragm used to protect photographic plate from secondary radiation and thus produce a sharper image (1902).[6]

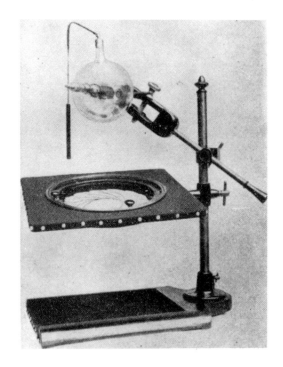

Iris type of diaphragm (Dessauer and Wiesner, 1903).[31]

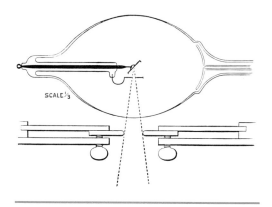

SCALE ⅓

Internal diaphragm tube of Rollins (1899).[3]

In the early nonfocused tubes, the entire tube was a source of x-rays of varying intensity. The production of focus tubes provided a source of concentrated x-rays from the target but still resulted in a large amount of less intense radiation being generated from other parts of the tube. To provide better quality radiographs, it was essential that this aberrant radiation not reach the plate or film. Initially, a diaphragm consisted of a small sheet of metal positioned between the tube and plate and containing a hole that permitted the focused beam of x-rays to emerge. The insertion of metal diaphragms with openings of various sizes permitted the diameter of the circular hole to be varied so that only a portion of the x-ray beam reached the part of the body to be examined. Another method was the "internal diaphragm" tube of William H. Rollins (1899), which contained a small ring in the tube just under the target area of the anode.[3] Other variations included a conical tube of lead open at both ends (1896), adjustable diaphragms of the shutter or iris type, and an adjustable metal diaphragm that could be pivoted in such a manner that on rotation a variety of openings cut in the metal could be swung under the tube and into the x-ray beam (1904).[4] Tousey (1910) described a "radiating cellular diaphragm," in which a cone was made containing a number of vertical

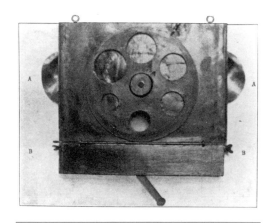

Exner's revolving aperture diaphragm (1904).[4]

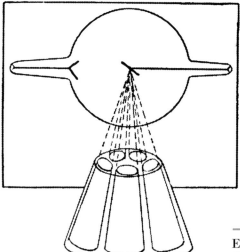

Example of Tousey's radiating cellular diaphragm (1910).[5]

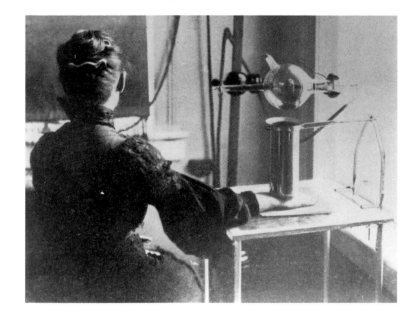

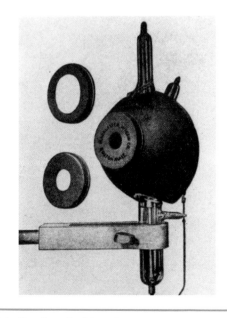

Radiographing the hand using the Beck diaphragm (1904). Note, however, the complete lack of shielding of the x-ray tube.[10]

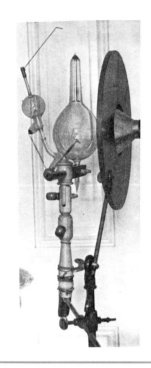

Stelwagon's x-ray shield (1904).[11]

cells that effectively made a number of small cones within a larger cone.[5] Although this device allegedly produced clearer images fairly free of fog, it also produced a number of extraneous and quite disconcerting lines in the image caused by the walls of the cells.

A. H. Pirie's "moving-slot" diaphragm (1913) consisted of a piece of flat lead containing a transverse slot that was moved during the exposure in such a way that a narrow x-ray beam covered the plate from top to bottom in successive strips.[7] Lewis G. Cole introduced the "double-slot" method in which a second piece of flat metal containing a larger transverse slot was placed beneath the patient and moved with the upper slot of Pirie so as to protect the plate wherever it was not exposed to the direct x-ray beam.[8] William D. Coolidge (1915) contributed the "hooded target," a molybdenum or tungsten shield placed around the focal spot to reduce the number of "extra-focal" rays that was reminiscent of Rollins' "internal diaphragm" tube reported more than a decade earlier.[9]

The use of aperture diaphragms led to a change in construction of the x-ray tubes. Initially, the glass used was uniformly thick. It was found, however, that greater intensity of radiation could be achieved by carefully grinding to a given thinness that small portion of the glass through which the x-ray beam was to pass.

Although the use of all these diaphragms was an admirable step in the right direction, the fact that the tube was unshielded permitted the secondary radiation from surrounding areas (walls, ceiling, room objects) to reach the sensitive emulsion on the photographic plate. To eliminate this source of scatter, metal or wooden boxes lined with lead were designed with an aperture to permit the x-rays to escape from the anode (or *anticathode*, as it was then called). At this aperture various types of stationary or adjustable diaphragms were fitted. By better controlling secondary radiation, there was substantial improvement in radiographic quality.

Early German workers attempted to confine the radiation not only to produce better radiographic results but also to protect the operator from the disastrous effects of radiation, which was becoming apparent before the end of 1896. Consequently, these workers used shielded tubes extensively. In the United States, however, virtually all American manufacturers provided few shielded tubes to protect the operator. The major

Friedlander shield with aperture diaphragms (Scheidel-Western catalogue, 1910).

Early wooden tube holder of Williams (1897).[12]

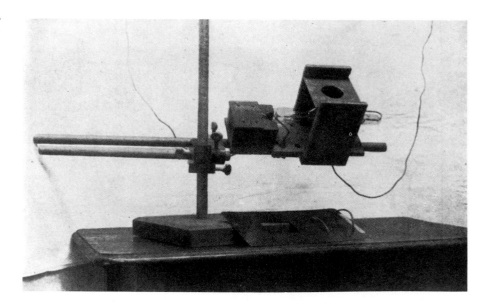

Early wooden tube holder of Williams (1897).[12]

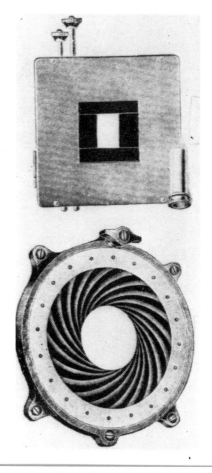

Two types of movable aperture diaphragms (Schall & Sons catalogue, 1914). *Top*, Shutter type. *Bottom*, Iris type.

proponents of the shielding technique were Francis H. Williams and his tube designer, William H. Rollins, who as early as 1898 used an adjustable revolving metal diaphragm in conjunction with an enclosed x-ray tube in a box lined with white lead.[12] Consequently, they were among the few early American radiographers who did not suffer from devastating radiation injury.

Heinrich Ernst Albers-Schoenberg (1904) was probably the earliest major advocate of the use of a cone mounted on a well-designed tube stand. He used cones of various sizes that were actually metal tubes lined with corrugated lead attached to the underside of an unshielded x-ray tube. In addition to restricting the size of the x-ray beam, the cone also served as a compression device to reduce the thickness of tissue irradiated and to restrict patient motion.[13] Preston M. Hickey modified the cone of Albers-Schoenberg to make it more adaptable to the American type of tube stand.[14]

An improved adjustable iris diaphragm introduced in the mid 1930s consisted of a number of steel and copper leaves arranged concentrically like the leaves in a lens iris diaphragm. It also was furnished with attachable cones, usually in the form of cylinders.

The value of aperture diaphragms and cones in reducing secondary radiation reaching the film was experimentally proven in a classic series of reports by Rex B. Wilsey and Millard D. Hodgson in 1921.[15,16] They clearly showed that the smaller the aperture diaphragm or cone, the better

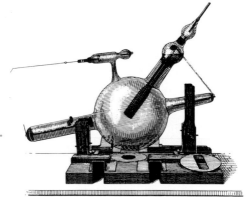

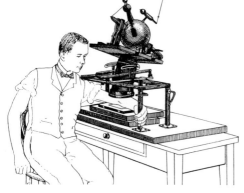

Early (1904) x-ray tube and aperture diaphragm of Albers-Schoenberg (*left*). Albers-Schoenberg tube holder and compression cylinder (*right*).[13]

142

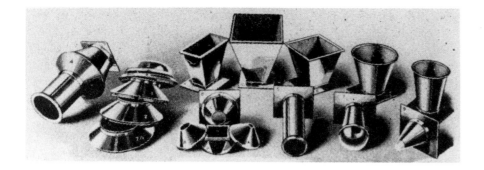

Various Hickey cones. (Kelley-Koett catalogue, 1916).

the definition solely resulting from the reduction in secondary radiation reaching the film and attributable to the smaller amount of tissue irradiated by the x-ray beam. As an example[16]:

> A kidney negative is taken at 25 inches target-film distance using a diaphragm that covers a 20-inch circle at the film. Let us assume that 8 inches of tissue are passed through. The result is a gray, foggy negative with very little detail, for one effect of the image-forming rays has been neutralized by the general fog produced by the scattered rays. A study of Mr. Wilsey's charts shows that under such conditions the scattered radiation reaching the film has a value equal to 88% of the effective radiation striking it. That is, only 12% of the exposure is image-forming—the rest is obscuring detail.

Over the years, the interest of radiographers in the use of aperture diaphragms and cones waxed and waned until the advent of the Potter-Bucky diaphragm, which produced remarkably improved radiographs, especially of thick parts of the torso. Ironically, for many years thereafter technicians blindly failed to use cones when a grid was employed. This was a mistake, for better radiographic quality could be produced by using a combination of cone and grid, especially with the use of higher kilovoltages.

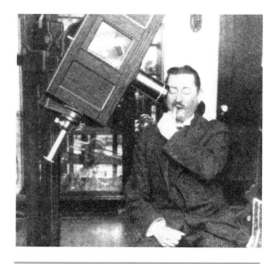

Lead-lined tube box and cylindrical cone in radiography of the teeth (1910).[5]

FILTERS

As early as March, 1896, William Francis Magie, Professor of Physics at Princeton, described the effectiveness of the aluminum filter. He was amazed to note that an obstacle to the x-rays actually improved the shadows that they cast. Apparently unwilling to trust his own judgment, Magie called in other witnesses to confirm it. "In the opinion of three observers, the interposition of a thin plate of aluminum between the vacuum tube and the fluorescent paper of the skiascope did not merely leave the fluorescence undimmed, but actually intensified it considerably."[17]

It was later shown that diagnostic x-ray beams are composed of photons with a broad spectrum of energies (polychromatic). Most of the low-energy photons are absorbed in the first few centimeters of tissue, and only the high-energy photons penetrate through the patient to form the radiographic image. The use of an aluminum filter to absorb a large portion of the low-energy photons resulted in a substantial decrease in patient dose. Removal of the low-energy photons also reduced the amount of scatter radiation generated in the patient and thus improved the radiographic image.[18]

For a discussion of George Pfahler's ingenious shoe-leather filter, see Chapter 11.

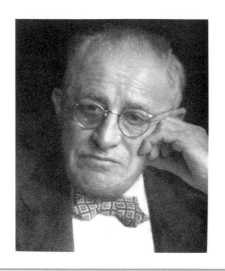

Gustav Bucky (1880-1963).[31]

GRIDS

Although aperture diaphragms and cones reduced scatter radiation by blocking out most of the undesirable rays coming from the x-ray tube and by decreasing the area irradiated by compression of tissues, these devices had no effect on the scattered radiation arising from the body itself as it lay interposed between the x-ray tube and the photographic plate. This cause of blurring of the radiographic image was first noted as early as February, 1896, by Arthur W. Wright of Yale, who made the first x-ray negative in the United States. As he noted,[19] "In some of the earlier experiments, the objects to be tested were separated from the sensitive plate by a screen of wood . . . Strong effects were produced easily, but the pictures had a blurred appearance." This blurring Wright correctly attributed to the "diffusing or scattering effect of the wood."

Otto Pasche of Switzerland was perhaps the first to suggest (in 1903) that the solution to blurring of the image lay in blocking the secondary rays by means of a device introduced between the patient and the x-ray plate, rather than inside the tube or between the tube and the patient.[20] He designed a movable diaphragm with a slit-shaped aperture, which travelled slowly across the plate to expose each portion of it successively to a thin rectangular beam of x-rays. Pasche actually used a pair of synchronized travelling-slit apertures—one between the x-ray tube and the patient, the other between the patient and the x-ray plate.

In 1913, the German radiologist, Gustav Bucky, reported the use of a stationary honeycombed grid-diaphragm (Gitter-Blende) to be placed between the patient and the plate.[21] The grid consisted of a metal lattice with cells oriented in such a way to permit primary rays emerging directly from the focal spot of the tube to pass through. However, secondary rays emitted at other angles by atoms in the body of the patient were blocked by being absorbed by the metal strips.[22] Unfortunately, Bucky's original grid had a major defect. To perform its function, the material composing the grid had to be of high atomic weight and therefore cast a marked shadow of the criss-cross configuration on the x-ray plate. Thus the price of eliminating the blurring was to superimpose an objectionable grid pattern that obscured most of the findings. Although Bucky[21] rationalized this problem by stating that "the network of white lines on the negative is of no disadvantage, but rather the contrary, since it may be used for the accurate measurement of the various organs," most radiologists disagreed and this initial grid never became popular.

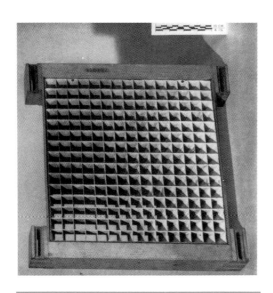

One of the first Bucky grids imported to the United States. Manufactured in 1913 in Germany by the Siemens & Halske Company, the grid measured 14½ inches × 14 inches × 2¼ inches.[31]

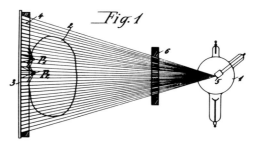

Principle of a grid from Bucky's German patent application (1913).

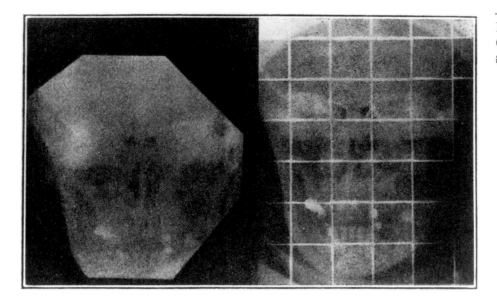

Initial example of the value of a Bucky grid (1913). *Left*, Without grid. *Right*, Using grid.[21]

Three researchers, acting independently of one another, soon tried in much the same way to solve the problem of the grid lines. The first was Bucky himself. Two months after his original patent application, Bucky applied for an additional German patent on a *moving* grid. The simple underlying theory was that if the grid were moved uniformly through the x-ray beam, so that each point on the photographic plate would lie in the shadow of the grid for the same length of time, the grid movement would in effect erase the shadow so that no disturbing lines would appear on the photographic plate.

The second researcher to conceive the same idea was Eugene W. Caldwell of New York. As Caldwell[8] wrote in 1917, "Immediately after the publication of the Bucky (stationary-grid) apparatus, I conceived the idea of moving the grid to get rid of the shadows of the grid and did a little experimenting in this direction." At the same time, however, Caldwell checked the patent applications and discovered that Bucky had already filed for a patent on a moving grid. Nevertheless, Caldwell continued experimenting and applied for a patent on a time switch connected to an automatic device for moving the Bucky grid.[23]

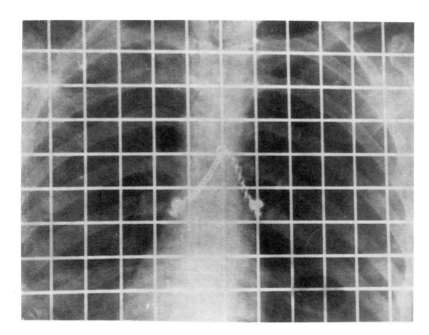

Bothersome grid lines from an early stationary Bucky grid (1919).[30]

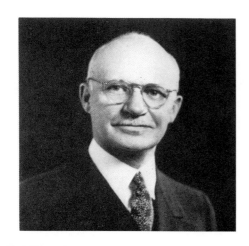

Hollis E. Potter (1880-1964).[31]

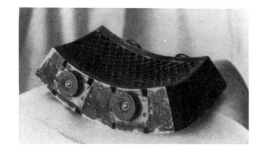

Original tubular diaphragm of Potter (1916).[27]

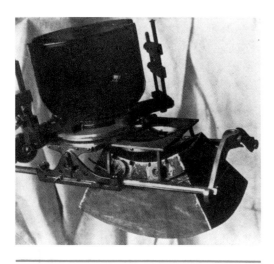

Diaphragm for experimental work fitted into tube stand (1916).[27]

Neither Bucky nor Caldwell presented a description of their moving grids in a medical publication. Thus a third researcher, Hollis E. Potter of Chicago, attacked the problem without knowing about the patent applications. He soon discovered the same basic solution as Bucky and Caldwell and presented his results at the February, 1915 meeting of the Central Section of the American Roentgen Ray Society (ARRS). At the September, 1916 meeting of the Society, Potter described the "Bucky diaphragm adapted to fluoroscopy," a rotating circular disk grid with strips placed radially that absorbed scatter radiation when rotated between patient and screen at the proper speed.[24]

None of the early moving grids designed by Bucky, Caldwell, and Potter was completely successful because of their criss-cross configuration. However, if the pattern of a criss-cross grid could not be completely erased from the plate by motion, what kind of pattern could be? Potter's simplest answer was a wire. When a wire was moved back and forth uniformly in the x-ray beam, at right angles to its own axis, no shadow was recorded on the plate. Next, Potter tried a lead strip, swung back and forth in the x-ray beam along an arc, in such a way that its flat sides always pointed directly to the focus area on the target. Again, this strip produced no shadow when moved uniformly. Finally, Potter tried a series of parallel strips similarly oriented and moved through an arc.[23] Although in theory such a device lacking cross-pieces should intercept only a portion of the blurring rays, Potter found to his surprise and delight that "the total amount of (blurring) rays suppressed by the parallel system was about the same as in the Bucky crossed grating, and it is far easier to build . . ."[8]

This device, now known as the Potter-Bucky grid or diaphragm (although it is in reality neither a grid nor a diaphragm), was introduced by Potter at the February, 1917 meeting of the Central Section of the ARRS. In addition to describing his invention, Potter[25] stressed the use of his device in "demonstration of the lumbar spine, hip joints and pelvis and particularly for calculi. In several cases where small urinary calculi in portly individuals were difficult of demonstration the results obtained . . . were so far superior as to justify almost any statement."

Following another radiological meeting where Potter again displayed negatives made with his moving parallel-strip grid, one radiologist stormed in anger and announced accusingly, "You've touched those negatives up!" He could not be convinced that so blur-free a negative could be produced with an x-ray tube.[23]

Although Potter's article was read before the ARRS meeting, it was not published because of a subsequent visit by Caldwell, who informed Potter that he and Bucky had designed and patented moving grids several years previously. According to Potter, "Up to this time I had never heard that Bucky had conceived the idea of making the grid invisible by movement and had only heard rumors that Caldwell was working on the Bucky diaphragm principle." Potter decided that it would be unfair to speak or write further on the grid diaphragm until the close of the war. Bucky should be given every chance to show any experimental results or any practical working apparatus.[8]

By 1920, Bucky had failed to make or report any practical progress; apparently the only radiologist using the grid principle was Albers-Schoenberg, who had a fixed cross-grid Bucky grating mounted for fluoroscopic work. As Potter wrote,[8,26]

I was placed in a position where it was beginning to look as if something were being held back from the profession. Numerous letters of inquiry were received urging that manufacturers make the apparatus available for general use . . . No one else working in this field of experiment had produced anything of practical value. Accordingly the article of February, 1917 was smoothed up and sent to this Journal.

An incidental effect of the Potter-Bucky diaphragm was to hasten the conversion from glass plate to film. The blurring of a plate by secondary rays, in the absence of a Potter-Bucky grid, increased rapidly with an increase in the size of the plate. Thus early radiologists were restricted to relatively small plate sizes (such as 4 × 5 inches) to hold blurring to a tolerable level. Following introduction of the Potter-Bucky grid, it became possible to secure images 14 × 17 inches or even larger with negligible blurring. But glass in these large sizes was so heavy, clumsy, and fragile that radiologists who wished to take advantage of the large size were forced to convert to film.[23]

Conversely, it was not until duplitized film was perfected to the point where it could reasonably displace glass plates that grid diaphragms could be used with facility or even with safety. The elimination of scattered radiation required more primary x-ray photons, which overtaxed the gas tubes and those Coolidge tubes with small capacity. Moreover, a short series of adequate exposures through the same skin areas involve the use of an erythema dose when corpulent individuals were being examined. The availability of duplitized film and the double-screen technique in 1920 paved the way for the widespread use of the grid diaphragm.[8]

The Potter-Bucky grid was marketed by General Electric in 1921, and its acceptance was immediate. Later that year, Rex B. Wilsey, of the Research Department at Kodak, made extensive quantitative measurements of scattered rays emerging from the deeper body tissues and confirmed that with the grid it was easily possible to remove more than 80% of the secondary radiation.[28]

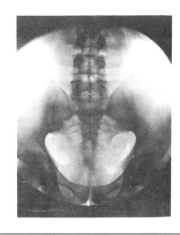

"Print of spine, etc., illustrating freedom from grid shadows obtainable by uniform motion of grid" (1920).[26]

Advertisements for x-ray diaphragms (AJR, January, 1922).

Ironically, at the end of World War I, the United States government confiscated about 1200 German patents and Bucky's patent was sold to the Chemical Foundation. It has been estimated that until that original antiscatter diaphragm patent ran out in 1933, about $4 million should have been paid to Bucky in royalties. He never received a penny.[29]

In one of his letters, Bucky wrote: "I emigrated to the United States in 1923. Being a newcomer, I did not want to start a controversy on priorities. My patents contained all the ideas ever built into the antiscatter diaphragm, except for minor constructive features. In spite of this fact, Potter's name always appears in connection with mine as co-inventor."[29]

An impartial assessment would seem to indicate that both Bucky and Potter should share the credit for the antiscatter device that bears their names. Clearly Bucky was the discoverer, but his grid principle had been virtually abandoned in his native Germany and elsewhere in Europe by the time Potter's perfected moving grid was popularized in the United States.

In 1923, Wilsey developed a focused grid composed of lead strips that were angled slightly so that they focused in space. In the 1960s, fine line grids (100 or more lines per inch) were introduced to eliminate the appearance of grid lines on images made with stationary grids. In the 1970s there was a renewal of interest in the concept of moving-slit radiography first suggested by Pasche (1903). Both linear and rotational slit motion were evaluated, but no commercial model was developed, probably because it was presumed that solid state digital radiographic devices would eventually dominate the radiographic field, and since scatter elimination would be an integral part of this equipment, there would be no need for scanning slit or grid devices.

Bibliography

Fuchs AW: On aperture diaphragms and cones. In Bruwer AJ (ed): Classic descriptions in diagnostic roentgenology. Springfield, Ill, Charles C Thomas, 1964.

References

1. Perry FL: Photographic experiments in Chicago with Röntgen rays. Western Elect 18: 73-77, 1896.
2. Robinson I: Zur Vereinfachung der Blendertechnik die Winkelblende. Fortschr Roentgenstr 8:183-191, 1905.
3. Rollins W: Roentgen light notes. Elec Rev 34:81, Feb. 8, 1899.
4. Exner E: Eine neue Hangeblende mit Rontgenrohre. Fortschr Roentgenstr 7:135-136, 1904.
5. Tousey S: Medical electricity and Röntgen rays. Philadelphia, WB Saunders, 1910.
6. Monell SH: System of instruction. New York, Harrison, 1902.
7. Pirie AH: A sliding diaphragm for improving the quality of skiagraphs. Amer Quart Roentgenol 3:142-145, 1916.
8. Potter HE: History of diaphragming Roentgen rays by use of the Bucky principle. AJR 25:396-402, 1931.
9. Coolidge W: AJR 2:881-892, 1915.

10. Beck C: Roentgen-ray diagnosis and therapy. New York, Appleton, 1904.
11. Allen CW: Radiotherapy and phototherapy including radium and high-frequency currents. New York, Lea Brothers, 1904.
12. Williams FH: The roentgen rays in medicine and surgery. New York, MacMillan, 1901.
13. Albers-Schoenberg HE: Technische Neuerungen. Fortschr Roentgenstr 7:137-149, 1904.
14. Hickey PM: The tubular diaphragm in roentgenology of the chest. Am Quart Roentgenol 1:14-22, 1906.
15. Wilsey RB: The intensity of scattered x-rays in radiography. AJR 8:328-338, 1921.
16. Hodgson MB: Remarks on the measurements of scatter radiation. AJR 8:338-339, 1921.
17. Magie WF: Am J Med Sci 111:251-255, 1896.
18. Trout ED, Kelley JP, and Cathey GA: The use of filters to control radiation exposure to the patient in diagnostic radiology. AJR 67:946-963, 1952.
19. Wright AW: Am J Med Sci 111:235-244, 1896.
20. Pasche O: Über eine neue Blendenvorrichtung in der Rontgentechnik. Deutsch Med Wschr 29:266, 1903.
21. Bucky G: A grating diaphragm to cut off secondary rays from the object. Arch Roentgen Ray 18:6-9, 1913.

22. Bucky G: Method of an apparatus for projecting röntgen images. US Patent No. 1,164,987, issued Dec. 21, 1915.
23. Brecher R and Brecher E: The rays: A history of radiology in the United States and Canada. Baltimore, Williams & Wilkins, 1969.
24. Potter HE: The Bucky diaphragm adapted to fluoroscopy. AJR 4:47-50, 1917.
25. Potter HE: The object secondaries in radiography. A practical working method for their suppression. Read at mid-winter meeting of Central Section, American Roentgen Ray Society, Cincinnati, February, 1917.
26. Potter HE: The Bucky diaphragm principle applied to roentgenography. AJR 7:292-295, 1920.
27. Potter HE: Diaphragming roentgen rays: Studies and experiments. AJR 3:142-145, 1916.
28. Wilsey RB: The efficiency of the Bucky-diaphragm principle. AJR 9:58-67, 1922.
29. Grigg ERN: The trail of the invisible light. Springfield, Ill, Charles C Thomas, 1965.
30. Weingaertner M: Physiologische und topographische Studien am Trachialbaum des lebenden Menschen. Arch Laryngol 32:1-88, 1919.
31. Fuchs AW: On aperture diaphragms and cones. In Bruwer AJ (ed): Classic descriptions in diagnostic roentgenology. Springfield, Ill, Charles C Thomas, 1964.

CHAPTER 10

Dark Adaptation and Image Intensification

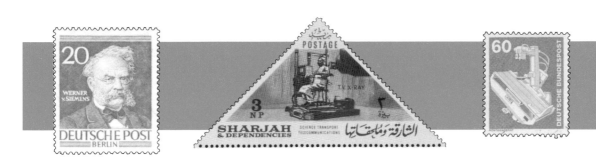

A major problem of fluoroscopy was the difficulty in producing an image of sufficient brightness that could be interpreted by the radiologist. Even with a darkened room and the mounting of the fluorescent screen in a light-tight box (as constructed by Salvioni and Edison), it was clear that the fluoroscopic screen yielded much less diagnostic information than the radiographic plate.

An early partial solution to the problem was *dark adaptation* (adjustment of the eyes over time to low levels of light). In a landmark paper published in 1899, Antoine Béclère explained the limited visual perception of the fluoroscopist in terms of the "Duplicity Theory" of retinal function, which stated that the rods and cones of the eye form two essentially independent receptor systems of different sensitivity and acuity. Béclère correctly attributed dark adaptation to physiological changes in the peripheral retina, rather than to dilation of the pupil as was generally believed. In this way, Béclère demonstrated that the perception of detail in fluoroscopy is ultimately limited by the anatomy and physiology of the human retina. The essential facts concerning dark adaptation were clearly stated by Francis H. Williams[2] in his classic textbook (1901). He stressed the need for the physician to remain in a dark room for about 10 minutes, and if necessary to go out, to wear dark glasses:

> After exciting the tube if it is uncovered, the eyes see nothing in the dark room except the green light in the tube itself; all else is black darkness; but after a few minutes the eyes begin to recognize objects in the room, and as soon as this can be done their ability to see other objects augments rapidly and within a few seconds, many things are seen that could not be recognized at first.

The use of red light in the fluoroscopic examining room to preserve the operator's dark adaptation was suggested as early as 1905, when Harry Waite advised,[3] "If the ordinary gas or electric light be screened

Fluoroscopy of the thorax (c. 1898).[14]

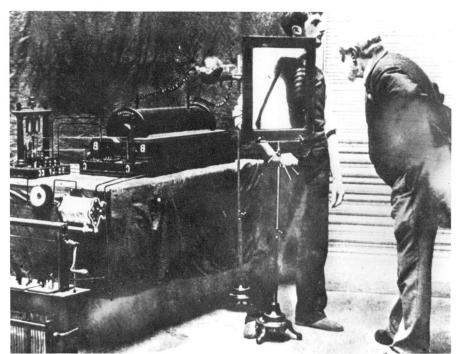

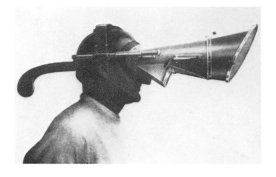

Surgical cryptoscope (1920). When using this 5-pound device, the fluoroscoping eye remained in the dark while the other eye was available for regular vision.

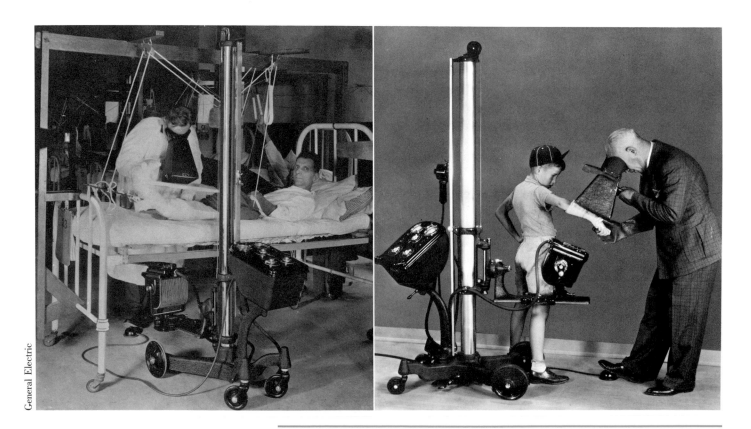

General Electric

Left, Mobile fluoroscopy of the leg at Cook County Hospital, Chicago. *Right*, Use of a hand fluoroscope with a mobile x-ray unit. Note that the physician is wearing lead gloves but no lead apron.

with dense ruby glass or several thicknesses of ruby fabric, sufficient light will be given for manipulating the apparatus without materially affecting the delicacy of the examination." As Tuddenham[4] noted, there appears to have been considerable resistance to the use of red light, as indicated in a 1910 article[5] stating that

> the x-ray worker will find great relief both to his eyes and temper if he will use a green light instead of the ordinary red light in his dark-room. For some people red light, as is well known, has a stimulating and irritating effect to the nervous system. A red light to a man acts like a red flag to a bull.

A major advance in fluoroscopy was the introduction of red adaptation goggles by Wilhelm Trendelenburg in 1916. He noted that spending time in a completely dark room before the fluoroscopic examination caused substantial inconvenience,[6]

> with the result that one unconsciously makes one's stay in the dark too brief and is then tempted, by overloading the tube, to obtain brightness objectively, which one should have obtained subjectively by an increased visual sensitivity. As opposed to this procedure, it would be of great value to have an effective method of preparing the eyes for fluoroscopy, which would not hinder the examiner in the performance of other work during the period of preparation of the patient for the examination.

As a visual physiologist himself, Trendelenburg noted that the brightness of the fluorescent light of an ordinary fluoroscopic screen was too weak to reach the threshold value for the cones in the fovea. Therefore it was essential to increase the sensitivity of the retinal rods by complete exclusion of light. Black glasses were unacceptable because, if the glasses were sufficiently dark to achieve their purpose, they would pre-clude the examiner from engaging in any useful activity during the period of adaptation. Because the retinal rods were relatively insensitive to longer wavelengths, the wearing of red goggles would permit the fluoroscopist to carry on essential activities without impairing his dark adaptation.

Manufacturers of fluoroscopic screens were continually improving the efficiency of their products. The fluorescent chemical used in fluoroscopic screens must emit light having a wave length to which the eye is most sensitive. This is in contrast to the intensifying screen, for which the color of the emitted light must be at its maximum intensity at the point of maximum sensitivity of the photographic emulsion. In addition, the fluorescent chemical for a fluoroscopic screen must be free from any of the observable lag. Until 1914, fluoroscopic screens were most commonly made of barium platinocyanide. This substance was extremely effective when freshly made but lost much of its fluorescing power if the screen was kept in an overheated room or subjected to intense x-ray bombardment. In that year, Carl V. S. Patterson discovered an entirely new fluorescent chemical, which had cadmium tungstate as its principal constituent. The resulting *Patterson Fluoroscopic Screen*, marketed in 1914, did not de-teriorate with use or age and almost immediately displaced all other screens.[7] In 1933, Leonard Levy and Donald W. West introduced a zinc-cadmium sulfide yellow-green fluorescent screen that doubled the degree of brightness.[8] However, 8 years later, W. Edward Chamberlain in his brilliant Carman lecture (1941) conclusively demonstrated that the poor performance of fluoroscopy was due not to any inherent imperfection of the

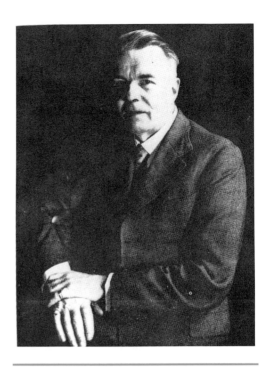

Wilhelm Trendelenburg (1877-1946).

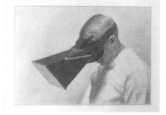

THE
PATTERSON
OPERATING FLUOROSCOPE

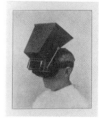

THIS PIECE OF APPARATUS IS OF USE WHEN THE OPERATING SURGEON DESIRES THE ASSISTANCE OF THE X-RAYS AND HAVE BOTH HANDS FREE. IT FITS ON THE HEAD BY MEANS OF ADJUSTABLE ELASTIC BANDS. AND IF, FOR ANY REASON, THE OPERATOR DE-SIRES NOT TO USE THE SCREEN IT CAN BE TILTED BACK AS SHOWN. WHEN IN THIS POSITION A PIECE OF RUBY GLASS AUTOMATICALLY FALLS DOWN IN FRONT OF THE EYE PIECE PROTECTING THE ACCOMMODATION OF THE EYES.
PRICE $45.00 COMPLETE EQUIPPED WITH PATTERSON FLUORO-SCOPIC SCREEN WITH LEAD GLASS PROTECTION.

THE PATTERSON SCREEN COMPANY
TOWANDA, PENNSYLVANIA, U.S.A.

Advertisement for the Patterson operating fluoroscope, which combined screen and red goggles in one device. When the fluoroscopic screen was raised, the protective red goggles dropped into place (AJR, 1918).

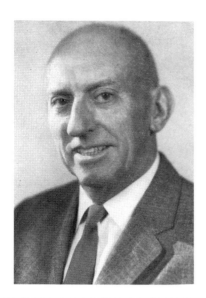

William Edward Chamberlain.

fluoroscope itself but rather to deficiencies of the human eye when operating at low levels of illumination.[9]

Chamberlain demonstrated that radiographs made with fluoroscopic screens in contact with the film exhibited much more detail than the same screens when used in fluoroscopy. Several years previously, Selig Hecht had shown that the human eye, when viewing fields having a brightness approaching that encountered in fluoroscopy, had a visual acuity or ability to perceive detail of only a small fraction of that occurring under normal lighting conditions.[10] Chamberlain reasoned that fluoroscopic performance should be substantially improved if the brightness of the screen were increased to levels at which the eye performs more satisfactorily. As a result of Chamberlain's discussion, extensive work began in the development of screen intensification for radiology.

At the brightness level at which radiographs are ordinarily viewed, the eye is capable of recognizing as discrete two contours separated by as little as ¹⁄₁₀₀₀ of an inch. As the brightness of an object is decreased, the visual acuity of the eye deteriorates. At about ¹⁄₁₀₀₀ of this intensity, cone vision is no longer effective, the color sense is gone, and the fovea centralis is no longer the most sensitive part of the retina. Only rod vision is now present, and the visual acuity is such that two contours must be separated by about ¹⁄₆₄ inch to be distinguishable. At the even lower light of the fluoroscopic range, however, a contour separation of about ¹⁄₃₂ inch is required. If one also considers the relatively low contrasts occurring in fluoroscopy, especially in thick body parts such as the abdomen, contour separation of more than ¹⁄₄ inch is necessary. Even this poor visual acuity could be acquired only by resorting to long periods (at least 20 minutes) of dark adaptation of the eye. Too short an adaptation time would greatly decrease the ability of the eye to perceive small objects.[11]

Fluoroscopic screens at that time converted about 30% of all the x-ray energy absorbed in the screen into visible light. Unfortunately, only about 15% of the incident x-rays were absorbed, the rest passing through without effect. Considering also the loss of some light within the screen, the gross efficiency of a fluoroscopic screen was about 3%. However, even a theoretically perfect fluorescent screen would be only about 30 times as bright as the ones in use at that time. Therefore to achieve the brightness gains of 100 to 1000 times required for optimal brightness, it was essential to develop some kind of amplification that injected energy from an external source into the system.[11]

The theory of screen intensification and the factors controlling the clarity of fluoroscopic vision were brilliantly elucidated by Russell H. Morgan.[12] He explained that "the diagnostic information provided by a fluoroscopic image is carried from the patient to the screen by the myriads of roentgen-ray photons which comprise the roentgen-ray beam . . . it is evident that fluoroscopic clarity is a function of the number of roentgen-ray photons falling on the screen during the fluoroscopic process." Therefore, "it may be reasonably concluded that if one wishes to see more fluoroscopically, one need only increase the milliamperage applied to the roentgen tube." Unfortunately, the resulting sharp increase in patient dose would be completely unacceptable.

> If one brightens the screen, not by increasing the milliamperage of the roentgen tube but by introducing into the fluoroscopic process a screen intensifier of one sort or another . . . no increase in clarity should occur. Even if the fluoroscopic screen is made brighter by a screen intensifier, the fact that the milliamperage on the roentgen tube, and hence, the number of roentgen-ray photons which take part

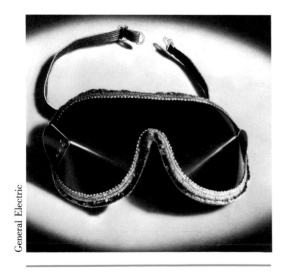

Fancy red goggles.

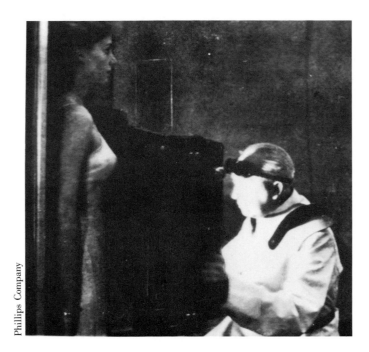

Phillips Company

Fluoroscopy as performed in the late 1940s before image intensification. Note the red goggles on the radiologist's forehead, ready to be flipped down over the eyes at the conclusion of the procedure to maintain the vital dark adaptation.

in the fluoroscopic process are not increased, indicates that no more diagnostic information is carried from the patient to the screen and hence no improvement in screen clarity can be expected. The only circumstance under which this reasoning will not be valid is one which occurs if the eye under the conventional fluoroscopic process does not utilize 100% of the information transmitted from the patient to the screen by the roentgen-ray beam's photons. Under such a circumstance, it might be possible by means of a screen intensifier to improve conditions in such a way that greater utilization of photon information could be effected.

Ralph Eugene Sturm and Morgan had previously shown that during conventional fluoroscopy the human eye utilizes the diagnostic information of only a small percentage (about 1% to 5%) of the roentgen-ray photons received at the screen.[13] If it were possible by the introduction of a screen intensifier to improve the efficient utilization of these photons, a considerable improvement in the diagnostic clarity of fluoroscopy could be employed. "For example, an improvement in the efficiency of the fluoroscopic process from 2% to 100% would effect an improvement in screen detail equivalent to that produced by an increase in the roentgen tube current from 5 milliamperes to 250 milliamperes."[12]

Morgan[12] emphasized that "if at conventional fluoroscopy, the eye utilized 100% of the information carried from the patient to the screen by roentgen-ray photons, no improvement in fluoroscopic clarity could be expected under any circumstances. It is only the fact that the eye utilizes a small fraction of the information carried by the roentgen beam that screen intensification holds promise of success."

The underlying principle of fluoroscopic image intensification is the acceleration of electrons emitted from a photosensitive surface in response to the action of x-ray photons. Although several different approaches were tried, only the electron-optical image intensifier became a commercial success. In this device, radiation from a conventional x-ray tube passes through the patient and impinges on a fluorescent screen mounted in contact with a window in the end of the instrument. In response to the light generated by the screen, a photoelectric layer on the

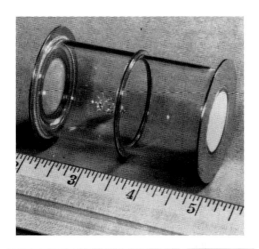

Photograph of the first pilot model of an x-ray image amplifier device (1948).[11]

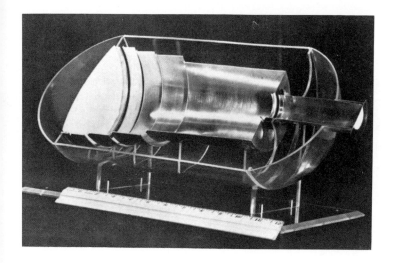

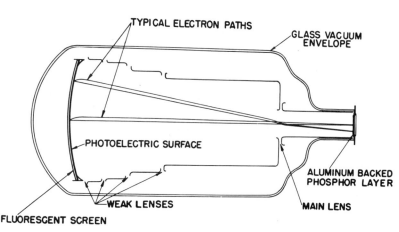

Left, Cut-away model and *right,* diagram of prototype image intensifier tube (1948). The mechanism of this tube is similar to the pilot model except that an inverted, reduced image is formed at a series of electrostatic cylinder lenses. The reduction in size produces another factor of 25 in brightness gain, bringing the total gain to 500. An optical magnifier (not shown) restores the size of the image to its original 5-inch diameter with no loss of brightness.[11]

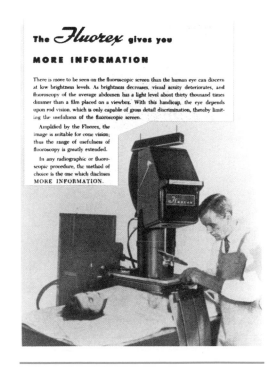

Advertisement for the Fluorex by Westinghouse, the first commercial image intensifier unit.[15]

inner surface of the window emits electrons having a spatial distribution proportional to the brightness of the screen. The electrons from the photoelectric layer are accelerated by a high potential placed across the highly evacuated tube and are focused by a constant magnetic field on a phosphor layer at the opposite end. This produces a visible image that is identical to the initial pattern on the fluorescent screen but which has a far greater brightness resulting from the acceleration of the electrons within the tube. The brightness is further increased by the fact that the size of the phosphor is small compared with that of the fluorescent screen. The observer views the intensified image appearing on the phosphor by means of a telescopic eyepiece or other optical system to bring the size of the image back to normal perspective.[12]

The first commercial image intensifier unit (Fluorex) was introduced by Westinghouse in 1953. However, its useful field was only about 3 inches in diameter,[14]

> not very attractive for routine fluoroscopy. To make matters worse, the system was supplied either with a viewing telescope (periscope), which displayed good images but poked the user in the eye whenever the fluoroscopic staging was moved, or with a monocular mirror viewer—an optical system with such a narrow viewing angle that the image could be viewed with only one eye, if one were fortunate enough to locate it at all.

More friendly binocular models were later introduced, although these were soon supplanted with the advent of television viewing of the images.

Another problem with early image intensifiers was the difficulty of mounting the systems on existing examination stands. Ceiling suspensions were provided to counterbalance the additional weight, but other stresses soon destroyed the spot-film device and its carriage.[14]

Larger intensifiers were introduced as solutions to the problem of small field size, but their weight proved to be far too much for existing tables. For example, an 11-inch system, introduced specifically as a cinefluorographic device, was so large that it could not be mounted on any existing examination stand. Several tables were built to accommodate the unit in an undertable mount, but these tables had to be installed over a pit excavated in the floor to accommodate the fluorographer and the entire aft section of the system.[14]

The age of practical imaging intensification began in 1962 with the introduction of a compact 6-inch system. Within a year, several firms announced tilting tables with internal counterbalancing for 6-inch and 9-inch systems, and imaging intensification became a routine diagnostic method.

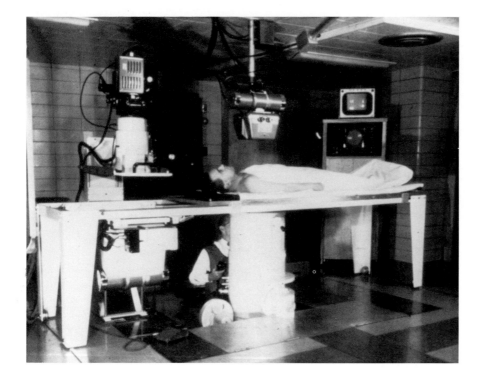

Fluorographer sitting "in the pit" to use the 11-inch image intensifier.[14]

In the early 1970s, a cesium iodide input phosphor was developed by Philips for image intensifier tubes. This phosphor provided the same improved absorption of diagnostic x-ray photons as was achieved with rare earth intensifying screens in radiography. Because much more of the cesium iodide material could be "packed" onto a given area of the input screen than was possible with other phosphors, it resulted in a decrease in patient dose and an increase in spatial resolution and has become universal in all image intensifier tubes.[15]

The development of image intensification completely revolutionized the use of fluoroscopy in clinical diagnosis. The fluoroscopic images were so bright that they could be viewed in an undarkened room without prior dark adaptation. Details could be seen that were invisible using conventional fluoroscopy. Image intensification permitted the development of cinefluorography, the recording of the fluoroscopic image on motion picture film or on magnetic tape, which previously had been limited by the inherent dimness of the fluoroscopic screen. Of major importance, the development of image intensification greatly decreased the x-ray exposure to both the patient and the examining physician.[16]

References

1. Béclère A: A physiologic study of vision in fluoroscopic examinations. Arch Electr Med 7:469-489, 1899.
2. Williams FH: The roentgen rays in medicine and surgery. New York, MacMillan, 1901.
3. Waite HF: A few points in the fluoroscopy of the chest. Arch Roentg Ray 9:141, 1904-1905.
4. Tuddenham WJ: Dark adaptation. In Bruwer AJ (ed): Classic descriptions in diagnostic roentgenology. Springfield, Ill, Charles C Thomas, 1964.
5. Butcher WE: Green light for the photographic dark room. Arch Roentg Ray 14: 168, 1909-1910.
6. Trendelenburg W: Adaptation glasses as an aid for fluoroscopy. Muenchen Med Wschr 63:245-246, 1916.
7. Fuchs AW: Radiographic recording media and screens. In Glasser O (ed): The science of radiology. Springfield, Ill, Charles C Thomas, 1933.
8. Levy LA and West DW: A new fluorescent screen for visual examinations. Brit J Radiol 6:404-410, 1933.
9. Chamberlain WE: Fluoroscopes and fluoroscopy. Radiology 38:383-412, 1942.
10. Hecht S: The dark adaptation of the human eye. J Gen Physiol 2:499-517, 1928.
11. Coltman JW: Fluoroscopic image brightening by electronic means. Radiology 51:359-367, 1948.
12. Morgan RH: Screen intensification: A review of past and present research with an analysis of future development. AJR 75:69-76, 1956.
13. Sturm RE and Morgan RH: Screen intensification systems and their limitations. AJR 62:617-634, 1949.
14. Angus WM: A commentary on the development of diagnostic imaging technology. RadioGraphics 9:1225-1244, 1989.
15. Krohmer JS: Radiography and fluoroscopy, 1920 to the present. RadioGraphics 9:1129-1153, 1989.
16. Brecher E and Brecher R: The rays: A history of radiology in the United States and Canada. Baltimore, Williams & Wilkins, 1969.

CHAPTER 11

Radiation Injury and Protection

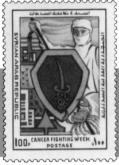

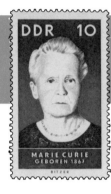

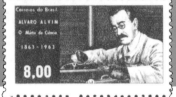

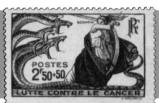

It is a curious thing, but it often happens, that nature appears to resent an intrusion into her secrets, and will sometimes make the intruder pay dearly. It was so in the case of x-rays; not only was that beneficent provision that we call pain (which tells us that something is wrong if there is time to remedy it) withheld, but the harm that was being done gave no warning, and thus was continued until after some weeks' interval the result of the accumulated indiscretions became apparent.

I will not pursue this unhappy subject further; enough to say that the most active and earnest of our workers were the worst victims, and the result was seen in empty chairs at our Councils and in the vanishing of familiar figures at our meetings. All honor to their memory. In most cases they gave their best ungrudgingly for the good of their fellow men.[1]

The many physicists, engineers, physicians, and lay experimenters working with x-ray photography in its earliest days took no deliberate measures to protect themselves, their assistants, or their patients from exposure to x-rays, since there was no reason to expect any adverse physical effects from radiation. What harm could there be from something that could not be seen, felt, tasted, heard, or detected in any way by the senses? The extent of radiation-induced injury to human tissues was not immediately obvious. Instead, the full picture was painfully synthesized from the anecdotal experiences of early workers in several countries over a period of 5 or more years.

As Percy Brown wrote in the opening statement of his classic biographical work[2]:

By the wave of a seemingly magical wand in the hand of a gentle German physicist, the prospect of a great new field to conquer was spread before a scientific world that charged upon it without perceiving, *for the moment*, the presence of the hostile force that lay in ambush. Enthusiasm was in the saddle, accoutered with the lance of investigation and the spurs of continued experimental revelation, but not yet with the shield and armor of protection.

Within 3 months after Roentgen's *Preliminary Communication*, reports dealing with physiological effects of x-rays began to appear in the literature. The earliest reports were concerned with possible damage to the eyes from the rays. Thomas A. Edison complained that his eyes were sore and red after working for several hours with his fluorescent tube, although he admitted that he was not certain that this effect could be specifically attributable to the x-rays.[3] William Morton stated that he saw brilliant flashes of light after he discontinued his experiments. Since he had worked with electrical lights for many years without injury, he inferred that the x-rays were injurious to the eye.[4] It was hard to determine, however, how much of Edison's and Morton's discomfort was due directly to the x-rays and how much to simple eye strain generated by peering for many hours at a dimly fluorescing screen.

Campbell-Swinton, however, reported that he and his associate had worked continuously with the Crookes tube for numerous hours and that neither had experienced any ill effects to their eyesight. He concluded that x-rays had no effect on the eye, either at the time of the experiment or afterward.[4]

Three weeks later, John Daniel, a physicist at Vanderbilt University in Nashville, wrote a letter to the editor of *Science* (March 23, 1896) calling attention to another unexpected phenomenon[5]:

> A month ago we were asked to undertake the location of a bullet in the head of a child that had been accidentally shot. On the 29th of February Dr. William Dudley and I decided to make a preliminary test of photographing through the head with our weak apparatus before undertaking the surgical case. Accordingly Dr. Dudley, with his characteristic devotion to the cause of science, lent himself to the experiment. A plate holder containing the sensitive plate was tied to one side of his head, with a coin between the plate and his head, and the tube was set playing on the opposite side of his head. The tube was about one-half inch distance from his hair, and the exposure was one hour. The plate developed nothing; but yesterday, 21 days after the experiment, all the hair came out over the space under the x-ray discharge. The spot is now perfectly bald, being two inches in diameter. This is the size of the x-ray field close to the tube. We, and especially Dr. Dudley, shall watch with interest the ultimate effect. The skin looks perfectly healthy, and there has been no pain or other indication of disorder. I called attention to the place before Dr. Dudley had himself noticed it, and we were both for some time at a loss to account for it, as we had no previous intimation of any effect whatever.

Some tongue-in-cheek responses to this letter in newspapers and technical journals suggested that x-rays might render daily shaving obsolete.

As more powerful x-ray equipment was introduced, accounts of more serious damage caused by the rays began to appear. Most of these involved the mucous membranes and the skin of the hands and face. The *Electrical Review* (August 12, 1896) reported the case of Herbert Hawks (working in the laboratory of Michael Pupin at Columbia University in New York, as well as giving x-ray demonstrations at the large department store of Bloomingdale Brothers)[7]:

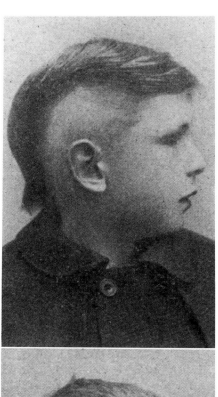

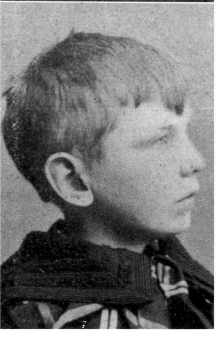

Effect of x-rays on the hair (Kolle, 1897). *Top*, Large area of hair missing from the side of a boy's head 3 weeks after an x-ray exposure of 40 minutes with the tube about 18 inches from the skull. The boy gave no history of pain, itching, or other signs of inflammation; all he knew was that on the previous night the hair had suddenly fallen out. *Bottom*, Appearance of the boy 4 months later. The new hair grew well and had been cut three times.[6]

. . . (who) has for the past few weeks been giving exhibitions in the vicinity of New York with an unusually powerful x-ray outfit. Mr. Hawks, during the afternoon and evening of each day for four days, was working around his apparatus for from two to three hours at a time. At the end of the four days, he was compelled to cease active work, owing to the physical effects of the x-rays upon his body. The first thing Mr. Hawks noted was a drying of the skin, to which he paid no attention, but after a while it became so painful it was necessary to stop all operations. The hands began to swell and assume the appearance of a very deep sunburn. At the end of two weeks the skin all came off his hands. The knuckles were especially affected, they being the sorest part of the hand. Among other effects were the following: the growth of the fingernails was stopped and the hair on the skin that was exposed to rays all dropped out, especially on the face and sides of the head. The hair at the temples has entirely disappeared, owing to the fact that Mr. Hawks placed his head in close proximity to the tube to enable spectators to see the bones of the jaw. The eyes were quite bloodshot and the vision considerably impaired. The eyelashes began to fall out and the lids to swell. The chest was also burned through the clothing, the burn resembling sunburn. Mr. Hawks' disabilities were such that he was compelled to suspend work for two weeks. He consulted physicians, who treated the case as one of parboiling.

Incredibly, after his enforced vacation, Hawks resumed exhibition of his x-ray apparatus! He tried to protect his hand, first with Vaseline and, when that failed to ward off the rays, with a glove. When the glove offered no protection, Hawks covered his hand with tinfoil as a more successful alternative. One month later, Hawks concluded that the effects seemed to

X-ray dermatitis (Gilchrist, 1897). Photograph showing extensive exfoliation of the epidermis.[8]

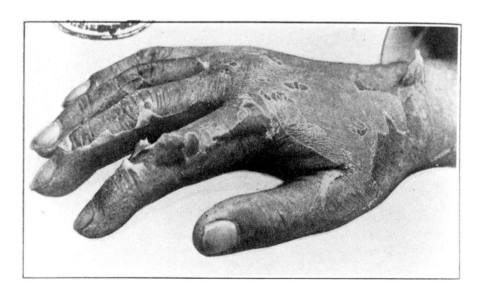

Carcinoma developing after an x-ray burn (1904).[9]

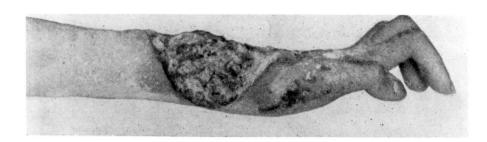

158

be confined to the skin and consisted of drying the oils in the skin, which produced the effects on hair and nails. He also noted that none of the effects were permanent; all disappeared when the skin became healthy again.[7]

Fred S. Jones of Minnesota soon reported the "particularly distressing case" of William Levy, who had been shot in the head by an escaping bank defaulter 10 years before. "The bullet had entered his skull just above the left ear, and had presumably proceeded toward the back of the head." Having heard about the x-rays, Levy decided to have his bullet located for possible removal. Since Jones was familiar with Daniel's and Dudley's experience at Vanderbilt, or with subsequent reports of epilation, he warned Levy that the experiment might cause him to lose his hair, but Levy was undeterred. He underwent x-ray exposure[11]:

> . . . from 8:00 in the morning until 10:00 at night. Exposures were made with a tube over his forehead, in front of his open mouth, and just behind his right ear. According to one account, the tube was actually placed inside his mouth. The current to the tube was estimated at 100,000 volts.
>
> The next day Mr. Levy began to notice a peculiar effect on his skin wherever it had been most exposed to the rays. And the hair on the right side of his head, which had been nearer the wire, began to fall out. In a few days the right side of his head was perfectly bald, his right ear had swollen to twice its natural size and presented the same appearance as if very badly frozen. Sores were visible on his head, his mouth and throat were blistered so that he could not eat solid food for three weeks, and his lips were swollen, cracked and bleeding. In fact the long exposure to the x-rays, while giving him no pain at the time, seemed to have produced very similar effects to a very severe burn.

Although this report was alarming, a follow-up story indicated that the "deleterious effects" were only temporary. However, not all x-ray burns healed so promptly. Cases were reported of prolonged exposure in which "every attempt to control the inflammatory action has failed." Serious damage from x-rays was reported from Edison's laboratory by Elihu Thomson,[12] who called these cases "severe, since they took place over the hands and arms of the victims, and made it necessary for them to

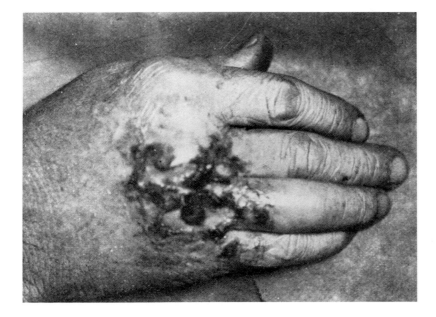

X-ray dermatitis (1912).[10]

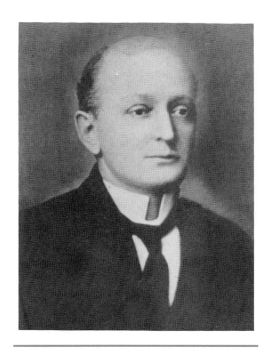

Clarence Dally (1865-1904), the first x-ray martyr.[2]

stop work altogether in connection with x-rays." The story goes that one of them was told by his physician that if he continued to work, it would be necessary to amputate his hands. It is probable that the worker threatened with amputation was Clarence Dally, the first x-ray martyr (see Chapter 4).

Soon reports appeared describing patients who suffered systemic reactions after x-ray exposure. David Walsh[13] of London described a patient who, in addition to dermatitis, "developed a high fever, languor and sluggish pupils resembling the picture of sunstroke, as well as diarrhoea and vomiting," which he interpreted as signs of "cerebral and gastric irritation." After he saw a second patient with postexposure colic and diarrhea, Walsh concluded that the x-rays produced a direct inflammatory reaction of the gastrointestinal mucous membrane.

Other examples of radiation injury to deeper tissues included "osteoplastic periostitis,"[8] inhibition of bone growth,[14] sterilization,[15] and hematological changes, including aplastic anemia.[16] Indeed, it was recommended that "all those who are employed in radiographic work or with radium have their blood examined periodically—say every six months—as by so doing the disease could be recognized at a very early stage, and probably be stopped."[17]

Although radiologists and others working professionally with x-rays were the victims of most radiation-induced cancers and deaths, some patients also were afflicted. One of them, a Massachusetts school teacher treated by Clarence E. Skinner, was dying of an incurable fibrosarcoma. For over 2 years, she received 136 x-ray treatments, and her "incurable" cancer was cured. However, 5 years later she developed severe pain and skin ulceration that was diagnosed as epidermoid carcinoma. Although cured of her fibrosarcoma, Skinner's patient now suffered from skin cancer in the area where she had been irradiated. After a series of additional operations and many months of suffering, the school teacher recovered again but unfortunately was lost to further follow-up.

Ironically, the medical literature of the early 1900s contains a number of cases in which patients suffering from skin cancers caused by x-ray burns were treated with additional x-rays in an effort to cure the cancers. Among them was Clarence Dally, whose physician justified this therapeutic approach as "applying the x-ray with the hope of undoing what the ray itself had done." As might be expected, this treatment approach failed, and amputation was required.

CAUSE OF RADIATION INJURIES

Although it was soon established that exposure to x-rays was associated with undesirable and dangerous physiological effects, during the next few years there was a lively debate concerning the *cause* of those effects. Hawks[7] declared that "as to what produces the burn, I think it is purely an electrical effect, and that the ray has nothing to do with it, except in a peculiar manner; the burn is such as would be produced by a combination of heat and light, as sunburn." W. M. Stine[18] concluded that "the effects are not due to the x-rays, but rather to ultra-violet rays, which are always present to a greater or less extent . . . It is noteworthy that such effects only result from exposure to the focusing tubes, when, owing to the concentration of energy, ultra-violet rays of considerable intensity must be produced." Nikola Tesla[19] was convinced that the harmful effects "are not due to the Roentgen rays, but merely to the ozone generated in contact

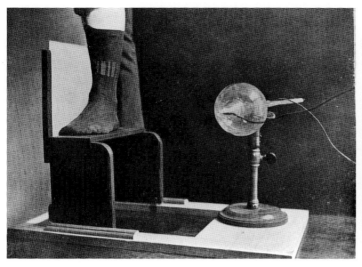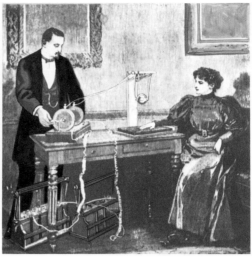

Examples of completely unshielded x-ray tubes. *Left,* Radiography of the ankle (Monell, 1902). *Right,* Radiography of the hand (Seguy, 1896).

with the skin. Nitrous acid might also be responsible, to a small extent. The ozone, when abundantly produced, attacks the skin and many organic substances most energetically." Edmund Kells, a New Orleans dentist, believed that radiation injury was caused by rays carrying infectious material from the surface. Therefore he recommended scrubbing the skin with soap and water before exposure. Other authors suggested that radiation injuries were caused by platinum particles from the x-ray tubes or by platinocyanides on the fluorescent screens. Among other things, red silk and thin rubber sheets were advocated as preventives! Even "personal idiosyncrasy" was considered. John Hall-Edwards[20] wrote, "There can be no doubt that some people are more sensitive to the rays than others and in my experience those are the most sensitive who are most easily burned by the sun. Fair people are, as a rule, more sensitive than dark ones, although there are some exceptions." Roentgen probably escaped injury because he conducted his experiments, which were mainly photographic, in a metal chamber used for eliminating extraneous light.

A Boston tubemaker, E. A. Frei, who had also begun manufacturing static machines, proposed a novel theory of how to avoid radiation burns. He noted that his x-ray dermatitis had been sustained when he was experimenting with induction coils; since switching almost exclusively to static machines, he had suffered no ill effects. When it was suggested that his hands had become "x-ray proof" as a result of the earlier burns, Frei

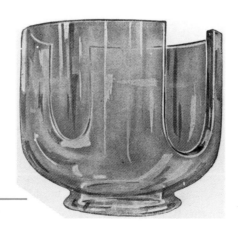

Leaded-glass tube shield (1912).[10]

Early leaden screen (1912).[10]

sought to disprove this explanation by performing new experiments on his previously unexposed left foot. After "treating" the foot for 30 minutes to 1 hour every 4 days, but allegedly experiencing no similar burns, Frei concluded that the damaging effect of x-rays was related to the induction coil and that x-rays were harmless when produced with a static machine.[21]

As an equipment manufacturer, Frei must have been familiar with the growing concern among physicians about the potential danger of x-ray examinations. As a maker of static machines, in addition to x-ray tubes, Frei may have thought it profitable to have the induction coil take the blame rather than the x-rays. As Frei wrote[21]:

> Many physicians bring forth the argument that the application of the x-rays might prove dangerous to their patients, that here a foot had to be amputated, there someone's fingernails dropped off, another has a sore of three months' standing, etc. Such arguments can be met with the above fact that the x-rays are not the direct cause of the trouble and with this fact established remedies could undoubtedly be found to reduce, if not entirely eliminate, the effect on the skin when coils are to be employed.

Charles L. Leonard of University Hospital in Philadelphia wrote that[22]:

> "The x-ray burn" is, therefore, not the result of the action of the x-ray, nor can it be produced by the x-ray; but the dermatitis produced as the result of the static current or charges induced in the tissues by the high potential induction field surrounding the x-ray tube. The therapeutic properties attributed to the x-ray do not belong to it, but are due to the static charges and currents induced in tissues, which have long been known to be capable of producing similar results.
>
> The x-ray per se is incapable of entering the tissues of a patient, and the dermatitis, which has been called an x-ray "burn" is the result of an interference of the nutrition of the part by the induced static changes.
>
> The patient may be absolutely protected from the harmful effects of the static charge by the interposition between the tube and the patient of a rounded sheet of conducting material that is readily penetrable by the x-ray—a thin sheet of aluminum, or gold-leaf spread upon cardboard, makes an effectual shield.

Elihu Thomson was the first x-ray worker to suggest that roentgen rays themselves might cause the adverse effects accompanying their use. He had developed the "Thomson Inductorium," an induction coil adapted especially for x-ray use and sold by General Electric in competition with Frei's static machine. By performing experiments on himself, Thomson not only established that the x-rays themselves caused the burns but also served to clear the reputation of his device.[23]

Thomson subjected his little finger to a 20-minute exposure to x-rays generated by a static machine and produced a severe reaction. When challenged that his dermatitis was merely the result of ultraviolet rays or brush discharges, Thomson refuted this possibility by describing his experimental design. He used a blue glass tube with a clear German glass window opposite the x-ray path. The fingers opposite the blue glass were not affected (since the glass was dense enough to absorb the x-rays). Only where the little finger was opposite the clear glass was it affected, and there was a sharp line of demarcation between that portion and the rest of the finger behind the blue glass. He concluded that the blue or purplish glass would have been transparent to ultraviolet rays but not to x-rays.

In addition to proving that the burns were due to the x-rays themselves, regardless of whether a static machine or an induction coil was used to generate them, Thomson also showed that the effect was cumulative by treating another finger with a series of short exposures over a period of many days.

The direct relationship between x-rays and the biological effects that followed prolonged exposure was unequivocally proved by the controlled experiments performed by Kienbock with irradiated rats (1900) and by William Rollins with guinea pigs 1 year later. In a note provocatively titled "X-Light Kills," Rollins[24] described an experiment in which he exposed two guinea pigs to x-rays for 2 hours each day. The animals were kept in grounded Faraday chambers to ensure that electrical fields or static charges were not responsible for the effects noted. One animal died on the eighth day of exposure, and the second died on the eleventh day. Skin burns, always associated with x-ray damage, were not noted.

On the basis of this experiment, which demonstrated the lethal effects of x-rays on a healthy mammal, Rollins offered three precautionary maxims to medical x-ray users:

1. Wear radio-opaque glasses.
2. Enclose the x-ray tube in a leaded (or other nonradiable) housing.
3. Irradiate only those areas of the patient of interest, and cover adjacent areas with radio-opaque materials.

For the most part, Rollins' report of the lethal effects of x-ray overexposure went unnoticed. However, an immediate reply came from Ernest A. Codman, a noted surgeon-radiologist. In an article titled "No practical danger from the x-ray," Codman[25] cited an experience of 10,000 exposures on 4,000 patients without a single case of hair loss or burns to the skin. In addition, Codman indicated that for all purposes, it was only necessary to keep one's hands away from the x-ray tube. He did admit, however, that some of the precautions suggested by Rollins might be necessary if exposures were continuous. Charging Rollins with being overly dramatic, Codman stated that "I believe that the comparatively small number of unfortunate cases which have been published circulated much farther than the immense number of fortunate cases, and have given the profession the idea that the process is a dangerous one *to the patient*."

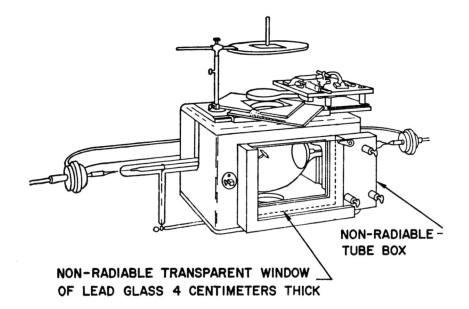

NON-RADIABLE TRANSPARENT WINDOW OF LEAD GLASS 4 CENTIMETERS THICK

NON-RADIABLE TUBE BOX

Nonradiable tube box (1902).[27]

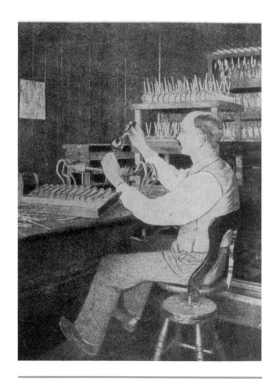

Dally "sealing off" incandescent lamps.[2]

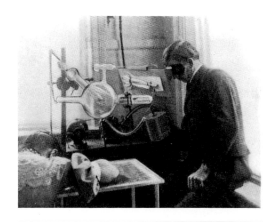

Fluoroscopy using Beck's osteoscope fastened to the fluoroscopic screen so that the operator can hold his hands at his side (1904).[32]

In the following issue of the *Boston Medical and Surgical Journal*, Rollins described the results of an experiment in which he exposed a pregnant guinea pig to x-rays. The fetus was killed, and Rollins expressed concern about exposure of pregnant women for pelvimetry or routine examinations. As an indirect reply to Codman, Rollins wrote[26]:

What people fear is uncertainty; therefore, when a new agent is employed in medicine it is important to determine its power by experiment on animals. When the worst is known, and the agent under control, we need not fear patients will object to its use. Nothing is gained by criticizing such experiments, for criticism is sterile while experiment is fertile. An experiment can only be discredited by another experiment.

One year later, Rollins[27] published a detailed description of another animal experiment in which guinea pigs exposed to x-rays were carefully protected from ultraviolet light and electrical induction and convection. The results conclusively demonstrated the lethal effects of total body irradiation. Rollins also pointed out the danger of radiation-induced cataracts and suggested that fluoroscopists wear leaded-glass goggles 1 centimeter thick.

Rollins developed numerous devices to provide for the safety of both operator and patient (see Chapter 4). As he wrote later (1903),[28] "That I have escaped injury is due to an early recognition of the dangerous nature of x-light and to the precautions recommended in earlier papers having been taken . . ."

In 1902, Codman collected and reported a review of the 147 patients whose accidental x-ray burns had been recorded.[29] The stimulus for this study was the case of a Doctor Weldon, who in 1899 purchased an x-ray machine from Otis Clapp & Son of Boston. Soon after installing the machine, Weldon tested it by "exposing himself for an x-ray picture of the hip-joint for 45 minutes, with the Crookes tube about 5 inches from the skin of his groin. A most intractable burn resulted, necessitating a severe operation, and producing disability for a year and a half."

Weldon sued the Clapp firm for $20,000 in damages, alleging that the company had warranted that its apparatus would not burn. Several of the country's foremost x-ray authorities, including Codman himself, testified on behalf of the manufacturer. Nevertheless, the physician was awarded $6,750 in damages by a US District Court on November 8, 1901.[29]

Codman concluded that the frequency of x-ray injuries had been much exaggerated by the medical press because of the wide publicity given to many early cases. Less than one half of his collected cases were "serious," and more than two thirds of the injuries occurred within the first 2 years of the use of x-rays. Codman failed to consider the possibility that x-ray injuries still occurred frequently but were no longer so uncommon as to warrant publication of each case. Among the dangerous conclusions Codman drew in this study[29] were that "there is no good evidence of injury to the deeper tissues without primary interference with the skin" and that "the static machine is somewhat less likely to produce injury than other forms of apparatus."

The makers of x-ray tubes (even more than patients and radiologists) were at extreme risk for radiation-induced injury. The process of exhausting the tube of its gases required that each tube be contained in an "oven" at a certain temperature. As the degree of vacuum increased through the action of a mercury pump, the "penetration" of the tube emanations became higher. Many ovens were inadequately constructed to resist or absorb this penetration, and thus there was much leakage of x-rays through their walls. The testing of the tube after its exhaustion was important work; it might represent a solid hour of exposure to x-rays unless the operator was sufficiently protected by the material used in the construction of the oven or by a shield between him and the oven. For the sake of easy accessibility, the windows of the oven were placed at face or mid-chest level. This led to many tube manufacturers sustaining severe radiation damage to the skin of the face, neck, and chest, as well as the hands.

The tube maker also made numerous demonstrations of the effectiveness of his wares. These demonstrations were almost always fluoroscopic, and this exposure added to that already sustained in the exhausting and "tuning" of the tubes produced an enormous cumulative effect in the skin of these x-ray pioneers.

The major danger to radiologists was fluoroscopy. Although a lead-glass protective device was designed for use in front of the eyepiece of the portable cryptoscope or fluoroscope, it did nothing to decrease the danger to the skin of the radiologist's hand held even momentarily as a testing gauge between the screen and the source of x-rays or of the hand that grasped the supporting handle of the instrument. The supporting hand, although not as directly in the beam of x-ray emanation, was generally as much exposed to the radiation around the Crookes tube as was the hand serving as a gauge of the level of x-ray penetration.

The novelty of the fluorescent screen in the form of the hand fluoroscope and the interest and enthusiasm it aroused tended to greatly prolong the exposure of the operator, who was always glad to demonstrate its wonders to the casual observer or to the patient and his physician. X-ray "exhibitions" were popular at fairs and similar gatherings and led to horrendous overexposures.

Shoe stores began to feature x-ray photographs of feet cramped by poorly fitted shoes. Fluoroscopes for fitting shoes soon were put on the market. The typical shoe-fitting fluoroscope consisted of a 50 kV x-ray tube operating at 38 mA through a 2-mm aluminum filter that was housed in a case lined with lead or steel and containing a fluorescent screen. The focal spot to skin distance was 7.5 to 20 cm. The unit was equipped with an opening for the customer's feet and three viewing openings so that the

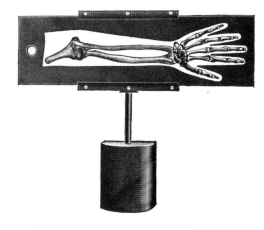

Osteoscope (1905). This instrument consisted of an articulated skeleton hand suitably mounted behind a small fluorescent screen, which served as a test object for assessing hardness of the x-ray beam. The fleshy parts of the hand were represented by suitably cut-out tin foil. The entire device ($25) was mounted on a holder surrounded by a metallic semicircle that afforded protection to the hand of the operator (Kny-Scheerer catalogue).[32]

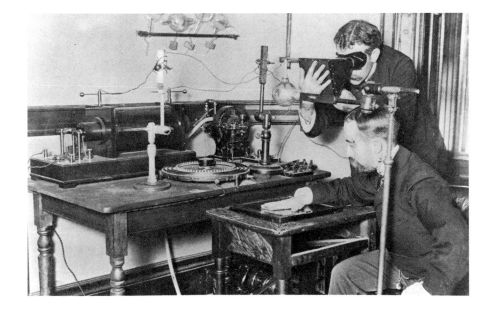

Dangerous practice of estimating the hardness of the x-ray beam by placing one's own hand between the tube and fluoroscopic screen before obtaining a radiograph of the patient's hand (1896).[30]

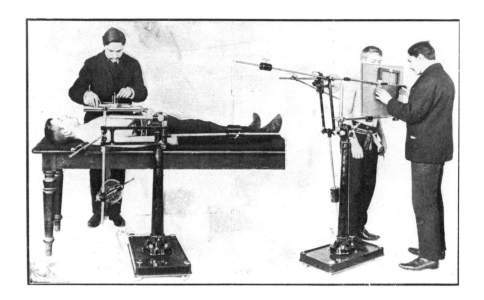

Dangerous technique of orthodiagraphy with an open fluorescent screen in horizontal (*left*) and vertical (*right*) positions (1907).[34]

customer, clerk, and one other person could observe the screen. A push-button automatic timer that could be set for any predetermined time was included in most installations. In actual use, the exposure time averaged about 20 seconds. However, since repeated exposures could be made by simply releasing and pushing the timer button, the unit could be operated as long as the viewer wished. More sophisticated models were equipped with three separate switches to provide different intensity levels—one for men, one for women, and one for children.

Although popular with customers, shoe-fitting fluoroscopes usually were inadequately maintained, and children who were fluoroscoped repeatedly when being fitted with new shoes received a substantial primary radiation dose to the feet (up to 116 r during a typical 20-second exposure) and secondary radiation to the gonads. Several cases were reported in which radiation-induced dermatitis developed in store employees who worked with improperly shielded x-ray machines. By the late 1950s the risk of damage to growing epiphyses and the possible induction of leukemia from the substantial radiation exposure of shoe-fitting fluoroscopes was generally recognized, and these devices soon disappeared.[35]

The open fluorescent screen was just as dangerous to its habitual user as the hooded fluoroscope. In its earlier forms, it was almost never covered with a thoroughly protective material such as lead-glass, since this would make the screen so heavy that it would be necessary to support it mechanically.

An accessory fluoroscopic procedure that was particularly hazardous to the x-ray pioneer was the process of tracing the outline of the "shadow" of any given organic structure (especially the heart) or a foreign body. Although some operators placed a rudimentary protective screen in front of the tube, there was virtually no protection of the fluoroscopist, especially when the tracing was made directly on the patient's skin (see Chapter 13).

The usual sequence of radiation-induced changes experienced by x-ray pioneers and demonstrated in some of the photographs of Mihran Kassabian of Philadelphia was (1) after some exposure, the skin became tanned, much as from the sun; (2) later, the skin cracked, fissured, and reddened, giving way to chronic roughening; (3) in time, skin cancer developed, leading to a succession of surgeries and progressive amputations; and (4) ultimately, the victim died of overwhelming metastases.[36]

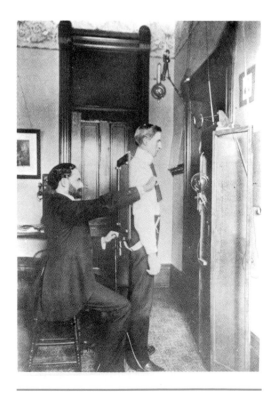

Dangerous practice of fluoroscopy using an open screen (1902).[33]

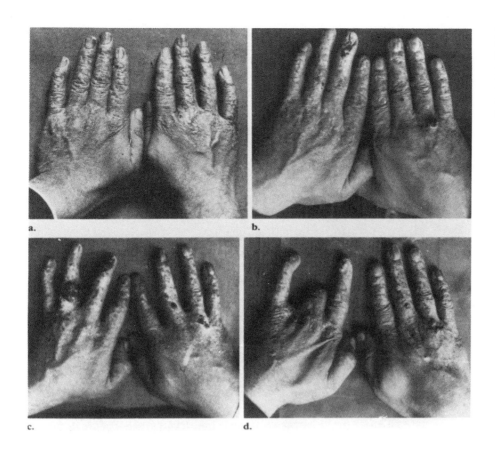

Sequential photographs of the hands of x-ray martyr Mihran K. Kassabian (1870-1910). *Top left and right*, 1903 and 1908. *Bottom left and right*, Unknown date, probably 1908 and unknown date, probably 1909.[38]

EARLY RADIATION PROTECTION

Most early radiologists assumed that if the initial effect of the x-ray—the burn or severe erythema—could be prevented, they and their patients would also be protected from the delayed effects of cancer and death. Since they had no method of measuring with any precision the dosages that they and their patients received, x-ray workers tended to rely on particular devices to prevent burns rather than on an overall program of radiation protection.

One protective device described by George E. Pfahler (1905) was the use of a filter. It had been previously shown that the rays from a Crookes tube were not homogeneous. Some were "soft" and mostly absorbed by the skin and other superficial tissues; the more penetrating "hard" rays were absorbed deeper in the body or passed all the way through it to strike the photographic plate beyond. Pfahler set out to find a filter that would strain out the soft, skin-burning rays while letting the others through, in much the same fashion as window glass strains out the ultraviolet rays of the sun that cause sunburn.

Pfahler also used the "principle of selective absorption," which implied that each material absorbs rays of a particular quality from the heterogeneous x-ray beam. For example, when an x-ray beam passes through an aluminum filter, soft rays are absorbed. If a second aluminum filter is then placed in the beam, little further absorption takes place, since the first filter has already removed most of the rays absorbable by aluminum. As a radiotherapist, Pfahler[37] noted that

> the rays which give us the most concern are those that affect the skin when we are treating deep-seated disease. If the law of selective absorption be correct, then the skin has a peculiar absorbing power.

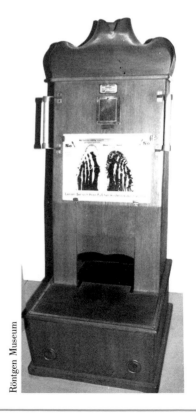

Röntgen Museum

Shoe fluoroscope.

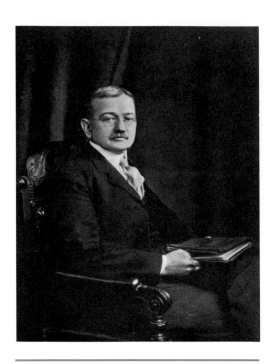

Charles L. Leonard (1861-1913).

Now, I reasoned that in order to filter out these harmful rays we must select a substance that resembles the skin as closely as possible. The substance resembling the skin most closely is leather. In order to make assurance doubly sure, I have selected the thickest leather possible, namely sole leather, which is about four times as thick as the human skin. Therefore the rays which pass through this leather should pass through the skin without affecting it in any way . . .

Pfahler's filter was a simple disk of sole leather 5 inches in diameter, soaked in water "in order to resemble the skin more closely." Although the Pfahler filter did provide considerable protection to the skin, a substantial part of this protection was overcome if a radiologist, relying on the filter, increased the dose too enthusiastically. As Henry K. Pancoast[38] reported at the 1906 meeting of the American Roentgen Ray Society (ARRS), "I have made general use of Doctor Pfahler's filter . . . and have found that as a rule from two to three times as much dosage could be applied when the wet filter was used as could formerly be done without it. But still a dermatitis could follow, and a very severe one, too."

An early editorial note[39] identified the *operator*, not his patient, as the person exposed to greater risk. By the 1907 meeting of the ARRS, the problem of radiation protection was becoming a major topic of concern. The deaths of Clarence Dally, Elizabeth Fleischman Ascheim, Lewis Weigel, Wolfram Fuchs, and a number of European x-ray workers were well known. A major paper, "Protection of Roentgenologists," was given by Charles L. Leonard[40] of Philadelphia, himself a victim of severe hand burns who died an x-ray martyr 6 years later. Leonard opened his talk by expressing concern about the misuse of x-rays by practitioners:

> . . . with little theoretical and no practical knowledge or experience. This is the grave danger of Roentgen therapy at the present time. Its mysterious and powerful action, its brilliant results, are leading many practitioners to attempt at employment in their own practices. The majority acquire no theoretical knowledge and their clinical experience is limited . . . Their results are necessarily poor and injure the name of Roentgen therapeutics. The practitioner should be warned against the employment unless he is willing to devote sufficient time to acquire technical knowledge and clinical experience. The general medical public should be warned not to entrust their patients to those inexperienced in employing it safely and effectively.

In therapeutic radiation, Leonard stressed that a particular hazard of inexperienced workers was the risk of *too small* a dosage. "The novice is fearful of producing ill effects and hence produces none. He prefers to employ inefficient dosage protracted over long courses of treatment rather than court invisible dangers."

Although trained and experienced radiologists could readily protect their patients, Leonard decried the fact that they were not doing enough to protect themselves from the rays.

> A seeming disbelief renders more experienced operators fearless. They are immune to its action. It may be dangerous for others but not for them. Because they cannot see immediate effects they cannot appreciate that any injury is being done. The earlier operators had the excuse of an ignorance that was common to the whole scientific world. They exposed themselves freely for experiment and scientific research. The injuries they suffered were not manifest for four or more years. The operator of to-day who has had only four or five years' experience, and has in a measure protected himself, feels

certain he will suffer no ill effects. His dose has been less powerful, it probably will not manifest its ill effects so speedily, but if he continues to expose himself to repeated though minute doses, the injury though slow in appearing may be more chronic in course and more resistant to treatment. The warning of past experience has not been heeded.

The principal protective measure that Leonard stressed was the use of protective shields around the tube to cut off stray or "vagabond" rays. "The only safe protection is metallic lead of at least a thickness known commercially as six pounds to the square foot over the active hemisphere of the tube." The remainder of the tube, except for the beam opening, should be encased in lead weighing at least three pounds per square foot. In addition, there should be a diaphragm to "cut off all secondary and vagrant rays to increase definition."

Leonard decried the practice of some radiologists who left their tubes unshielded but moved behind a lead screen before activating the tube. Perhaps from personal experience, Leonard knew that this strict procedure was often not followed and led to large amounts of unnecessary exposure. "The practice of some operators of working behind a lead screen with an open or semi-protected tube is unsafe, because familiarity breeds carelessness, and while the occasional exposure might not result in visible injury, such exposures will certainly become more frequent, with results that are certain to be serious." The only solution was to have protection built into the apparatus itself.

Leonard also criticized equipment manufacturers for their alleged safety devices. Although some were apparently safe, "others are of questionable value, while others are totally valueless and by engendering a false sense of security lead the operator into grave danger."

After Leonard's presentation, Russell H. Boggs[41] of Pittsburgh spoke before the ARRS, stressing the importance of maintaining sufficient distance between the tube and the patient and the value of an adequate filter. However, during the discussion period that followed, several participants warned of excessive caution.

W. S. Laurence of Memphis, Tennessee, stated[42]:

It seems to me that there is no such thing as absolute protection, unless you go to an adjoining town and operate by telephone. Then the question is, how much protection is it wise to take? I believe that there is a point of tolerance in the human body to the x-ray as there is to other injurious agents. We all know that tobacco in certain quantities will kill the individual, but if one will limit himself to a certain number of cigars a day he can smoke and still live to be old and die from some other cause than tobacco poisoning . . . I am sure that the body will tolerate a certain amount of x-ray energy, either the direct or the secondary ray. For that reason I do not believe that it is necessary to clothe ourselves in armor or to leave the city and operate our apparatus from a distance. To work without protection is foolhardy and inexcusable, but I believe attempts at absolute protection have been carried to rather absurd extremes.

Eugene W. Caldwell of New York, who had already had one operation for cancer of the hand a few months before, argued against surrounding the tube with lead.[43] As he remarked,

Undoubtedly we should avoid all unnecessary exposure, but I believe there has been undue alarm over the dangers of the secondary rays, and that we are not warranted in sacrificing facilities for observing and controlling our tubes in order to exclude the last vestige of

THE KNY-SCHEERER COMPANY, NEW YORK.
Telegraphic Address: EXRAY—NEW—YORK.

MACALASTER-WIGGIN COMPANY 25

Radiation protection devices in 1905 (Kny-Scheerer catalogue). Advertisement for protective gloves, apron, and penetration gauge (1907) (Macalaster-Wiggin catalogue).

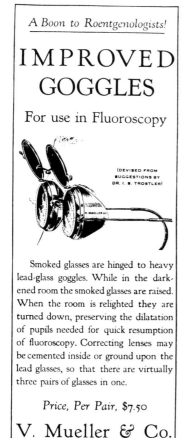

Advertisement for improved goggles for use in fluoroscopy (AJR, 1914).

Protection for X-Ray Operators.

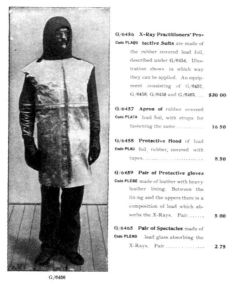

G/6456   X-Ray Practitioners' Pro-
Code PLAQU tective Suits are made of
the rubber covered lead foil, described under G/6454. Illustration shows in which way they can be applied. An equipment consisting of G/6457, G/6458, G/6459 and G/6465... $30 00

G/6457   Apron of rubber covered
Code PLATA lead foil, with straps for fastening the same..........   16 50

G/6458   Protective Hood of lead
Code PLAU foil, rubber, covered with tapes....................   8 50

G/6459   Pair of Protective gloves
Code PLEBE made of leather with heavy leather lining. Between the lining and the uppers there is a composition of lead which absorbs the X-Rays. Pair.......   5 00

G/6465   Pair of Spectacles made of
Code PLENG lead glass absorbing the X-Rays. Pair...............   2 75

G/6456

ALL OUR PRODUCTS ARE GUARANTEED AND BEAR OUR TRADE MARK FOR IDENTIFICATION

X Ray Protective Gloves

No. 102.   Code Word, Sonoras.   Price per pair, $5.00

These gloves are made of rubber in combination with an opaque substance and they effectually cut off the burning rays. They are the only gloves which give the operator the free use of his hands.

X Ray Protective Apron

No. 103.   Code Word, Sonore.   Regular size, Price, $8.50
Extra large size, reinforced, Price, $10.00
These aprons are made of the same material as the gloves and are an effectual protection for all parts of the body.

Penetration Guage

No. 104.   Code Word Grotesque.   Price, $5.00

This guage may be used with any fluoroscope, to measure the penetration of the X-Rays. Ten fields are provided, the density increasing in geometrical progression. Seven of these, measured at 18 inches on a 12 inch coil, and with a tube to withstand the voltage, will take a hip joint of a 200 lb. adult in 2 minutes. It can be carried in the pocket.

secondary radiation. It is well known that overexposure to sunlight may produce very disastrous results, but it does not follow from this that we must live in darkness . . . I think that a screen which will protect the photographic plate so well that only a little fog is shown on development after two or three weeks' exposure in the position occupied by the operator is practically safe, even if all the secondary rays are not excluded.

Caldwell may have fallen victim to his own faulty reasoning, since he died of radiation-induced injury 11 years later.

Although there was no agreement on the need for x-ray safeguards, many radiologists had begun to take precautions. Aprons, jackets, gloves, and ray-proof goggles were recommended for all x-ray work. Protective coverings for the operator became so extreme that, according to Deane Butcher, the German Roentgen expert was "encased from Schnurrbart to foot in a veritable suit of armour."[44]

Rome Wagner, a major tube manufacturer, adopted the use of a primitive "film badge." As he noted at the 1907 meeting of the ARRS[43]:

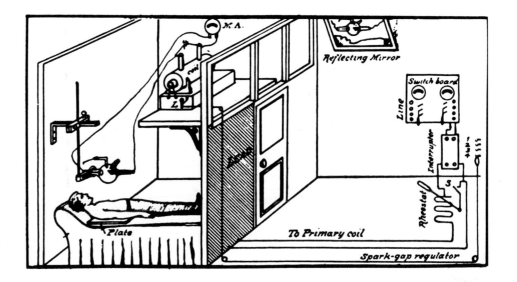

Design for leaded room for operator's protection (1907).[46]

One of the most difficult things about this work is to determine what absolute protection is . . . Every operator knows how to protect the photographic plate, but he never stops to consider the protection of himself in the same way. The thing is to know whether you have exposed yourself during the day . . . I concluded that I would not take chances with any ray that would affect a photographic plate, so I carry one in my pocket, and in the evening, after the day's work, I develop this film to see whether I have been exposed to the ray. Once in awhile I find that I have, and then I try to figure out where I have been exposed. Now I often go for a week without any exposure; in fact, only seldom is the film affected. I believe that this plan is a good one because you need not worry about being exposed when you have not been exposed.

Unfortunately, Wagner's precautions came too late, and he died an x-ray martyr less than 6 months later.

As Deane Butcher wrote, "It is too late to begin to adopt precautions when the hands begin to show signs of burning. The mischief is done, and is probably irreparable."[44] Nevertheless, for many years the protection of x-ray workers was rudimentary or nonexistent, and injuries and death continued.

The most dramatic statement of the danger of x-radiation was a paper presented to the Royal Society of Medicine (1908) by John Hall-Edwards, a victim of severe radiation injury resulting in radiation osteitis, necrosis, and cancer, which necessitated the amputation of both hands.[20] He exhibited photographs and radiographs of his hands, both before and after amputation, and was an outspoken advocate for the need for stringent precautions. Three years later, the *Archives of the Roentgen Ray* printed a remarkable series of 23 radiographs made by Ernest Wilson (an x-ray martyr) of his own right middle finger, covering the 6-year period from before his initial amputation to the final operation in 1910. They presented a complete picture of radiation osteonecrosis, complicated by osteomyelitis and malignant transformation.[47] These horrible complications among prominent x-ray workers were critical factors in the movement toward establishing strict standards for adequate radiation protection.

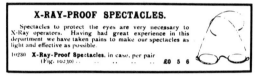

X-RAY-PROOF SPECTACLES.

Spectacles to protect the eyes are very necessary to X-Ray operators. Having had great experience in this department we have taken pains to make our spectacles as light and effective as possible.

10230 X-Ray-Proof Spectacles, in case, per pair
(Fig. 10230) £0 5 6

Advertisement for x-ray proof spectacles[46] (1910).

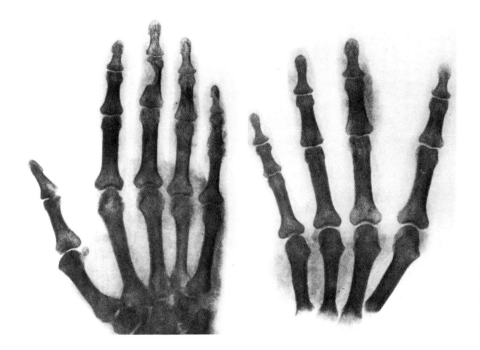

Radiographs of the amputated left hand and wrist (*left*) and right four fingers (*right*) of John Hall-Edwards, which he published in 1908 to illustrate the effect of prolonged x-ray exposure on bone.[20]

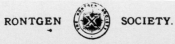

RONTGEN SOCIETY.

Recommendations for the Protection of X-ray Operators.

The harmful effects produced by X-rays are cumulative and do not generally appear until some weeks or months after the damage has been done. It is to be noted that X-rays of any degree of hardness are capable of producing ill effects, although it is commonly supposed that soft rays only are harmful.

It is undesirable that any X-ray treatment should be carried out except under the direction of a qualified medical practitioner experienced in X-ray work.

All X-ray tubes must be provided, when in use, with a protecting shield or cover which prevents the access of rays to the operators and which encloses the tube, leaving an adjustable opening only sufficiently large to allow the passage of a sheaf of rays of the size necessary for the work in hand. Even with this shielding the operator may not be completely protected in all cases (e.g., especially in screen work), and the use of movable screens, gloves and aprons is recommended.

Operators should be warned that shields obtainable commercially are often ineffective and tests of their opacity should be made.

Whenever possible the cubicle system should be used for X-ray treatment and the operator should be able to make all adjustments from a protected space.

When screen examination is required it is essential that the screen should be covered with thick lead glass of proved opacity and that the screen should be independently supported and not held in the hands of the operator. If the hands are so used they should be properly protected.

The hand or any portion of the body of the operator should never be used to test the hardness or quality of the X-ray tube; any simple form of penetrometer can be easily arranged for this purpose.

November 1915

First British code of practice for the protection of x-ray operators (1915).

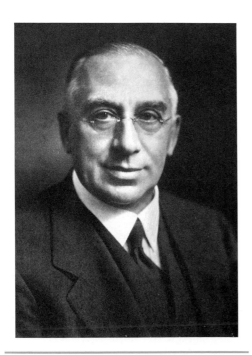

George W. C. Kaye (1880-1941).

The demands of World War I overwhelmed existing x-ray facilities and operators, resulting in a large number of poorly trained x-ray workers who did not fully realize the potential of radiation danger and failed to provide adequate protection. In addition, Army x-ray units were of relatively primitive design, using induction coils and gas tubes with low output, which necessitated long exposures. This situation led the Röntgen Society (1915) to promulgate *Recommendations for the Protection of X-ray Operators*, the first British code of practice.

The final impetus to the establishment of strict radiation protection guidelines was the death from aplastic anemia of another British radiologist, Ironside Bruce. In a long letter to *The Times of London* (March 29, 1921), Robert Knox eulogized his dead colleague and attempted to calm the anxiety of the public about the safety of x-rays. Knox urged the adoption of more stringent protective measures for both radiologists and the public. Almost immediately after publication of this letter, the British X-ray and Radium Protection Committee was formed to tackle the formidable task of drawing up recommendations for the manufacture and use of radium and roentgen ray apparatus that would make it impossible for a reasonably careful worker to injure himself. The Committee recognized three sources of danger: excessive exposure to x-rays, high-voltage risks from exposed electrical conductors, and undue exposure to toxic gases produced by coronal discharge. Without measurement techniques or any background knowledge of radiobiology, the Committee members applied their energy to defining pragmatically sensible precautions for the x-ray operator, including such areas as lead shield thickness for x-ray tubes, hours of work, and periodic blood checks. In July, 1921 a "Preliminary Report" was issued, the first set of recommendations to be established by any country.[48] The American Roentgen Ray Protection Committee, although founded 6 months earlier than its British counterpart, did not publish its similar set of recommendations until September, 1922.

Some radiologists and equipment makers strongly criticized the Recommendations and accused them of being unnecessarily drastic. The Committee's efforts to provide adequate protection against stray radiation were deprecated as heavy, clumsy, and costly. Many radiologists complained that they were being overly restricted. Soon, however, the heavy lead protection was replaced by safer devices such as the self-protected x-ray tube, in which the full thickness of lead protection laid down by the Protection Committee was incorporated into the tube itself. Additional technical improvements included shock-proof tubes and insulated high-tension cables and transformers immersed in oil. By the mid-1930s, x-ray tubes were no longer enclosed in glass globes with naked high-tension wires and Snook rectifiers. The objections to protective measures had been overcome; patients no longer suffered skin burns or depilation, and all operators wore aprons and gloves.[49]

Another valuable contribution of the recommendations was to pressure hospitals to replace old, unsafe apparatus and to provide satisfactory working conditions in x-ray departments. In the early days, any dark, disused cellar was considered good enough for x-ray work, and the availability of adequate ventilation was rarely considered. The National Physical Laboratory (under superintendent, George W. C. Kaye) became a source where manufacturers could have their apparatus tested and certified as complying with the standards recommended by the Protection Committee. This led to the condemnation and rebuilding of many unsatisfactory radiology departments. As Kaye wrote, "Up to 1920, almost all radiology departments were deplorably housed, often in permanently darkened, crowded and unhygienic cellars, whereas the light, roomy, cheerful and well-ventilated departments of today are frequently a source of justifiable pride to the parent hospitals."[50]

International collaboration between radiologists was inaugurated in 1925 at the First International Congress of Radiology in London. Although recommendations from both the British and the American Protection Committees were considered by the delegates, the discussions were inconclusive. Three years later at the Second Congress in Stockholm, the International X-ray and Radium Protection Committee (IXRPC) was established with Stanley Melville and Kaye as joint secretaries. The latest recommendations of the British Protection Committee were accepted with a few minor modifications.

MARTYRS MEMORIAL

In 1936 the German Röntgen Society, at the suggestion of Hans Meyer of Bremen, erected a monument to the x-ray and radium martyrs of all nations. The monument stands beside the radiology department of St. George's Hospital in Hamburg, the hospital of Heinrich Albers-Schoenberg, the celebrated x-ray pioneer who died from radiation injuries in 1921. Inscribed on the column are the names of x-ray and radium workers of many nationalities who died before 1936, as well as the following inscription written by Kaye:

> To the Röntgenologists and Radiologists of All Nations, Doctors, Physicists, Chemists, Technical Workers, Laboratory Workers, and Hospital Sisters who gave their lives in the struggle against the diseases of mankind. They were heroic leaders in the development of the successful and safe use of x-rays and radium in medicine. Immortal is the glory of the work of the dead.

At the unveiling ceremony of the Martyrs Memorial, the famed French pioneer, Antoine A. Béclère, spoke the following eloquent words:

> I come to bow with reverence before this monument which was piously erected to the victims of x-rays and radium. I come to salute their memory, and honor their sufferings, their sacrifices and their premature deaths. I come also to pay homage to the generous thought of which this monument is an expression . . .
>
> All these victims acquitted their task, humble or exalted, and with the same devotion. All have acquired equal merit, all have equal right to honor. These noble martyrs did not speak the same language, did not belong to the same country, they were of different races and religions. Forgive me, I am wrong—they were all of the same race, the race of brave people; they were all faithful to the same religion, the religion of duty. They were all devoted to the mission of fighting, at the peril of their lives, the same enemies, illness and suffering, with the aid of the marvelous weapon which Röntgen gave to medicine, without fear that this weapon was double-edged and, wielded, as it was, without the precautions now in use, would one day wound and kill them.
>
> The great name and the celebrated name of Röntgen formed part of your national inheritance of which you are naturally proud. You might, without incurring criticism, have reserved this monument for the victims of German nationality alone. You did not desire this, and so the names of those who in all civilized countries have devoted and sacrificed their lives to a common ideal, are here fraternally united in a common homage.

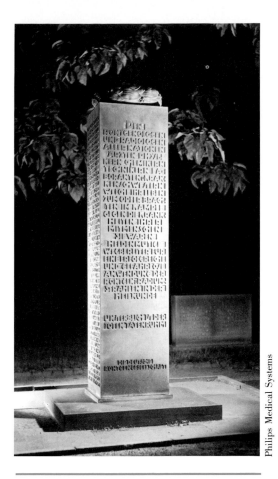

Philips Medical Systems

Monument to x-ray and radium martyrs in Hamburg, Germany.

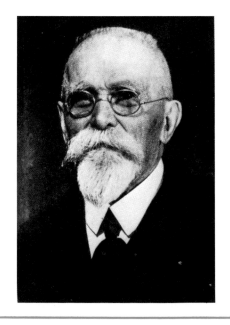

Antoine A. Béclère (1856-1939).

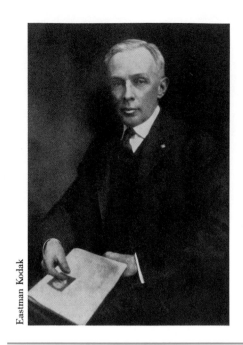

Percy Brown (1875-1950).

In the same year, Percy Brown, an eminent Boston radiologist, published the classic *American Martyrs to Science through the Roentgen Rays*. The work contains biographical accounts of 28 prominent x-ray workers who died of radiation injury. Ironically, one story with which Brown was intimately connected was omitted from the book; Brown himself died of x-ray-induced cancer in 1950 after years of painful suffering.

RADIATION PROTECTION IN THE NUCLEAR AGE

In the summer of 1942, behind locked and guarded doors of the University of Chicago's Metallurgical Laboratory, Enrico Fermi and his fellow physicists were only a few months away from activating the world's first nuclear reactor or "atomic pile." They had calculated the amount of radiation of various kinds that would emerge from atomic piles of various sizes and designs and knew at least approximately how thick a shield of lead, concrete, or other materials would be needed in each instance to reduce this radiation to any desired level. However, before the shielding could be designed, it was essential to know the level of ionizing radiation that could prudently be permitted in the working areas around the pile. This policy decision became the responsibility of the Health Division under the leadership of Robert S. Stone of the University of California. Rather than being satisfied with the official "tolerance dose" recommendations, Stone (with Simeon T. Cantril, a fellow radiologist of the Health Division) launched a comprehensive review of all previously published studies on radiation hazards and safeguards.

The first effort to determine a "safe" or "harmless" dose of radiation was by William Rollins in 1902 (see Chapter 4), who suggested that the amount of radiation should be limited to that which would "fog a photographic plate following 7 minutes of contact exposure." For more than 2 decades, no attempt was made to more precisely define the safe radiation dose.

The first individual to recommend a numerical maximum exposure level based on empirical evidence was probably Arthur Mutscheller. In a landmark 1925 paper,[51] the American physicist noted that "the results of inadequate protection against the harmful effects of overdosage with Roentgen rays that has been reported in the past, are so appalling that search for protective standards is one of the most important problems in Roentgen ray physics and Roentgen ray biology . . . In order to be able to calculate the thickness of the protective shield, there must be known

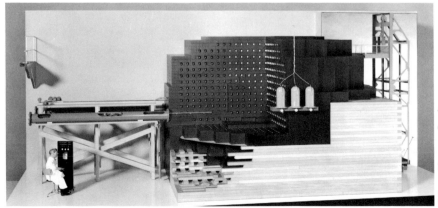

Model of Fermi's first nuclear reactor.

the dose which an operator can, for a prolonged period of time, tolerate without *ultimately* suffering injury."

To solve this problem, Mutscheller visited "several typically good installations" where radiology was being practiced in the New York City area and observed that radiologists and technicians at these laboratories had not suffered any ill effects. On this basis, he decided that the measured levels of radiation in these laboratories were safe and therefore constituted a recommended maximum exposure level. Mutscheller concluded "it seems that under present conditions and standards accepted at present, it is entirely safe if an operator does not receive every 30 days a dose exceeding 1/100th of an erythema dose, and from the present status of our knowledge, this seems to be the tolerance dose for all conditions of operating Roentgen ray tubes for roentgenography, roentgenoscopy, and therapy." Translated into 1942 terminology, Mutscheller's proposed tolerance dose was roughly equivalent to 0.2 roentgen (r) per day.

Mutscheller himself realized the roughness of his estimate, stressing that it was derived "from the average of a limited number of typical examples and is perhaps not sufficiently checked biologically; so it may happen that in the future this dose will be changed either to a larger or a smaller practical tolerance dose."

Mutscheller's new concept was well received, and several other researchers in the United States and Europe repeated his measurements in their own and a few neighboring installations. In Kaye's influential 1928 textbook on radiology, the eminent British physicist averaged these various rough estimates and announced his own recommendation that was close to Mutscheller's.[52] In 1934 the International X-ray and Radium Protection Commission accepted Kaye's recommendation that 0.2 r per day be adopted as the tolerance dose for radiation workers—the daily dose to which workers could be exposed year after year without damage. Two years later (1936), the US Advisory Committee on X-Ray and Radium Protection recommended that the tolerance dose be cut from 0.2 to 0.1 r per day. When members of the Committee were subsequently asked why they had halved the recommended tolerance dose, they indicated that "this was done because it was felt that with the more penetrating radiations from higher voltage machines coming into more general use, a smaller surface dose was necessary." By 1942, Stone was convinced that the generally accepted tolerance-dose recommendations "rested on rather poor experimental evidence" and that it was all too clear that "the scientific data . . . were very limited."

Were the levels of radiation to which radiologists and their assistants were being exposed really entirely safe? Although the incidence of radiation dermatitis had been drastically reduced, a wide range of evidence indicated that radiologists were in fact being damaged by the radiation they were then receiving.[53] The results of a questionnaire sent to all radiologists indicated that there was a much greater-than-normal incidence of sterile marriages and congenital anomalies in their offspring.[54] In 1927, Herman J. Muller, one of America's foremost geneticists, showed conclusively that radiation of the gonads in fruit flies produced mutations that were manifest in subsequent generations. Studies in mice and other mammals confirmed that the number of mutations produced was strictly proportional to the dose administered. Muller concluded his report[55] with an eloquent plea for radiological caution: "We must remember that the thread of germ plasm which now exists must suffice to furnish the seeds of the human race even for the most remote future. We are the present custodians of this all-important material, and it is up to us to guard it carefully and not contaminate it for the sake of an ephemeral benefit to our own generation."

Initial studies had suggested that presumably trivial exposures to ionizing radiation might also increase the risk of leukemia or other forms of cancer. In 1942, Dunlap published an extensive review on the effects of radiation on hematopoietic tissue and included a report of 24 cases of human leukemia.[56] The first epidemiological study of radiation and leukemia was published 2 years later by Henshaw and Hawkins.[57] This classic study indicated that leukemia occurred in the physician population 1.7 times more frequently than the general population. In a letter to the editor of the *Journal of the American Medical Association*, Herman C. March pointed out that the primary reason for the previously reported twofold increase in leukemia among physicians was the inclusion of radiologists. When radiologists were excluded from the physician study population, the leukemia incidence was approximately the same as the general population.[58] Six years later (1950), March published the results of an expanded study that indicated that radiologists had a 10 times higher risk for developing leukemia than a control group consisting of all other physicians.[59]

The early concept of a "tolerance dose" had assumed a threshold response by humans to radiation. Only exposures in excess of the recommended dosage limits would result in injury, whereas lower levels of permissible exposure were considered to be entirely safe. The studies of radiation-induced genetic damage and the increased incidence of leukemia suggested that long-term latent radiation effects followed a linear, nonthreshold, dose-response relationship. If this were true, radiation exposure should be maintained at an even lower level than was currently acceptable. No longer could radiation protection be limited to individuals. As increasingly larger groups of persons would be exposed to ionizing radiation in the atomic age, the exposure to society at large must be considered. No tolerance dose could be considered safe because even the smallest radiation exposure was presumed to be accompanied by a finite probability of latent physiological effect. As Stone[60] perceptively noted, ". . . for the individual there is very little cause for worry, but for the future of the human race, with an ever increasing application of radiations, there is a real problem."

Accordingly, Stone recommended (and the Metallurgical Laboratory adopted) three basic policy decisions: (1) the generally accepted tolerance dose of the US Advisory Committee on X-ray and Radium Protection was to become the Metallurgical Laboratory ceiling above which no radiation exposures would be authorized; (2) the doses actually delivered to personnel would be held as far as possible below this ceiling; and (3) despite other urgent war-time demands, a relatively large-scale research program was to begin without delay, under Metallurgical Laboratory auspices, to secure the missing data needed for prudent future decisions. As Stone remarked, "It was agreed at that time (1942) that we would be given the opportunity to check our calculations by experiments and so establish the tolerable limits of exposure on solid ground."

Stone's strict requirements were successful. The atomic pile shield was designed with such a sufficient margin of safety that the emitted radiation in the control room was at a level too low to be measured. Similarly, when Stone was asked to recommend the amount of plutonium to which workers at Oak Ridge and Hanford might prudently be subjected, he succinctly recommended "The only safe procedure is to see that *none* of it is inhaled or ingested."

New Standards

In 1946 the US Advisory Committee on X-Ray and Radium Protection (formed in 1931) was changed to the National Committee on Radiation Protection and Measurements (NCRP). Under the leadership of Lauriston S. Taylor, the NCRP was a private organization of scientific experts specializing in radiation science that formulated recommendations for radiation control. The Committee, renamed the Council in 1964, is now purely advisory, and its recommendations carry no legal status. However, they are usually adopted by state and federal agencies and codified into law.

With evidence mounting that only acute radiation responses were of the threshold type and that long-term somatic and genetic consequences were of the nonthreshold type, the old term *tolerance dose* was replaced by the term *maximum permissible dose*. Although many felt that this term was equally objectionable, it was defined as "the dose of ionizing radiation that in the light of present knowledge is not expected to cause appreciable bodily injury to a person at any time during his lifetime."[61] The 0.2 or 0.1 r per day pre-war ceilings for occupational exposure established in 1934 and 1936 were cut to 0.3 r per week and then to 5 r per year—roughly a tenfold reduction from the 0.2 r per day level.

In addition to a value for the whole body of occupationally exposed persons, maximal permissible doses were also recommended for specific organs such as the gonads, the bone marrow, and the lenses of the eye. The maximum permissible doses were translated into maximum permissible concentrations for radioactive substances in air, water, milk, and other foodstuff. Furthermore, the principle was recognized that doses received by persons not employed at places where ionizing radiation is used (e.g., neighbors) should also be limited to an amount one tenth that of the maximum permissible dose for employees.

In recognition of the cumulative genetic effect, some maximum permissible doses were not set for daily, weekly, or even annual exposure, but rather for an individual's accumulated exposure from conception until age 30. For types of exposure likely to be experienced by large proportions of the population, the 30-year cumulative dose to the gonads was set at 5 r, substantially less than the 900 r permitted during a 30-year period under the old 0.1 r per day tolerance dose.

Radiology Responds

Before World War II, there was little concern with the dose of ionizing radiation delivered to a patient during the making of a diagnostic x-ray film. Fluoroscopic examinations delivered hundreds of times as much radiation with no apparent harm, and doses thousands of times as large were routinely administered in radiation therapy. Except for a few geneticists like Muller, the risk that any given patient or his remote descendants might be damaged during medical radiography was too implausible to be considered. However, during the late 1940s it became apparent that even though the risk to a single patient, or to all the patients treated in 1 year by a single physician, was hardly of concern, the cumulative exposure of the population as a whole could be significant and that risk could be substantially lowered by decreasing the exposure during each of the tens of millions of radiographic exposures each year.

Radiologists began paying attention to many dose-reducing techniques that had been suggested years earlier but were infrequently used in clinical practice. Substantial reductions in radiation dose to internal organs could be achieved merely by increasing the tube kilovoltage to 85 or higher, rather than the 60 to 70 kV that was customarily used for many diagnostic exposures before World War II. Filtration of the beam to strain out undesirable low-energy radiation, as well as tight coning to limit the volume of tissue irradiated, combined with faster film, better development, and the general use of intensifying screens all resulted in decreased radiation exposure. The widespread use of phototimers dramatically decreased the incidence of underexposed or overexposed studies requiring repeat examinations. Image intensification permitted significant lowering of the radiation dose during fluoroscopic procedures.

Another substantial mechanism for decreasing radiation exposure to the population was the elimination of radiation therapy for benign conditions. Before World War II, radiation was considered the treatment of choice for more than 100 benign conditions. Glasser's classic text listed 96 skin diseases from acne to warts that dermatologists typically treated with radiation.[66] In 1941 and 1942 the *Year Book of Radiology* included abstracts from the world's radiological literature indicating the use of radiation for a broad and bizarre spectrum of conditions, including bursitis, staphylococcal and other infections, pulmonary and other forms of tuberculosis, hyperthyroidism and hyperparathyroidism, angina pectoris, late sequelae of syphilis (including dementia and tabes), sinusitis, Raynaud's disease, many forms of arthritis and rheumatism, high blood pressure, glaucoma, conjunctivitis and other diseases of the eye and its surrounding tissue, persistent nosebleed, psoriasis, herpes simplex, ileitis, asthma, hay fever, peritonitis, and salivary fistulas. Several papers even reported on the value of radiation of the ovaries for an array of menstrual difficulties, infertility, and other "functional disorders of the female." It was even recommended that if a child had one leg longer than the other, the longer leg should be irradiated to curb further growth and thus achieve symmetry. The radiation doses administered for these questionable purposes were substantial, sometimes totalling hundreds of roentgens.

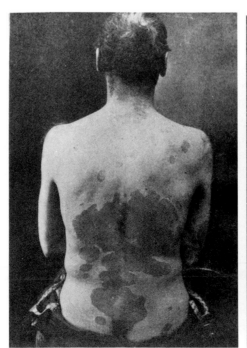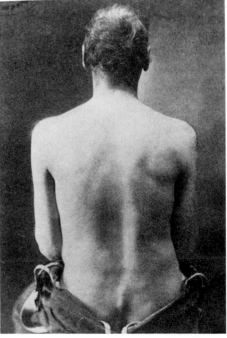

Radiation therapy for benign conditions (1904). *Left*, Pretreatment and *right*, post-treatment photographs of the back of a patient with psoriasis.[9]

By the early 1960s, radiation treatment for benign disease had dramatically decreased. In part, this reflected the development of alternate forms of therapy. The sulfa drugs, penicillin, and other antibiotics and chemical agents made radiation unnecessary for a wide range of infections, and the introduction of cortisone and other steroid drugs provided an alternative to radiation for many inflammatory conditions. Nevertheless, much of the credit for the elimination of radiation treatment for benign disease must go to radiation therapists and dermatologists, who voluntarily relinquished a portion of their traditional practice in exchange for the new philosophy of protection against radiation hazards.

Radiation therapy for benign conditions was now limited to cases that failed to yield to alternative modes of therapy and to conditions in which the medical benefits clearly outweighed the hazards. Much greater attention was paid to selecting proper radiation, such as soft rays for skin conditions to minimize the dosage to internal organs, and to limiting the volume of tissue irradiated.

Concomitant with the decreased radiation exposure in diagnostic and therapeutic radiology, the 1960s saw the introduction of new radioisotopes that delivered much smaller doses than those commonly used in the 1950s while achieving the same or superior diagnostic results. The development of isotopic "cows" led to the widespread availability of radionuclides such as technetium-99m with their short half-lives.

During the 1950s, leaded gloves and aprons finally received widespread acceptance among radiologists and technologists. Although early reports of the benefits of these protective devices had appeared in the literature,[63,64] it was clear that these precautionary measures were infrequently employed. One of the most bizarre rationalizations for not wearing protective apparel during examination of the barium-filled stomach was that the barium itself provided adequate shielding for the ungloved hand when positioned in the middle of the radiation field. As Cilley and associates[65] concluded in their series of five articles (1934-35): "In a routine examination of both the stomach and the colon, the examiners wear no protective devices whatsoever. In spite of the fact that these examiners have sustained multiples of the tolerance dose with impunity, we nevertheless advocate no change whatever in the accepted method of protection." These reports came from the Mayo Clinic, and it is not surprising that leaded protective apparel did not become required at that facility until many years later.

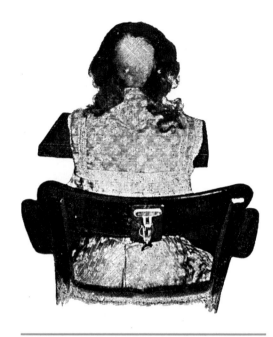

Radiation therapy for favus capillitii (1904). After 3 weeks of x-ray therapy, the patient's hair fell out, revealing a smooth, shining back of the neck.[62]

Government-Practitioner Cooperation[66]

During the 1950s and early 1960s, there was a new appreciation of the possibility that long-term biological effects might be induced by relatively small amounts of radiation. A primary impetus for this concept was apprehension about the consequences of the above-ground testing of nuclear weapons by the United States and the Soviet Union. Ordinary citizens became worried that a harmful agent, undetectable by the senses, might contaminate the environment in trace amounts and find its way into their bodies via air, water, and food. Thus "radiation protection" had taken on a new meaning, expanding to include the public and those who were occupationally exposed. This reflected a broad societal trend toward recognition of the importance of low-level environmental contamination from a host of harmful agents such as the fear of certain pesticide residues, which was the focus of Rachel Carson's 1962 classic *Silent Spring*.

In response to these concerns the Public Health Service of the United States, in cooperation with state and local health agencies, undertook a nationwide program to monitor air, water, and foodstuff for radioactive fallout. Since most Americans, even at the height of nuclear weapon testing, received far more radiation exposure from diagnostic x-ray procedures than from fallout, it seemed reasonable that the government should also try to minimize unnecessary exposure from this ubiquitous source as well.

It soon became clear that the problem of unnecessary radiation exposure from diagnostic x-ray procedures had three distinct facets: equipment (Is the machine capable of producing images with minimum radiation exposure of the patient?); techniques (Is the operator using the machine so as to minimize patient exposure?); and clinical judgment (Is the x-ray examination clinically useful?).

In the program's early days, the emphasis was on upgrading existing x-ray machines, ensuring that they had at least rudimentary collimation and filtration. Many dental machines used in that era were not equipped with collimators, so that they produced excessively large beams that irradiated a patient's thyroid gland and other tissues in the head and neck far beyond the edges of the film. In a joint federal-state program, tens of thousands of dental machines were evaluated in dentists' offices and were retrofitted with simple lead washers, thus reducing the beam size to the area of clinical relevance.

It was also important to motivate and train users of x-ray machines to keep the exposure of their patients to a minimum. In an era when many general-purpose radiographic units still had sets of heavy, cumbersome, fixed-aperture collimators and no beam-finding lights, strong motivation was needed to overcome the operator's natural inclination to use the largest collimator under all circumstances. Therefore a variety of educational initiatives were undertaken, often in cooperation with professional organizations. The following concepts were stressed: use a technique chart rather than guessing at exposure settings, collimate to the area of clinical interest, use the proper filtration, use a gonad shield when appropriate, use fresh developer in a light-tight darkroom, and develop the film according to the manufacturer's time and temperature recommendations rather than relying on the "dip-and-look" method.

In 1968, passage of the Radiation Control for Health and Safety Act gave the government authority to establish and enforce manufacturing performance standards for radiation-emitting devices. The congressional hearings that led to the passage of the Act were driven chiefly by concern about certain models of color television sets that had been found to emit excessive levels of x-radiation. The first standard for diagnostic x-ray equipment was promulgated in 1974. Since it was applied at the manufacturing stage, the standard allowed for the prevention of safety-related problems rather than relying on subsequent corrections in the field.

In the early 1970s the traditional inspections of diagnostic x-ray machines carried out by the states were supplemented by a sophisticated pair of joint programs between the Public Health Service and the state radiation control agencies. The first program, Dental Exposure Normalization Technique (DENT), was intended for dentists, and the second, Breast Exposure Nationwide Trends (BENT), was for physicians conducting mammographic examinations. Although participation was voluntary, nearly all the physicians and dentists involved agreed to participate once the programs had been endorsed by their local professional societies. The remarkable effectiveness of these programs was illustrated by pilot tests of the DENT program in several states, which noted a 40% overall reduction in patient exposure from dental x-rays.

The area of clinical judgment was not addressed until the late 1970s when the American College of Radiology and the government joined in a long-term effort to develop and disseminate "referral criteria" for certain x-ray procedures. These criteria were formulated by expert panels of radiologists and clinicians representing the appropriate specialties and were intended to provide voluntary guidance to clinicians on the indications for the various x-ray procedures. Criteria were published and widely distributed on x-ray pelvimetry, routine chest radiographic screening, presurgical chest radiography, skull radiography after trauma, and dental radiography. The impetus toward developing effective referral criteria was affected by two societal trends in the United States—the demand for cost effectiveness by government and third party payers and the need for a consensus concerning acceptable medical practice during an age of accelerating medical malpractice litigation.

As Mark Barnett concluded in his perceptive article, "Whatever improvements have occurred in medical x-ray protection can be attributed in large measure to the extraordinary degree of cooperation over the past few decades between the Federal government, the states, the health professions and the x-ray industry. Their joint efforts could well serve as a model for progress in other areas."

Bibliography

Barnett M: The evolution of federal x-ray protection programs. RadioGraphics 9:1277-1282, 1989.

Brecher E and Brecher R: The rays: A history of radiology in the United States and Canada, Baltimore, Williams & Wilkins, 1969.

Burrows EH: Pioneers and early years: A history of British radiology, Channel Islands, England, Colophon, 1986.

Bushong SC: The development of radiation protection in diagnostic radiology, Cleveland, CRC Press, 1978.

Nauman JD: Pioneer descriptions in the story of x-ray protection. In Bruwer AJ (ed): Classic descriptions in diagnostic Roentgenology, Springfield, Ill, Charles C Thomas, 1964.

References

1. Gardiner JH: President's address. J Röntgen Society 12:1-10, 1916.
2. Brown P: American martyrs to science through the Roentgen rays. Springfield, Ill, Charles C Thomas, 1936.
3. Dyer FL, Martin TC, and Meadowcroft WH: Edison: His life and inventions. Harpers 2:581, 1929.
4. Editorial comment: Nature (London) 53:421, March 5, 1896.
5. Daniel J: Letter. Science 3:562, March 23, 1896.
6. Kolle FS: The effect of x-rays on the hair. Elect Engineer 23:267, 1897.
7. Hawks HD: The physiologic effects of the Roentgen rays. Elect Engineer 22:276, September 16, 1896.
8. Gilchrist TC: A case of dermatitis due to the X-rays. Bull Johns Hopkins Hosp 18:17-23, 1897.
9. Allen CW: Radiotherapy and phototherapy including radium and high-frequency currents. New York, Lea Brothers, 1904.
10. Martin JM: Practical electro-therapeutics and x-ray therapy. St. Louis, The CV Mosby Co, 1912.
11. Jones FS: Elect Rev 29:17, October 21, 1896.
12. Thomson E: Letter. Boston Med Surg J 135:610-611, 1896.
13. Walsh D: Deep tissue traumatism from Roentgen ray exposure. Brit Med J 2:272-273, 1897.
14. Perthes G: Cited by Colwell HA and Russ S: X-ray and radium injuries. London, Oxford University Press, 1934.
15. Albers-Schoenberg H: Cited by Henshaw PS: Biologic significance of the tolerance dose in x-ray and radium protection. J Nat Cancer Inst 1:789-805, 1941.
16. Gavazzeni S and Minelli S: L'Autopsia d'un radiologo. La Radiologia Medica 1:66-71, 1914.
17. Larkins FE: A case of acute aplastic anaemia. Arch Radiol Electrotherapy 25:380-382, 1921.
18. Stine WM: Effect on the skin of exposure to Roentgen tubes. Elect Rev 29:250, 1896.
19. Tesla N: On the hurtful actions of Lenard and Roentgen tubes. Elect Rev 30: May 5, 1897.
20. Hall-Edwards J: On x-ray dermatitis and its prevention. Proc Roy Soc Med 2:11-34, 1908.
21. Frei GA: X-rays harmless with the static machine. Elect Engineer 22:651, 1896.
22. Leonard CL: The x-ray "burn:" Its production and prevention. NY Med J, p 18, July 2, 1898.
23. Thomson E: Roentgen ray burns. Amer X-ray J 3:451-453, 1898.
24. Rollins W: X-light kills. Boston Med Surg J 144:173, 1901.
25. Codman EA: No practical danger from the x-ray. Boston Med Surg J 144:197, 1901.
26. Rollins W: Notes on x-light. Boston Med Surg J 144:221, 1901.
27. Rollins W: Non-radiable cases for x-light tubes. Elect Rev 40:795-799, 1902.
28. Rollins W: Notes on x-light: the effect of x-light on the crystalline lens. Boston Med Surg J 148:364, 1903.
29. Codman EA: A study of the cases of accidental x-ray burns hitherto recorded. Phila Med J 9:438-442, 1902.
30. Morton WJ and Hammer EW: The x-ray. New York, American Technical Book Co, 1896.
31. Pusey WA and Caldwell EW: The practical application of roentgen rays in therapeutics and diagnosis. Philadelphia, WB Saunders, 1904.
32. Beck C: Roentgen-ray diagnosis and therapy. New York, Appleton & Lange, 1904.
33. Monell SH: A system of instruction in x-ray methods and medical uses of light, hot-air, vibration and high-frequency currents. New York, Pelton, 1902.
34. Kassabian MH: Roentgen rays and electro-therapeutics. Philadelphia, JB Lippincott, 1907.
35. Williams CR: Radiation exposures from the use of shoe-fitting fluoroscopes. N Engl J Med 241:333-335, 1949.
36. Murphy WA: Introduction to the history of musculoskeletal radiology. RadioGraphics 10:915-943, 1990.

37. Pfahler GE: A roentgen filter and a universal diaphragm and protecting screen. Trans Amer Roentgen Ray Soc 217-224, 1906.

38. Pancoast HK: Amer Quart Roentgen 1:67, 1906.

39. Editorial: J Röntgen Soc 1:47, 1905.

40. Leonard CL: Protection of roentgenologists. Trans Amer Roentgen Ray Soc 95-102, 1907.

41. Boggs RH: Protection of patient during roentgen exposure. Trans Amer Roentgen Ray Soc 103-109, 1907.

42. Laurence WS: Discussion. Trans Amer Roentgen Ray Soc 117-118, 1907.

43. Caldwell EW: Discussion. Trans Amer Roentgen Ray Soc 111-112, 1907.

44. Butcher WD: Protection in x-ray work. Arch Roentgen Ray 10:38-39, 1906.

45. Wagner R: Trans Amer Roentgen Ray Soc 161-170, 1908.

46. Mould RF: A history of x-rays and radium. 1980.

47. Scott SG: Notes on a case of x-ray dermatitis with a fatal termination. Arch Roentgen Ray 15:443-444, 1910-11.

48. British X-Ray and Radium Protection Committee: Preliminary report. J. Röntgen Soc 17:100-103, 1921.

49. Andran GM: The society and x-ray protection. Radiography 37:157-165, 1971.

50. Kaye GWC: The story of protection. Radiography 6:41-60, 1940.

51. Mutscheller A: Physical standards of protection against Roentgen ray dangers. AJR 13:65-71, 1925.

52. Kaye GWC: Roentgenology: Its early history, some basic principles, and protective measures. New York, Hoeber, 1928.

53. Carman RD and Miller A: Occupational hazards to the radiologists with special reference to change in the blood. Radiology 3:408-413, 1924.

54. Hickey PM: A report analyzing the results of the questionnaire sent out to radiologists, under the direction of the sex committee of the National Research Council. AJR 18:458-462, 1927.

55. Muller HJ: The effect of Roentgen rays upon the hereditary material. In Glasser O (ed): The science of radiology. Springfield, Ill, Charles C Thomas, 1933.

56. Dunlap CE: Effects of radiation on normal cells: Effects of radiation on the blood and the hemopoietic tissues, including the spleen, the thymus and the lymph nodes. Arch Path 34:562-608, 1942.

57. Henshaw PS and Hawkins JW: Incidence of leukemia in physicians. J Nat Cancer Inst 4:339-343, 1944.

58. March HC: Leukemia in radiologists, correspondents. JAMA 135:179, 1947.

59. March HC: Leukemia in radiologists in a 20-year period. Amer J Med Sci 220:282-285, 1950.

60. Stone RS: The concept of a maximum permissible exposure. Radiology 58:639-642, 1952.

61. NCRP Report No. 17: Permissible dose from external sources of ionizing radiation. National Bureau of Standards, H.B. No. 59, 1954.

62. Freund L: Elements of general radio-therapy. New York, Rebman, 1904.

63. Kaye GWC: Some fundamental aspects of Roentgen rays and the protection of the Roentgen ray worker. AJR 18:401-409, 1927.

64. White TN, Cowie DB, and Delosmer AA: Radiation hazards during roentgenoscopy. AJR 19:639-641, 1943.

65. Cilley EIL, Kirklin BR, and Leddy ET: The dangers of roentgenoscopy: Methods of protection against them. IV. A detailed consideration of the doses received by the fingers of the examiner. AJR 33:390-396, 1935.

66. Barnett M: The evolution of federal x-ray protection programs. RadioGraphics 9:1277-1282, 1989.

DEVELOPMENT OF CLINICAL RADIOLOGY

O, Röntgen, then the news is true,
  And not a trick of idle rumour,
That bids us each beware of you,
  And of your grim and graveyard humour.

We do not want, like Dr. Swift,
  To take our flesh off and to pose in
Our bones, or show each little rift
  And joint for you to poke your nose in.

We only crave to contemplate
  Each other's usual full-dress photo;
Your worse than "altogether" state
  Of portraiture we bar *in toto!*

The fondest swain would scarcely prize
  A picture of his lady's framework;
To gaze on this with yearning eyes
  Would probably be voted tame work!

No, keep them for your epitaph,
  these tombstone-souvenirs unpleasant;
Or go away and photograph
  Mahatmas, spooks, and Mrs. B-s-nt!

Punch, January 25, 1896

CHAPTER 12

Chest Radiology

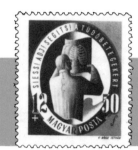 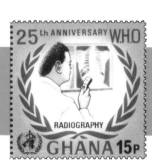 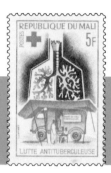 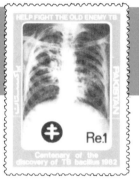

Soon after Roentgen's discovery, fluoroscopy of the chest became an established clinical procedure. The most comprehensive early discussion of the use of x-rays in thoracic diseases was presented by Francis H. Williams of Boston at the May, 1897 meeting of the Association of American Physicians. After initially describing the effects of x-rays on organic substances in isolation, Williams detailed the x-ray appearance of normal human anatomy and physiology before describing the findings in various pathological states[1]:

> To use the Roentgen rays successfully in practice it is first essential that the physician become familiar with the appearances in the fluoroscope which present themselves in health by examining a number of healthy persons of different ages and weights. This applies particularly to the thorax, and the picture of this part of the body, when seen on the screen of a large fluoroscope, presents so much that it should be studied systematically. The trunk appears lighter above than below the diaphragm, and the rise and fall of this muscle, which is dark in the fluoroscope, are distinctly seen. The chest is divided vertically by an ill-defined dark band, which includes the back bone, on each side of which the lungs, forming the brightest part of the picture, are crossed by the darker ribs; this band varies in width according to the intensity of the light, narrowing as this becomes stronger; with a strong light the vertebrae from the neck to the heart are made out. The pulsating heart is seen, especially the dark ventricles, the outlines of the venae cavae and of the pulmonary artery, and under favorable conditions the lighter right auricle. A small portion of one side of the arch of the aorta may be observed in the first intercostal space to the left of the sternum. After this general view has been taken the outline of the lungs should be noted during full inspiration and expiration, and the excursion made by the diaphragm during quiet breathing and during full inspiration and expiration.

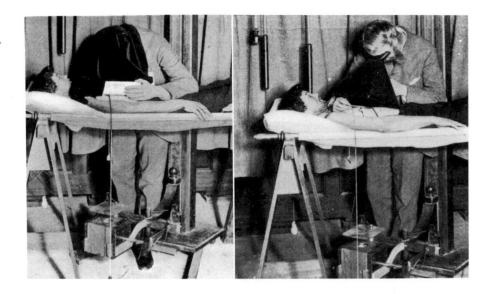

Method of examining the whole thorax (*left*) with a large open screen measuring 30 × 35 cm (1901).[2] Method of drawing outlines on a patient's skin (*right*) while looking through the fluoroscope (1901).[2]

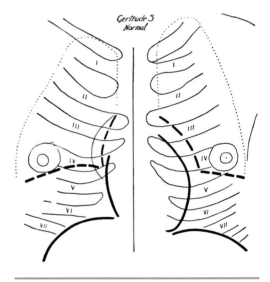

Gertrude S
Normal

Diagram of x-ray outlines of a normal chest (1901). The heavy lines indicate the position of the part in deep inspiration, the broken lines in expiration, the dotted line shows the limit of the bright pulmonary area.[2]

The lungs usually appear brighter during deep inspiration; in younger persons brighter than older persons, as the tissues of the former are more easily penetrated by the rays. In the stout, the lungs appear darker than in the thin, because the outlines are dull, as it were, by a thicker layer of tissues, which contain much water. It has seemed to me that the right apex is normally larger than the left apex. The normal brightness of the lungs and the normal outlines of the clavicles and ribs should be observed, for, as we note different degrees of pallor by reference to our standard of color in health, in the same way it is necessary to know the normal amount of light which should penetrate any given part in order to recognize variations from the normal. The eye must be trained in the use of the x-rays as is the ear for auscultation and percussion.

Williams stressed the importance of bilateral examination for comparing normal with diseased tissue[1]:

In making examinations of the lungs, changes in the amount of light seen in the fluoroscope should be carefully observed: for example, whether or not one lung is darker than the other. In pathological conditions the indications of change in density, shown usually by diminished brightness, may be estimated by comparing the two sides and observing whether the outlines of the organs and whether the ribs and clavicles are more clearly seen on one side than on the other. When both sides are diseased, the opportunity for direct comparison with the normal is lost, and one is obliged to depend on the recollection of the normal in an individual of the same build.

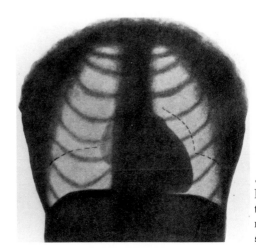

Diagram showing the heart and the outline of the diaphragm of a normal chest, as seen in the fluoroscope during full inspiration (1897).[1]

Evaluation of diaphragmatic movement was another vital part of the examination. Williams noted that the diaphragm in six men with healthy lungs moved an average of 2¾ inches on the right and 2½ inches on the left. In eighteen patients with tuberculosis, the average movement of the diaphragm was 1¼ inches. He also noted that in health the diaphragm was less sharply defined in expiration than in inspiration.

Williams stressed correlation of the radiographic appearance with the pathological findings. As he wrote, "In order to get further suggestions in regard to the possibilities of the x-ray examinations in diseases of the lungs, I took a number of radiographs of healthy and diseased lungs just after death, which were removed from the body and put over a photographic plate."

Williams next turned to his experience in patients with pulmonary tuberculosis. To eliminate bias in all cases, he examined patients with the fluoroscope before any knowledge of the physical examination. Later, he compared his own radiological findings in each case with the physical examination of the referring physician. He concluded that "we can detect an abnormal condition of the lung in some cases of tuberculosis earlier by means of the fluoroscope than by auscultation and percussion. In most cases of pulmonary tuberculosis the fluoroscope enables us to estimate the amount of lung involved better than any other method of examination."

Characteristic radiographic findings included:

> a diminution in the volume of the diseased lung shown by the position and movement of the diaphragm [and] an increase in density by diminution in the normal brightness, the degree and extent varying in accordance with the increase in, and extent of, the density. The lung may become so dense that no more rays pass through it than through the liver. The brightness of light in the lungs indicates the amount of air in the chest. The diaphragm lines may be partially or wholly obliterated, as well as the outline of the heart.

In patients with pneumonia, Williams performed fluoroscopy not only during the active stage of the disease but also during the period of convalescence. As he noted, by observing the patients at intervals of 2 or 3 or more days, "as they improve, we may see the dark areas become lighter and lighter, and finally disappear; and we may see the excursion of the diaphragm, which has been restricted and restricted on the lower side, become gradually longer as the lungs clear up . . ."

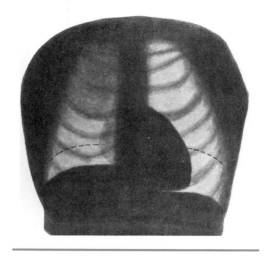

Williams' diagram illustrating tuberculosis of the lung (1897).[1]

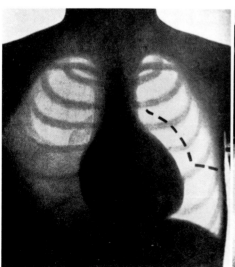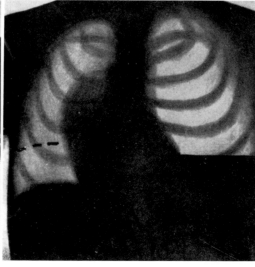

Williams' diagrams illustrating various chest diseases. *Left*, Pleurisy with a small effusion (1901.[2] *Right*, Hydropneumothorax (1901).[2]

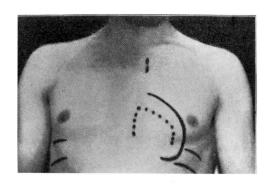

Williams' diagram illustrating emphysema (1901).[1]

Williams also noted that in patients with pleurisy and effusion the amount of fluid could be estimated by the amount of light that passed through the thorax. In large effusions, no more rays passed through it than through the liver, and the outlines of the diaphragm, ribs, and heart were obliterated on the side of the effusion. A smaller amount of fluid enabled the outlines of some of the upper ribs to be seen and only outlines low down in the thorax were ill defined. The fluoroscope also assisted him in distinguishing between an effusion and a thickened pleura.

In emphysema, Williams observed fluoroscopically that

> the lungs are unnaturally clear and their volume is increased; the dilated right auricle and pulmonary artery are observed, and the whole enlarged heart is seen more clearly than normal, although by percussion its true outline cannot be determined; it is also seen to lie lower than in health, and in the later stages in a more vertical direction. The diaphragm is seen to be lower than normal and the excursion which it performs between deep inspiration and expiration to be less than normal.

Williams observed a number of patients with hydrothorax and pulmonary edema and concluded that these conditions were more frequent than had been supposed:

> On first examining a patient of this class, his condition being unknown, I was surprised to find how difficult was the passage of the rays, and when I saw that the picture of the patient's thorax under fluoroscopy was unusually dark, supposed something was wrong with my Crookes tube; but after trying another I realized that the patient's chest was denser than normal; the tube was not at fault. I have examined a number of cases which illustrate the aid the fluoroscope renders in congestion or oedema of the lungs; this instrument showed that one of these conditions was present when it was not made by physical signs, and it thus assists the physician to recognize the interference that may occur in the pulmonary circulation in cardiac or renal disease.

After detailing the radiographic findings in pneumothorax and aneurysms and describing the appearance of the heart, Williams[1] summarized his experience with fluoroscopy of the chest:

> The normal brightness of the chest having been observed in the fluoroscope, the departure from the normal in two directions may be noted by comparison. First, a given part of the chest may be darker than normal on account of the obstruction offered to the passage of the rays, which is due to the *increase* of density that occurs in tuberculosis, pneumonia, infarction, oedema, congestion of the lungs, aneurisms, new growths, or to fluid in the pleural and pericardial sacs, that occurs in pleurisy with effusion and pericarditis with effusion; the distribution, location, and amount of this increase in density which the fluoroscope shows, assists us in some cases to distinguish between these diseases or conditions. Second, a given part of the chest may be brighter than normal, because it is *more* permeable than in health by the rays on account of the diminution in density, due in the case of emphysema to increase in the amount of air in the lungs, or, in the case of pneumothorax, to increase in the amount of air entering the thorax and displacing the lung.

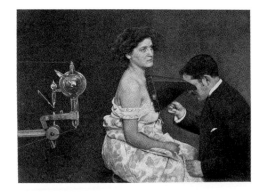

Fluoroscopy of the chest (1910). Note the total lack of shielding of the x-ray tube.[4]

Other pioneer radiologists made important contributions to the fluoroscopic evaluation of the chest. Bouchard in Paris was the first to publish the fluoroscopic observations in patients with pleural effusions. He addressed the problem of distinguishing between the different appearances produced by pleuritic effusions and congestion of the lungs. "When opacity of great extent is not accompanied by displacement of the mediastinum, it is more probably caused by pulmonary infiltration than by pleural effusion. On the contrary, if the opacity becomes gradually more pronounced from above downward, and if the heart is displaced, whilst the other side is transparent, there is probably effusion."[3]

In England, Hugh Walsham produced impressive radiographs of cavitating and miliary tuberculosis,[5] as well as thoracic aneurysms.[6] In the United States, Augustus W. Crane produced an exhaustive treatise on the application of fluoroscopy to the respiratory system.[7]

By the end of the century, C. M. Moullin in an address to the Röntgen Society wrote[8]:

> to such an extent has the fluorescent screen been improved, and so easy has investigation with it been made, that it is probable that some day the examination of a patient's chest with it will be considered as much a matter of routine and as little to be neglected in all doubtful cases as an examination with the stethoscope is at the present time. Valuable as are the indications given by the ophthalmoscope in obscure disease of the brain, they are not to be compared with those which can be obtained by systematic and skilled use of the fluoroscent screen in diseases of the heart and lungs.[8]

Although fluoroscopy had been used almost exclusively up to that time, reports of radiation dermatitis and the first death attributable to the effects of radiation emphasized the hazards of the technique and it was almost abandoned. Fortunately, the decline of fluoroscopy was concurrent with the steadily improving quality and decreased exposure time of radiographic plates.[9] In 1901, Hugo von Ziemssen and Hermann Rieder published a beautiful atlas illustrating the results of chest radiographs made with exposures of 1 second or less. Examples of this "instantaneous skiagraphy," which permitted chest radiographs to be obtained without respiratory or cardiac movements, were presented at the 1902 ARRS meeting in separate papers by Henry Hulst[10] and Mihran Kassabian.[11]

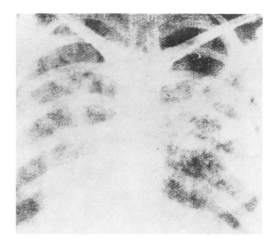

Miliary tuberculosis (1901).[5]

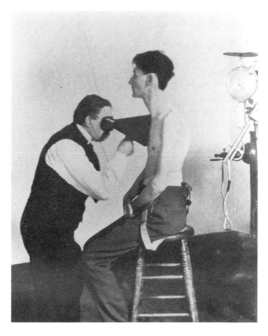

Fluoroscopy of the chest performed as a "screening" examination for pulmonary tuberculosis. The operator is Rudis-Jicinsky, the first secretary of the ARRS.

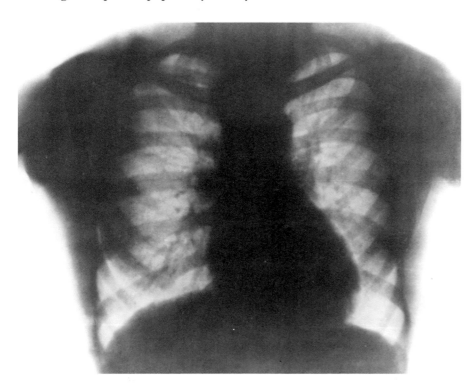

Instantaneous radiograph of an adult chest (1900).[12]

189

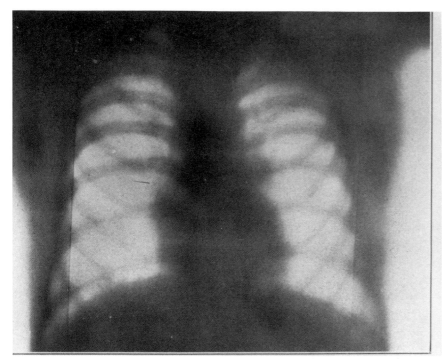 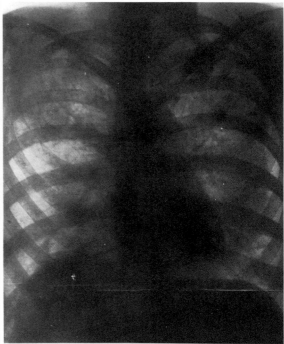

Instantaneous radiographs (1902). *Left*, Normal chest.[11] *Right*, Tuberculosis.[10]

Although some doubters were convinced that rapid-exposure radiography would not become popular because of the hazard to tubes (which at $20 apiece were not to be sacrificed lightly), the technique rapidly gained favor. Pfahler's demonstration of "tubercules the size of a pin head" indicated that it was possible to obtain plates of remarkably good technical quality despite the imperfections of the available gas-tube equipment.[9]

The development of the Coolidge hot-cathode x-ray tube and intensifying screens led to a dramatic expansion in chest radiography as increasingly clear and detailed radiographs permitted improved lesion detection and differential diagnosis. The radiographic evaluation of tuberculosis continued as a major focus of interest. Clinicians generally agreed that the chest radiograph was superior to physical examination alone for detecting and characterizing pulmonary tuberculosis, and sanatoriums began performing x-ray examinations on all admitted patients. In 1910, Lewis Gregory Cole observed[13]:

> considering the large percentage of cases in which tuberculosis is found at autopsy when only a few gross sections are made of the specimen, and the fact that the Germans say that 98% of all adults have or have had a tuberculous lesion of the lung, and that 93% of children reacted to the cutaneous tuberculin test, it is not a question of who has tuberculosis, but what is the variety and extent of the lesion and is it active or inactive. If pulmonary tuberculosis can be diagnosticated radiographically as early and accurately as now appears, and if one can state with a reasonable degree of certainty the variety of the lesion and whether it is active or inactive, and can determine with absolute certainty whether the process is advancing, held in check, or resolving, it seems that the question of the diagnosis of incipient pulmonary tuberculosis is solved.

Extensive correlation of radiographic and pathological findings, especially by H. Kennon Dunham,[14] eventually led to the development of radiographic criteria for the diagnosis of tuberculosis. Systems were proposed for classifying tuberculosis in terms of the x-ray findings,[15] and

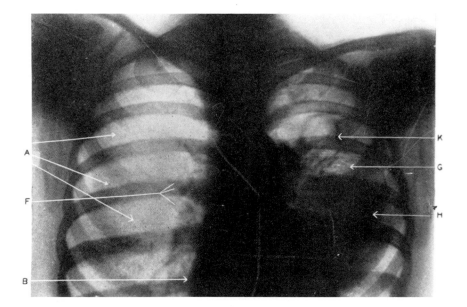

Tuberculosis (1910). In this patient with typical symptoms, physical signs indicated only a slight involvement. There is a left mid-lung infiltrate (*G*) with a consolidation below it (*H*) and a 3-cm cavity above it (*K*). On the right, there is a mottled infiltrate (*F*). *A*, Normal lung markings; *B*, normal heart.[3]

in 1917 the first edition of *Diagnostic Standards and Classification of Tuberculosis* was published.[9]

Continued refinements in the differential diagnosis of pulmonary tuberculosis led to the emergence as discrete disorders of other pulmonary lesions that produced somewhat similar yet distinct radiographic findings. Among these were the large group of inhalation changes in the lung known generally as the *pneumoconioses.* The initial radiographic studies of pneumoconiosis were made by the South African Miners' Phthisis Commission (1916). Silicosis was already a compensable disease in South Africa, and thus the establishment of objective radiographic criteria for its diagnosis was of utmost importance.[9]

During the next two years, three major American studies[16-18] reviewed the radiographic findings in pneumoconiosis; the latter two developed schemes for radiographic classification.

Lanza and Childs[17] reported the results of a clinical and radiographic study sponsored by the United States Public Health Service and the Bureau of Mines that investigated 433 cases of "miners' consumption" among the zinc miners in Missouri.[16] As summarized in an extensive review of the pneumoconioses by Henry K. Pancoast and Eugene P. Pendergrass (1925), the progress of the condition was divided into the following three stages[19]:

First Stage: The root shadows are denser and more extensive, and they show nodules; the trunk shadows are increased in density and breadth, with numerous punctate deposits of varying size along them; the appearance is symmetrical on both sides at first, but not so later; there is no difference in diaphragmatic excursion.

Second Stage: In addition to the foregoing there are found fairly symmetrical small, circumscribed, dense areas throughout both lungs, and later larger masses accumulate, usually at the lower part of the upper third, about the root shadows; the domes of the diaphragms seem accentuated.

Third Stage: This differs from the second only in the extent of lung involvement, indicated by increased numbers of deposits and more massive groupings. They then go on to describe more advanced fibrotic changes, with heart, vessel and tracheal dis-

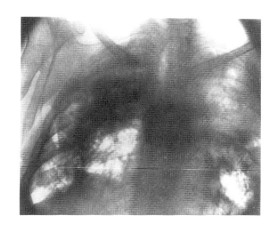

Pneumoconiosis in a coal miner who worked 30 years inside the mines (1918). "Extreme fibrosis of the third stage, with greatest density in the subapical regions where it simulates consolidation. Emphysema at bases; bronchiectasis on left side; diaphragm almost fixed. Intense dyspnea but repeated sputum examination negative."[18]

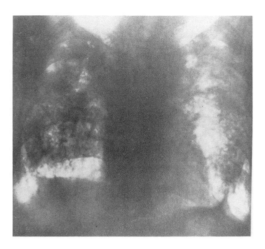

Pneumoconiosis in a potter with a 45-year occupational history (1918). "Almost complete fixation of diaphragm (intense dyspnea). Hilus shadows increased; linear markings obscured; emphysema bases; dense mottling becoming conglomerate, especially toward apices; extreme diffuse fibrosis, with bands to diaphragm, and heart and vessels drawn to the left; bronchiectatic cavities both subapical regions. Repeated sputum examinations negative."[18]

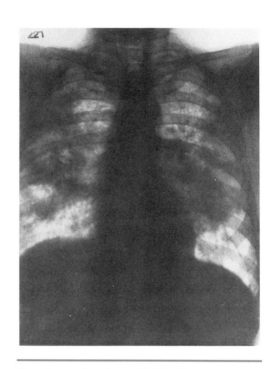

Granite-worker lung (1921). Extensive patchy disease following long-term exposure. The physical examination was essentially normal.[20]

placement and restricted diaphragmatic excursion which they were inclined to ascribe to a tuberculous complication, but which we now know may be due entirely to advanced silicosis, although tuberculosis may be a factor. This classification, with a few minor changes, answers the purpose admirably today (eight years later).

Other major contributions to the understanding of pneumoconiosis were the extensive series on dust inhalation in the granite industry by Jarvis[20] and Sparks' study of asbestosis.[21] Jarvis stressed the value of serial radiography to evaluate changes in the lungs over a considerable period of time. In 1930, the first International Labour Office (ILO) classification of the radiographic appearance of pneumoconiosis was published as part of the recorded proceedings of an international conference on silicosis held in Johannesburg, South Africa. Since then, periodic updates of the classification have appeared.

The radiographic appearance of primary carcinoma of the lung and pulmonary metastases was described in a series of papers published between 1918 and 1920. As early as 1912, Adler observed[22]:

it was not very long ago that A. Frankel wrote that x-rays were of little service in the diagnosis of lung tumors. Since then the x-rays have become a most remarkable and efficient aid to diagnosis in general, and there exists the well-founded hope of their increasing efficacy as further improvements in apparatus and advances in technique are made . . . The hope may reasonably be entertained that with the systematic and proper application of the x-rays to the exploration of the chest, the diagnosis of lung tumor may be assured when no other means will have equally certain results.

In 1917, F. B. McMahon and Russell Carman[23] described in detail the radiographic appearance of primary carcinoma of the lungs and bronchi and offered differential points in distinguishing these "rare" tumors from other intrathoracic conditions: "in most instances the roentgen findings in primary carcinoma of the lungs are pathognomonic of the disease, and may be the first to suggest the exact nature of the pulmonary lesion." They recognized three types of the disease: infiltrative, miliary, and mixed, "which correspond to the gross pathological groupings." A striking feature common to all tumors "and one of considerable diagnostic importance is the absence of practically any increase in mediastinal density."

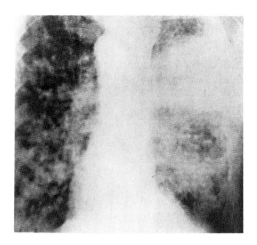

Primary carcinoma of the lung (1918). Multiple areas of increased density extending throughout both lungs, with a massive area involving the base of the upper right lobe.[23]

McMahon and Carman noted:

the presence of extensive pleural involvement in primary carcinoma of the lung renders the interpretation of the roentgenogram correspondingly more difficult, but not impossible. The presence of large pleural effusions tends to completely mask the roentgenographic picture and conceal the underlying and principal pathological condition in the lung. A second roentgen examination is necessary after thoracentesis. Fortunately these latter two conditions rarely occur until the terminal stages of the disease.

In a subsequent report, Arthur Christie (1921) cautioned that although[24]:

there is a certain roentgen picture that is practically pathognomonic of primary carcinoma of the lungs, there are certain other conditions so closely resembling it that constant watchfulness is necessary to avoid mistakes. It is essential in every case to interpret the roentgenogram in the light of these symptoms, the physical findings, and especially the mode of onset and course of the disease. Unfortunately, like malignant disease in other parts of the body, tumors of the lung may be almost or quite symptomless."

Christie observed that primary lung carcinoma was apparently much more common than previously believed. He decried the feelings of some that "it is not very important whether we make an actual diagnosis or not, because the patient is doomed anyway," for he thought that

it is a matter of great importance to the patient. Aside from the question of scientific accuracy in diagnosis, it is of great moment to the patient whether he is going to be moved around from here to there as a tuberculosis patient for the rest of his life, with the final destruction of false hopes that he may get well, or whether it is definitely known from the beginning that he has a malignant disease.

Four years later (1925), Ross Golden reported the bronchostenosis and resulting atelectasis caused by carcinoma of the lung. He described the reverse S-shaped curve (S sign of Golden) on frontal views in patients with collapse of the right upper lobe in whom the upper, laterally concave segment of the S was formed by the elevated minor fissure, whereas the lower medial convexity was produced by the tumor mass that caused bronchial narrowing and was responsible for the collapse.[25]

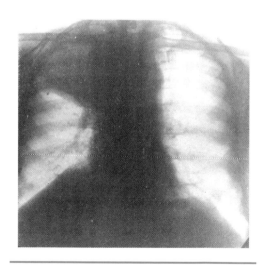

S sign of Golden (1925). "The area of the right upper lobe is occupied by a dense shadow with a sharply defined concave lower margin. The upper lobe has become atelectatic."[25]

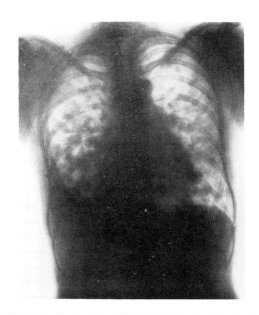

Pulmonary metastases (Crane, 1918). Multiple nodules in both lungs.[26]

As Augustus W. Crane wrote (1918)[26]:

One of the substantial contributions of roentgenology to clinical medicine is the ready diagnosis of pulmonary metastasis in malignant disease. In pre-roentgen days carcinoma or sarcoma of the lungs was reported almost exclusively from post-mortem findings. The diagnosis could rarely be final in the absence of an autopsy, and the frequency of pulmonary invasion was a matter of statistical conjecture. But now the diagnosis can be made at an early stage by the x-ray plate with a precision unexcelled by the roentgen diagnosis of any other pulmonary lesion. The detection of a pulmonary metastasis is of decisive surgical importance. The question of the nature of the primary lesion, the question of operability and the question of prognosis are thus settled. For this reason the x-ray examination of the lungs has been established as routine in some surgical clinics in cases of suspected malignancy anywhere in the body.

One year later (1919), George Pfahler[27] noted that pulmonary metastases often were not suggested clinically "because of the general good condition of the patients and the indefinite symptoms which this disease produces." He stressed the early recognition of pulmonary metastases[27]:

as a guide in the treatment. In some instances it will prevent a mutilating operation, and I am hoping in the future that its early recognition may lead to the early institution of some form of constitutional treatment which is as yet undiscovered. I am sure that at present many patients are operated upon with the hope of complete recovery at a time when there is already distinct metastasis in the lungs and mediastinum.

Pfahler observed that "metastatic malignant disease of the lung is common, and should always be looked for in connection with advanced malignant disease. A roentgen examination of the chest should be made in every case of carcinoma of the breast referred for operation or roentgen therapy."

The frequent involvement of the lungs and mediastinum in patients with Hodgkin's disease, lymphosarcoma, and leukemia was reported by Byrl Kirklin and Hans Hefke (1931). However, they noted that the x-ray examination "does not permit a precise diagnosis of any one of these diseases" and suggested that they all be considered as one group "which might be called either lymphoblastoma or malignant lymphoma."[28]

Le Roy Sante stressed the importance of serial radiography, especially in patients with lobar pneumonia. After initially appearing as a homogenous consolidation, "during the stage of resolution the shadow becomes mottled and irregular, complete resolution being effected often in a very short time—three days. The average time for resolution is seven to ten days after the crisis. The persistence of shadow or failure of resolution after fourteen days is distinctly pathological, and suggests some complicating lesion."[29] Sante listed the most frequently encountered pulmonary complications following pneumonia as (1) dry pleurisy with thickening of the pleura; (2) pleural effusion, either serous or purulent, and either general or local; (3) plastic serofibrinous pleurisy; (4) chronic interstitial pneumonia or fibrosis; and (5) lung abscess.

A major topic of radiological interest at this time was "pulmonary atelectasis." Numerous reports described acute and chronic collapse of the lung that was either spontaneous or related to inspired foreign bodies, benign or malignant bronchial tumor, and tuberculosis.[9] The definitive work on the appearance of lobar and segmental collapse of the lung was a

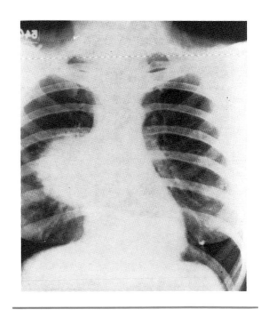

Hodgkin's disease (1931). Extensive involvement of the right hilum.[28]

of the ramifying bronchi. An English writer has considered them to be the lines of the interlobular pleura. For the sake of establishing the meaning of these tracings, a number of experiments was made. A cadaver was chosen, which was injected with the ordinary lead solution of the anatomic laboratory, as fully as possible, the solution being injected at different intervals so as to distend thoroughly the vessels. The cadaver was allowed to dry out, so that the tissues did not present much fluid. An exposure was then made with the plate next to the dorsal side of the thorax, under conditions to accentuate the contrast of the injected vessels. On comparing this plate with the normal chest of the young adult, it will be seen that there is a marked similarity between the vague tracings of the living subject and the representation of the pulmonary vessels of the cadaver.

After describing additional studies of differential injections of the bronchi and blood vessels, Hickey concluded that "from these experiments it would seem to the writer that the tracings which we often see in the midst of the pulmonary tissue *usually* represent ramifications of the pulmonary vessels."

Attempts to visualize the pulmonary circulation in living subjects date from the same era as the early injection studies on cadavers. Franck and Alwens (1910) and Heuser (1919) demonstrated the pulmonary vessels following the intravenous injection of contrast material (see Chapter 13). Perhaps the first intentional study of the pulmonary arteries in a living man was reported by Dunner and Calm (1923) in Berlin. Although their single illustration showed only the left brachial and axillary veins up to the first rib, Dunner and Calm[48] noted that "if one compares the films taken before and after the injection, it is readily recognized that the structures of the lungs, only slightly visible before injection, are much clearer and more apparent on the second exposure." Thus they concluded that "it is possible to demonstrate the pulmonary vessels in the living human being in some instances to the point that the vessel and the side branches are seen like in an anatomical preparation when the vessel is injected."[48]

To assess changes in the pulmonary circulation with pneumothorax, Adolf Lindblom of Sweden (1928) performed intravenous injections of water-soluble material in rabbits and obtained an excellent set of radiographs using serial films and short exposures.[49]

The technical breakthrough permitting effective pulmonary arteriography was the work of Werner Forssmann, who in 1929 first catheterized the human heart, initially in cadavers and then in himself (see Chapter 13). Using this technique for catheterizing the right atrium, Moniz, de Carvalho, and Lima (1931) performed the first true pulmonary arteriography (angiopneumography) by demonstrating that "injections of sodium iodide directly into the right ventricle, auricle and jugular vein produced good visualization of pulmonary arteries and veins."[50] Lopo de Carvalho became the chief proponent of this technique, writing voluminously on this subject for many years thereafter.[51] The development of safer contrast agents that could be injected in much larger quantity permitted demonstration of the pulmonary vasculature by direct contrast injection into a cubital vein without the use of a cardiac catheter.

The selective injection of contrast material into a pulmonary artery was a natural outgrowth of the development of selective angiocardiography. Although used as early as 1933 in animals, Bolt and Rink in 1951 were among the first to perform selective pulmonary arteriography in humans.[52] By placing the catheter far peripherally, they obtained arte-

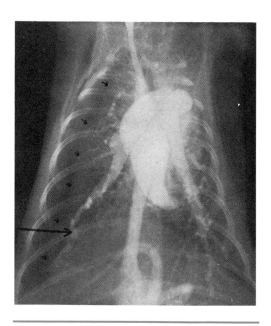

Pulmonary arteriography in rabbits (1928). Pneumothorax with collapse of the right lung 6-days-old. Superb visualization of the vascular tree after the injection of contrast material into a vein in the ear.[49]

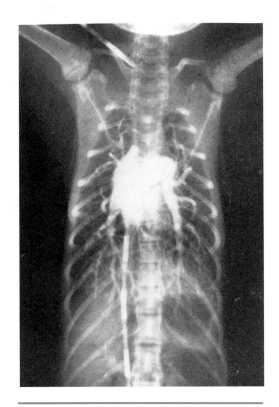

Angiopneumography of a monkey (1931). Injection of an 80% solution of sodium iodide into the right auricle by catheterization of the inferior vena cava.[50]

rial, capillary, and venous delineation simultaneously. An extension of this procedure was wedge pulmonary arteriography, described by Bell and coworkers in 1958 for study of the terminal arteries.[53]

Although selective arteriography produced clearer opacification of the pulmonary vascular tree than did peripheral venous or intracardiac injection, some authors argued that in most cases this technique was neither necessary nor desirable since it involved additional effort, excluded information about the other portions of the lungs, and might be associated with a higher complication rate. Other workers stressed that diseased segments of the arterial tree caused blood to be shunted away from that segment, so that a venous or intracardiac injection tended to opacify comparatively normal branches remote from the disease rather than the area of interest.[54]

Although pulmonary arteriography currently is performed almost exclusively to investigate thromboembolic disease of the lung, it previously was used for many other purposes. These included detection of congenital abnormalities of the pulmonary vascular tree (e.g., agenesis or coarctation of the pulmonary artery; arteriovenous malformations; intralobar pulmonary sequestration[55-59]; anomalous pulmonary venous drainage[60]; investigation of the resectability of bronchogenic carcinoma[61,62]; differentiation of mediastinal masses[63]; guide for extirpative surgery for bullous emphysema[64]; and even the assessment of active pulmonary hemorrhage.[65]

PHOTOFLUOROGRAPHY

An interest in the public health became a major force in medicine in the 1930s. There was a "desire to provide a simple, inexpensive, and yet reasonably accurate method for the surveying of large numbers of individuals for the presence of tuberculosis or other diseases of the lungs."[66] This idea was not new; x-ray surveys had been made in South Africa in 1911 and two of the old regiments of World War I had been similarly screened. Ironically, the Surgeon General opposed screening all recruits at that time for several reasons, including the expense and the problem of storing the plates. Although the radiograph was clearly the ideal medium for detecting incipient tuberculosis, mass x-ray surveys with conventional techniques were impractical. The solution was the development of photofluorography as a practical technique.[9]

Within a year of Roentgen's discovery of x-rays, at least three articles described methods for photographing the image on a fluorescent screen.[67-69] J. Mount Bleyer stressed that[68]:

> one of the most important advantages that the photofluoroscope presents over the roentgen method of photographing, is that curves, corners, and angles are no obstacle to it, while an object in the Roentgen photography must always be in direct contact on a flat plate containing the sensitized plate, the reason being that the Roentgen rays must be applied directly on the surface of the object, while with the photo-fluoroscope it may be taken at a short distance.

Of more relevance to future developments was the comment by John MacIntyre that[69]:

> we have yet no means of bringing Röntgen rays to a focus, but the thought occurred to me that instead of using large plates to cover half

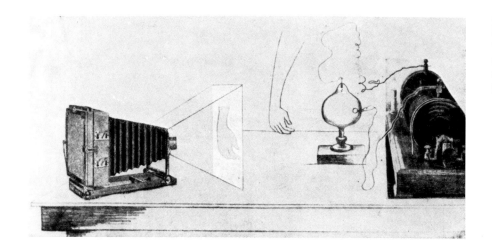

of the body, one might photograph the shadows as seen on the fluorescent screen by means of the camera . . . By this new method we may be able to reduce a picture of a large portion of the human body to magic-lantern slide size right away.

In 1911, Eugene Caldwell[9] experimentally demonstrated beyond question that the camera could record much more than the eye could see on the fluorescent screen. Nevertheless, more than 20 years would pass before the practical application of photofluorography to clinical problems.

Priority for the earliest large-scale clinical application of photo-fluorography goes to Manoel de Abreu of Brazil, who used the technique "in order to obtain records at a moderate expense and thereby make possible obligatory thoracic examinations of the general public."[70] He described "Roentgen-photography" as "a method for collective mass examinations, permitting the achievement of a large and never before realized social investigation for the purpose of detecting tuberculosis under ordinary living and working conditions." He added that "only a vast number of statistics in which will be included large human groups in terms of dwelling quarters, provinces, schools, factories, social classes, cities, neighborhoods, and rural zones will permit a rational orientation regarding prophylactic measures." In the past, "two methods of x-ray analysis have been available for the thoracic survey of large groups of individuals. One, radiography, is expensive and impractical, while the other, fluoroscopy, requires the services of a considerable number of skilled specialists (about 150 per million examinations per annum)." In contrast, photography of the fluoroscopic screen could "permit practical chest surveys of large groups effectively and have a low cost." De Abreu preferred 35-mm film because it was easily available and inexpensive (about one cent per record): "We are convinced that the small image, 2.4 cm square, has a perfection of detail completely adequate for a diagnostic survey."

After three years' experience, de Abreu reported that[71]: "collective fluorography is universally accepted . . . The objections with which we had to contend at the beginning were principally that since the initial roentgenological indications of tuberculosis are frequently very vague, fluorography would not show sufficient detail to demonstrate early tuberculosis, and that fluoroscopy in various planes was essential to diagnosis. Also, the wear and tear on x-ray tubes from the exposures on a large scale would make the procedure expensive." In answer to these possible disadvantages, de Abreu recorded Hans Holfelder's remark that "for the first

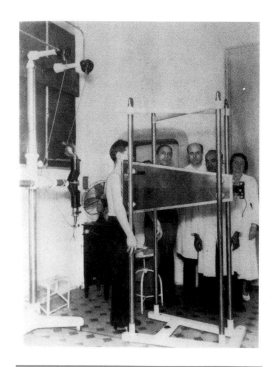

Roentgen-photography apparatus (1937).[71]

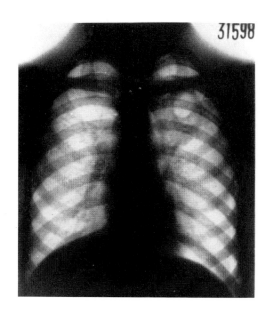

Photofluorogram in patient with tuberculosis (1939) shows left upper lobe cavity with previously undiagnosed disease.

time in practice, a means has been found which, in my opinion, is capable of settling the problem of the proper position of roentgen diagnosis in the battle against tuberculosis," as well as R. Vaccarezza's comment that "its application in social work I consider one of the greatest medical conquests of recent time."

After a visit to de Abreu in Brazil, D. O. M. Lindberg introduced 35-mm photography in the United States in 1938. However, as Hollis Potter observed that same year, "these very small films can be economically taken but must, of course, be enlarged before they can be interpreted." Two years later, in collaboration with Douglas and Birkelo, Potter reported that "the most desirable objective in photography of the fluoroscopic image should be the production of a small film—small enough to constitute real economy in its use, and yet large enough to be readily interpreted without enlargement, or at least no greater enlargement than that provided by a simple reading glass."[66] Their solution was the use of a 4 × 5 inch film, which could be obtained at a rate of slightly more than one per minute. When compared with full-sized films obtained in 1,610 persons, the "miniature chest films" had only a 2.6% error in detecting 271 cases with active tuberculous lesions.

During World War II, photofluorography was used by the US Army for routine induction chest x-ray examinations. As Alfred de Lorimier, Director of the Department of Roentgenology at the Army Medical School in Washington, DC, observed, there were[72]:

> several reasons for obtaining more complete examinations (of the chest) in the present mobilization. There must be obviated, first of all, any unnecessary dissemination of diseases such as pulmonary tuberculosis. The hospitalization rates (soldier-days-lost) must be reduced as compared with the last great mobilization (World War I). Finally, and equally important to our country as a whole, the Government must be protected against false claims due to lesions not associated with the Service. This latter aspect does not imply that just compensation will not be recognized for actual service-connected lesions. In short, these experiences have enforced a policy of examination which should serve both epidemiological and legal purposes.

Experimental studies showed that the best screening results were obtained using stereoscopic 4 × 5 inch films. Stereoscopy was recommended because of its easy viewing, causing less visual and mental fatigue. In addition, it provided for (1) the separation of parenchymal density from overlying soft tissue densities and from osseous densities such as are referable to the ribs and spine, (2) the distinguishing of peribronchial irregularities that may be due to involuntary movements of the pulmonary vessels or to actual changes in the lymphatics or fibrous tissues, and (3) control against defective artifacts, which may occur either because of transient changes in radiographic performance or improper handling of the film. In addition, stereoscopy was

> particularly important when hundreds of cases must be studied in a day and when the films may serve for legal evidence. Certainly, a two film record showing duplication of evidence should be irrefutable. It is merely important that the second projection be made after shifting of the x-ray tube, whereby the incident x-ray beam has changed from one point source to another. It is not mandatory that these images be studied by third-dimensional viewing though that, too, is favored.

Single emulsion x-ray films, rather than the conventional duplitized type were recommended because they increased sharpness of detail and

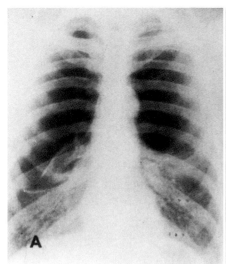
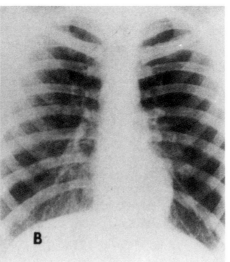

Military photoroentgenograms (1942).
A, Massive bilateral pneumothorax.
B, Normal-appearing chest.[72]

decreased contrast characteristics. Kilovoltages higher than those conventionally used for chest radiography were favored to reduce exposure times, contrast effects on the image, and the punishment imposed on the x-ray tubes.

Storage and durability were also critical factors in a wartime environment. The use of miniature films rather than standard 14 × 17 inch films reduced storage requirements from ⅙ (in the case of the 4 × 5 inch films) to approximately 1/150 (in the case of 35-mm films). One reason for preferring a stereoscopic pair of 4 × 5 films instead of a single 35-mm film was the fear that small cut films were more likely to be lost during the prolonged period during which pension claims were filed and eventually adjudicated.

The development of automatic cameras by Recordak and Fairchild was a major advance in making possible the routine use of photofluorography.[73] However, an even more significant technical advance making possible the routine use of this technique in large-scale survey work was the development of Russell H. Morgan of automatic x-ray exposure control.[74] As Morgan noted, the photofluorographic process

> requires the fulfillment of certain criteria not usually encountered in general radiography. For example, the procedure must be conducted rapidly in order to permit the examination of large numbers of subjects in a reasonable interval of time, and, in addition, it must be extremely simple in order to reduce to a minimum the operating personnel. The number of repeat examinations due to technical failure of any kind obviously must be small, and, finally, the standard of uniformity between films must be maintained at an extremely high level if the films are to yield a maximum of diagnostic information.

His solution was the photoelectric timing mechanism, or phototimer:

> This device completely automatizes the photofluorographic process, so that the technician is required merely to place the subject before the x-ray machine and to close the exposure switch; time-wasting adjustments of equipment are entirely eliminated. Furthermore, the photoelectric timing mechanism, by its inherent design, terminates x-ray exposure at the instant when a film has received the proper quantity of radiation to insure correct exposure. Excellent uniformity of radiographic quality thereby is assured, and repeat examinations due to technical failure are infrequent.

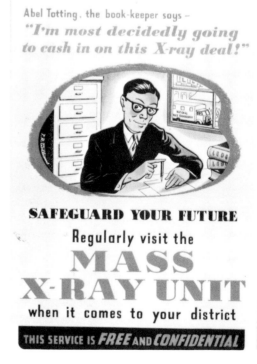

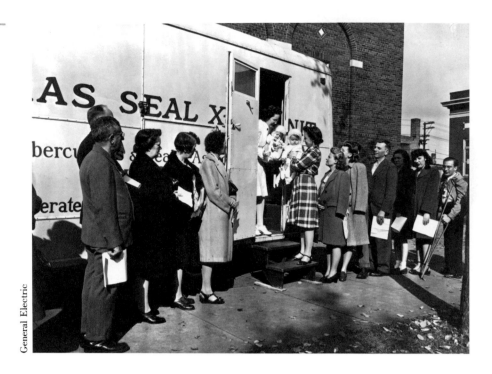

General Electric

Minnesota residents lined up for tuberculosis screening outside a mobile chest unit.

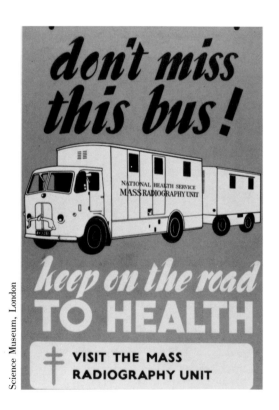

Science Museum, London

Subsequent modifications of this device made it applicable for general radiographic procedures.

POST–WORLD WAR II ERA

The experience of Allied forces in a variety of war zones led to increased interest in previously inconsequential tropical diseases. The pulmonary manifestations of fungal diseases were widely discussed in the literature. In the United States, interest in coccidioidomycosis reflected the presence of military installations in the San Joaquin Valley. Other evidence of the war was seen in discussions of the pulmonary findings in blast injuries and poison gas inhalation.[9]

By the beginning of the postwar decade, bacterial pneumonias had become rarities, the conquest of tuberculosis through specific antibiotic agents was at hand, and thus radiologists could focus their attention on new diagnostic problems, most notably carcinoma of the lung. Although this entity had been discussed in the radiological literature for more than 30 years, the radiologist's interest in its specific diagnosis had remained largely academic because thoracic surgery was hazardous and little progress had been made in the treatment of the disease since Graham's first successful pneumonectomy for carcinoma in 1933. Immediately following the war, however, men with extensive experience in military thoracic surgery returned to civilian practice, the old chemotherapeutic agents were augmented by antibiotics, and a new knowledge of anesthesia and of postoperative management was applied to this clinical problem. As thoracic surgery rapidly developed, carcinoma of the lung came to be regarded as a curable neoplasm. Thus significant effort focused on the establishment of specific radiographic criteria for the diagnosis of bronchogenic carcinoma. In the course of these intensive studies, new entities including pulmonary adenomatosis and pleural mesothelioma were characterized, but no consistent pathognomonic criterion of pulmonary malignancy was found.[9]

204

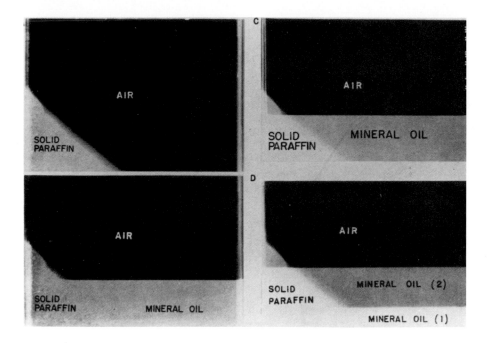

Experiment illustrating the basic principle of the silhouette sign for localizing intrathoracic densities (1950). "*A,* Paraffin wedge in front carton; empty rear carton. *B,* Paraffin wedge and mineral oil in front carton; empty rear carton. *C,* Paraffin wedge in front carton; mineral oil in rear carton. Note obliteration of the border of the paraffin shadow in *B* (silhouette sign) and its preservation in *C. D,* A small amount of mineral oil was poured into the carton containing the paraffin wedge (*1*) and a larger amount into the other carton (*2*). The direction of the central ray was reversed. Note the presence of the silhouette sign below the lower fluid level and the absence of the sign above it. Photographs were not retouched."[75]

Despite the advent of surgical therapy for the disease, the death rate from lung cancer continued to mount at an alarming rate. This led to interest in the early detection of such lesions by mass photofluorographic screening. Initial results of these screening surveys were discouraging, especially in view of reports by Garland[94] and others indicating the relatively high error rate in interpreting chest radiographs. Studies indicating the inadequacies of conventional radiographic techniques for demonstrating certain types of intrathoracic lesions led to the use of controversial high kilovoltage techniques for diagnostic chest radiology.[9]

The rapid advances in thoracic surgery made it increasingly more important for radiologists to be able to provide precise segmental localization of pulmonary disease. As Benjamin and Henry Felson wrote in their classic 1950 article,[75]

> This has required that the roentgenologists use any method which may serve to localize disease processes within the thorax. The earliest method of localization was by means of stereoscopic films. Later, combined postero-anterior and lateral roentgenograms were employed. More recent refinements in this direction have included oblique views, laminagraphy, bronchography, etc. It is often helpful, if possible, to determine the exact location of a pulmonary density from the postero-anterior film alone.

Adapting an observation of Robbins and Hale in their series of articles on lobar and segmental collapse, the Felsons[75] coined the term silhouette sign "to indicate obliteration of a portion of the cardiovascular silhouette by adjacent disease." They noted that "the same effect (the silhouette sign) is produced by any radiopaque intrathoracic shadow, whether it be of pulmonary, pleural, or mediastinal origin."

Three other classic signs were introduced to aid in the diagnosis of pulmonary embolism. Westermark (1938) described local pulmonary oligemia distal to a large vessel embolus,[76] and Aubrey Hampton (1940) illustrated his famous "hump," a convex pleural-based mass with the shape of a truncated cone convex toward the hilum.[77] In 1950, the "plump hilus" sign (enlargement of the ipsilateral main pulmonary artery as a result of pulmonary hypertension or distention of the vessel by bulk thrombus) was described by Felix Fleischner, the famed Boston radiologist in whose honor the international chest radiology society is named.[78]

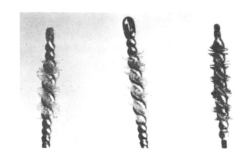

Types of brushes for bronchial studies (1966).[86]

INTERVENTIONAL PROCEDURES

As early as 1883, Leyden[79] performed the first transthoracic aspiration lung biopsies to isolate organisms in three cases of pneumonia. During the 1930s, a number of publications indicated that fine-needle aspiration (18-gauge or less) was a safe method for studying the bacteriology of pneumonias.[80] Sappington and Favorite (1936) reviewed the results of fine-needle lung aspiration performed before that time in over 2,000 patients with pneumonia and found only one procedure-related death.[81]

The use of transthoracic needle aspiration biopsy for the diagnosis of cancer was also first described during the 1930s. Martin and Ellis (1930) gave a detailed description of the technique of aspiration biopsy, while Blady (1939) stressed the importance of fluoroscopic guidance for biopsying tumors in obscure locations (hilar regions, mediastinal and juxtacardiac portions of the lungs, anterior and posterior mediastinum), small lesions (less than 5 cm in diameter), masses situated at depths greater than 10 cm, and tumors in close proximity to important vital structures (large vessels, esophagus, heart).[82] Later investigators used large-bore cutting needles to obtain histological samples of cancerous lesions and diffuse lung disease, although this technique was associated with far more major complications than reported with fine-needle aspiration of pneumonias.[79]

Modern fluoroscopically guided transthoracic fine-needle aspiration became popular following publication of the work of Dahlgren and Nordenstrom,[83] who in 1966 reported a high degree of safety and success in diagnosing cancer using this technique. The high diagnostic yield and low complication rate prompted radiologists who had previously not attempted lung biopsy to try this procedure. The successful use of fine-needle aspiration of the lung depended on two major developments: high-resolution image intensification and improved cytological techniques. With the advent of image intensification, the procedure could be performed in a fully lighted room rather than in the dark, and both the patient and the fluoroscopic image could be monitored at the same time. Improved cytological diagnosis made it possible to identify tumor cells in the minute samples provided by fine-needle aspiration. Thus large-bore histological needle techniques and their associated complications were no longer essential for cancer diagnosis.[79]

Bronchial brushing (1964). *a*, Frontal projection shows a mass near the right hilum. *b*, Lateral projection shows the brush inserted into the coin lesion via a Metras catheter.[85]

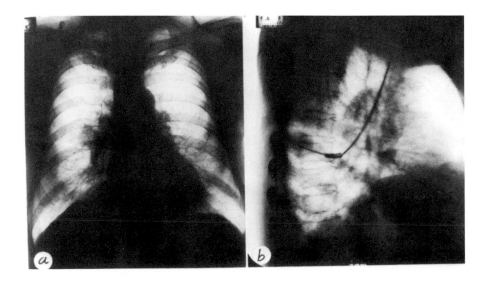

As with needle aspiration biopsy, the popularization of bronchial brushing as a diagnostic technique was closely linked to the development of image intensifiers and progress in cytodiagnostic procedures.[84] In 1964, Hattori and coworkers[85] first described the use of metal and nylon bronchial brushes in diagnosing 13 of 14 carcinomatous nodules using fluoroscopically guided, preformed transoral catheters. In the United States, Fennessy (1966) introduced fluoroscopically controlled bronchial brush biopsy using a transnasal technique.[86] Another approach was the use of the Seldinger technique (see Chapter 25) to selectively catheterize the bronchial tree by introducing a radiopaque catheter through the cricothyroid membrane and subsequently maneuvering it into various primary and secondary bronchi under fluoroscopic control.[87,88] The use of preformed catheters proved to be time-consuming because guidewires had to be inserted and the catheter had to be changed to enter various parts of the bronchial tree. The development of controllable pleuridirectional brushes and catheters led to greater popularity of the technique.[84] A multidirectional controlled-tip catheter, introduced by Rabinov and Simon[89] in 1969, made it easier to catheterize peripheral bronchi and substantially reduced the time required to brush multiple regions of the lungs.

Various devices were developed for obtaining biopsy specimens through bronchial catheters. Steel and nylon brushes, augers, curettes, and biopsy forceps were designed to help improve the diagnostic yield of bronchial brush biopsy.[84]

A further advance was the development by Ikeda and associates[90] of a flexible fiberbronchoscope (1968) that allowed direct visualization and biopsy of lesions of the central bronchial tree. These 4- to 5-mm diameter bronchoscopes could be advanced into segmental bronchi to obtain biopsy specimens with forceps or brushes. However, because these early fiberbronchoscopes were considerably larger than the controllable radiological catheters available at that time and their motion more restricted, radiologists continued to employ the smaller nonfiberoptic controllable catheters.[3]

Of the two interventional procedures, transthoracic needle aspiration biopsy has a higher yield than bronchial brushing in the diagnosis of cancer (95% vs 70%). Although somewhat time-consuming and more stressful for the patient than needle aspiration, bronchial brushing has a significantly lower morbidity rate, is especially useful in evaluating cavitary lesions and peripheral consolidations, and is the preferred biopsy technique when bleeding is likely to occur or when abnormal pulmonary function makes pneumothorax resulting from needle aspiration an unacceptable risk.[84]

NEWER IMAGING MODALITIES

Although the plain chest radiograph remains the major screening technique because it is easy to obtain and relatively inexpensive and sensitive, only cross-sectional studies can distinguish among structures that are superimposed on conventional radiography. The advent of computed tomography (CT) revolutionized radiological imaging of the thorax because its wide dynamic range permits the display of the entire spectrum of thoracic densities (lungs, soft tissues, bones) with a single exposure. Its superior contrast sensitivity allows the detection of mediastinal vessels and lymph nodes embedded within surrounding fat, and the use of

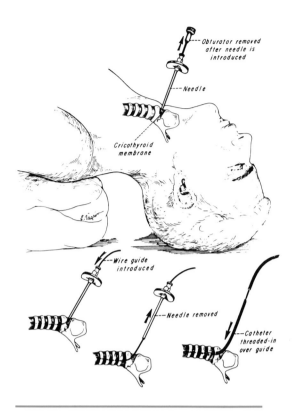

Introduction of a catheter through the cricothyroid membrane and into the trachea using a modified Seldinger technique (1964).[87]

207

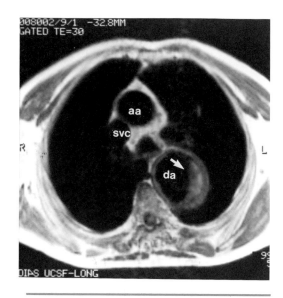

908002/9/1 -32.8MM
GATED TE=30
R
aa
svc
da
L
DIAS UCSF-LONG

MRI of thoracic aneurysm. Transverse scan with cardiac gating permits differentiation of a large mural thrombus (*arrow*) from the signal void of rapidly flowing intraluminal blood in the descending aorta (*da*). *aa*, ascending aorta; *svc*, superior vena cava.[93]

intravenous contrast material permits the distinction between mediastinal vessels and nonvascular processes. More recent improvements in the spatial resolution of CT have resulted in images of such excellent anatomical detail that diffuse pulmonary parenchymal disease can be evaluated. The major limitation of CT is that only a small part of the thorax is demonstrated on each slice. The inability of the patient to precisely reproduce the same degree of inspiration on sequential scans means that a small pulmonary lesion could possibly be missed between sections. In addition, the axial plane may be of less value in displaying longitudinally oriented structures (such as the aorta) or in assessing structures that primarily fall in the same plane of section (such as the diaphragm). These limitations may be overcome by the direct sagittal and coronal imaging offered by magnetic resonance (MR). The mediastinum is ideally suited to MR imaging because of the inherent contrast between the bright signal intensity of mediastinal fat and the signal void produced by flowing blood within the heart and mediastinal vessels. Because it requires no intravenous contrast, MR imaging is especially valuable in differentiating enlarged nodes from vessels in patients with bronchogenic carcinoma and lymphoma (although its poorer spatial resolution may result in blurring of the edges of individual discrete nodes and suggest that they represent a single large mass). In the future, MR angiography may become of value in differentiating vascular from nonvascular mediastinal masses and in the noninvasive imaging of patients with suspected pulmonary embolism.

References

1. Williams FH: The Röntgen rays in thoracic diseases. J Am Med Sci 114:665-687, 1897.
2. Williams FH: The roentgen rays in medicine and surgery. New York, MacMillan, 1901.
3. Bergonie M and Carriere M: The use of the fluoroscope in pleuritic effusions. Arch Roentgen Ray 4:67-75, 1899.
4. Tousey S: Medical electricity and Röntgen rays. Philadelphia, WB Saunders, 1910.
5. Walsham H: Discussion on the use of Röntgen rays in the diagnosis of pulmonary tuberculosis. Trans Brit Congr Tuberc (1901) 3:267, 1902.
6. Walsham H: The diagnosis of thoracic aneurism by the roentgen rays. Arch Roentgen Ray 6:70-74, 1901.
7. Crane AW: Skiascopy of the respiratory organs. Phila Med J 1:154-170, 1899.
8. Nature 60:426, August 31, 1899.
9. Tuddenham WJ: Fifty years of progress in roentgenology of the chest. AJR 75:459-467, 1956.
10. Hulst H: Skiagraphy of the chest. Trans Amer Roentgen Ray Soc 89-94, 1903.
11. Kassabian MK: Instantaneous skiagraphy of the thoracic organs. Trans Amer Roentgen Ray Soc 95-100, 1903.
12. Rieder H: Arch Roentgen Ray 5:1900.
13. Cole LG: The radiographic diagnosis and classification of early pulmonary tuberculosis. Am J Med Sci 140:29-53, 1910.
14. Dunham HK: The relation of the pathology of pulmonary tuberculosis to the roentgen findings. AJR 4:280-283, 1917.

15. Heise FH and Sampson HL: The classification of pulmonary tuberculosis, with a comparative analysis of the different methods employed. AJR 5:139-144, 1918.
16. Boardman WW: Pneumoconiosis. AJR 4:292-299, 1917.
17. Lanza AJ and Childs SB: Roentgen-ray findings in miner's consumption, based upon a study of 150 cases. U.S. Public Health Bull 85, January 1917.
18. Pancoast HK, Miller TG, and Landis HRM: A roentgenologic study of the effects of dust inhalation upon the lungs. AJR 5:129-138, 1918.
19. Pancoast HK and Pendergrass EP: A review of our present knowledge of pneumoconiosis, based upon roentgenologic studies, with notes on the pathology of the condition. AJR 14:381-423, 1925.
20. Jarvis DC: A roentgen study of dust inhalation in the granite industry. AJR 8:244-258, 1921.
21. Sparks JV: Pulmonary asbestosis. Radiology 17:1249-1257, 1931.
22. Adler I: Primary malignant growths of the lungs and bronchi. London, Longman, 1912.
23. McMahon FB and Carman RD: The roentgenological diagnosis of primary carcinoma of the lung. Am J Med Sci 155:34-47, 1918.
24. Christie AC: The diagnosis of primary tumors of the lung. AJR 8:97-103, 1921.
25. Golden R: The effect of bronchostenosis upon the roentgen-ray shadows in carcinoma of the bronchus. AJR 13:21-30, 1925.
26. Crane AW: Pulmonary metastasis. AJR 5:479-482, 1918.

27. Pfahler GE: Malignant disease of the lungs, its early recognition and progressive development, as studied by the roentgen rays. AJR 6:575-579, 1919.
28. Kirklin BR and Hefke HW: Roentgenologic study of intrathoracic lymphoblastoma. AJR 26:681-690, 1931.
29. Sante LR: A study of lobar pneumonia and its pulmonary complications by serial roentgenographic examination. AJR 10:351-366, 1923.
30. Robbins LL and Hale CH: The roentgen appearance of lobar and segmental collapse of the lung: A preliminary report. Radiology 44:107-114, 1945.
31. Robbins LL and Hale CH: The roentgen appearance of lobar and segmental collapse of the lung. II. The normal chest as it pertains to collapse. Radiology 44:543-547, 1945.
32. Robbins LL and Hale CH: The roentgen appearance of lobar and segmental collapse of the lung. III. Collapse of an entire lung or a major part thereof. Radiology 45:23-26, 1945.
33. Robbins LL and Hale CH: The roentgen appearance of lobar and segmental collapse of the lung. IV. Collapse of the lower lobes. Radiology 45:120-127, 1945.
34. Robbins LL and Hale CH: The roentgen appearance of lobar and segmental collapse of the lung. V. Collapse of the right middle lobe. Radiology 45:260-266, 1945.
35. Robbins LL and Hale CH: The roentgen appearance of lobar and segmental collapse of the lung. VI. Collapse of the upper lobes. Radiology 45:347-355, 1945.

36. Lubert M and Krause GR: Patterns of lobar collapse as observed radiographically. Radiology 56:165-182, 1951.

37. Samuel E: Bronchography. In Bruwer AJ (ed): Classic descriptions in diagnostic radiology. Springfield, Ill, Charles C Thomas, 1964.

38. Springer K. Prager Med Wschr 31:162, 1906.

39. Waters CA, Bayne-Jones S, and Rowntree LG: Roentgenography of the lungs. Roentgenographic studies in living animals using intra-tracheal injection of iodoform emulsion. Arch Int Med 19:538-549, 1917.

40. Jackson C: The bronchial tree: Its study by insufflation of opaque substances in the living. AJR 5:454-455, 1918.

41. Lynah HL and Stewart WH: Roentgenographic studies of bronchiectasis and lung abscess after direct injection of bismuth mixtures through the bronchoscope. AJR 8:49-61, 1921.

42. Sicard JA and Forestier J: The radiologic examination of the bronchopulmonary cavities by means of intra-tracheal injections of iodized oil. J Med Franc 13:3-9, 1924.

43. Rigler LG: The development of roentgen diagnosis. Radiology 45:467-502, 1945.

44. Ballon DH: Lipiodol in the diagnosis of bronchopulmonary lesions by the bronchoscopic method. Arch Otolaryng 3:401-422, 1926.

45. Dunbar JS, Skinner GB, Wortzman G, and Stuart JR: An investigation of effects of opaque media on the lungs with comparison of barium sulfate, lipiodol, and Dionosil. AJR 82:902-926, 1959.

46. Nadel JA, Wolff WG, and Graf PD: Powdered tantalum as a medium for bronchography in canine and human lungs. Invest Radiol 3:229-238, 1968.

47. Hickey P: The interpretation of radiographs of the chest. Trans Amer Roent Ray Soc 5:136-140, 1905.

48. Dunner L and Calm A: X-ray examination of blood vessels, especially the vessels of the lung in the living man. Fortsch Roentgenstr 3:635-636, 1923.

49. Lindblom AF: A roentgenologic study of the distribution of blood in the rabbit lung during treatment with artificial pneumothorax. Acta Radiol (Stockh) 9:147-154, 1928.

50. Moniz E, de Carvalho L, and Lima A: Angiopneumography. Presse Med (Paris) 39:996-999, 1931.

51. Figley MM: Angiopneumography. In Bruwer AJ (ed): Classic descriptions in diagnostic radiology. Springfield, Ill, Charles C Thomas, 1964.

52. Bolt W and Rink H: Selective Angiographie der Lungengefabe bei Lungentuberkulose. Schweiz Z Tuberk 8:380-392, 1951.

53. Bell A, Shimomura S, and Taylor JA: Wedge pulmonary arteriography. Application in congenital and acquired heart disease. Circulation 18:691, 1958.

54. Fraser RG and Pare JAP: Diagnosis of diseases of the chest. Philadelphia, WB Saunders, 1989.

55. Arvidsson H, Karnell J, and Moller T: Multiple stenoses of the pulmonary arteries associated with pulmonary hypertension diagnosed by selective angiocardiography. Acta Radiol 44:209-216, 1955.

56. Clairborne TS and Hopkins WA: Aorto-pulmonary artery communication through the lungs. Report of a case. Circulation 14:1090-1092, 1956.

57. Ingram MD, Hudson GW, and Davis TJ: Aplasia of the lung. With angiocardiographic demonstration of anomalous pulmonary circulation. AJR 64:409-413, 1950.

58. Madoff IM, Gaensler EA, and Streider JW: Congenital absence of the right pulmonary artery: Diagnosis by angiocardiography and cardiorespiratory studies. N Engl J Med 247:149-157, 1952.

59. Smith HL and Horton BT: Arteriovenous fistula of the lungs associated with polycythemia vera: Report of a case in which the diagnosis was made clinically. Amer Heart J 18:589-592, 1939.

60. Dotter CT, Hardisty NM, and Steinberg I: Anomalous right pulmonary vein entering the inferior vena cava: Two cases diagnosed during life by angiocardiography and cardiac catheterization. Amer J Med Sci 218:31-36, 1949.

61. Amundsen P and Sorensen E: Angiocardiography in intrathoracic tumors with particular reference to the question of operability. Acta Radiol 45:185-198, 1956.

62. Steinberg I and Finby N: Great vessel involvement in lung cancer: Angiocardiographic report on 250 consecutive proved cases. AJR 81:807-813, 1959.

63. Thompson SA: Differential diagnosis by means of intravenous contrast medium of two cases simulating aneurysm of the pulmonary artery. AJR 46:646-649, 1941.

64. Muscall L and Duffy RW: Surgical treatment of bullous emphysema: Contributions of angiocardiography. Dis Chest 24:489-499, 1941.

65. Wagner RB, Baeza DR, and Stewart JE: Active pulmonary hemorrhage localized by selective pulmonary angiography. Chest 67:121-125, 1975.

66. Potter HE, Douglas BH, and Birkelo C: The miniature x-ray chest film. Radiology 34:283-291, 1940.

67. Battelli A and Garbasso A: Concerning the rays of Roentgen. Il Nuovo Cimento 4:40-61, 1896.

68. Bleyer JM: On the photo-fluoroscope. Laryngoscope 1:1-20, 1896.

69. MacIntyre J: Experiments on röntgen rays; the introduction of the use of the camera to reduce the size of plates. Nature 55:64-65, 1896.

70. de Abreu M: Roentgen-photography. Procedure and apparatus for roentgen-photography. Pulmonary tuberculosis. Social surveys. Radiography and Radioscopy. Large scale roentgen-photography. Rev Ass Paulista Med 9:313-324, 1936.

71. de Abreu M: Collective fluorography. Radiology 33:363-371, 1939.

72. de Lorimier AA: Mass roentgenography of the chest for the United States Army. Radiology 38:462-472, 1942.

73. Moseley RD: Photofluorography. In Bruwer AJ (ed): Classic descriptions in diagnostic roentgenology. Springfield, Ill, Charles C Thomas, 1964.

74. Morgan RH: The automatic control of exposure in photofluorography. Public Health Rep 58:1533-1541, 1943.

75. Felson B and Felson H: Localization of intrathoracic lesions by means of the posteroanterior roentgenogram: The silhouette sign. Radiology 55:363-373, 1950.

76. Westermark N: On the roentgen diagnosis of lung embolism. Acta Radiol 19:357-372, 1938.

77. Hampton AO and Castleman B: Correlation of postmortem chest teleroentgenograms with autopsy findings: With special reference to pulmonary embolism and infarction. AJR 434:305-326, 1940.

78. Fleischner FG: Unilateral pulmonary embolism with increased compensatory circulation through the unoccluded lung. Radiology 73:591-597, 1959.

79. Greene R: Transthoracic needle aspiration biopsy. In Athanasoulis CA, Greene R, Pfister RC, and Roberson GH (eds): Interventional radiology. Philadelphia, WB Saunders, 1982.

80. Woolf CR: Applications of aspiration lung biopsy with a review of the literature. Dis Chest 25:286-301, 1954.

81. Sappington SW and Favorite GO: Lung puncture in lobar pneumonia. Am J Med Sci 191:225-234, 1936.

82. Blady JV: Aspiration biopsy of tumors in obscure or difficult locations using roentgenoscopic guidance. AJR 42:515-524, 1939.

83. Dahlgren S and Nordenstrom B: Transthoracic needle biopsy, Chicago, Year Book, 1966.

84. Greene R: Bronchial brush biopsy. In Athanasoulis CA, Greene R, Pfister RC, and Roberson GH (eds): Interventional radiology. Philadelphia, WB Saunders, 1982.

85. Hattori S, Matsuda M, Sugiyama T, and Matsuda H: Cytologic diagnosis of early lung cancer: Brushing method under x-ray television fluoroscopy. Dis Chest 45:129-142, 1964.

86. Fennessy JJ: Bronchial brushing in the diagnosis of peripheral lung lesions. AJR 98:474-481, 1966.

87. Steckel RJ and Grillo HC: Catheterization of the trachea and bronchi by a modified Seldinger technic: A new approach to bronchography. Radiology 83:1035-1037, 1964.

88. Moskowitz M and Freihofer A: Seldinger brush biopsy: A synthesis of techniques. Chest 57:426-427, 1970.

89. Rabinov K and Simon M: A new selective catheter with multidirectional controlled tip. Radiology 92:172-173, 1969.

90. Ikeda S, Yanai N, and Ishikawa S: Flexible bronchofiberscope. Keio J Med 17:1, 1968.

91. Baron RL et al: Computed tomography in the evaluation of mediastinal widening. Radiology 138:889-901, 1981.

92. Eisenberg RL: Diagnostic imaging in surgery. New York, McGraw-Hill, 1987.

93. Thoeni RF and Margulis AR: Introduction. In Eisenberg RL: Diagnostic imaging: An algorithmic approach. Philadelphia, JB Lippincott, 1988.

94. Garland LH: Studies on the accuracy of diagnostic procedures. AJR 82:25-38, 1959.

CHAPTER 13

Cardiac Radiology

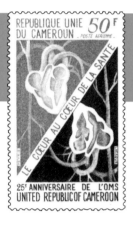
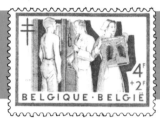
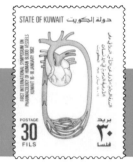
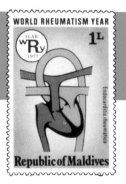

The history of cardiac radiology can be conveniently divided into four eras that are based on technological achievements. According to a masterful, unpublished study by Ronald P. Seningen and Richard G. Lester in 1970,[1] during the pioneer period (1895-1912) the early radiologists peering at dim images of the heart produced by gas tubes were concerned primarily with general observations of the outside of the heart and laid the foundation for quantitative cardiac measurements. The second era began in 1913 with Coolidge's invention of the hot-cathode x-ray tube. This more powerful source permitted detailed visualization of the cardiac contours. The hallmarks of this era were extensive cardiac measurements, basic observations of abnormalities in the size of the heart and its specific chambers, the detection of cardiac calcifications, the rise and fall of interest in kymography, and the beginnings of angiocardiography. The third era began in the early 1930s with the introduction of practical methods of angiocardiography that led to serious investigation of the internal anatomy of the living heart and great vessels. This extremely fruitful period paralleled the early phases of cardiac surgery.

The fourth era began with the introduction of the electronic image intensifier in 1952. Paralleling the advances of more refined intracardiac surgery made possible by the advent of extracorporeal circulation, this period has been characterized by critical evaluation of the internal anatomy of selected areas within the heart, study of the coronary arteries, an awareness of physiological parameters, and the explosive development of cardiac isotope techniques.

PIONEER ERA

Less than 1 year after the discovery of x-rays, Francis H. Williams of Boston published two papers concerning the use of radiology in cardiac

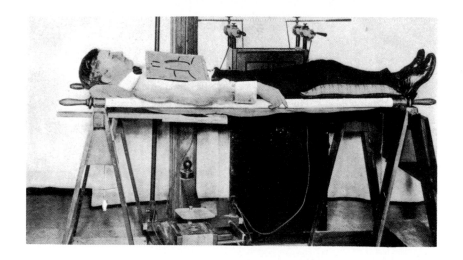

diagnosis. The first was read before the Association of American Physicians on April 30, 1896. Williams[2] reported that

> the first medical case I examined was that of a man with an enlarged heart (seven inches in transverse diameter). I found that the outline of the heart as seen from the front of the body through the fluoroscope corresponded in a general way to the outline drawn on the skin with percussion as a guide. It was interesting to note that the heart could be made out through the man's waistcoat and two shirts.

Williams' second paper[3] noted that "the constant motion of the heart and diaphragm interfere with the use of radiography but renders fluoroscopy all the more valuable."

Williams was the first to describe the fluoroscopic findings in pericardial effusion and defined differences in pulsations between this disease and cardiac enlargement. By the end of 1898, Williams had studied virtually all cardiac diseases recognized at that time and had described quite accurately the radiographic features of pericardial effusion, intrathoracic aneurysm, and cardiac hypertrophy.[4] In the following year, Williams compared the radiologically and percussion-determined cardiac size with postmortem specimens in 546 cases. He concluded that the x-ray offered the best means for determining heart size and that radiographic examination was especially valuable for demonstrating the left border of the heart in cases of enlargement or displacement.

A quantitative estimation of "normal" cardiac size was offered by Albert Abrams (1902),[6] who noted that the "Right heart measures 3 cm from median line, and left heart, 8.5 cm from median line; total, 11.5 cm." However, Abrams did not consider the overall size of the chest or of the individual. In Germany, Levy-Dorn related the width of the heart to the height of the individual. Williams stressed the importance "not only to obtain the size of the heart as a whole, but also the size of the right heart as compared with the left."

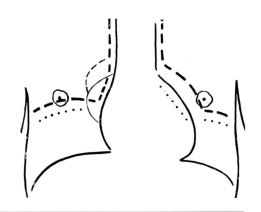

Diagram of movements of the heart, blood vessels, and diaphragm (1901). "The full lines are in deep inspiration, the broken lines in expiration; the dotted lines just below the broken ones represent the position of the diaphragm in ordinary inspiration. The line of large and small dots inside the left border of the heart shows the position of the left border in systole, the full line in diastole, during full inspiration."[5]

Thoracic aneurysm (1897). "The curved line in the upper part of the patient's left chest, and the curved line on his right chest indicate the outline of the aneurysm as seen in the fluoroscope. The lower curved line on the left chest marks the outline of the heart; the lowest curve on the right front, part of the outline of the diaphragm; the dotted line, the cardiac area as determined by percussion."[111]

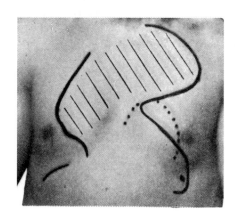

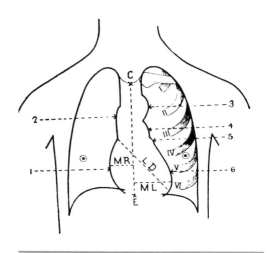

Orthodiagram of the normal heart (1909).[7]
LD, Longitudinal diameter; *MR* and *ML*,
total transverse diameter; *1*, right atrial
curve; *2*, curve of the great vessels; *3*, arch
of the aorta and its descending limb; *4*,
pulmonary artery; *5*, left atrial curve; *6*,
left ventricular curve.

In the United States, quantitation of the normal relationship between heart size and body size was first pioneered by Thomas Claytor and Walter Merrill. In 1909, they noted that "from our observations it appears that the size of the heart depends more upon the body-weight than upon the body-height." They proposed a method of approximation of the heart area based on 70% of the product of the longitudinal diameter and the transverse diameter.[7] The last "measurement pioneers" were Van Zwaluwenburg and Warren. Realizing the importance of knowing what chamber of the heart was of abnormal size, they considered the oblique diameter as an approximate dividing line between the atrial and ventricular areas. "Since distension of the auricular area is a marked feature in a mitral lesion, the ratio (auricular area/ventricular area) should be larger than normal in mitral disease."[8]

The major controversy during the pioneer era was whether the determination of cardiac size and contour was better demonstrated by fluoroscopy or film radiography. In 1902, Friedrich Moritz introduced the technique of *orthodiagraphy*. This method consisted of tracing the shadows of the margins of the heart and great vessels on a thin sheet of transparent paper that was affixed to the fluoroscopic screen. An accurate delineation of the cardiac border was assured by the use of a thin-slit screen, and distortion was practically eliminated by a long focal-screen distance. The paper tracing became a permanent record of cardiac size and contour.[4]

As Claytor and Merrill described in their classic paper[7]:

> Skiagrams or Rontgen-ray shadows of the internal organs are always enlarged and distorted to a greater or less extent. To overcome this distortion and to outline the internal organs in their exact size, parallel instead of divergent rays should be used, and these parallel rays should be perpendicular to the reading screen. It is impossible to obtain parallel Rontgen rays directly from our Crookes tube, so that in the effort to overcome this difficulty the orthodiagraph has been developed.
>
> The working principle may be outlined as follows: A pneumatic pen, the centre of the anticathode of the Crookes tube, or source of the Rontgen rays, and the centre of a small fluorescent screen are so

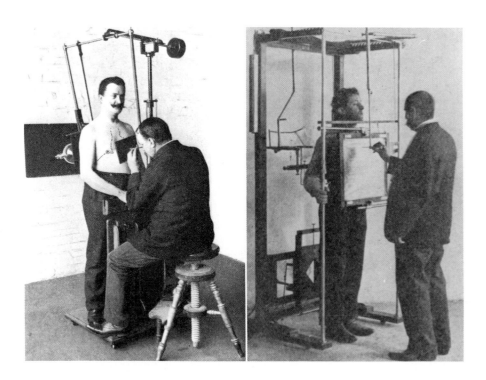

Technique of orthodiagraphy. *Left*, Albers-Schoenberg (1903). *Right*, Tousey (1910).

mounted on arms that they are in a straight line. These arms are attached to a carriage which, while allowing all motions in one fixed plane, will keep the straight line perpendicular to the plane. Thus, the pencil of rays coming from the tube, through a small circular aperture in a lead diaphragm, to the centre of the screen, while it may be moved over a considerable surface, will always occupy parallel positions.

In using the machine it is only necessary to move the carriage so that the lead spot in the centre of the screen touches the edge of the shadow to be outlined; a mark is made with the pneumatic pen on the sheet of paper, which is clamped upon a drawing-board fixed behind the tube. The lead spot is then moved to a new position along this edge and a second mark made. In this way the process is continued until the entire shadows are outlined. Then, upon removing the sheet from the machine, these marks, when connected will give the exact size of the object casting the shadow.

According to Claytor and Merrill, the major advantage of the orthodiagram was that, when completed, it

is intelligible to any one who takes the trouble to inform himself upon the topographical anatomy of the interior of the thorax. The lines are clearly marked and the object is outlined in its exact position with regard to its surrounding landmarks—the ribs, the sternum, the liver, the diaphragm—and its size may be determined and compared with the normal. On the other hand, the skiagram usually requires long experience to interpret correctly. A shadowy distorted outline is often all that can be made out. This may mean much to the expert, but practically nothing to the ordinary physician, who must accept the statement of another and is often but half convinced. The fluoroscope, as ordinarily used, allows of no photographic or diagrammatic record.

An additional advantage was the rapidity with which the orthodiagram could be made since the time (and expense) required for the development of a plate was avoided.

At about the same time, the danger to the radiologist of long fluoroscopic seances for study of the heart was recognized. By 1905, radiographic technique had advanced to such a degree that Kohler could introduce teleroentgenography (tube-patient distance of 2 m) for accurate measurement of cardiac size. However, the exposure time of one-half second for radiography of the heart was still too long, and blurring of the cardiac borders on chest radiographs was accepted as a necessary evil.[4]

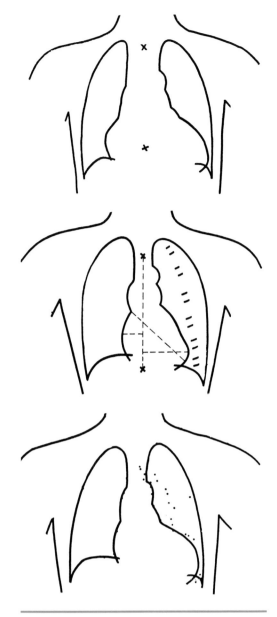

Orthodiagrams of Claytor and Merrill (1909). *Top,* Aortic insufficiency; *middle,* mitral stenosis; *bottom,* mitral insufficiency.[7]

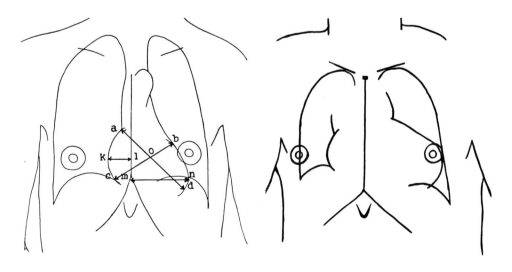

Orthodiagrams of Van Zwaluwenburg and Warren demonstrating various dimensions of the heart shadow (1911). "*Left,* Right-median (MR) or greatest perpendicular distance from the right border to the median line (*k-l*); left-median (ML) or similar measurement to the left (*m-n*); total transverse (*TT*) equals the sum of k-l and m-n; long diameter (*l*) measured from the auriculovenous junction to the apex, *a-d*; and transverse distance, measured from the left auriculoventricular junction to the auriculohepatic angle, *b-c. Right,* Chronic interstitial nephritis and cardiac failure. MR is equal to 6.1 cm; ML is 13.3 cm; and l is 19.3 cm."[8]

THE SECOND ERA

Coolidge's invention of the hot tungsten cathode and tungsten target (1913) provided radiologists with a more powerful source of x-rays that permitted critical study of cardiac size, contour, pulsations, and calcifications. As early as 1916, Charles R. Bardeen[9,10] produced the first of several reports in which he related the area and volume of the heart to height, weight, and sex. In calculating the area, Bardeen made use of a planimeter, an engineering instrument that automatically computed the area of the heart when it was moved around the outline of the cardiac silhouette. Bardeen's calculations could be performed using orthodiagraphy or teleroentgenography. In the latter case, "6% is then subtracted from the square area to make the correction necessitated by the divergence of the Rontgen-rays."[11] The time-consuming method of Bardeen and the need for extra planimeter equipment were too much to ask of most practitioners, who merely wanted some general radiographic information about heart size in their patients. Consequently, in 1919, C. Saul Danzer of New York popularized the cardiothoracic ratio. He found that "the normal heart is usually less than half the greatest diameter of the thorax."[12] The normal range was considered 39% to 50%. Allowing for a 2% "margin of safety" above the upper limit, Danzer considered a ratio of 53% or more to be definitely pathological and evidence of "hypertrophy." Three years later, Karshner and Kennicott[13] criticized this method because it ignored variation in the position of the diaphragm—a problem that has troubled users of cardiothoracic ratio ever since.

For 20 more years, controversy raged over whether linear diameters, frontal areas, or volume calculations were more valuable in estimating normal and abnormal heart size. In 1939, Comeau and White[14] demonstrated that these various measurements were woefully inadequate, primarily because the wide range of normal heart size and shape was impossible to correlate with such external factors as height, weight, and body surface area. Three years later (1942), Ungerleider and Gubner[15] sagely noted that "innumerable measurements have been proposed for the estimation of the size of the heart, and this has resulted in general confusion and skepticism about all measurements." Their cardiac nomogram, culminating 40 years of measurement, enabled calculation of frontal heart area from the long and broad cardiac diameters. Comparison was made with values predicted from measurements of body height and weight. Putting the entire controversy in perspective, Ungerleider and Gubner stated that:

> measurements are not to be regarded as final, but should be employed to complement careful study of the individual cardiac chambers by fluoroscopic examination; and the diagnostic significance of cardiac enlargement should always be considered in relation to the associated clinical observations.

At this stage of development, cardiac radiology faced two major problems: acceptance by clinicians (who were at the same time faced with multiple instruments for cardiac examination) and the question of exactly what was offered by radiographic methods in cardiac examinations.

In a classic 1919 editorial, Augustus W. Crane[16] noted that cardiac radiology

> is not a generally accepted or much used method. Internists are perhaps superabundantly supplied with instrumental means of examining the heart. The stethoscope, percussion hammer, the sphygmograph or polygraph, the blood pressure manometers and the elec-

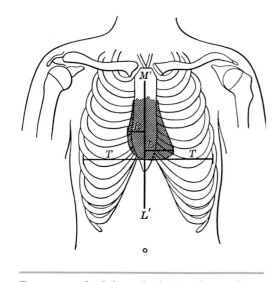

Danzer method for calculating the cardiothoracic ratio (1919).[12] "*ML'*, Midline; *R*, distance from M'L' to right border (fourth space); *L*, distance from M'L' to left border (fifth space); R + L = *TH* (transverse diameter of the heart); *TT*, transverse diameter of the thorax; *CT*, cardiothoracic ratio = TH/TT."[12]

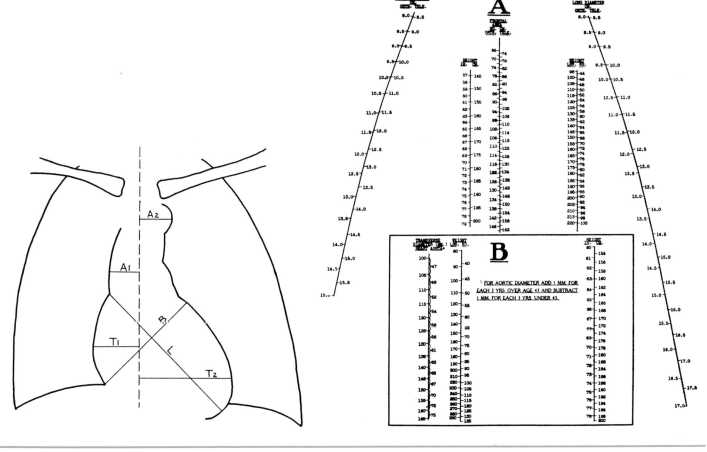

trocardiograph somewhat deter the internist from feeling the need of another and more elaborate instrument. Many able and successful men admit the importance of these instruments for purposes of research but use the stethoscope merely as a sanitary convenience, holding that the palpating finger and the ear are the only necessary instruments for the examination of the heart.

Crane considered it ironic that

in no department is the x-ray revision of internal medicine more inevitable and less acceptable to internists than in the examination of the chest. Barium or bismuth for the alimentary tube, oxygen or carbon dioxide for pneumoperitoneum, sodium iodide or thorium for the urinary tract, suggests the technical requirements of later x-ray work, but the chest without any preparation excepting a full breath provided perfect conditions for x-ray study from the beginnings of clinical roentgenology. The work below the diaphragm has met with enthusiastic reception; the x-ray examination of the lungs has won a tardy recognition; but the examination of the heart by screen or plate is apparently still on trial.

Crane then cited the statement of Sir James Mackenzie, the prominent senior editor of *Oxford Medicine:*

The inspection and palpation of the movements of the heart and the percussion of the heart's dullness give a far more valuable indication of the size of the different chambers of the heart than an x-ray examination. Indeed I am doubtful if any x-ray examination of the heart has ever thrown the slightest light upon any cardiac condition.

Ungerleider and Gubner method of measuring heart size (1942). "*Left,* Diameters for measuring the size of the heart. A_1 to A_2, Transverse diameter of the aortic arch; T_1 to T_2, transverse diameter of the heart; L, long diameter of heart; B, broad diameter of heart. *Right,* Nomograms for frontal cardiac area, transverse diameter of the heart, and the aortic arch. The values for actual (or predicted) area are read at the point at which a straight line extending from the long and broad diameters (or weight and height) intersects the cardiac area scale. Orthodiagram values are on the left, teleroentgenogram values on the right. In the lower nomogram, the predicted transverse diameter of the heart (left side of the scale) or aortic arch (right side of scale) is obtained as an extension of a straight line connecting height and weight. A correction for age, as indicated, is necessary for the aortic diameter. Values exceeding 10% above the predicted for any of these measurements are abnormal."[15]

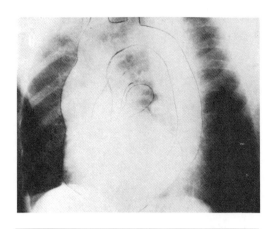

Left oblique posteroanterior view with outline drawn in (1930). "The tortuous aorta is dilated in the lower portion of the ascending arch. There is extreme right and left ventricular enlargement. The left auricular appendage is dilated. Wassermann reaction negative; blood pressure, 220/140. Clinical diagnosis: arteriosclerotic and hypertensive heart disease, chronic nephritis."[18]

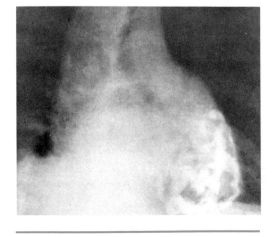

Pericardial calcification (1923).[23]

Although Crane admitted that in many areas of cardiology "the x-ray cannot claim to be a substitute for a clinical examination," he maintained that

> the heart signs which can be demonstrated only by the x-ray are the form of the heart, the pulsation of each chamber separately, calcifications of the pericardium or aorta, small aneurysms and dilatation of the thoracic aorta . . . We do not mean that the x-ray screen can or should replace the stethoscope. On the contrary, the best screen work can only be done in collaboration with auscultation. The practice of listening to the heart sounds while making a screen observation should be routine.

Nevertheless, Crane concluded that although "we do not undervaluate clinical methods, but such is the supremacy of the eye and such the importance of things seen that the Rontgen-ray image will take an assured precedence as diagnostic evidence."

In a letter to Crane published just after the editorial, Van Zwaluwenburg complained that

> my irritation is altogether in consequence of the failure of the medical profession to recognize the value of this method of cardiac examination. Undoubtedly men have not wished to take the time to learn the trick or to do the work when other more immediately profitable work was at hand. Besides, few roentgenologists have the necessary preparation in medicine to interpret their findings when they get them . . . The orthodiagram is so little known that the medical examiner at Camp Custer confused it with the electrocardiogram, and it went through three medical hands without detection.

Reiterating the importance of experience, Van Zwaluwenburg added that "it is a matter of sad experience that I have never succeeded in teaching a student to inscribe the same (orthodiascopic) figure that I see . . . At first a man 'goes wild' on the numerous shadows of the lower thorax, all of which are moving in synchronism with the pulse beat, but in time he learns to see a figure that for him at least is normal. Whether or not this is the actual outline of the heart is another question."

A simple determination that the heart was enlarged had limited clinical value. To predict the underlying pathological abnormality, it was essential to develop a technique for evaluating the cardiac contour and develop signs of specific chamber enlargement. As early as 1922, Rolla G. Karshner and Robert M. Kennicott[13] noted that "the typical forms of heart silhouette, such as the . . . boxing glove heart of mitral stenosis, the round heart of mitral regurgitation, snub-nose or shoe-shaped heart of aortic regurgitation, the water bottle shadow of pericardial effusion, have long been accepted among orthodiagraphers and require no comment." At this time, most American descriptions of the cardiac contour were based on the frontal projection. Although the value of oblique projections had been mentioned several years previously (1918) in France by Vaquez and Bordet,[17] a standardized oblique position for the radiographic study of the heart and great vessels was not generally accepted in the United States until the work of O'Kane, Andrew, and Warren in 1930.[18] These authors stressed that

> the left oblique posteroanterior teleroentgenographic (or orthodiagraphic) technique . . . offers the only way of comparing the right and left ventricular size without interference of overlapping auricular shadows. Area measurements are more accurate than those in the posteroanterior view and give a better index of cardiac volume. The great vessels can be measured and studied to greater advantage than from any other single aspect.

To obtain this view, they fluoroscopically positioned the patient with the apex pointing directly toward the examiner. Using many illustrations of thoracic dissections of cadavers, the authors illustrated the anatomical basis for the various measurements possible with this technique.

Ralston Paterson of Toronto pointed out the differential diagnostic value of the anatomical relation of the esophagus and bronchi (especially the left bronchus) to the left atrium in cases of suspected mitral valve disease.[19] Enlargement of the right ventricle and inflow and outflow tracts was illustrated by Nemet and Schwedel,[20] while the entire subject of cardiac contour was well summarized by Roesler[21] in 1934.

The importance of cardiac calcification was first recognized during this period. Although Rudis-Jicinsky had shown "calcarous deposits" at heart valves in 1902,[22] later observers concluded that "these must have been on his negatives, as they are not at all clear on the figure in his article." In describing the first American case of pericardial calcification, or as he termed it, *pericarditis calculosa*, James B. Case[23] (1923) wrote, "Rarely does the Rontgen-ray examiner stumble on to anything more interesting and startling than the revelation of a calcarous deposit in the pericardium." One year later (1924), Cutler and Sosman described endocardial, myocardial, and pericardial calcification in a patient with a history of rheumatic fever.[24] Calcification in the aortic and mitral valves was reported in 23 cases by Sosman and Wosika in a 1933 review.[25] Over the next 10 years, many radiologists reported the detection of cardiac calcifications, stressing that they were most easily found on fluoroscopy and difficult to record on films. The most prolific of these authors was Merrill Sosman, who in 1943 published his technique for locating and identifying pericardial and intracardiac calcifications because "very little of the techniques have been incorporated in textbooks of radiology and cardiology."[26] One of his major points was that

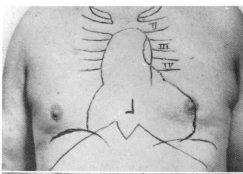
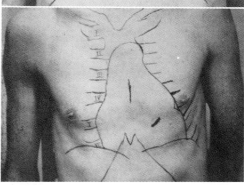

Calcification in aortic and mitral valves (1933). *Top*, Orthodiagram traced on the chest of a patient with aortic stenosis and calcification demonstrates the typical silhouette with the valve low and almost in the midline. *Bottom*, Orthodiagram in a patient with mitral disease with calcification shows the typical silhouette with the valve low and well to the left.[25]

> no roentgenologist should be content to examine a patient for heart disease by films alone. Roentgenoscopy is the much more important part of the examination, and the more one does, of course, the greater facility and skill he acquires. Roentgenograms rarely add anything if the roentgenoscopy is carefully and thoroughly done, but they do furnish a permanent record and a check on the roentgenoscopic findings. They may, however, add important details in the lungs, ribs, spine, or other structures outside the heart.

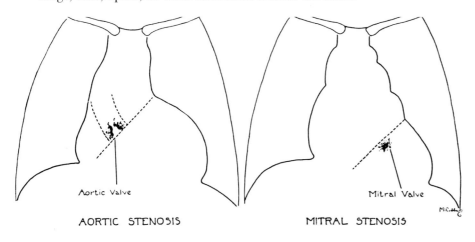
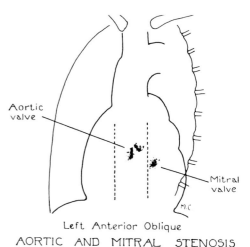

Sosman's technique for locating and identifying intracardiac calcifications (1943). *Left*, Diagram of a posteroanterior projection shows the marked difference in position between calcification in the aortic valve (*left*) and mitral valve (*right*). *Right*, Diagram of a left anterior oblique projection shows the different positions of calcification involving the aortic and mitral valves.[26]

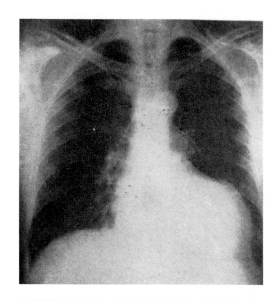

Left ventricular aneurysm (1934). Unusually well-marked localized bulging in the upper portion of the left ventricle.[29]

Hypertensive heart (1929). *Left,* Practically normal heart (slight hypertrophy of left ventricle) in a patient with blood pressure of 158/100. *Right,* Marked left ventricular hypertrophy with rounded apex in a patient with blood pressure of 170/110.[31]

Although radiographic signs of acquired heart disease were recognized by the early orthodiagraphists, for almost 20 years few articles on the subject appeared in the American literature. In 1925, Ledbetter, Holmes, and White,[27] when writing on the value of radiography in determining the cause of aortic regurgitation, noted that "in a survey of the literature it becomes evident that the chief study of the heart and aorta by the x-rays is of foreign origin." By the end of the second era of cardiac radiology, the radiographic aspects of acquired heart disease had been well described. Changes in the appearance of individual chambers in stenosis and insufficiency of the aortic and mitral valves were comprehensively discussed by David Steel in 1930.[28] Drawing on earlier work by Assmann in Germany, Steel emphasized that hypertrophy causes a change in shape, whereas dilatation produces a change in size of the heart.

Four years later (1934), Steel described the radiographic appearance of cardiac aneurysms.[29] Expanding on the work of Sezary and Alibert in France (1922), Steel described the paradoxical ventricular movements, writing that "when the other portions of the ventricle are in systole, the weakened wall of the aneurysm dilates, and hence during ventricular systole the aneurysm shows expansion." Like Sosman, Steel emphasized the importance of fluoroscopy:

> The absence of roentgenologic evidences of an aneurysm does not rule out the latter. It is quite evident that a careful fluoroscopic examination in the various degrees of rotation is most essential, and it seems probable that with a more careful search the cases (of cardiac aneurysm) will be more commonly diagnosed.

The radiographic changes in various cardiac chambers for disorders of all four valves of the heart were well summarized by Sosman in 1939.[30] He also stressed the frequency of calcification in diseased valves. The "hypertension roentgenogram" was discussed in detail by Arthur M. Master (1929). He described the characteristic cardiac appearance secondary to long-standing hypertension as "an enlarged heart, an hypertrophied left ventricle, and an apparently dilated but actually tortuous aorta, with a prominent aortic knob."[31]

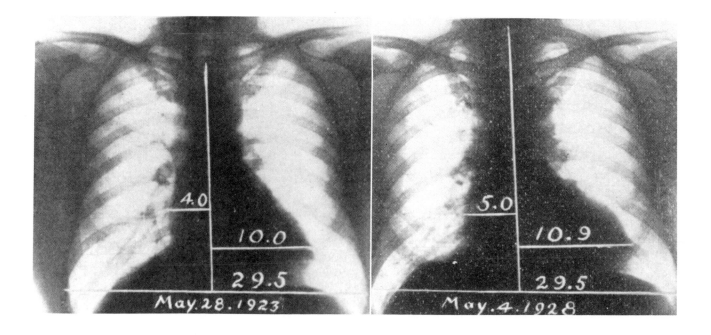

Unlike acquired heart disease, congenital cardiac defects were generally relegated to the storehouse of medical curiosities, with one striking exception.[4] In 1898, W. Zinn of Germany described a case of patent ductus arteriosus in which the clinical diagnosis was confirmed by the fluoroscopic evidence of enlargement of the pulmonary artery.[32] Thereafter the pulsatile dilated pulmonary artery segment in patent ductus was termed the *cap of Zinn*. There was little impetus toward the radiographic diagnosis of congenital diseases of the heart because there were no surgical means of correcting them. After the first successful ligation of a patent ductus arteriosus by Robert E. Gross (1938) at the Peter Bent Brigham Hospital in Boston, the x-ray diagnosis of this congenital anomaly became more popular. Five years later (1943), Donovan, Neuhauser, and Sosman summarized the radiographic signs of the first 50 surgically verified cases from that hospital.[33]

Coarctation of the aorta was the only other congenital cardiovascular disease for which radiographic criteria were established. In 1930, Walter E. Fray[34] noted that "the diagnosis of coarctation is rarely made during life, though post-mortem experience would indicate that this condition is not extremely uncommon . . . The roentgenologist has an excellent opportunity to make this diagnosis, entirely unaided by clinical or laboratory data." Fray outlined direct signs (defect in the aortic arch in the posteroanterior and left anterior oblique views) and indirect signs (left ventricular hypertrophy, dilatation of the ascending aorta, and rib erosions) that related to the obstruction of aortic flow and the subsequent development of collateral circulation.

The second era of cardiac radiology saw the extensive development of *kymography*, a technique for recording on radiographic film the movements of the silhouettes of an organ, especially the heart. First described by Sabat of Poland in 1911,[35] kymography was independently reported 2 years later by Gott and Rosenthal of Munich.[36] As they wrote, "The study of the natural movements of the heart has received little attention. This is so because no method exists by which the pulsations, which are too rapid for the human eye and which are not synchronous in all sections of the heart, could be recorded . . . Our goal was to record the pulsating movements of various heart sections in the form of curves." The single-slit method utilized a lead screen with a horizontal aperture about 10 mm in width. The screen was placed between the radiographic film and the patient, while the slit and the x-ray tube were centered over the organ to be studied. During the radiographic exposure, the film was moved at a uniform rate of speed, usually 4 to 5 cm per second, with the direction of the movement being at right angles to the slit in the lead screen. The resultant radiograph presented a continuous shadow of the contour of the organ in a series of bands or waves that represented the movements of its silhouette.[37] The multiple-slit method proved more satisfactory because it permitted simultaneous visualization of several points along the edge of an organ. In the United States, this technique was introduced by Crane, who preferred to call the method "roentgenocardiography."[38] Crane noted the similarity of kymography to the electrocardiogram:

> The electrocardiogram . . . is a tracing obtained on a strip of photographic film which moves across a slit. Running at right angles to this slit is a very fine metallic filament which vibrates with the electric currents excited by the heart muscle. An electric light behind the filament prints the vibrations on a moving film. A microscope is arranged so as to magnify these vibrations and thus yield a tracing having the requisite amplitude.

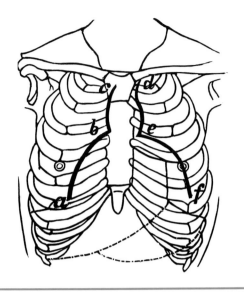

Patent ductus arteriosus (1898). *abef*, Outer contour of ventricle and atrium; *ed*, contour of dilated pulmonary artery; *bc*, contour of aorta.[32]

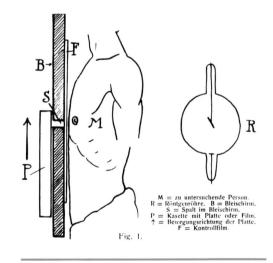

Kymography (1912). *M*, Patient to be examined; *R*, x-ray tube; *B*, lead shield; *S*, slit in lead shield; *P*, plate holder for film or photographic plate; *F*, control film; *arrow*, direction of motion of plate.[36]

219

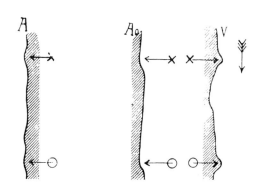

Kymography (1912). "Tracings of the right auricle (A), aorta (Ao), and left ventricle (V) of a 38-year-old man. The ventricular and auricular curves were taken through the same horizontal slit so that the points correspond directly. The slit used to record the aortic pulse was located much higher but for ease of comparison has been shifted so that the synchronous points on all three curves fall on the same horizontal line."[36]

In the case of the roentgenocardiogram the wire filament is replaced by the edge of the heart muscle itself and the light is replaced by the roentgen ray. There is no other essential change. No microscope is required.

In the electrocardiogram we deal with the electrical changes in the heart; in the sphygmogram or polygram we deal with pressure variations within the blood-vessels; but in the roentgenocardiogram we deal directly with the movements of the heart muscle. The electrocardiogram is stated to give a record of both auricles contracting as a unit and of both ventricles contracting as a unit . . . But the roentgenocardiogram is capable of giving a separate record of the muscle movements of each chamber of the heart. In this respect it stands unrivaled.

Kymography was valuable in the study of cardiac physiology and for diagnosis of certain cardiac abnormalities and pericardial disease, as well as the differentiation of extracardiac from paracardiac masses. Its greatest use was in the diagnosis of adhesive and constrictive pericarditis, pericardial effusion, neoplasms in the region of the heart, and certain instances of aneurysm and cardiac infarction.[37] A later development was the electrokymograph, an electrical apparatus used with a conventional medical fluoroscope to produce detailed records of the motions of the heart borders or of the great vessels.[39] This device produced a sharply defined and easily read wave form that could be amplified electronically and record as many successive cardiac cycles as desired.[37]

Near the close of the second era, the famed cardiologist, Paul Dudley White, summarized the state of cardiac radiology from the point of view of the clinician in an address to the thirteenth annual meeting of the American Roentgen Ray Society (1929):

> It is wise to include routinely a roentgen examination in the analysis of every cardiovascular patient but it is essential that it be made accurately and interpreted intelligently by an experienced person.

Kymography technique of Crane (1916). "*Left*, Roentgenocardiograph on x-ray table. *Right*, Demonstration of the slit bars and carriage which holds the cassette."[38]

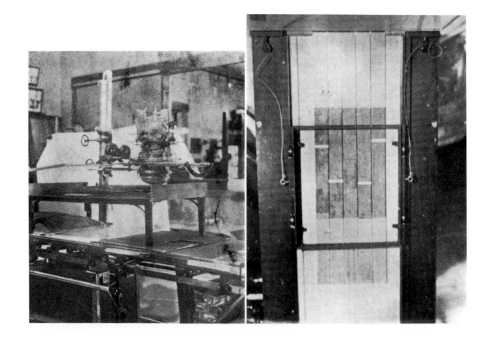

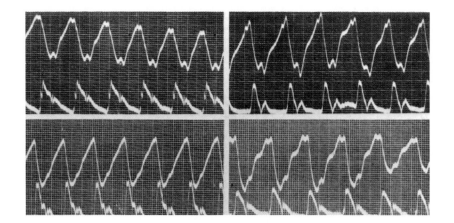

Sometimes errors in technique and interpretation render the procedure a serious handicap in diagnosis rather than a help and in a considerable percentage of cases examined routinely throughout the countryside at the present time it would for this very reason be more helpful to omit roentgen-ray study than to include it. This fact is true of all other methods of examination and is by no means limited to the roentgenological procedure . . . The roentgen rays provide a method for the demonstration of moderately or far advanced pathology only . . . Serious and indeed fatal heart disease may be present with no indication of trouble on roentgen examination.

White added that "the roentgenologist or internist using the roentgen rays should state what he sees in the way of structural changes and not attempt to make an etiological diagnosis . . . It is safer and wiser in the end not to diagnose too much from the roentgen examination."

In the journal article that was published several months later, White added a "later note" to "balance against the limitations of roentgen study in heart disease its special advantages, even though they are better known and recognized." The "six particular points on which the usefulness of the roentgen ray and cardiovascular diagnosis is based" were[41]:

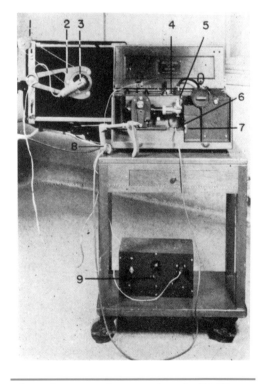

1. The roentgen ray affords by far the most accurate measurements of heart size and of heart shape that we possess in the clinic.
2. In the presence of obesity, emphysema, and other complications which render physical examination of the heart very imperfect, the roentgen ray affords sometimes the only means of determining heart size and shape.
3. Surprising and unexpected findings like pericardial calcification or aneurysms of the aorta are sometimes revealed by roentgen study alone, and in themselves justify a routine employment of this method of examination whenever possible.
4. The size of the aorta and of the left auricle, and even sometimes of the left ventricle, can be determined only by the roentgen ray.
5. Abnormalities of the hilus shadows and of the pulmonary artery are important findings to be discovered only by the roentgen ray.
6. Roentgen-ray observation of peculiarities of the actual pulsation of the heart and great vessels is alone worth the trouble of applying this method of study."

As Seningen and Lester[1] exclaimed, "Cardiac radiology had come of age!"

THE THIRD ERA

The hallmark of the third era of cardiac radiology, extending from the early 1930s through the early 1950s, was the development of angiocardiography. Improved techniques for passing vascular catheters and obtaining rapid serialized exposures, combined with the development of tolerable contrast agents, made it possible to seriously investigate the inside of the heart, rather than merely assess its external features.

Primitive attempts to visualize the vascular system began several months after the discovery of x-rays. As early as January, 1896, Hascheck and Lindenthal[42] injected the severed hand of a cadaver

> . . . through the arteria brachialis (with) Teichmann's mass, which consists essentially of chalk and therefore, in a manner similar to bones, promised to be impenetrable to x-rays . . . The digital and interosseous arteries and their anastomoses were clearly recognized . . . (but) the superficial vessels could not be differentiated from the deeper rami.

Less than 1 month later, in Italy, Uberto Dutto[43] injected a paste of calcium sulfate through the brachial artery of a cadaver to obtain an excellent representation of the arterial vascular system of the hand. In the United States, William J. Morton[44] wrote,

> The arteries and veins of dead bodies may be injected with a substance opaque to the x-ray, and thus their distribution may be more accurately followed than by any possible dissections. The feasibility of this method applies equally well to the study of the other structures and organs of the dead body.

The first human angiocardiogram was probably performed by Mihran K. Kassabian of Philadelphia. In his 1907 book, Kassabian[45] wrote,

> I have studied the blood vessels of infants and adults by injecting into them a substance opaque to the x-rays. The substance used is a concentrated emulsion of bismuth subnitrate, a strong solution of litharge (red oxide of lead), or metallic mercury. In order to demonstrate sharply the arterial tree, the injection must be done carefully and slowly.

Roentgen picture of an amputated hand filled with Teichmann's mixture (January, 1896).[42]

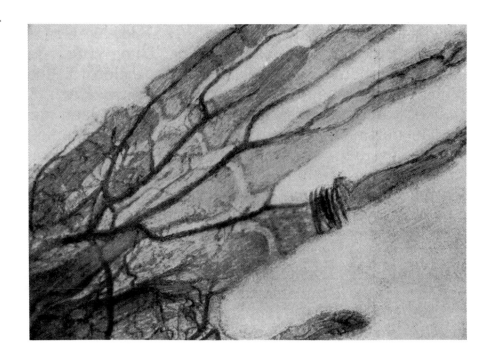

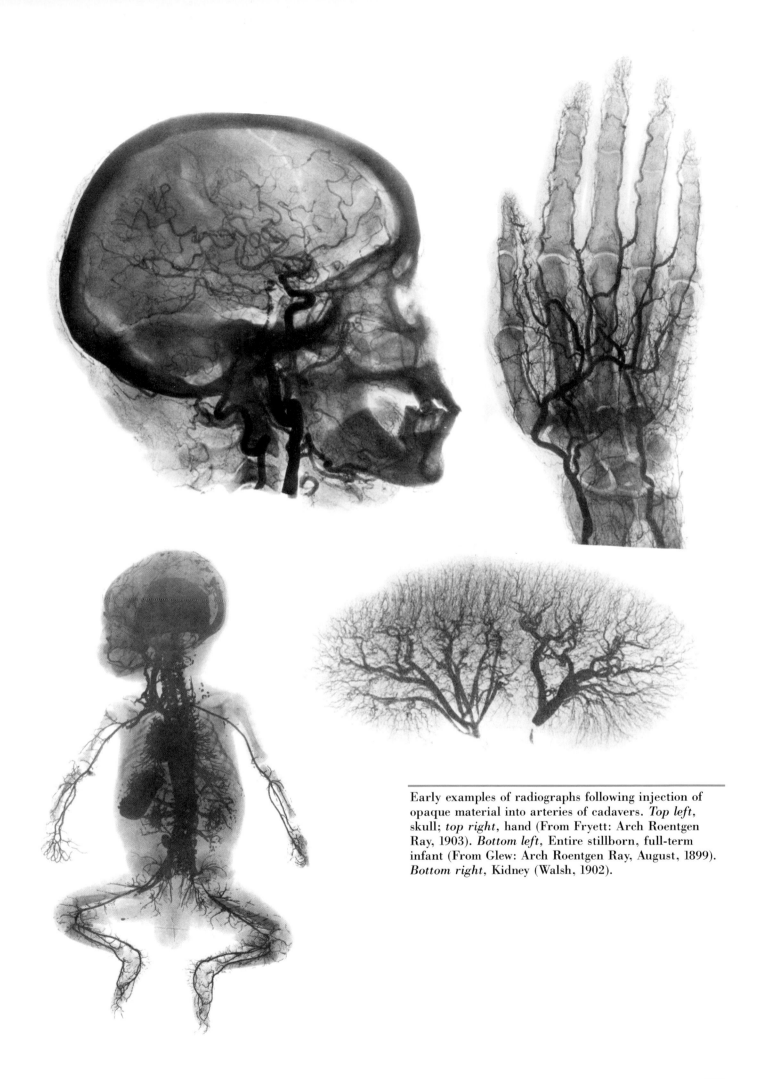

Early examples of radiographs following injection of opaque material into arteries of cadavers. *Top left*, skull; *top right*, hand (From Fryett: Arch Roentgen Ray, 1903). *Bottom left*, Entire stillborn, full-term infant (From Glew: Arch Roentgen Ray, August, 1899). *Bottom right*, Kidney (Walsh, 1902).

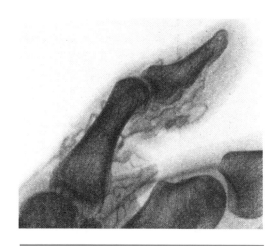

One of the first angiograms of peripheral blood vessels (1924). Arterial circulation of the thumb.[49]

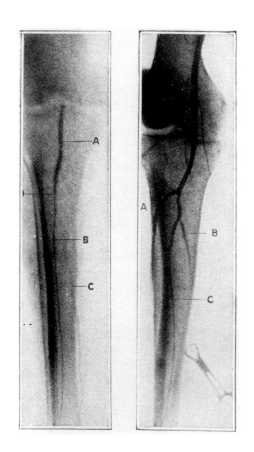

One of the first femoral arteriograms in humans (1924). After the injection of sodium iodide, there is visualization of the popliteal (A), posterior tibial (B), and peroneal (C) arteries.[50]

In vivo angiocardiography was first performed fluoroscopically in 1910 by Franck and Alwens of Germany.[46] These investigators injected an oil-bismuth suspension intravenously and observed the opaque media passing through the heart and into the lungs, an amazing accomplishment considering that they were using a gas tube as the x-ray source. Nine years later (1919), Carlos Heuser of Argentina was the first to perform angiography and angiocardiography in a living human.[47] As he wrote, after injecting a potassium iodide solution into an arm vein, "In a child with lesions of congenital syphilis, I have seen the iodide in a radiograph of the heart. To those who have hospital services, I commend this method, for here is a new method for examining the pulmonary artery and vein."

Unaware of Heuser's previous work, Jean-Athanase Sicard and Jacques Forestier of Paris made similar observations 4 years later using oil-based Lipiodol. After injecting this substance in the antecubital vein,[48]

> the passage of the opaque drops is perfectly visible on the screen, quite slow in the superficial veins and accelerating progressively in the axillary vein. The transit to the pulmonary capillaries is complete in 3 to 4 minutes. The stopping of the oily drops in the capillary mesh takes only 6 to 8 minutes, and sometimes provokes coughing spells without dyspnea. Within 10 minutes, the whole amount has crossed the capillary network and is carried into the greater circulation without causing trouble.

In 1923, Berberich and Hirsch[49] obtained the first angiograms of peripheral blood vessels and introduced halogen compounds as contrast media when they injected 20% strontium bromide into the arteries and veins of the arm and hand. One year later (1924), Barney Brooks[50] reported the intraarterial injection of sodium iodide as a means of demonstrating the vessels of the lower extremity in man. His arteriograms were of excellent technical quality and detailed precise arterial anatomy, as well as atherosclerotic changes. Five years later (1929) in Portugal, dos Santos, Lamas, and Pereira-Caldas applied the techniques used by their countryman, Egas Moniz, for cerebral arteriography (see Chapter 18) to peripheral studies and obtained satisfactory angiograms in various disorders of the lower extremities.[51] At the same time, they announced their method for clearly visualizing the abdominal aorta and its branches by the insertion of a long needle through the left paravertebral region in the back to pierce the aorta, and the injection directly into it of a concentrated solution of sodium iodide.

The most dramatic early angiocardiogram was performed by Werner Forssmann, who in 1929 inserted a "well oiled ureteral catheter" into the antecubital vein of his own arm and maneuvered it into the right atrium. For his first attempt, Forssmann[52] asked a colleague to puncture the vein. However,

> after a week, I undertook another experiment alone . . . I administered local anesthesia, and, since venapuncture with a thick needle in one's own body is technically very difficult to accomplish, I performed a venosection on my left elbow vein and passed the catheter without resistance its entire length of 65 cm. This length seemed to me after measuring on the surface of the body to be equal to the distance from the left elbow to the heart . . . I examined the position of the catheter by means of a mirror which was held by a nurse in front of a fluoroscopic screen . . . The length of the catheter was not sufficient for it to be inserted further.

Forssmann regarded this method as useful for intravenous injections, such as the administration of gallbladder and kidney contrast media. He closed his first article with "Finally, I would like to point out that the method which I have employed opens numerous prospectives on new possibilities on the study of metabolism and of cardiac activity, which I am now pursuing."

Over the next 2 years, Forssmann continued his investigations. In addition to using the cardiac catheter for physiological experiments, Forssmann conceived the idea of visualizing the chambers of the heart by the injection of contrast material through his "heart-probe." After obtaining satisfactory cardiograms of the chambers of the right side of the heart in dogs, Forssmann again experimented on his favorite subject—himself. He injected 20 cc of 25% sodium iodide in his own right atrium via a catheter in a vein at the left elbow[53]:

> Shortly after the injection there was a slight sensation of dizziness which disappeared quickly again. Only during a period of one and one-half days when the iodide salt was being excreted was there slight stuffiness of the nose and unpleasant sensations of taste. The films showed only good opacification of the pulmonary vessels, but it was otherwise unsatisfactory. Under any circumstances, the experiment gave proof that this was a safe diagnostic method.

Forssmann later repeated this experiment using Uroselectan, the new organic iodide contrast developed by Moses Swick (see Chapter 17). This material and the improved variations that soon followed were far safer than inorganic sodium iodide, and for years they remained the major contrast agents for the opacification of the interior of the heart.

Forssmann's momentous achievements ironically fell victim to conservative medical politics. When he asked Professor Sauerbruch, also of Berlin and the world's leading thoracic surgeon, whether any use could be made of this new technique of cardiac catheterization, either for therapeutic or diagnostic purposes, Sauerbruch's reaction was that he ran a "clinic for patients, not a circus." Forssmann was barred from any further important hospital appointments and had difficulty in obtaining suitable work. Twenty years later he was discovered working as a general practitioner in a small town in the Rhine valley. Fortunately, Forssmann's originality and personal heroism achieved international recognition when he shared the Nobel Prize for Medicine in 1956 (with the Americans, André Cournand and Dickinson Richards) for their pioneering work in introducing diagnostic cardiac catheterization.[53]

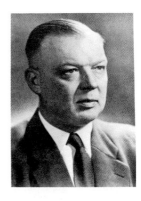

Werner Forssmann (1904-1979).

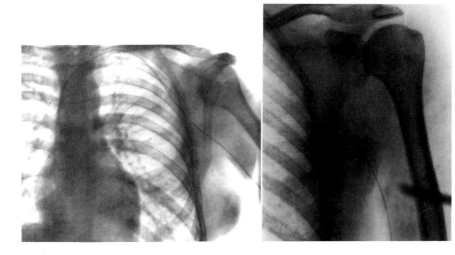

Forssmann's first cardiac catheterization on himself (1929). The ureteric catheter is seen extending from his left arm into his right atrium.[52]

225

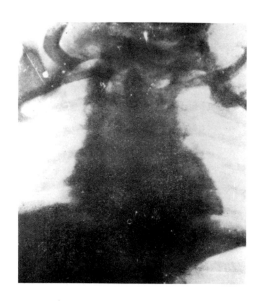

First attempted angiocardiogram (1931). Only the superior vena cava and right atrium are visualized.[56]

Pulmonary arteriography ("angiopneumography") was first described by Moniz, de Carvalho, and Lima in 1931.[54] Using the Forssmann technique for catheterizing the right atrium, they injected sodium iodide to demonstrate the pulmonary arterial tree. Subsequently, they established the accurate interpretation of the hilar shadows and lung markings. After a few years experience, the Lisbon group found that they could obtain the same results without the use of a catheter by simply injecting contrast material directly into a cubital vein[55] (see Chapter 12).

The first successful application of angiocardiography (the name they gave the procedure) as a practical diagnostic method was reported in 1937 by Castellanos, Pereiras, and Garcia.[56] Using this technique in infants and children, they radiographically defined the pathological anatomy of a large number of congenital heart malformations, primarily septal defects. The illustrations contained in their publication only showed the chambers on the right side of the heart, except in cases with right-to-left shunts where the pathophysiology allowed the contrast material to be carried in high concentration to the left side of the heart. The Cuban pediatricians succeeded because they pioneered (1) the use of a large needle, actually a Lindemann trocar, (2) the fast-emptying syringe, "of a sufficiently great interior diameter so that a strong push on the plunger permits the whole quantity to be injected in a short time," and (3) rapid injection, with an upper limit of 1½ to 2 seconds.[57] They also, in essence, introduced biplane rapid-injection angiocardiography:

> Initially, we obtained the antero-posterior and lateral views on separate days . . . However, we soon thought of using a special arrangement requiring that a single injection of opaque medium . . . using two tubes . . . it is necessary to place one plate behind the patient and the other vertically on the left side; the cones limit the exposure to only the corresponding radiographic plate.

Using the 50% concentration of Per-Abrodil then available, they were successful in opacifying the heart in small children. They did not succeed in larger children and did not even attempt the procedure in adults, although they suggested that more concentrated solutions (up to 70%) would probably solve the problem.

Their paper concluded,

> the principle objective of angiocardiography in the living individual is to aid the pediatrician and the radiologist in the anatomic diagnosis of the congenital cardiac lesions of infancy, especially of those which are accompanied by cyanosis and affect principally the right heart. It does not pretend to replace the auxiliary methods which we are using today such as kymography, teleradiography, orthodiascopy, electrocardiography, phonocardiography, etc., but we believe it to be another auxiliary method of investigation of great value and high objectivity, permitting in many an anatomic diagnosis to be made with a security not available with other procedures . . . *Angiocardiography* in the living individual is *not an experimental method*; it is a *clinical method*, perfectly standardized, which can and should be used as a routine procedure in congenital cardiopathies in hospitals, clinics, and radiologic laboratories.

Angiocardiography came of age with the publication in 1938 of the remarkable work of George P. Robb and Israel Steinberg[58] in which they announced that they had succeeded in visualizing for the first time all the

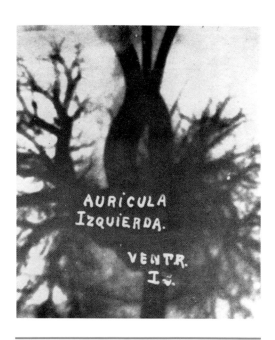

Postmortem angiocardiography (1931). Demonstration of the pulmonary vessels, left side of the heart, and thoracic aorta and its branches.[56]

chambers of the heart, as well as the aorta. Robb had gained wide experience in the determination of the circulation time and had used, among other testing agents, brilliant vital red dye that he found to pass through the heart and lungs in a high concentration. This led him to believe that an adequate concentration of a substance opaque to x-rays was similarly passed en masse through the heart and great vessels following peripheral intravenous injection.[57] Robb and Steinberg formulated their technique while unaware of the work of Castellanos in Cuba. Their original features were

1. A highly concentrated radiopaque solution to increase the opacifying power of the injected dose (initially 70% skioden, later 70% diodrast)
2. An oversized lumen (12 gauge) of needle and syringe-tip, to speed up the rate of injections
3. Inspiration during injection to draw the opaque material from the arm veins into the vena cava and heart
4. Ether and cyanide circulation time measurements, to synchronize opacification and roentgenography

This last development permitted the opacification of selected heart chambers and vessels to coincide with the timing of the radiographic exposures. The frontal position was used to study the pulmonary circulation, while the oblique position proved more advantageous for examination of the heart and the aorta.

In the summary of their paper, Robb and Steinberg wrote:

No longer must roentgenographic evidence of disease depend upon change in the silhouette of the entire heart or the distortion of adjacent structures. Instead, each chamber and great vessel can be visualized separately, and the nature and degree of abnormality ascertained. Exact mensuration of the heart thus becomes a possibility. At the same time, the circulation time of the blood to the various parts of the cardiovascular system can be determined objectively. Characteristic changes were observed in congenital, rheumatic, pulmonary, hypertensive, and syphilic heart disease . . . This method promises to be of practical value in the differential diagnosis of heart disease, the recognition of early organic change, and the exclusion of heart disease in the normal.

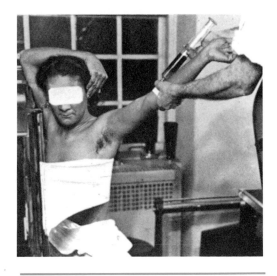

Early angiocardiography technique (1939). Right anterior oblique position, immediately before injection (viewed from the side). Syringe containing opaque contrast material is attached to the needle-stopcock unit. Note the column of blood above the contrast and the position of the injector's hands.[58]

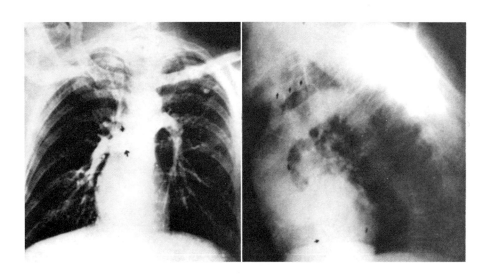

Angiocardiography (1939). *Left*, Contrast film at 3 seconds shows the left branch of the pulmonary artery pulled up by a tuberculous process. Note the decreased vascularity to the upper lobes. *Right*, Extreme left anterior oblique position 11 seconds after beginning of injection. Enlargement of the left ventricular cavity and wall and dilatation and uncoiling of the aorta. The lower dart denotes the interventricular septum; the upper three darts indicate the innominate, left common carotid, and left subclavian arteries.[58]

Just 1 year before Robb and Steinberg's extensive report, the era of practical cardiac surgery began with the first successful ligation of a patent ductus arteriosus by Robert Gross of Boston. The next decade saw dramatic advances in the surgical treatment of cardiac disease. This served as a strong stimulus to the development of angiocardiography, which was needed to supply much of the detailed anatomical and physiological diagnostic information that made the surgical advances possible and practical. Numerous papers described the angiocardiographic findings in virtually all the congenital and acquired lesions of the cardiovascular system.

Important technical achievements complemented the diagnostic advances. The first automatic angiocardiographic injection device was reported in 1938 by Castellanos and co-workers.[59] Another important advance was the development of a technique for direct intracardiac contrast injections. In 1946, Alejandro Celis of Mexico described the fluoroscopic localization of a catheter (inserted via the external jugular vein) in the upper part of the right atrium or right ventricle, through which he injected organic iodide contrast media.[60] Two colleagues, Ignacio Chavez and Normo Dorbecker, applied Celis' technique and assessed its diagnostic value. They pointed out such disadvantages of the peripheral injection method as "(1) the relatively long distance that the opaque substance must travel from the antecubital veins to the heart, (2) too much dilution of the opaque substance with nonopaque blood, and (3) a shunt of the opaque material to undesirable veins." In outlining the advantages of their intracardiac injections, they wrote that "to avoid these defects it is necessary (1) to put the opaque substance in the place where it is needed, if possible; (2) to fill the part to be visualized completely; and (3) to inject the substance very rapidly to avoid too much dilution." The illustrations provided in their report confirmed their excellent results.[61] In a few years, the development of image intensification allowed much more precise catheter placement within the heart, and selective angiocardiography became a progressively more widespread procedure.

Successful angiocardiography required a method for obtaining rapid sequence exposures of the opacified heart.[57] "In general, there are three basic types of apparatus: (1) those for photofluorography with the cine or modified miniature camera; (2) those for fast continuous changing of cassettes; and (3) those for rapid direct radiography on large roll film."

As Thompson, Figley, and Hodges (1949) wrote,[62]

Any specialized device designed for use in the radiographic study of cardiac circulation must meet four basic requirements of performance if the potential value of such examination is to be fully realized:

1. Individual exposures must be sufficiently brief to stop effectively the movement of cardiac walls and the advancing column of opacified blood. Exposures as rapid as one-sixtieth of a second are desirable; exposures which exceed one-twentieth of a second approach the allowable maximum.

2. Ability to provide multiple exposures in extremely rapid sequence is necessary if the entire cycle of cardiac circulation is to be observed. Within the beating heart, events occur so rapidly that an exposure rate of 4 per second may well be considered to be a minimum requirement.

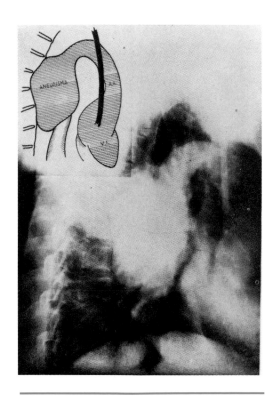

Direct intracardiac contrast injection (1947). Huge aneurysm of the thoracic aorta.[61]

3. Roentgenographic images must be brilliant and clearly detailed if they are to be interpreted with the degree of accuracy which an examination of this type requires.
4. Apparatus used for angiocardiography must be automatic and dependable in operation. A rapid burst of automatically timed and spaced exposures is required to record the fleeting circulation of the opaque mass from vena cava to the descending aorta.

Cineangiography, the photographic recording of the fluoroscopic image of the opacified chambers of the heart and great vessels, was introduced by Stewart and associates in 1939.[63] Although they initially used a 16-mm cine-camera, they soon developed a 35-mm camera with a motor that rotated a new section of film into position automatically after each exposure. This method obviated the problem of precisely timing exposures to coincide with the movement of opaque contrast material into the desired chambers of the heart and great vessels. As Sussmann and associates wrote,[64] "there is no need to depend upon the circulation time except where there is reason to suspect prolongation. Furthermore, since direct inspection of fluoroscopic screen is possible while the camera is operated, exposures may be continued until part or all of the circuit is completed." To reduce the amount of radiation received by the patient, Watson and Weinberg introduced a synchronized lead shutter to interrupt the x-ray beam during the time occupied by the movement of the film.[65] Thus the patient was exposed only during the time necessary to actually make each picture.

Limitations of photofluorography included the high capital expense of the equipment, the substantial radiation dose to the patient, the inability to properly view the miniature film without special equipment, and the poor detail and quality of the small films when compared with those obtained by direct radiography.[57]

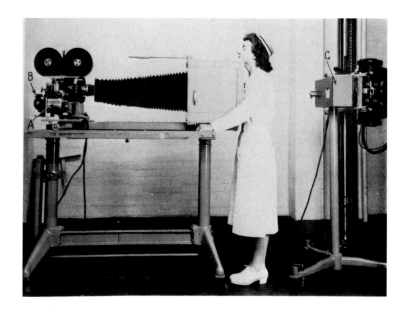

35-mm cinefluorography unit (1948). The camera on the left has a drive motor (B) and a repeater motor (A). The lead shutter mechanism (C) is placed between the x-ray tube and subject.[65]

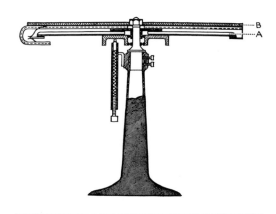

First cassette changer, the "radiocarrousel" of Pereira-Caldas (1934). *A*, Large metal wheel in which six 24 × 30 cm cassettes were set in frames about the periphery. *B*, Round disk covered by a sheet of lead in which an exposure opening was cut. X-ray exposures could be made at the rate of 1 per second by manually rotating the wheel to successively bring the cassettes under the exposure opening.[57]

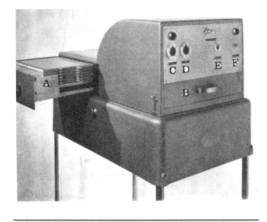

Automatic "seriograph" (1949). *A*, Loading drawer; *B*, removing drawer; *C*, line switch; *D*, timer switch; *E*, foot switch; *F*, button switch.[68]

First radiographic table for simultaneously exposing standard cassettes in vertical and horizontal magazines (1948).[57]

The prototype unit for rapidly changing cassettes was the "radiocarrousel" of Pereira-Caldas introduced in 1934.[66] This consisted of a large wheel with six 24 × 30 cm cassettes that were sequentially rotated manually under the exposure opening at a speed of 1 per second. The platform could be tilted at right angles for examinations in the erect position. In the same year, Moniz developed the "escamoteur," which contained two cassettes on top of each other.[67] After the first cassette (lying in a lead tray) was exposed, it was manually pulled to a receiving bin, with the underlying second cassette pushed up into place by a set of springs. One year later (1935), Sanchez-Perez began modifying the escamoteur principle, which eventually evolved into an electrically driven "seriograph" that could be automatically controlled and was capable of shifting eight cassettes at intervals ranging from 0.5 to 2.0 seconds.[68]

Another approach was the "tautograph," a motor-driven chain-conveyer system that brought 11 × 14 inch cassettes from the magazine into filming position. This was the first device in which the shifting of cassettes and the roentgen exposures were synchronized with a self-cocking grid, with the entire equipment fully automated and controlled from a single push-button. Any number of cassettes could be exposed at the rate of one per second. However, like most cassette changers then available, this did not expose films fast enough, was large and cumbersome, and could not be adapted easily to existing equipment.[57]

In Stockholm (1948), Axen and Lind[57] developed the first fast continuous cassette changer for taking radiographs in two planes at right angles to each other. Their device had a capacity of ten 12 × 12 inch cassettes for each magazine and exposed them at half-second intervals.

A machine for rapidly starting and stopping large roll film for direct radiography (the "cinematograph") was first demonstrated by Howard Ruggle in 1925.[69] As described by Chamberlain and Dock (who made the first cardiac x-ray "movies" in the United States using the machine),[70] in Ruggle's cinematograph, the device could take fifteen 8 × 10 films per second and was primarily used for making measurements and recording relative movements of portions of the heart during various phases of the cardiac cycle. Its major disadvantages were that it was "necessarily quite noisy" and had to be operated in a room lighted only by a safe light.

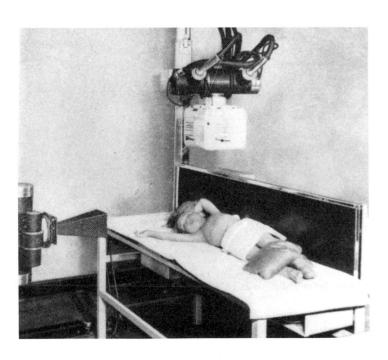

During the next two decades, sporadic attempts were made to improve the roll-film device. In 1948, Wendell G. Scott[57] developed the "rapidograph," a compact unit that was mounted to the underside of a radiographic table so that the magazine could be removed for reloading. The radiographic exposure and momentary stoppage of the film were synchronized with a fast self-cocking grid. The whole unit was automated so that with the closing of one switch a series of x-ray exposures could be made on 78 feet of film at half-second intervals (a speed nearly twice as great as those of most cassette changers of the period). To keep the cost of production down, they selected a film size of 9½ × 9½ inches that was already available.[57]

In 1949, Thompson, Figley, and Hodges[62] constructed a roll-film device permitting 11 × 11 inch exposures at rates from 2 to 6 per second. In the same year, Gidlund[71] of Sweden developed a new apparatus for taking two-plane radiographs, utilizing larger roll-film (12 × 12 inch exposures) and speeds of up to 8 per second.[71]

The main disadvantage of large roll film was the inconvenience of loading the magazine and processing the long strips of film, especially in departments that had been mechanized for cut film. This problem was addressed by Rigler and Watson (1953),[72] who designed a device in which the roll film was transported in intermittent fashion by a Geneva drive piercing the film edge by sharpened phonograph needles. After the exposure, an automatic cutting knife transformed the roll film into cut film, which was stored in the receiver bin and could be more easily processed.

At the end of the third era, angiocardiography was clearly the glamorous modality in the diagnosis of cardiovascular disease. Nevertheless, Sosman (and others) stressed that "the ultimate objective of all of these very complicated and sometimes dangerous procedures is to learn enough about these conditions so that we can go back and refer our knowledge to the original, simple, uncomplicated examination and know more about what we are seeing and finding." Thus in many cases a combination of the simple and specialized radiographic techniques was necessary for a complete diagnosis of congenital and acquired heart disease.[57]

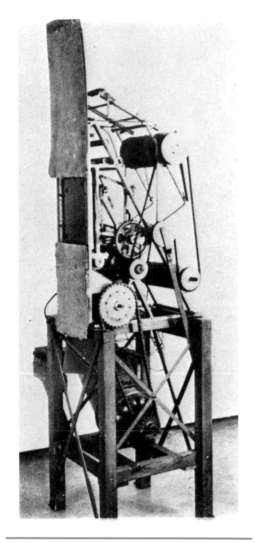

Ruggles cinematograph (1925). This was the first apparatus for using a large roll film for rapid continuous x-ray exposures.[69]

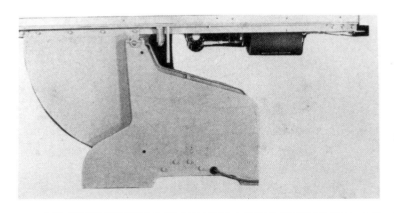

"Rapidograph" of Scott (1948). This device for obtaining a continuous series of exposures at half-second intervals was constructed by taking the war surplus magazine of a Fairchild A-5 aerial camera and converting it for radiographic purposes by installing intensifying screens, devising a new drive shaft, and attaching it to a speed reducer motor.[57]

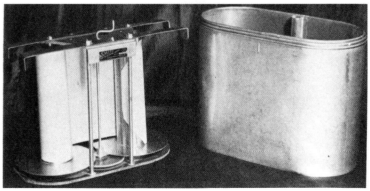

Automatic developing outfit for processing long strips of 9½-inch roll film (1951). By placing stainless steel bars across the top of these units (as shown in the photograph), they may be suspended in conventional 10-gallon solution tanks. In actual work, many technicians preferred to develop these strips with film by hand in regular darkroom tanks. In most instances, the strips were not sufficiently long to warrant the time consumed in mounting them in the developing outfits. An electric motor that fit on top of the crank between the spools could be used for continuous operation.[57]

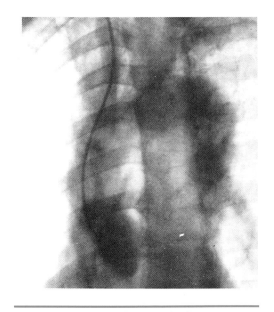

First in vivo contrast study of the coronary arteries (1933). Excellent visualization of the entire thoracic aorta, as well as the coronary artery system.[73]

Thoracic aortography (1948). Contrast injected through a radial artery catheter threaded into the bulb of the aorta demonstrates the ascending aorta, the arch and brachiocephalic vessels, and the descending aorta.[75]

THE FOURTH ERA

The modern era of cardiac radiology began with the development of image intensification in the late 1940s and early 1950s (see Chapter 10). Using image intensification, movies of the fluoroscopic image (cinefluoroscopy) either with film or with magnetic tape were of far better quality. Catheters could be more easily and precisely placed within specific areas of the cardiac chambers. Other practical advantages included the ability to see images that were previously barely visible, the opportunity to view the images in an undarkened room, and a substantial reduction in radiation exposure to both patient and radiologist.

At almost the same time, the development of a mechanical pump oxygenator for extracorporeal circulation permitted the development of delicate *intracardiac* surgery. Cardiac surgery soon expanded to include operative procedures on the coronary artery. The first in vivo contrast studies of coronary arteries were reported independently by Rousthoi[73] and by Reboul and Racine[74] in 1933. Applying Rousthoi's animal experiments to man, Radner introduced a catheter into the radial artery and guided it under fluoroscopic control via the subclavian artery into the ascending aorta, where three exposures were made after the rapid injection of contrast material.[75] According to Dotter and Frische,[76] the credit, if not the priority, for widely applied coronary visualization belongs to Gunnar Jonsson,[77] who published many beautiful reproductions showing all of the major coronary arteries following the injection of liberal doses of concentrated contrast material through a catheter inserted far down the ascending aorta, "preferably with the tip down by the semilunar valves."

Although the coronary arteries could be visualized by the injection of contrast material into the aortic root, there was little control over the disposition of contrast agent, "with the result that during systole most of it is swept up the ascending aorta into the systemic arteries while only a small fraction reaches the coronary vessels."[76] In addition, only after the availability of image intensification was it possible to accurately define the position of the catheter tip and to fluoroscopically observe the opacification of the tiny vessels to the heart. Among the first deliberately produced coronary arteriograms in humans were those reported by Thal, Lester, Richards, and Murray in 1957.[78] Although using a nonselective aortic root injection via a catheter introduced into the brachial artery via an arteriotomy, they concluded that "from the surgical standpoint, this technique has great potentialities both in the selection of patients for surgical treatment and in demonstrating the type of surgical procedure best indicated."

Many modifications of this procedure were subsequently employed. Increased filling of the coronary artery was attempted by decreasing the cardiac output at the time of arteriography by temporary occlusion of the inferior vena cava or by increasing the intrabronchial pressure. Occlusion of the ascending aorta by the use of a rapidly inflatable and deflatable balloon was attempted to increase the delivery of contrast material to the coronary arteries.[76] Some experimenters even used acetylcholine to produce controllable cardiac arrest during coronary arteriography, although this resulted in a loss of flow of contrast material into the smaller coronary radicals and was thus abandoned.

Following the report by Miller, Hughes, and Kolff (1957)[79] of successful opacification of the coronary artery in dogs by injection in the coronary sinuses near the coronary ostia, this "semiselective" method was applied in humans by Sones and co-workers in 1958.[80] After observing that in some cases the catheter had actually entered the coronary artery without adverse effect, they began to selectively catheterize the coronary arteries under fluoroscopic control from the brachial artery. This selective technique eliminated the need to inject large doses of contrast material in the ascending aorta, which generally caused superimposition of the opacified aortic root and the descending thoracic aorta on the coronary vessels and often resulted in obscuration of the margins and proximal portions of the coronary arteries.[81] Four years later (1962), Sones and Shirey[82] reported a success rate of 95% in performing bilateral selective catheterization and coronary opacification in more than 1,000 attempts.

Percutaneous transfemoral selective coronary arteriography was first performed in 1961 by Ricketts and Abrams.[81] They used "preshaped opaque polyethylene catheters, one designed to enter each coronary artery." Six years later (1967), Melvin Judkins developed "catheters of soft, moldable material preshaped to conform to the anticipated anatomy" so that "the coronaries may be catheterized with startling consistency and ease."[83] This technique has subsequently become the most widely applied method of coronary arteriography throughout the world.[84]

As cardiac surgery progressed, it became crucial to understand the altered hemodynamics of the underlying condition in addition to defining the abnormal anatomy. The tip of the angiographic catheter became more than a mere conduit for the passage of contrast material into the cardiac

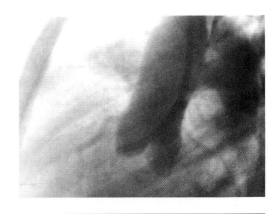

Visualization of the two coronary arteries (1948). The sinus of Valsalva and the semilunar valves are also seen in this patient with a patent ductus arteriosus.[77]

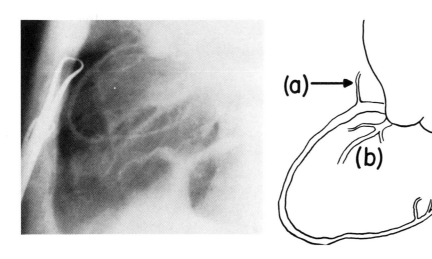

Early coronary arteriogram (1957). *Left*, Radiograph and *right*, diagram of a lateral projection showing the right coronary artery in detail. The cardiopulmonary branch (*a*) is clearly demonstrated as is the anterior descending branch of the left coronary artery (*b*).[78]

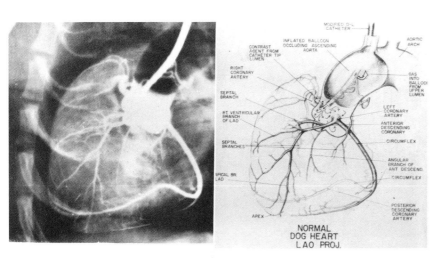

Selective coronary arteriography using the occlusion technique (1958). *Left*, Radiograph and *right*, labelled diagram of a left anterior oblique projection of a dog made during complete occlusion of the ascending aorta by a balloon peripheral to the site of injection.[76]

233

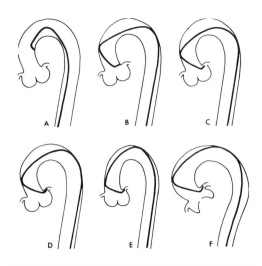

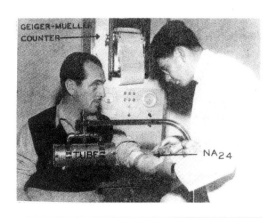

Left coronary catheter technique (1967). "The guide is removed as the catheter is advanced through the proximal descending thoracic aorta. *A*, Catheter is maneuvered to a "relaxed" position in the aortic arch, cleared, and the patient turned 20 degrees RPO. *B*, Catheter is advanced slowly until (*C*) it drops into the coronary orifice. The spring afforded by the secondary bend holds the tip in the coronary orifice. Note the catheter position and the reasons for "catheter arms" of varying lengths when used in (*D*) medium, (*E*) small, and (*F*) poststenotic (large) aorta."[83]

Radiocardiography technique (1949). The shielded Geiger counter tube is in front of the precordium. The Geiger-Mueller counter is shown in the background. The radioactive sodium (*24NA*) is injected directly into the antecubital vein.[90]

chambers. Pressures were recorded and blood samples obtained to measure the concentration of gas or dye for determination of flow, shunts, and valve areas. As these physiological parameters became increasingly important, the role of the radiologist in angiocardiography began to decrease. In some departments, all or the majority of this work was done by cardiologists or cardiac surgeons; in others, the specialists worked with cardiac radiologists.

The information accumulated on the abnormal anatomy and physiology of acquired and congenital heart disease led to the "physiologic interpretation" of plain radiographs. For example, Shanks and Kerley (1951) called attention to the now well-known "A," "B," and "C" lines as seen in silicosis.[86] Three years later (1954), Fleischner and Reiner wrote the first American paper for recognizing Kerley's "B" lines as evidence for acute long-standing recurrent pulmonary congestion in patients with mitral stenosis.[87]

Richard Lester (1958)[88] introduced the concept of physiologic interpretation of plain films based on pulmonary vascularity in congenital heart disease.

> Roentgenologic evaluation of congenital heart lesions is the most important single tool available . . . A classification has been devised that permits an objective division into three groups on the basis of roentgenologic criteria. Left-to-right shunts and admixture lesions are found in patients with increased pulmonary vascularity; left-sided and right-sided stenotic lesions, myocardial lesions, and acquired lesions are found in patients with normal pulmonary vascularity; and right-to-left shunts are found in patients with decreased pulmonary vascularity.

Two years later, Owings Kincaid added a fourth group consisting of "congenital lesions producing pulmonary venous hypertension owing to obstruction of pulmonary venous flow."[89]

Nuclear Cardiology

A major development of the modern era has been the introduction of radioactive isotopes for the study of cardiovascular physiology and disease. In 1949, Prinzmetal and associates[90] described "radiocardiography" for the detection of intracardiac shunts and other disturbances of intracardiac blood flow. In this technique, radioactive sodium (*24Na*) was injected intravenously and a continuous graphic recording of intracardiac radioactive blood concentration was obtained by use of a specially constructed ink-writing Geiger-Mueller counter.

Three years later (1952), Pritchard and colleagues used *131I*-labeled human serum albumin, assayed with a well-counter, to determine cardiac output in humans.[91] The measurement of coronary blood flow using isotope techniques, first described by Waser and Hunzinger in 1953,[92] has been estimated in three ways:

> (1) by measuring how fast an isotope which is injected into the blood is taken up by the myocardium; (2) by following a bolus of tagged blood as it flows through the coronary vessels; and (3) by measuring the rate at which a freely diffusable inert gas is washed out of the heart muscle by the blood.

Ross and co-workers (1964)[93] used a precordial counter to record the disappearance of solutions of *133Xe* or *85Kr*, which had been injected

234

directly into the coronary arteries through an arteriographic catheter. As they summarized,

> This method has two major advantages over the existing methods of measuring human myocardial blood flow. Firstly, the right and left coronary circulation can be studied separately, this being the only method whereby the right circulation can be studied in man. Secondly, anatomical and physiological correlations are readily available as arteriography is an essential feature of the method.

A radioisotope scanning method to visualize the intracardiac blood pool was reported by Rejali, MacIntyre, and Friedell in 1958.[94] Wagner and associates (1961) stressed the value of cardiac blood pool scans in the differentiation between pericardial effusion and cardiac dilatation.[95] Their four criteria of pericardial effusion were:

> (1) . . . zone of decreased radioactivity separating the cardiac blood pool from the lung fields; (2) . . . marked separation of hepatic and cardiac blood pools on the cardiac scan; (3) . . . in patients with pericardial effusion, the cardiac blood pool was normal in size on the scanning image, in contrast with enlargement observed in patients with cardiac dilatation; and (4) with pericardial effusion, the ratio of cardiac diameter measured by photoscan to cardiac diameter measured by routine roentgenogram . . .

was significantly smaller than with cardiac dilatation. Five years later (1966), Bonte and Curry[96] described the advantages of the newly developed ^{99m}Tc as a label on albumin for cardiac blood pool scans.

In addition to evaluating pericardial effusions, intracardiac blood pool scanning was used to demonstrate aneurysms of the thoracic and abdominal aorta, to differentiate aneurysms of the aorta from mediastinal and abdominal masses, and occasionally to visualize neoplasms and thrombi of the cardiac walls that might encroach on the blood pools. However, as Rejali and co-workers[94] stressed in their initial paper,

> it should be emphasized that although fairly sharp delineations may be obtained on our scanograms, visualization of the blood pools by angiography, by the very nature of the process, is much sharper and superior in detail. Whenever fine detail is essential, angiocardiography is, therefore, of distinct advantage.

An extension of the blood pool scanning technique using "gating" permitted assessment of ventricular function and ejection fraction. After the injection of a tracer, an ECG-triggered switch, or "gate," was used to select a specific portion of the cardiac cycle during which the display oscilloscope or computer would accept data.[97] The gate concept was introduced in 1969 by Mullins and associates, who used it to collect a single end-diastolic image to assess ventricular volume.[98] Strauss (1971), Zaret (1973) and co-workers acquired an end-diastolic image for 200 to 400 beats, moved the gate position relative to the R wave, and collected an end-systolic image over an additional 200 to 400 beats. By comparing these two static images, they could calculate the left ventricular ejection fraction and assess regional wall motion. The introduction of high-speed computers led to the development of the multigated acquisition (MUGA) technique, which permitted acquisition of images through most or all of the cardiac cycle. In this procedure, the R wave trigger initiated the recording of image data into the first frame of the computer memory for a preset time. Then data were recorded into the second frame for the same preset time and so on. When the next R wave occurred, the gate reset, data were recorded into the first frame once again, and the entire process

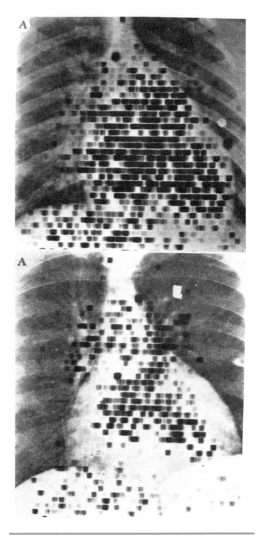

Radioisotope scanning for suspected pericardial effusion (1961). *Top,* Normal intracardiac blood pool. *Bottom,* Large pericardial effusion in a patient with myxedema.[95]

of recording into sequential frames was repeated. Data from corresponding parts in each cycle were added together into the computer memory until sufficient counts were recorded. The frames could then be replayed as an endless-loop cinematic display. The final result depicted an "average" cardiac cycle gleaned from the data of 100 to 600 cardiac cycles.[97]

The radionuclide detection of intracardiac and extracardiac shunts in congenital heart disease was reported in 1957 by Greenspan, Lester, and Marvin.[99] Following the injection of ^{131}I-labeled human serum albumin, externally placed scintillation counters positioned over the heart and femoral artery recorded time-concentration curves. An analysis of their shapes permitted detection of left-to-right and right-to-left shunts without the need for arterial puncture associated with conventional dye-dilution curves. More rapid studies with minimal radiation exposure were reported by Braunwald and associates (1962) using the inhalation of [85]Kr.[100]

A pressing clinical problem was to identify patients with coronary artery disease before myocardial infarction and irreversible damage. Myocardial perfusion studies were based on the Sapirstein principle,[104] which stated that if a tracer is almost totally extracted by an organ and rapidly cleared from the blood by other tissues on the first pass, then the regional distribution of the tracer in the organ is flow related. When applied to the heart, this meant that the uptake of tracer was initially proportional to myocardial blood flow. On later scans, the distribution would be altered by the ongoing processes of equilibrium.

Early work on myocardial perfusion imaging centered on $^{43}K^+$. Initial studies showed that perfusion through stenotic arteries at rest might become inadequate when myocardial oxygen demands were increased, as during exercise. Several investigators evaluated various isotopes of potassium and its analogs, rubidium and cesium. Eventually, it was clear that the best radionuclide was [201]Tl (thallium-201), which had a higher extraction and retention by the myocardium and was more suitable for imaging because of its low-energy gamma radiation and relatively lower hepatic and gastric uptake. Produced by a cyclotron, ^{201}Tl was commercially supplied as the chloride salt with a half-life of 73 hours (decaying by electron-capture to mercury-201).[97]

At first, thallium perfusion images were acquired after two separate injections. The initial set of images was usually obtained immediately after injection of the radionuclide at peak exercise to define blood flow under conditions of stress. The second set was acquired immediately after injection at rest, at least 3 days later (to reflect the 73-hour half-life of the tracer). Defects in uptake seen on both sets of images were thought to represent zones of scarring, while those seen on exercise scans but not on scans obtained at rest were thought to represent stress-induced ischemic zones. It was soon shown that some thallium defects noted at rest filled in if the imaging were carried out long enough after injection, and it was believed that these represented zones of chronic underperfusion. Thus it became apparent that the two-injection technique might not adequately differentiate ischemic but viable from nonviable myocardium unless the late images were obtained.[97] Pohost and colleagues (1977) suggested that sequential imaging for 1 to 6 hours after a single dose of thallium injected during exercise could differentiate between ischemia and infarction or scar.[102] They also noted that defects related to ischemia would resolve in time, calling this phenomenon *redistribution*, and that

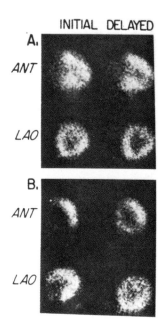

INITIAL   DELAYED

A.
ANT

LAO

B.
ANT

LAO

Thallium-201 myocardial imaging (1980). A, Normal images immediately after exercise (*INITIAL*) and 4 hours later (*DELAYED*). Note the homogeneous distribution of tracer except for the apical and apical-inferior segments, where activity can normally be slightly lower. B, Abnormal study. Note the inferior and apical defects in the initial anterior (*ANT*) view and the septal and apical-inferior defects in the initial left anterior oblique view (*LAO*). There is complete redistribution into the septal and apical-inferior segments (transient defect), partial redistribution into the inferior segment, and no redistribution into the apical defect (persistent defect).[103]

defects related to scar or infarction would persist. The single-dose technique offered substantial advantages over the double-injection method. In addition to probably being more physiological, it achieved a 50% reduction in radionuclide administration (decreasing both radiation exposure and cost to the patient) and required only a single patient visit.[103]

Nuclear medicine studies also could be performed to detect acute myocardial infarction. Studies by D'Agostino (1964) and Shen and Jennings (1972) showed that calcium was deposited in irreversibly damaged myocardial cells in a crystalline structure suggesting hydroxyapatite. These early observations led Bonte and associates (1974) to evaluate whether ^{99m}Tc-pyrophosphate (PYP) might be capable of identifying irreversibly damaged myocardial cells on the basis of pyrophosphate complexing with calcium in crystalline forms. Their results showed that pyrophosphate scintigraphy was a sensitive indicator of acute myocardial infarction.[104] Unlike previous radiotracers used for myocardial imaging (cesium, potassium, rubidium), which normally distributed in well-perfused and healthy myocardium and showed an infarction as a cold area in a hot field, PYP resulted in a hot spot on a cold background, since it concentrated in the abnormality rather than in the adjacent normal myocardium. The PYP study might be positive as early as 12 hours after the onset of acute infarction, although the sensitivity at that time was relatively low. Serial studies indicated that the radionuclide concentration within an acute myocardial infarction reached a peak at 48 to 72 hours and then gradually diminished over the next 2 weeks.[105]

NEWER IMAGING MODALITIES

Single photon emission computed tomography (SPECT) has become the preferred imaging technique for ^{201}Tl myocardial perfusion studies. By focusing on a thin slice of the heart, tomographic imaging minimizes overlying and underlying isotope activity and results in substantially better image contrast than can be achieved with planar techniques. Another advantage of SPECT is its three-dimensional nature as images are obtained from multiple projections around the heart. When viewed in a cine format, the image of the heart rotating in space can aid in interpretation. In addition, the image set can be reoriented to display the heart in other perspectives, permitting superior localization of perfusion defects in the myocardium.[106]

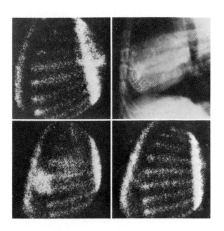

Infarct-avid myocardial scanning (1974). *Top left,* Lateral scan of the chest of a dog made 1 hour after the intravenous administration of technetium pyrophosphate. Only normal skeletal distribution is seen. *Top right,* Chest radiograph made immediately after instillation of metallic Hg into branches of the anterior descending artery. *Bottom left,* Lateral scan made 24 hours later after repeat isotope administration shows intense localization of radioactivity at a site presumably representing a myocardial infarction. *Bottom right,* Eight days later, repeat study after tracer administration shows no abnormal uptake. Serial scans had shown persistent localization only through the fourth day after infarction.[104]

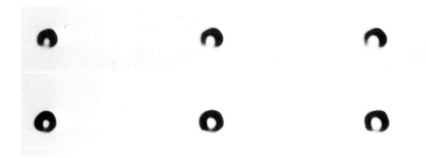

SPECT scanning. The stress views (*top*) show a posterior wall infarct. On the rest study (*bottom*), there is minimal reperfusion that is probably related to collateral flow.

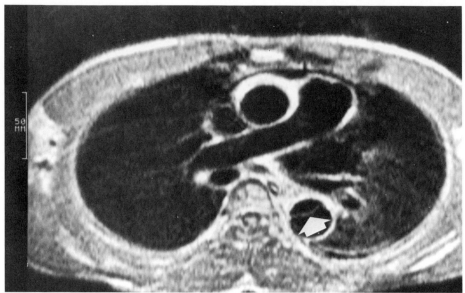

MR imaging of aortic dissection. Axial scan at level of main and right pulmonary arteries clearly shows the intimal flap (*arrow*) in the descending aorta.[110]

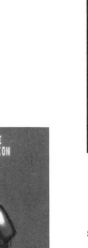

PET scanning. *Left*, Myocardial blood flow study using radioactive ammonia demonstrates a lack of blood flow in the upper left portion of the image (10 o'clock to 12 o'clock positions), which corresponds to the ischemic cardiac apex in this patient. *Right*, Fluorine-18 deoxyglucose metabolism study in the same patient demonstrates active, viable myocardium in that same area, confirming that this patient could obtain major benefits from interventive therapy. There is clearly viable myocardium in the hypoperfused area of the heart.[107]

Positron emission tomography (PET) using highly extracted tracers such as rubidium and ammonia is a rapidly advancing technology for distinguishing areas of reduced blood flow in the myocardium. By providing a regional metabolic map of the heart based on the distribution of substrates of myocardial metabolism, PET scanning can aid in distinguishing viable, ischemic myocardium from myocardial necrosis or scar. Imaging the myocardial blood pool can assess regional wall motion and detect abnormal wall thickening.[107,108]

Magnetic resonance (MR) imaging will be playing an increasingly important role in the evaluation of the heart and great vessels. Because of its ability to display anatomical detail, its tomographic and multiplanar nature, and the lack of need for intravenous contrast material, MR imaging is already an established technique for the evaluation of congenital heart disease, cardiac tumors, and disorders of the aorta and pericardium. Using fast scanning and a cine format, MR can evaluate ventricular function and the regurgitation of blood across heart valves. In the future, MR spectroscopy may permit the detection of abnormal metabolic activity in various cardiac conditions.[109]

For a brief discussion of echocardiography, see Chapter 26.

Bibliography

Seningen RP and Lester RG: History of cardiac radiology. Unpublished report, 1970.

References

1. Seningen RP and Lester RG: History of cardiac radiology. Unpublished report, 1970.
2. Williams FH: Notes on x-rays in medicine. Trans Assoc Amer Physicians 11:375-382, 1896.
3. Williams FH: A method for more fully determining the outline of the heart by means of a fluoroscope together with other uses of this instrument in medicine. Boston Med Surg J 135:335-337, 1896.
4. Fulton H: Sixty years of cardiovascular roentgenology. AJR 76:657-663, 1956.
5. Williams FH: The Roentgen rays in medicine and surgery. New York, MacMillan, 1901.
6. Abrams A: Roentgen rays in pulmonary disease. JAMA 38:1142-1147, 1902.
7. Claytor TA and Merrill WH: Orthodiagraphy in the study of the heart and great vessels. Am J Med Sci 138:549-562, 1909.
8. Van Zwaluwenburg JG and Warren LE: The diagnostic value of the orthodiagram in heart disease. Arch Int Med 7:137-152, 1911.
9. Bardeen CR: A standard of measurement in determining the relative size of the heart. Anat Rec 10:176, 1916.
10. Bardeen CR: Estimation of cardiac volume by roentgenology. AJR 9:823-832, 1922.
11. Crane AW: The Bardeen method of estimating cardiac volume. AJR 6:48-49, 1919.
12. Danzer CS: The cardiothoracic ratio: An index of cardiac enlargement. Am J Med Sci 157:513-521, 1919.
13. Karshner RG and Kennicott RH: A practical method of roentgen examination of the heart based upon a study of one hundred consecutive normal and abnormal cases. AJR 9:305-314, 1922.
14. Comeau WJ and White PD: An evaluation of heart volume determinations by the Rohrer-Kahlstorf formula as a clinical

method of measuring heart size. Am Heart J 17:158-168, 1939.

15. Ungerleider HE and Gubner R: Evaluation of heart size measurements. Am Heart J 24:494-510, 1942.

16. Crane AW: The heart, the x-ray and the internist. AJR 9:323-329, 1922.

17. Vaquez H and Bordet E: The heart and the aorta. Paris, Baillière, 1918.

18. O'Kane GH, Andrew FD, and Warren SL: A standardization roentgenologic study of the heart and great vessels in the left oblique view. AJR 23:373-383, 1930.

19. Paterson R: The value of roentgenologic study of the esophagus and bronchi in cases of heart disease, especially mitral disease. AJR 23:396-408, 1930.

20. Nemet G and Schwedel JB: Roentgenographic studies of the right ventricle. Am Heart J 7:560-573, 1932.

21. Roesler H: Relation of shape of heart to shape of chest, with special reference to antraposterior dimension and morphology of various normal heart types. AJR 32:464-486, 1934.

22. Rudis-Jicinsky J: Skiagraphy as in art. Trans Am Roentgen Ray Soc 3:57-65, 1903.

23. Case JT: Pericarditis calculosa. JAMA 80:236-240, 1923.

24. Cutler EC and Sosman MC: Calcification in the heart and pericardium. AJR 12:312-320, 1924.

25. Sosman MC and Wosika PH: Calcification in aortic and mitral valves. AJR 30:328-348, 1933.

26. Sosman MC: The technique for locating and identifying pericardial and intracardiac calcifications. AJR 50:461-468, 1943.

27. Ledbetter PV, Holmes GW, and White PD: The value of the x-ray in determining the cause of aortic regurgitation. Am Heart J 1:196-212, 1925.

28. Steel D: Roentgenological and pathological findings in some of the valvular lesions. AJR 23:384-389, 1930.

29. Steel D: The roentgen diagnosis of cardiac aneurysms. JAMA 102:432-436, 1934.

30. Sosman MC: Roentgenologic aspects of acquired valvular heart disease. AJR 42:47-59, 1939.

31. Master AM: Characteristic electrocardiograms and roentgenograms in arterial hypertension. Am Heart J 5:291-299, 1929.

32. Zinn W: Persistence of the ductus arteriosus Botalli. Berl Klin Wschr 35:433-435, 1898.

33. Donovan MS, Neuhauser EBD, and Sosman MC: The roentgen signs of patent ductus arteriosus. AJR 50:293-305, 1943.

34. Fray WW: Roentgenologic diagnosis of coarctation of the aorta (adult type). AJR 24:349-362, 1930.

35. Sabat B: A radiographic method of recording movements of the diaphragm, heart, and aorta. Lwowski Tygodn Lek 6:395-396, 1911.

36. Gott T and Rosenthal J: Method of recording heart movements by means of x-rays (roentgen kymography). Muenchen Med Wschr 59:2033-2035, 1912.

37. Ritvo M: Kymography in roentgenology. In Bruwer AJ (ed): Classic descriptions in diagnostic roentgenology. Springfield, Ill, Charles C Thomas, 1964.

38. Crane AW: Roentgenology of the heart. AJR 3:513-524, 1916.

39. Henny GC and Boone BR: Electrokymograph for recording heart motion utilizing the roentgenoscope. AJR 54:217-229, 1945.

40. Henny GC, Boone BR, and Chamberlain WE: Electrokymography for recording heart motion: Improved type. AJR 57:409-416, 1947.

41. White PD: Observations on the clinical value of the roentgen ray in the diagnosis of cardiovascular disease. AJR 23:353-357, 1930.

42. Haschek E and Lindenthal OT: A contribution to the practical use of the photography according to Rontgen. Wiener Klin Wschr 9:63-64, 1896.

43. Duto U: Rendiconti della Reale Accademia dei Lincei 5:129-130, 1896.

44. Morton WJ: The x-ray or photography of the invisible and its value in surgery. New York, American Technical Book Co, 1896.

45. Kassabian MK: Roentgen rays and electrotherapeutics. Philadelphia, JB Lippincott, 1907.

46. Franck O and Alwens W: Kreislaufstudien am Rontgenschirm. Munchen Med Wchnschr 57:950, 1910.

47. Heuser C: Pieloradiografia con ioduro potasico y las inyecciones intravenosas de ioduro potasico en radiografia. Semana Med (Buenos Aires) 26:424, 1919.

48. Sicard JA and Forestier G: Injections intravasculaires d'huile iodee sous contrôle radiologique. C R Soc Biol (Paris) 88:1200-1202, 1923.

49. Berberich J and Hirsch S: Die Röntgenographische Darstellung der Arterien und Venen am Lebenden. Muenchen Klin Wschr 2:2226-2228, 1923.

50. Brooks B: Intra-arterial injection of sodium iodid. JAMA 82:1016-1019, 1924.

51. Dos Santos, Lamas M, and Pereira-Caldas J: L'arteriographie des membres de l'aorte et de ses branches abdominales. Bull Mem Soc Natl Chir 55:587-601, 1929.

52. Forssmann W: Die Sondierung des rechten Herzens. Klin Wschr 8:2085-2087, 1929.

53. Forssmann W: Ueber Kontrastdarstellung der Hohlen des levenden rechten Herzens und der Lungenschlagader. Muenchen Med Wschr 78:489-492, 1931.

54. Moniz E, de Carvalho L, and Lima A: Angiopneumographie. Presse Med 39:996-999, 1931.

55. de Carvalho L, Moniz E, and Saldanha A: The visibility of the pulmonary vessels (angiopneumographie). J Radiol de'Electrol 16:469-480, 1932.

56. Castellanos A, Pereiras R, and Garcia A: La angiocardiografia radio-opaca. Arch Soc Estud Clin (Habana) 31:523-596, 1937.

57. Scott WG: The development of angiocardiography and aortography. Radiology 56:485-519, 1951.

58. Robb GP and Steinberg I: Visualization of the chambers of the heart, the pulmonary circulation, and the great blood vessels in man. AJR 41:1-17, 1939.

59. Castellanos A, Pereiras R, and Vazquez-Paussa A: On a special automatic device for angio-cardiography. Bol Soc Cuba Pediatr 10:209, 1938.

60. Celis A: A preliminary note on a personal method of angiocardiography. Revista Med Hosp Gen 8:1101-1110, 1946.

61. Chavez I, Dorbecker L, and Celis A: Direct intracardiac angiocardiography: Its diagnostic value. Am Heart J 33:560-593, 1947.

62. Thompson WH, Figley MM, and Hodges FJ: Full cycle angiocardiography. AJR 53:729-737, 1949.

63. Stewart WH, Breimer CW, and Maier HC: Cineroentgenographic diagnosis of congenital and acquired heart disease. AJR 46:639-640, 1941.

64. Sussman ML, Steinberg MF, and Grishman A: Multiple exposure technique in contrast visualization of the cardiac chambers and great vessels. AJR 46:745-747, 1941.

65. Watson JS and Weinberg S: A 35-mm unit for cinefluorography. Radiology 51:728-732, 1948.

66. Pereiria-Caldas J: Artériographies en série avec l'appareil radio-carrousel. J Radiol Electrol Med Nucl 18:34-39, 1934.

67. Moniz E: Evolution of the technique of cerebral angiography. Progr Med 46:1777-1781, 1934.

68. Sanchez-Perez JM and Carter RA: Time factor in cerebral angiography and an automatic seriograph. AJR 62:509-518, 1949.

69. Ruggles HE: X-ray motion pictures of the thorax. Radiology 5:444-448, 1925.

70. Chamberlain WE and Dock W: The study of the heart action with the roentgen cinematograph. Radiology 7:185-189, 1926.

71. Gidlund AS: New apparatus for direct cineroentgenography. Acta Radiol 32:81-88, 1949.

72. Rigler LG and Watson JC: A combination film charger for rapid or conventional radiography. Radiology 61:77-80, 1953.

73. Rousthoi P: Über Angiokardiographie. Vorläufige Mittelung. Acta Radiol 14:419-423, 1933.

74. Reboul H and Racine M: La ventriculographie cardiaque expérimentale. Presse Med 1:763-767, 1933.

75. Radner S: Thoracal aortography by catheterization from the radial artery. Acta Radiol 29:178-180, 1948.

76. Dotter CT and Frische LH: Visualization of the coronary circulation by occlusion aortography: A practical method. Radiology 71:502-523, 1958.

77. Jonsson G: Visualization of the coronary arteries. Acta Radiol 29:536-540, 1948.

78. Thal AP, Lester RG, Richards LS, and Murray MJ: Coronary arteriography in arteriosclerotic disease of the heart. Surg Gynec Obstet 105:457-464, 1957.

79. Miller EW, Hughes CR, and Kolff WJ: Angiography of the coronary arteries in the live dog. Cleveland Clin Q 24:41-48, 1957.

80. Sones FM, Shirey EK, Proudfit WL, and Westcott RN: Cine-coronary arteriography (abstract). Circulation 20:773, 1959.

81. Ricketts HJ and Abrams HC: Percutaneous selective coronary cinearteriography. JAMA 181:620-624, 1962.

82. Sones FM and Shirey EK: Cine coronary arteriography. Mod Concepts Card Dis 31:735-738, 1962.

83. Judkins MP: Selective coronary angiography. Radiology 89:815-824, 1967.

84. Abrams HC: Introduction and historical notes. In Abrams HC (ed): Vascular and interventional radiology. Boston, Little, Brown, 1983.

85. Grainger RG: Intravascular contrast material: The past, the present, and the future. Brit J Radiol 55:1-18, 1982.

86. Shanks SC and Kerley P: A text-book of x-ray diagnosis by British authors in four volumes. Philadelphia, WB Saunders, 1951.

87. Fleischner FG and Reiner L: Linear x-ray shadows in acquired pulmonary hemosiderosis and congestion. N Engl J Med 250:900-905, 1954.

88. Lester RG, Gedgaudas E, and Rigler LG: Method of radiologic diagnosis of congenital heart disease in children. JAMA 166:439-443, 1958.

89. Kincaid OW: Approach to the roentgenologic diagnosis of congenital heart disease. JAMA 173:639-647, 1960.

90. Prinzmetal M, Corday E, Spritzler RJ, and Fleig W: Radiocardiography and its clinical applications. JAMA 139:617-622, 1949.

91. Pritchard WH, MacIntyre WJ, Schmidt WC, Brofman BL, and Moore DJ: The determination of cardiac output by a continuous recording system utilizing iodionated (I-131) human serum albumen. II. Clinical studies. Circulation 6:572-577, 1952.

92. Love WD: Isotope technics in clinical cardiology. Circulation 32:309-315, 1965.

93. Ross RS, Ueda K, Lichtlen PR, and Rees JR: Measurement of myocardial blood flow in animals and man by selective injection of radioactive inert gas into the coronary arteries. Circ Res 15:28-41, 1964.

94. Rejali AM, MacIntyre WJ, and Friedell HL: A radioisotope method of visualization of blood pools. AJR 79:129-137, 1958.

95. Wagner HN, McAfee JG, and Mozley JM: Diagnosis of pericardial effusion by radioisotope scanning. Arch Int Med 108:679-684, 1961.

96. Bonte FJ and Curry TS: The radioisotope blood pool scan. AJR 96:690-697, 1966.

97. Bakal CA and Strauss HW: Radionuclide imaging. In Morganroth J, Parisi AF, and Pohost GM (eds): Noninvasive cardiac imaging. Chicago, Year Book, 1983.

98. Mullins CB, Mason DT, and Ashburn WL: Determination of ventricular volume by radioisotope angiography. Am J Cardiol 24:72-78, 1969.

99. Greenspan RH, Lester RG, and Marvin JF: Isotope circulation studies in congenital heart disease. Radiology 69:106-107, 1957.

100. Braunwald E, Goldblatt A, Long RTL, and Morrow AG: The krypton-85 inhalation tests for the detection of left-to-right shunts. Brit Heart J 24:47-54, 1962.

101. Sapirstein LA: Regional blood flow by fractional distribution of indicators. Am J Physiol 193:161-168, 1958.

102. Pohost GM, Zir LM, Moore RH, et al: Differentiation of transiently ischemic from infarcted myocardium by serial imaging after a single dose of thallium-201. Circulation 55:294-302, 1977.

103. Okada RD, Boucher CA, Strauss HW, et al: Exercise radionuclide imaging approaches to coronary artery disease. Am J Cardiol 46:1188-1203, 1980.

104. Bonte FJ, Parkey RW, Graham KD, et al: A new method for radionuclide imaging of myocardial infarcts. Radiology 110:473-474, 1974.

105. Lyons KP, Olson HG, and Aronow WS: Pyrophosphate myocardial imaging. Semin Nucl Med 10:168-177, 1980.

106. Guiberteau MJ (ed): Nuclear cardiovascular imaging: Current clinical practice. New York, Churchill Livingstone, 1990.

107. Akin JR: Positron emission tomography (PET): The future is now. In Gooding CA and Margulis AR (eds): Diagnostic radiology. Berkeley, UC Press, 1990.

108. Merhige ME and Rowe RW: Positron emission tomography—an introduction. Practical Cardiology 14:51-67, 1988.

109. Edelman RR and Hesselink JR (eds): Clinical magnetic resonance imaging. Philadelphia, WB Saunders, 1990.

110. Ovenfors CO and Godwin JD: Aortic aneurysms and dissections. In Eisenberg RL (ed): Diagnostic imaging: An algorithmic approach. Philadelphia, JB Lippincott, 1988.

111. Williams FH: Thoracic aneurysm, J Am Med Sci 114:665-687, 1897.

CHAPTER 14

Skeletal Radiology

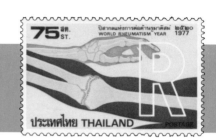
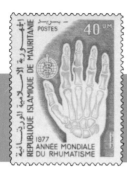
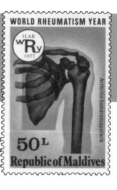
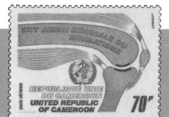

The first decade of radiology was dominated by musculoskeletal imaging. The earliest application of x-rays to the skeleton was to detect and characterize fractures and dislocations. As the *Boston Medical and Surgical Journal*[1] reported less than 1 year after Roentgen's discovery,

> Oberst, of Halle, has for several months examined every fracture in his hospital service by means of the Röntgen rays. He finds, as a result of his observation, that without anesthetizing the patient, or subjecting the broken limb to manipulation, it is possible to make an exact diagnosis of the position, nature, and direction of fractures, and of the amount of deformity. He, therefore, employs anesthesia only in cases where painful manipulations are necessary to correct faulty positions of the ends of the bones. He thus avoids that experience common to almost all surgeons, the etherization of cases with a negative result, and also the danger of fresh hemorrhage or laceration of tissues from stirring up the fractured ends.

Several reports described clinically unsuspected fractures, especially near joints, that could only be demonstrated radiographically ("x-ray fractures").

> It not infrequently happens that even an extensive injury to the osseous framework may be, and sometimes is, mistaken for a more simple lesion. That many cases of actual fracture, particularly at or near the articulating portion of the long bones, have gone unrecognized and untreated, is evidenced by the well-known popular saying that "A sprain is ofttimes worse than a fracture." This saying is well founded on the fact that, when a fracture has been diagnosed as a sprain, and treated as such, it usually results in an exuberance of callus that, almost invariably, causes subsequent impairment of function.[2]

A major advantage of radiography was that it could be performed through an ordinary plaster bandage without needing to remove a splint.[4]

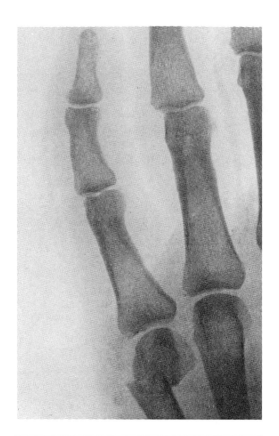

Fracture of the head of the fifth metacarpal (1901).[3]

This technique also substantially altered the concept of fracture healing[5]:

> The Roentgen ray has demonstrated that the former exact coaptation which was supposed to be obtained when a fracture was reduced, was and is often only a beautiful idea on the part of the attending medical man; in other words, that perfect reduction of a fracture is rarely secured, and that nature is, indeed, very kind in taking care of our surgical shortcomings. It is obviously improper, therefore, to criticize the setting of a fracture as shown by a good radiograph, from the standpoint of our old ideas. Criticism of radiographs of fractures should be made only with a full understanding of what radiography has revealed in the healing of these breaks. It is obvious that such knowledge and understanding is not possessed by the laity; and it is, therefore, a great injustice, to ever submit a radiograph of a fracture to a jury of lay minds.

In patients with fractures, radiographs were valuable for assessing the effectiveness of fracture treatment, since "these cases more than any others lead to medico-legal difficulties. If a physician can show a radiograph of the bones in good position in his splints it is the best possible evidence. On the other hand, nothing could be more convincing to the jury than a picture of the bones in bad position. A radiograph is almost a necessary record of a fracture."[4]

Conversely, other investigators[1] found that

> the so-called ideal or perfect union after fracture is rarer than has been generally believed . . . in almost all oblique fractures union takes place with more or less overriding of the fractured ends, a slight degree of which might escape simple manual examination, as the outline of the fragments is obscured by the callus, which is larger

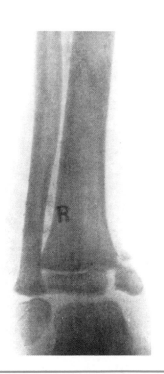

Fracture of the distal tibial epiphysis (1901). R, The point opposite which the light was placed and the right leg.[3]

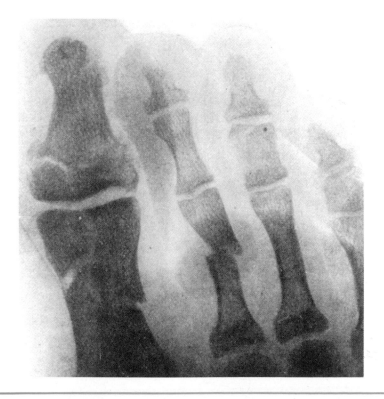

Fractures of both phalanges of the great toe and the proximal phalanx of the second toe (1901). Two of these fractures were unsuspected before the radiograph was made.[3]

in proportion to the amount of overriding. In bones which are deeply covered-in by soft parts, it is possible for a considerable deformity to escape even careful observation . . . For a correct understanding of the symptoms which frequently persist after union of a fracture, a correct knowledge of the position of the ends of the bones is, however, of the greatest importance, and this knowledge the Röntgen rays enable us to possess.

Improper setting of a fracture could lead to deformity and secondary joint disease. One observer[2] questioned, "How many of these diseased joints could have been averted by the (radiographic) recognition of the true nature, and the proper treatment of the initial lesion?"

Nevertheless, the role of x-ray examinations in evaluating skeletal disease was met with considerable skepticism. An editorial in *The Medical News* stated[6]:

> As far as our present knowledge goes, the positive advantages to medicine seem to be limited to three conditions: fractures, dislocations and tumors of bones, encysted bullets, needles or pieces of glass in the tissues, and earthy calculi. In the first class of conditions, its advantages would appear to be slight unless great advances upon present powers and methods can be made . . . it is questionable how much help can be obtained by such crude and blurred shadow pictures as can at present be obtained. In recent cases of fracture or dislocation, the delay and discomfort to the patient necessarily involved in the application of the method would be practically an insuperable objection to its use for purposes of diagnosis.

This generally negative view of the value of x-rays was reflected in the *Report of the Committee of the American Surgical Association of the Medico-Legal Relations of the X-rays*, published in 1900. This long and

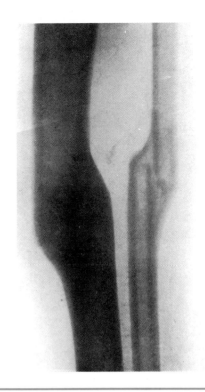

Healed fractures of the tibia and fibula 2 years after the original injury (1901).[3]

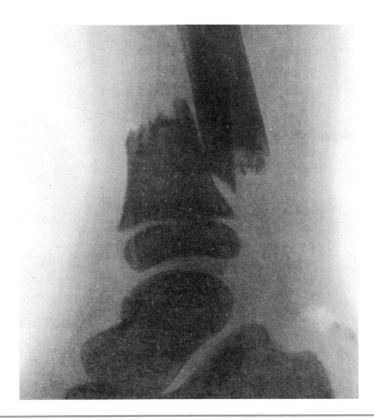

Fracture of the distal tibia and fibula (1901). Lateral view shows no apposition of the fracture fragments.[3]

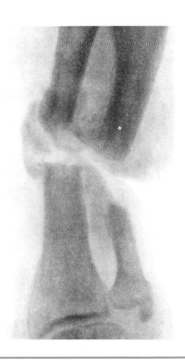

Ununited fracture and necrosis of bone (1901). After falling 40 feet from a house, the patient's radius was fractured at its midportion and there was backward dislocation of the elbow. Examination obtained 5 months later shows "necrosis of bone for about 3.5 centimetres."[3]

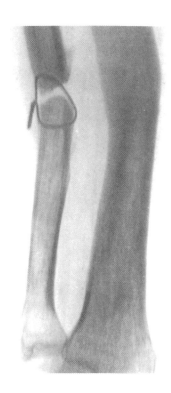

Postoperative radiograph of a fractured forearm (1896). This 3½ minute exposure shows the ends of the ulna approximated by silver wire.[7]

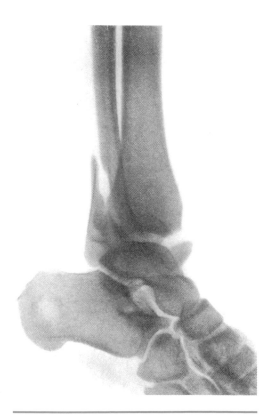

Pott's fracture of the ankle (1900).[12]

fascinating document,[8] consisting primarily of complaints by members who had been sued for malpractice on the basis of x-ray evidence, concluded that "the routine employment of the x-ray in cases of fracture is not at present of sufficient definite advantage to justify the teaching that it should be used in every case." The American Surgical Association's position was only reversed 13 years later (1913), when its committee on fractures recommended the routine use of x-rays in all cases of fractures and dislocations.[9]

In a review of recent progress in the treatment of fractures, which appeared in the same journal in July 1896, McCosh omitted all mention of the use of x-rays.[10] Four years later (1900), the new edition of Bigelow's classic, *The Mechanism of Dislocations and Fracture of the Hip*, failed to include even a single radiograph.[11] However, in that same year, Carl Beck published *Fractures, With an Appendix on the Practical Use of the Röntgen Rays*.[12] Dedicated to Roentgen "without whose discovery much of this book could not have been written," this was the first textbook on the diagnosis and treatment of fractures based on the routine use of x-rays.

By 1904, Martin I. Wilbert[2] enunciated the general opinion that

while it must be admitted that the x-rays, even at the present time, will not indicate the exact nature of all of the possible injuries to the extremities, they do, when properly applied, invariably show all serious lesions of osseous structure and, in a number of cases, will indicate correctly the nature and extent of the injuries to the soft parts; particularly when this injury involves the denser portions of the tendons. It is reasonable, then, for us to assert that precision and exactness of diagnosis, without incurring any additional risk of injuring surrounding tissues, are practically impossible without the use of the x-rays, and that without a complete and correct diagnosis of an injury, the accompanying treatment must necessarily be entirely a matter of chance.

In the early days of radiology, only fluoroscopy was performed for the detection of fractures and the assessment of subsequent therapy. As Russell Boggs observed in the discussion of Wilbert's paper,

There are many x-ray workers in all sections of the country who depend too much on the fluoroscope in the examination of a fracture. It is far better not to make any examination at all than to use the fluoroscope. It is very unreliable. In the last year I examined a number of shoulder joint fractures with the fluoroscope and in only one case was I able to make a diagnosis. In five cases in which a fluoroscopic examination was made the attending physician told me that he did not want to put the patient to the expense of having a radiograph made. In three cases chloroform was given and attempts made to reduce a dislocation where no dislocation existed.

In response, Wilbert noted that

I discarded the fluoroscope for diagnostic purposes a long time ago, and for various reasons. I found that so far as diagnosis is concerned it is absolutely useless, and the X-ray plates we use are so cheap that there is no excuse for not having a radiograph of every case that comes to our institution. The plate is filed away and we have a complete record of every case to which we can refer at any time. These records become more valuable every day because patients who have been treated in our hospital four or five years ago are continually coming back with new injuries.

A fascinating insight into the world of a pioneer radiographer is the retrospective review of Charles Thurstan Holland of Liverpool, England,

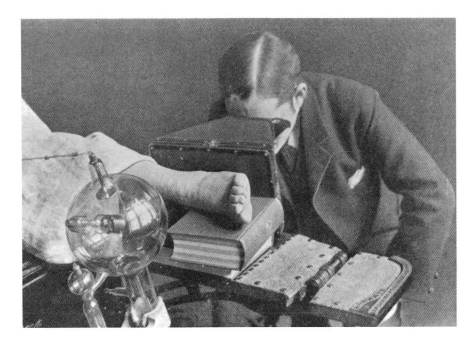

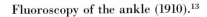

Fluoroscopy of the ankle (1910).[13]

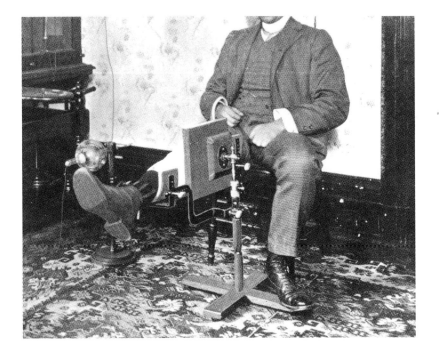

Radiography of the knee with the inner side on the plate (1902). "Tube leveled at twenty inches with access of rays striking centre of knee and plate. With different adjustments of the curved supports, any part of the leg may be postured at any angle or in extended or partly flexed fixture."[14]

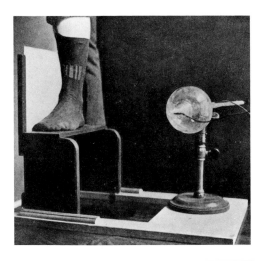

Radiography of the ankle (1902). The tube (with no shielding) "is fixed centrally with the focus at right angles to the part. The plate-holder and foot-rest are adjustable to distance in the path of the rays, but cannot move out of axis." To obtain correct exposure of the ankle, "slide it to twenty inches from the anode, place the foot in position, insert the film or plate, press the part against it, and make the exposure."[14]

who described a series of 261 photographic plates he made from May through December of 1896.[15] Almost all of Holland's examinations were musculoskeletal, primarily to locate foreign bodies, to diagnose fractures and dislocations, to study various congenital deformities, and to develop a series of children's hand images to elucidate normal growth and development. Specific pathological conditions radiographed by Holland included rheumatoid arthritis, hypertrophic osteoarthropathy, tuberculous arthritis, enchondroma, osteochondroma, and rickets.[9]

The special problems of skeletal radiology in children was addressed by Preston Hickey, who in 1903 observed that "in considering radiographs of the joints of children it is most important to have a thorough knowledge of the epiphysis."[16] Demonstrating a radiograph of a normal elbow, he noted that the olecranon "has been repeatedly mistaken for a fracture, even by those whose surgical skill is excellent." Therefore Hickey recommended the use of comparison views: "To avoid mistakes the injured joint should be compared with the corresponding sound joint of the same child."

Radiography of the hand (1901). The part is supported on a thin pine board, which rests on the horses, and is placed along the side of the stretcher.[3]

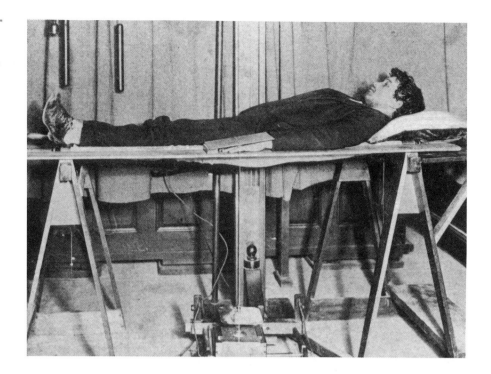

Hickey also stressed the importance of knowledge of the temporal development of the skeleton, which had been described 5 years earlier by John Poland.[17] Gilbert P. Girdwood[18] summarized Hickey's paper,

> As he suggested such a radiographic history of bone development may be very useful for comparison with diseases of bone in children of the same age. It will also give you an idea as to whether the development is progressing normally in children who are backward in their growth, children who are the victims of the diseases of malnutrition.

Girdwood then indicated the importance of determining the precise age of a child, especially in medicolegal questions.

> For instance, a child who was born as a posthumous child or is the heir to a large sum of money or to a title, may have here a very important piece of evidence that is positive and must be accepted as such.

Most of the early advances in skeletal radiology occurred in Europe, especially in Germany. A major force was Alban Köhler, who published his first monograph on bone disease in 1910.[19] Among his many subsequent writings was the classic text, *Roentgenology*, which appeared in 1910 and was translated into English in 1928 by Arthur Turnbull of Glasgow.[20]

The development of Coolidge's hot-cathode tube, especially the fine-focus type cooled by water, and the movable grid made possible striking refinements in diagnosis, especially in deeper and heavier skeletal structures. Hickey stressed the importance of lateral radiography of the spine. As he noted,[21]

> On account of the technical difficulties encountered in making plates laterally, most of us have been content to make stereoscopic plates in the anteroposterior direction. The difficulties which arise embrace, first, the problem of suitable penetration, and, second, the natural exaggeration due to the distance of the examined part from the plate. Thanks to the improvement in tubes in the last few years, we for-

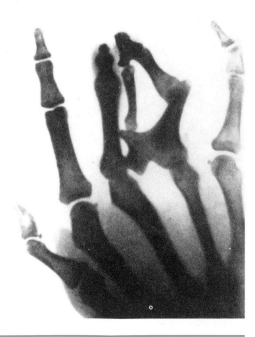

Congenital deformity of the hand in an adult woman (1896). The radiograph was obtained with a 2-minute exposure using a 3-inch coil.[15]

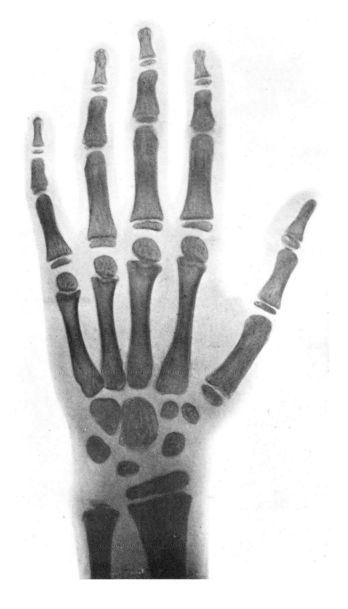

Hand and wrist for bone age. Skiagram of Poland's son, aged 8 years and 5 months, taken in April, 1896 by Alan A. Campbell-Swinton.[17]

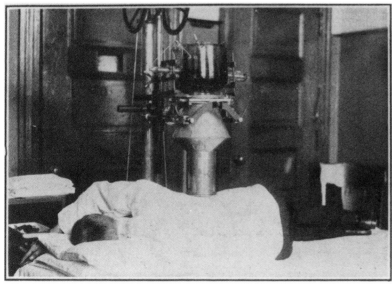

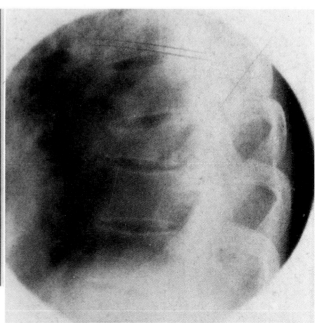

Lateral radiography of the spine (1917). *Left*, Use of an extension diaphragm to minimize distortion. *Right*, Lateral plate of a compression fracture.[21]

tunately now have apparatus at our disposal which afford sufficient penetration for an adequate length of time to satisfactorily radiate the body from side to side. Of course, the use of screens furnishes an additional means with which to accomplish this purpose . . . The second technical point, distortion, can be obviated by increasing the distance between the tube and the patient.

In summarizing the value of the lateral projection, Hickey stressed that "many lesions of the spine which are inconspicuous or almost unobservable on the antero-posterior plate, will show a good clear reading on the lateral view of a definite pathology and consequently a lateral examination of the spine should be made a routine laboratory rule."

In 1911, Fraenkel[22] made a comprehensive study of tumors of the spinal column. Over 12 years, he made sagittal sections of the spinal column and subsequent radiographs of 150 patients who were dying of carcinoma. Fraenkel described two types of secondary bone metastases, osteoclastic and osteoplastic, which could be detected in about 20% of patients in his study. Although metastases could involve any part of the spinal column, Fraenkel found that the most frequent location was in the lower dorsal and upper lumbar regions. Six years later (1917), George Pfahler[23] indicated that one reason vertebral metastases

> cannot be more thoroughly studied is because of the difficulty of making a careful Roentgen study of this portion of the spinal column, and the roentgenogram is the only means of making an accurate diagnosis. The lower dorsal and the upper lumbar vertebrae are the most difficult of all to demonstrate clearly, and in order to demonstrate clearly the early changes of malignant disease fine details are, of course, essential.

Nevertheless, Pfahler warned against confining the radiographic study to any particular portion of the spinal column because the whole column must be carefully examined. He stated that to exclude bony metastases a study of the entire skeleton should be made and repeated at intervals while the patient was under treatment and until all symptoms or evidence of the disease had disappeared.[23] As a corollary, he indicated that "rheumatic pains occurring in the presence of malignant disease should always suggest metastatic carcinoma in the spinal column or other bones and demand a thorough Roentgen study."

In 1918, while addressing the differential diagnosis of bone tumors, Frederick H. Baetjer stressed that "the essential thing is to determine whether the growth is malignant or benign. If that point can be determined the surgeon will be given the information that he wishes." Nevertheless, he added[24]:

> It is well to go beyond that and, if possible, determine the character of the growth belonging to these two great classes. We have found the following set of cardinal points of greatest assistance in establishing the correct diagnosis. These are: *first*, invasion; *second*, bone production; *third*, point of origin; *fourth*, condition of the cortex. Of course it is not always possible to establish the presence of these four points, but practically with every tumor that we see we will be able to find one of these groups in which to place it. By so doing we can automatically rule out a number of growths. The establishment of one such point will almost inevitably give a clue to one or more other points and thus eventually establish the diagnosis.

The radiographic appearance of multiple myeloma involving the skeletal system, producing extensive bone destruction resembling carcinomatosis, was apparently first described by William Evans in 1919.[25]

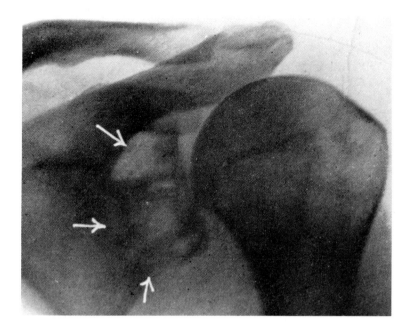

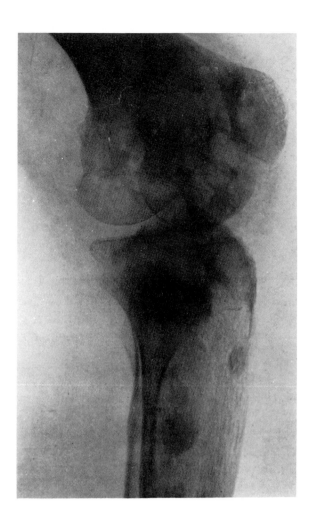

Skeletal metastases (1917). *Left*, Metastatic carcinoma involving the glenoid process, with an early focus of disease in the greater tuberosity of the humerus. *Right*, Advanced carcinomatous metastases about the knee joint.[23]

A classic article on osteomyelitis was published in 1919 by Baetjer[26] (who with Waters, authored the first American book that dealt solely with the radiographic appearance of musculoskeletal disease).[27] After he described the various portals of entry of infection, Baetjer stressed the importance of noting several radiographic findings:

(1) the place where the infection started; (2) the character of the destructive process; (3) the path of extension, that is, spreading equally in all directions or following the path of least resistance; (4) the character and situation of new bone production; and (5) the condition of the cortex, whether it is intact, destroyed as a whole or pierced by sinuses, expanded or not.

He concluded that careful study of the plate not only provided the correct diagnosis but also gave further information to the surgeon. The radiograph could determine the extent of the disease, as well as the presence or absence of a sequestrum and an involucrum, factors significantly affecting the operative approach. Baetjer warned,[27]

Our diagnosis is based upon bone destruction and production, arising from infection. If any other cause has been added to the infection, particularly surgical interference, we may draw erroneous conclusions, because our apparent bone destruction may not be due to disease but may be the result of the surgeon's currette; and furthermore, our new bone production may take place in the normal bone through which the surgeon passed to reach the infection. It is always well to know beforehand in any bone lesion whether there has been surgical interference. One should always be extremely guarded in giving a diagnosis in such a case.

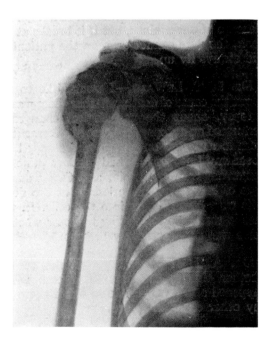

Multiple myeloma (1919). Extensive destruction of the upper end of the humerus, with involvement of the clavicle, scapula, and ribs.[25]

249

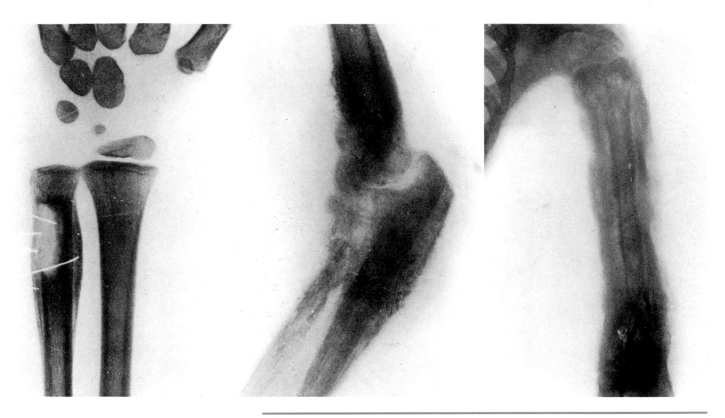

Osteomyelitis (1919). *Left*, Infection starting in the medullary cavity with periosteal bridging and new bone. *Middle*, Joint infection spreading to involve the heads of all three bones about the elbow. *Right*, The entire shaft of the humerus is a sequestrum, with dense new bone forming the involucrum.[26]

In 1911, Roland Hammond addressed the role of radiology in the classification of chronic joint disease.[28] He described both atrophic and hypertrophic forms of chronic joint disease and urged "the careful Röntgen diagnosis of all obscure joint affections coupled with a careful clinical examination, for both are essential and neither alone will give the complete and accurate picture." In outlining the problem of etiology, Hammond wrote:

> most cases of chronic joint disease in which some bacteriologic agent cannot be demonstrated, are shown to be due to faulty metabolism. The absorption of putrefactive substances from the intestinal tract, especially the colon, cause a deposition in and around the joints, of insoluble substances which act as irritants to the delicate synovial membrane. The auto-intoxication resulting from the absorption of products of incomplete metabolism is often found to rest on a simple mechanical basis. Ptosis of the viscera, especially the stomach and colon, allows the food to stagnate, and torsion and partial occlusion of the intestines resulting from the ptosis permit the delay in the passage of food and so favor the absorption of toxins from the alimentary tract.

A major advance in musculoskeletal radiology was the development of body-section imaging. By eliminating superimposed shadows caused by structures above and below the region of interest, conventional tomography offered much greater detail than could be obtained from plain radiographs and allowed diagnoses to be made with much greater certainty (see Chapter 24). From 1940 to 1975, conventional tomography was easily the most advanced and precise technique for imaging diverse disorders of the musculoskeletal system.[9]

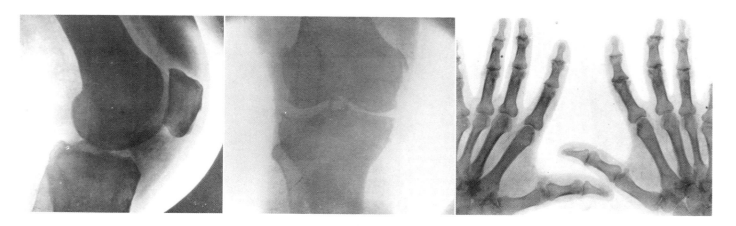

Chronic joint disease (1911). *Left*, Villous arthritis. Thickening of soft parts beneath the patella without bony changes. *Middle*, Hypertrophic arthritis. Note lipping on both the femur and tibia. *Right*, Mixed atrophic and hypertrophic arthritis.[28]

ARTHROGRAPHY

In 1905, Werndorff and Robinsohn were the first to describe examination of the internal structures of the knee after the insufflation of air into the joint.[29] In the following year, Hoffa used oxygen as the contrast material for knee arthrography.[30] However, pneumoarthrography gained little acceptance as a useful diagnostic tool until about 35 years later. The major disadvantage of this technique was the uncomfortable distension of the knee that resulted with the large quantities of gas used, as well as the possible hazard of air embolism. Because the difference in density between the relatively radiolucent cartilage and the surrounding air was not very great, interpretation of the resulting radiographs could be difficult.[31]

In the early 1930s, positive-contrast arthrography was introduced using diiodized contrast material of the "iodoxyl" type. However, positive-contrast arthrography had limited applicability at that time because the available contrast agents caused synovial irritation and pain. The technique became more popular with the development of urographic contrast media, which did not produce these complications. However, an important disadvantage of positive-contrast arthrography was that excess contrast material drained into the dependent portion of the knee where it could partly cover and obscure, rather than outline, the meniscus.[31]

In 1933, Bircher first performed double-contrast arthrography using a combination of gas and positive contrast material.[32] However, it did not come into extensive use until the introduction of nontoxic contrast material. In 1964, Ricklin and coworkers[33] introduced fluoroscopic spot-filming, a technique that was later popularized by Freiberger[31] in the United States.

The major advantage of double-contrast arthrography was that the meniscus, which was thinly coated with positive contrast agent, was also surrounded by air. The major disadvantage was that, as in air arthrography, large quantities of air could cause embolization, and excess contrast material could obscure portions of the meniscus. These disadvantages were overcome by Andren's and Wehlin's[34] development of the horizontal x-ray beam technique, which used small quantities of air and positive-contrast material. Excess positive-contrast material drained into the dependent portion of the knee, away from the portion of the meniscus under

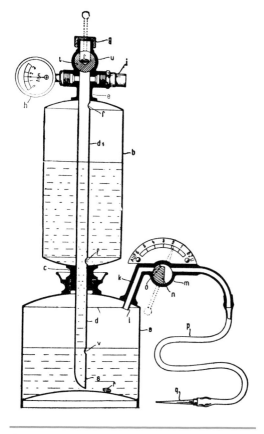

Oxygen pneumoarthrography (1906). Complicated device for production of oxygen. Introduction of a catalyst tablet into the bottom jar filled with 3% hydrogen peroxide initiated a reaction that produced oxygen in the upper portion of the jar. When the valve was opened, gas flowed out into the tubing to the knee joint.[30]

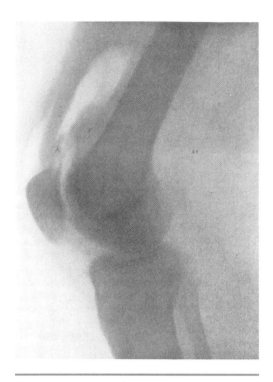

Pneumoarthrography (1906). Prominent synovial thickening representing tuberculous involvement.[30]

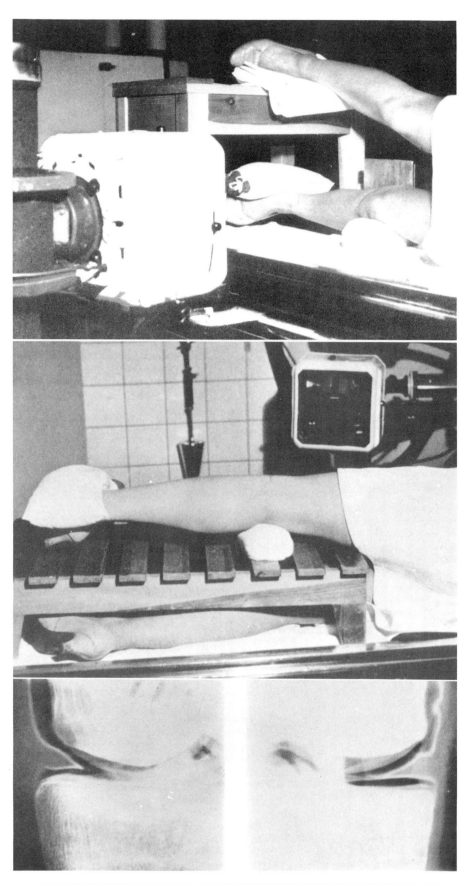

Double-contrast arthrography of the knee using a horizontal x-ray beam (1960). Equipment and position of patient during examination of (*top*) medial and (*middle*) lateral meniscus. Examples of normal medial meniscus in its (*bottom left*) anterior and (*bottom right*) middle aspects.[34]

examination. Simultaneously, air rose to envelop the part of the meniscus being studied. Since small quantities of air and positive-contrast material were being used, the patient was comfortable during the procedure and could resume his usual activity as soon as the examination was completed.[31]

In most centers, magnetic resonance (MR) imaging has replaced arthrography as the modality of choice for imaging the knee and other joints. Multiplanar thin section sequences using surface coils can produce excellent spatial and contrast resolution in studies that are quick and do not require either ionizing radiation or the injection of contrast material.[35]

NEWER IMAGING MODALITIES

In the early 1970s, with the development of technetium compounds containing pyrophosphate and diphosphonate, radionuclide bone scanning became the major imaging technique for the early detection of skeletal metastases. This modality was extremely valuable in confirming the presence of skeletal lesions that were suspected clinically but not demonstrated on conventional studies. However, although radionuclide bone scanning was highly sensitive, it had a low specificity. A region of increased radionuclide uptake could reflect a broad spectrum of benign and malignant conditions. In addition, false negative studies could result from increased uniform and symmetrical uptake attributable to diffuse metastatic disease or with myeloma or metastases from certain anaplastic

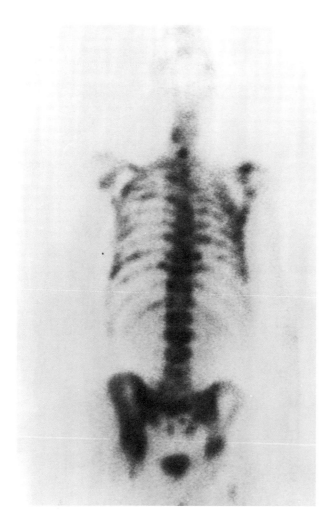

Screening radionuclide bone scan. Multiple focal areas of radionuclide uptake in the axial skeleton, representing metastases from prostate carcinoma. The patient complained of left hip pain and had no previously known metastases.

CT of osteogenic sarcoma. Scan obtained at the level of the femoral heads shows destruction of the left ischium that was seen on plain radiographs. In addition, the CT scan demonstrates a large soft-tissue mass (*arrows*) in an area covered by the gluteus maximus muscle and separated from the rectum. The mass was not clinically palpable.[36]

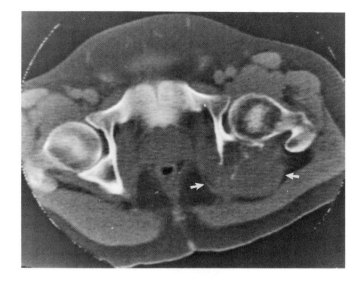

MR imaging of skeletal tumors. *Left*, Synovial sarcoma about the knee. Coronal T1-weighted scan showed a lobular mass (*m*) arising in the soft tissues adjacent to the lateral aspect of the femur (*F*). Note that the tumor is invading the overlying fat (*arrow*). *T*, Tibia. *Right*, Chondrosarcoma of the femur. Note how the T1-weighted image clearly delineates the caudal extent of tumor involvement of the high-signal marrow.

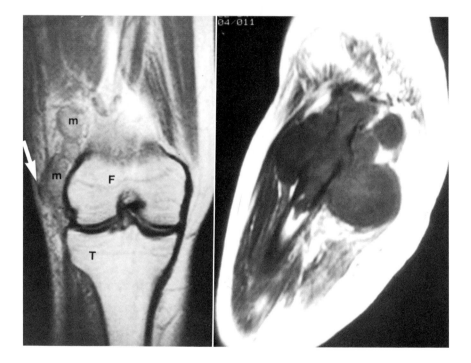

tumors that stimulate little host response and thus may not produce any focal area of increased uptake of radionuclide.

By the late 1970s, computed tomography (CT) became the major modality for evaluating virtually all musculoskeletal diseases, with the exception of screening for bony metastases. Conventional tomography was almost totally eliminated. The ability of CT to provide exquisite bone detail revolutionized the characterization and staging of bone tumors and facilitated the treatment of fractures in anatomically complex regions such as the pelvis. More recently, magnetic resonance (MR) imaging has become the dominant imaging method for the investigation of soft-tissue masses, internal derangements of joints, and alterations in bone marrow.[9]

References

1. Röntgen rays in the treatment of fractures. Boston Med Surg J 135:534-535, 1896.
2. Wilbert MI: A comparative study of fractures of the extremities. Trans Amer Roentgen Ray Soc 195-204, 1904.
3. Williams FH: The roentgen rays in medicine and surgery. New York, MacMillan, 1901.
4. Codman EA: Practical medical use of the x-ray. Boston Med Surg J 135:50-51, 1896.
5. Hickey PM: The interpretation of radiographs. J Mich State Med Soc 3:496-499, 1904.
6. Editorial: Medical News, February 22, 1896.
7. MacIntyre J: Demonstration on the Röntgen rays. Glasgow Med J 45:277-281, 1896.
8. Report of the Committee of the American Surgical Association on the Medico-Legal Relations of the X-rays. Trans Am Surg Assoc 18:429-461, 1900.
9. Murphy WA: Introduction to the history of musculoskeletal radiology. RadioGraphics 10:915-943, 1990.
10. McCosh AL: Resume of recent progress in surgery: The treatment of fractures. Medical News 69:46-48, 1896.
11. Peltier LF: The impact of Röntgen's discovery upon the treatment of fractures. Surgery 33:579-586, 1953.
12. Beck C: Fractures, with an appendix on the practical use of the Rontgen rays. Philadelphia, WB Saunders, 1900.
13. Tousey S: Medical electricity and Rontgen rays. Philadelphia, WB Saunders, 1910.
14. Monell SH: A system of instruction in x-ray methods and medical uses of light, hot-air, vibration and high-frequency currents. New York, Pelton, 1902.
15. Holland CT: X-rays in 1896. Liverpool Med Chir J 45:61-77, 1937.
16. Hickey PM: The development of the skeleton. Trans Amer Roentgen Ray Soc 4:120-125, 1903.
17. Poland J: Skiagraphic atlas showing the development of the bones of the wrist and hand. London, Smith, Elder & Co, 1898.
18. Girdwood GP: Discussion. Trans Amer Roentgen Ray Soc 4:125-126, 1903.
19. Kohler A: Knochenerkrankungen im Roentgenbilde. Wiesbaden, Bergmann, 1901.
20. Kohler A: Röntgenology (translated by Turnbull). New York, William Wood, 1929.
21. Hickey PM: Lateral roentgenography of the spine. AJR 4:101-106, 1917.
22. Fraenkel E: Ueber Wirbelgeschwulste im Rontgenbilde. Fortschr Roentgenstr 16:245-257, 1910-11.
23. Pfahler GE: The roentgen diagnosis of metastatic malignant disease of bone, with special reference to the spinal column. AJR 4:114-122, 1917.
24. Baetjer FH: Differential diagnosis of bone tumors. AJR 5:260-264, 1918.
25. Evans WA: Multiple myeloma of bone. AJR 6:646-649, 1919.
26. Baetjer FH: Osteomyelitis. AJR 6:259-263, 1919.
27. Baetjer FH and Waters CA: Injuries and diseases of the bones and joints. New York, Hoeber, 1921.
28. Hammond R: Chronic joint disease from a roentgenologic standpoint. Amer Quart Roentgenol 3:124-131, 1911.
29. Werndorff R and Robinsohn I: Kongressverhandl Deutsch Gesellsch Orthop Chir, pp 9-11, 1905.
30. Hoffa A: Über Röntgenbilder nach Sauerstoffeinblasung in das Kniegelenk. Berlin Klin Wschr 43:941-945, 1906.
31. Freiberger RH, Killoran PJ, and Cardona G: Arthrography of the knee by double contrast method. AJR 97:736-747, 1966.
32. Bircher E: Über Binnenverletzungen des Kniegelenkes. Langenbecks Arch Klin Chir 177:290-359, 1933.
33. Ricklin P, Ruttimann A, and Del Buono MS: Die Meniskuslaesion. Stuttgart, Thieme Verlag, 1964.
34. Andren L and Wehlin L: Double-contrast arthrography of the knee with horizontal roentgen ray beam. Acta Arthop Scand 29:307-314, 1960.
35. Stoller DW, Genant HK, and Crues JV: MR imaging of the knee. In Edelman RR and Hesselink JR (eds): Clinical magnetic resonance imaging. Philadelphia, WB Saunders, 1990.
36. de Santos LA, Bernardino ME, and Murray JA: Computed tomography in evaluation of osteosarcoma. AJR 132:535-540, 1979.

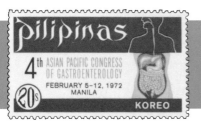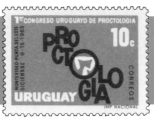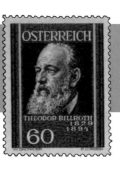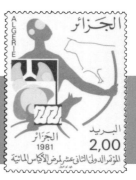

CHAPTER 15

Gastrointestinal Radiology

The use of x-rays to study the gastrointestinal tract began a few months after Roentgen's discovery. Unlike many other areas in radiology, pre-Roentgen methods of examining the intestinal tract, such as gas insufflation and sounding, were immediately applicable. In addition, bismuth, which had been used therapeutically for years, was found to be an excellent contrast agent. Unfortunately, although the means of delineating the intestinal tract were available, adequate equipment to demonstrate these agents (e.g., powerful x-ray tubes, fingertip diaphragming methods, integration of tube and screen movements in three dimensions, tilt tables, spot-film methods, and comfortable protective clothing) was not in existence. The primitive radiological examinations of the gastrointestinal tract were laborious, tiring, not without danger to the participants, and often utterly disagreeable to the unfortunate patient. As late as 1916, Hirsch[2] wrote that "until recently the esophagus was outlined for this (contrast) examination by the insertion into its lumen of sounds, bougies, rubber tubes filled with shot, chains, by inflation of rubber bags filled with bismuth, etc." An even more unpleasant technique for examination of the stomach was Turck's "gyromele," an instrument composed of a mop on the end of a long cable, rotated by an old-fashioned egg beater mechanism. By applying bismuth salt emulsion to the mop and passing it down the esophagus and into the stomach, both these organs could be coated with radiopaque material.

The first "gastrointestinal study" was probably performed by Wolf Becher (March 26, 1896), who opacified the stomach and a portion of the intestine of white mice and guinea pigs by injecting them with "liquor plumbi subacetici." As he wrote,[3]

> The property of such solutions (salts of various metals) in being impermeable to x-rays offers a means of obtaining photographs of the internal hollow organs of animals through the use of roentgen procedures. One needs only to introduce into a hollow organ a solution of the metal salt in such an amount that the walls of the organ are somewhat distended.

256

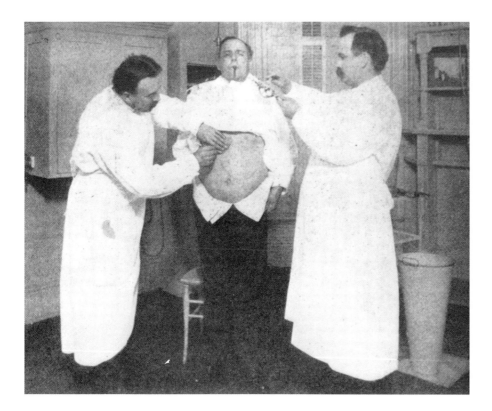

Turck's gyromele (1901). Palpation of the vibrations of the rotating cable within the stomach permitted outlining of its contour on the abdominal wall. The assistant on the patient's left rotates the "egg beater," while the physician on the patient's right outlines the vibrations.[1]

One month later (April 30), Carl Wegele suggested the introduction of a thin metal wire into the lumen of a long pliable Boas gastric tube so that the position of the tube could be demonstrated radiographically as it bent around the greater curvature and moved up to the pylorus.[4] By placing a small coin over the umbilicus, both the metal of the wire and the coin would show in the photograph and thus give some idea of the location of the stomach. However, it would give no impression of the size of the organ since the tube would only show the margin of the greater curvature. The first radiographic image using this technique was published 1 year later (April 22, 1897) by E. Lindemann,[5] who stated that "we have here an adequately reliable method for determining the boundaries of the stomach."

A demonstration of the inferior border of the stomach was important in those days to make the diagnosis of gastroptosis (Glenard's disease), an "abnormally low position of the stomach." There was much discussion in the literature regarding the position of the greater curvature or the pylorus relative to the umbilicus and whether this finding was related to the presence of underlying disease. This is one reason why a metal marker is seen on the umbilicus in many early radiographs. Some authorities argued that the vertical stomach that plunged below the level of the umbilicus was abnormal, while others just as strongly insisted that this vertical appearance was the normal and not merely the embryonic position of the stomach.

A variety of techniques were employed to show the inferior gastric margin. Max Einhorn, the developer of the "string test" and the duodenal tube, attempted to transilluminate the stomach after introducing a capsule containing a small amount of radium bromide.[6] Other less extreme methods included inflating the hollow organs with air or oxygen to visualize their contours on the fluoroscopic screen or x-ray plate and the swallowing of various types of capsules containing a variety of opaque media.[5]

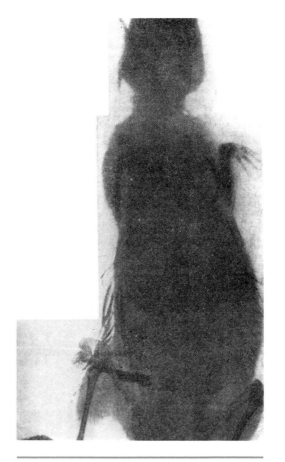

First "gastrointestinal study" (1896). Opaque contrast can be seen within a portion of intestine that, without freeing it from its attachments, was laid out transversely at the level of the knee joint of a hind leg of a guinea pig.[3]

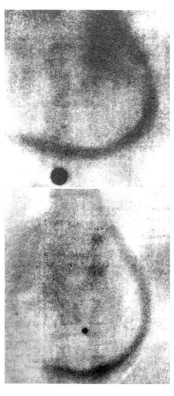

Gastroptosis (1897). *Top,* Normal examination with opaque gastric tube (outlining the margin of the greater curvature) lying above a coin placed over the umbilicus. *Bottom,* In another patient, the position of the greater curvature lies two fingerbreadths below the navel, indicating "a sinking of the stomach due to atony without dilatation."[5]

John C. Hemmeter (June, 1896) introduced the use of an "intragastric, deglutable, elastic-rubber bag" filled with plumbic acetate. The bags

can be made strong enough to hold sufficient of the solution to distend the adult stomach and at the same time can be swallowed easily or pushed down, after they are folded over a thin esophageal tube. When the bag, which has exactly the shape of the stomach, has reached the cavity of the organ, the plumbic acetate solution can be slowly filled in through the mouth by means of the esophageal tube until the bag is distended far enough to closely apply itself to the gastric walls.

After marking the umbilicus by a coin (as suggested by Wegele), "a photograph taken in this manner would give, not only a part of the stomach, but the entire organ and show its location and size. After the exposure the solution of plumbic acetate would have to be removed by aspiration, for which a stomach-pump would be useful for speedy evacuation."[7] In a curious addendum to the article, Hemmeter described the corrosive effect of the plumbic acetate on the bag and suggested that a solution of bone powder might be "a proper substance with which to distend the intra-gastric bag" before taking a radiograph.

Strauss (September, 1896) is said to have been the first to describe the use of gelatin capsules containing a radiopaque material to identify the greater curvature of the stomach by means of a fluoroscope.

Rumpel (April 20, 1897) was apparently the first to report radiographs of a segment of the gastrointestinal tract opacified by a *bismuth solution.*[8] He poured 300 ml of a 5% suspension of bismuth subnitrate into a patient's dilated esophagus by means of a tube and observed it fluoroscopically. Many other radiologists must have had the opportunity to discover accidentally the value of bismuth as a contrast medium, since during the 1890s and early 1900s, bismuth compounds were often prescribed as a gastric ulcer remedy in doses so large that 60 grams of bismuth might well have been found in the stomach at one time.[9] As George Pfahler recalled much later, in 1897, while examining plates of a patient's abdomen for another condition, he "incidentally (noted) the photographic plate showed bismuth in the stomach which had been taken therapeutically." But following in the footsteps of his Philadelphia colleague, Arthur Goodspeed, who had made an x-ray plate in 1890 without knowing it, Pfahler[10] added regretfully, "I did not follow through and failed to show the value of bismuth meals in the study of the gastrointestinal tract." Charles Leonard (1897) noted that he had washed out a patient's stomach, instilled an ounce of bismuth, and made the diagnosis of gastroptosis in 1897. Indeed, the bismuth-laden stomach had dropped so low that the x-ray plate showed "the area of the stomach through the bones of the pelvis." At a scientific meeting later that year, Leonard explained that "by filling the hollow organ with opaque liquids, as emulsions of bismuth in the stomach . . . their exact area can be readily determined."[11]

Another early observation that unfortunately was not followed up was that of David Walsh, the first Honorary Secretary of the Röntgen Society of London. As he wrote in 1897,

For a fortnight before being skiagraphed he (the patient) took 5 grains of bismuth three times a day. The result shows a faint outline of the stomach and colon, with some coils of small intestine and sigmoid flexure. It seems fair to assume that this result may—in part, at any rate—be attributed to the opaque bismuth present in the intestine.

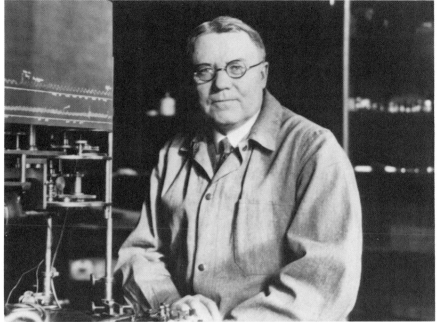

With happy memories of our work together Walter B. Cannon

Walter Bradford Cannon (1871-1945).

WALTER BRADFORD CANNON

The towering figure in early American gastroenterology was Walter Bradford Cannon, who described the basic physiology of the gastrointestinal tract. Cannon and Albert Moser, a fellow first-year student at Harvard, approached Professor H. P. Bowditch, the head of the Department of Physiology, to ask for a research project. Having already heard of the new penetrating rays, Bowditch suggested an experiment to study the swallowing mechanism in animals after ingestion of a substance opaque to x-rays. As Cannon later recalled[13]:

> Our first observation was made on December 9, 1896, when we watched globular pearl buttons pass down the esophagus of a dog.
> . . . then we procured a goose and made for it a box so arranged that the long neck reached up through the cover. A high cardboard collar was then attached to the top of the box in such a way that it could be closed in front when surrounding the goose's neck. Thus the goose, with the appearance of using the most stylish neckwear, presented to the fluoroscopic screen a very satisfactory extent of esophagus. At the meeting of the American Physiological Society in Boston, December, 29, 1896, the phenomenon of deglutition (swallowing) as exhibited by the goose when swallowing capsules containing bismuth subnitrate was informally demonstrated to the members by means of the Roentgen rays. This was, I think, the first public demonstration of movements of the alimentary canal by use of the new method.

Ten days later, Cannon and Moser employed "bismuth subnitrate mixed with food (in this case a bread mush) to render the swallowed mass visible." After completing their studies of the esophagus, they observed the action of the stomach with the same bismuth meal.[9]

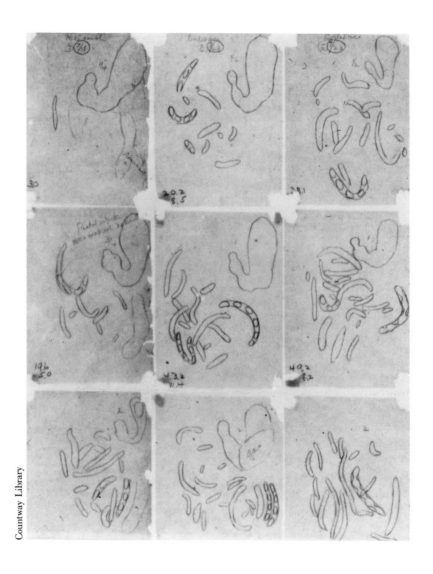

Photograph of original tracings from Cannon's studies on gastrointestinal motility.[15]

By April, 1897, Cannon was using bread soaked in warm water and mixed with bismuth subnitrate for studying peristalsis in the cat's stomach. To make illustrations for his classic 1898 paper[14] Cannon placed toilet paper over the fluoroscopic screen and traced an outline of the stomach at various times after the bismuth meal.

Within five minutes after a cat has finished a meal of bread, there is visible near the duodenal end of the antrum a slight annular contraction which moves peristaltically to the pylorus; this is followed by several waves recurring at regular intervals. Two or three minutes after the first movement is seen, very slight constrictions appear near the middle of the stomach, and, pressing deeper into the greater curvature, course slowly toward the pyloric end. As new regions enter into constriction, the fibers just previously contracted become relaxed, so that there is a true moving wave, with a trough between two crests. When a wave swings round the bend in the pyloric part the indentation made by it deepens; and as digestion goes on the antrum elongates and the constrictions running over it grow stronger, but, until the stomach is nearly empty, they do not entirely divide the cavity.

After the antrum has lengthened, a wave takes about 36 seconds to move from the middle of the stomach to the pylorus. At all periods of digestion the waves recur at intervals of almost exactly ten seconds. So regular is this rhythm that many times I have been able to determine within two or three seconds when a minute had elapsed simply by counting six similar phases of the undulations as they passed a given point. It results from this rhythm that when one wave is just beginning, several others are already running in order before it . . . The number of waves during a single period of digestion is larger than might possibly at first be supposed. In a cat that finished eating 15 grams of bread at 10:52 a.m., the waves were running continuously at 11 o'clock. The stomach was not free from food until 6:12 p.m. During that time the cat was fastened to the holder at intervals of half an hour and the waves were always observed, following one another in slow and monotonous succession. At the rate of 360 an hour, approximately 2,600 waves passed over the antrum during that single digestive period.

Cannon next addressed the working of the pyloric valve. Was food ejected through this sphincter into the duodenum, or did it merely drop through the pyloric valve in response to gravitational forces? Cannon learned that the food was ejected with considerable force and that the function of the pyloric valve was far more selective than had been anticipated:

In cats fed with bread mixed with subnitrate of bismuth, 10 or 15 minutes elapse after the first constriction in the antrum before any food can be seen in the duodenum. When food does appear it is spurted through the pylorus and shoots along the intestine for 2 or 3 centimeters.

Not every constriction-wave forces food from the antrum. On one occasion, about an hour after the movements began, three consecutive waves were seen, each of which squirted food into the duodenum. The pylorus remained closed against the next eight waves, opened for the ninth but closed once more against the tenth and eleventh . . . In this irregular way the food continued passing from the stomach . . .

When a hard bit of food reaches the pylorus, the sphincter closes tightly and remains closed longer than when the food is soft . . . On one occasion, the sphincter was seen to open only seven times in 20 minutes following the arrival of a hard particle of food at the pylorus. The conclusion may therefore be drawn that hard morsels keep the pylorus closed and hinder the passage of food into the duodenum.

Cannon was fascinated by the fact that the wavelike constrictions of the stomach were amazingly sensitive to emotional states. On one occasion, as Cannon was watching the rhythmic undulations coursing regularly over the stomach, the cat

suddenly changed from her peaceful sleepiness, began to breathe quickly, and struggled to get loose. As soon as the change took place, the movements in the stomach entirely disappeared; the pyloric portion relaxed and presented a smooth rounded outline. I continued observing, and stroked the cat reassuringly. In a moment she became quiet and began to purr. As soon as this happened, movements commenced again in the stomach; first a few constrictions were visible near the end of the antrum then a few near the sharp bend in the lesser curvature, and finally the waves were running normally from their habitual starting place.

By holding the cat's mouth closed between the thumb and last three fingers and covering her nostrils with the index finger, she could be kept from breathing. At the first sign of discomfort the fingers were removed. This experiment was repeated a great many times on different cats, and invariably the evidence of distress was accompanied by a total suspension of the motor activities of the stomach . . . It has long been common knowledge that violent emo-

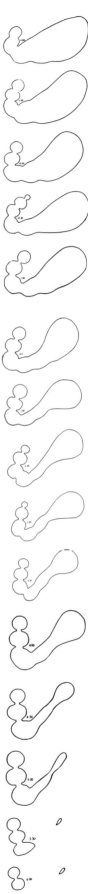

Peristalsis studies of Cannon (1898). Changes in the appearance of the stomach at half-hour intervals, from the time of eating until the stomach is nearly empty.

tions interfere with the digestive process, but that the gastric motor activities should manifest such extreme sensitiveness to nervous conditions is surprising.[14]

It is interesting to note the comments of Merrill Sosman when Cannon sought his advice on a draft of his Caldwell lecture in 1934.[16] Sosman noted that talking about specific foods often increased peristaltic activity and resulted in opening of the pylorus. "Women as a rule respond to salads, pickles, and desserts. Men as a rule respond to roast beef, ham and eggs, or mince pie and ice cream."

In July, 1898, Cannon and Moser published their work on the radiographic examination of the esophagus.[17] They concluded that there was a difference in swallowing according to the animal and the food used. "In man and the horse liquids are propelled deep into the esophagus at a rate of several feet a second by the rapid contraction of the mylohyoid muscles. Solids and semi-solids are slowly carried through the entire esophagus by peristalsis alone."

With the crude equipment they had available, Cannon and Moser were less successful in examining the esophagus in man[17]:

> The thickness of the thorax, the distance of the esophagus from the surface, and the relation to dense tissues, render the observation of a swallowed mass difficult, especially when the mass is in rather rapid motion. The few observations which we have to report were made on a 7-year-old girl placed in the sitting posture. Gelatin capsules containing bismuth were used for solids, and were traced to a point below the heart. The motion was very regular, and apparently due to peristalsis, for the bolus descended without a hitch or irregularity of any kind.

Unfortunately, Cannon received severe burns on his knee from sitting close to the x-ray tube. His gonadal dose must have been huge, "and it was little wonder that the Cannons, keenly desirous of starting a family, had no children until the administrative duties of the department, assumed in 1906, had taken Cannon away from much of his radiologic research on the digestive tract."[15] In 1931, 23 years after he had stopped his exposure to x-rays, Cannon developed severe itching and diffuse "fiery red papular cutaneous lesions." A biopsy revealed mycosis fungoides. Cannon eventually died in 1955 of lymphatic leukemia.

OTHER PIONEERS

Jean-Charles Roux and Victor Balthazard in France studied the motor function of animal and human stomachs using a 15% to 20% suspension of bismuth subnitrate in water or syrup. They concluded that[18]:

> in man, as in the dog, and as in the frog, from the functional point of view, the stomach is divided into two distinct regions: the largest part serves as a reservoir for ingested food; and the prepyloric part is the sole motor organ of the stomach, which, by its vigorous peristaltic movements, gradually propels into the duodenum the material which has accumulated in the stomach.

In his classic text (1901), Francis H. Williams described his experiences with the x-ray examination of the gastrointestinal tract.[19] He appeared to be the first to stress the importance of patient preparation before an examination of the stomach. "First, a good movement of the patient's bowels should be secured on the day before, and on the morning

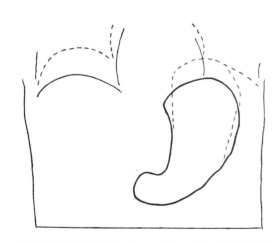

Fluoroscopic tracing a 7-year-old girl showing the outline of the stomach 1 hour after a meal of bread and milk containing subnitrate of bismuth (1901). The full horizontal line is at the level of the iliac crests; the full lines at right angles to it are the outlines of the body; the other full lines indicate the position of portions of the diaphragm, heart, and stomach during full inspiration. Broken lines show the position in expiration.[19]

on which the observations are to be made, in order to diminish the obstruction to the rays and allow the bismuth to be seen as clearly as possible. Second, the stomach should be free from food." In addition to offering a number of drawings showing changes in the stomach from peristalsis, Williams predicted the future of gastrointestinal radiology:

> Thus we see that if bismuth is given, an outline of the stomach, its position in inspiration and expiration and some peculiarities of shape may be noted; likewise changes in rapidity with which digestion proceeds in different individuals may be watched. After various characteristics belonging to the stomach in health have been established, the presence of abnormal conditions of this organ, such as some cases of malignant disease, will perhaps be more readily recognized than at present. The constant presence of a darkened area in the stomach, for example, may suggest the thickening of its walls due to malignant disease; some displacements or adhesions may be recognized as well as hourglass contractions, or an unusual delay of the digestive process.

Up to this time, the x-ray examination of the gastrointestinal tract was a fluoroscopic procedure designed primarily to depict the topographical anatomy and motor activity. Hermann Rieder stressed the use of large doses of bismuth compounds (initially mixed in food or water, later as a pure thick paste) to produce radiographs of the digestive tract. Although the idea of examining the gastrointestinal tract by opaque meals was certainly not new at the time of the publication of Rieder's pioneer papers[20,21] in 1904 and 1905, "he succeeded where none of his predecessors had, in obtaining sharp, contrast-rich, roentgen pictures of the digestive tract filled with opaque material and he also succeeded even in his first publications in tracing these pictures back to a corresponding anatomical basis."[22] Rieder used fluoroscopy very little, depending largely on a series of plates to indicate the peristalsis and general form of the stomach. He also called attention to the appearance of the small intestine and later even of the colon following the ingestion of the bismuth mixture, which became popularly known as the "Rieder meal."

Rieder and his co-workers developed the technique of "bioroentgenography," which was defined as "the preparation of a sufficient number of successive roentgenograms of an organ in situ during the course of a single cycle of its characteristic movements."[23] They noted that

> the fluoroscopic procedure, in contrast to the photographic one, reveals only indistinctly or not at all details which are here very

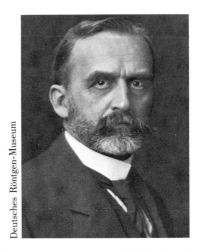

Deutsches Röntgen-Museum

Hermann Rieder (1858-1932).

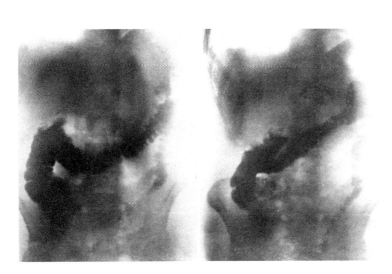

Rieder meals (1905). Two of the 30 illustrations of radiographs taken at varying intervals following bismuth meals.[21]

263

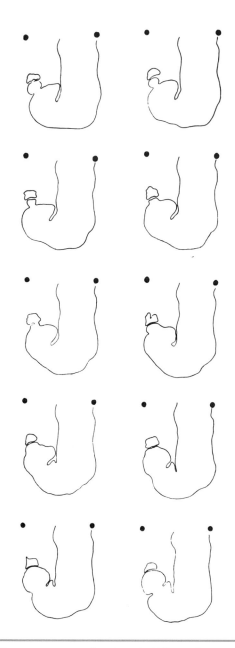

Bioroentgenography (1909). Effect of peristalsis on the contour of the stomach.[23]

essential. With a fluoroscopic screen the course of movement cannot be observed simultaneously at all points. The movements are often so rapid that the eye cannot carry out an analysis of the movement process in the available time.

When analyzing the appearance of the chest during deep inspiration and expiration, they obtained 12 radiographs in the course of a single phase using an exposure time for each individual picture of only a fraction of a second: "Visible markings on the pictures were made by lead pellets, which serve as fixed reference points for a comparison of the pictures of different stages in respiration."

THE AGE OF BARIUM

The widespread use of bismuth compounds as contrast material for gastrointestinal radiology soon ended. Cases were reported of poisoning after the use of bismuth subnitrate (from the reduction of the nitrate to highly toxic nitrite). The neutralization of all free and organically combined hydrochloric acid by bismuth carbonate was also considered objectionable. In addition, bismuth salts were expensive.

A variety of substances were recommended as substitutes for bismuth salts. These included the insoluble salts of heavy metals (especially those of iron), thorium compounds, and zirconium oxide. But all these substances had drawbacks, primarily bad taste and expense.

Carl Bachem and Hans Gunther (1910) set out to find a gastrointestinal contrast agent that would be nontoxic, inexpensive, easy to make, and still produce pictures rich in contrast. They settled on pure barium sulfate, which they administered in the form of a chocolate drink. "Barium sulfate is tasteless and odorless, and when mixed with some sort of food is quite agreeable to take."[24] The mixture they selected (kept on hand as a finely divided powder) contained 150 g of barium sulfate along with 15 g of cornmeal, 15 g of sugar, and 20 g of cocoa. The meal was prepared by first stirring it in a little water, heating it briefly (10 minutes) in 500 ml of water, and then cooling it. As a stable mixture, the barium solution could be used for divided doses. Bachem and Gunther emphasized that barium sulfate could also be administered in other forms as were bismuth salts, "thus it can be given as wafers, capsules, as an emulsion, a shake mixture (for enemas and esophageal examinations), or as a paste analogous to Beck's bismuth paste for the visualization of fistulas, etc."

A great deal of credit for the introduction and popularization of barium sulfate as an excellent and perfectly safe opaque contrast agent for gastrointestinal examinations should go to Paul Krause of the University of Bonn, at whose instigation Bachem and Gunther tested and proved its value. A major interest of Krause was to investigate radiopaque materials used clinically as contrast agents whenever injurious effects from such materials were reported. Thus when a single death was attributed to the use of barium sulfate, Krause made an extremely thorough investigation, including a world-wide survey, which showed that among 120,000 examinations in which this compound had been used, there had been no instance of any harmful effects.

It should be noted that Cannon reported on the virtues of barium for opacification of the gastrointestinal tract as early as 1904, 6 years before it was introduced in Europe. In his initial experiments in 1896, Cannon used both bismuth and barium but eventually selected bismuth for his

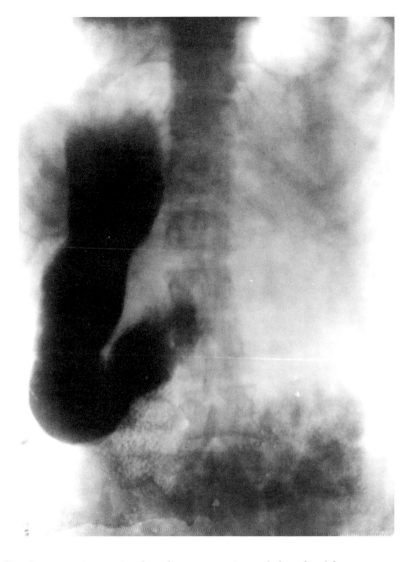

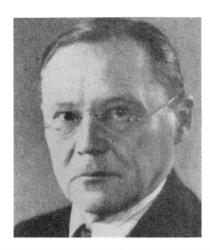

Above, Hans Gunther (1884-1956). *Left*, First published barium study (1910) of the stomach and proximal small intestine.[24]

studies because it was in the pharmacopeia and thus he felt more assured of being able to consistently obtain a purified product.

The final conversion from bismuth to barium was hastened by the onset of World War I (1914), which cut American radiologists off from their European sources of bismuth.

FLUOROSCOPY VS RADIOGRAPHY/ DIRECT SIGNS VS INDIRECT SIGNS

The major controversy in gastrointestinal radiology revolved around the respective merits of fluoroscopy and radiography. Roentgen had discovered almost simultaneously both the fluorescent effects of x-rays on a screen coated with crystals and the photographic effect on a sensitive emulsion. Early equipment produced such a low quantity of x-rays that an exposure time of 30 minutes or more was required for obtaining radiographs of thick portions of the body, such as the abdomen. A moving organ could not be effectively demonstrated on a photographic plate. Thus in the earlier reports fluoroscopy was clearly the method of choice. As Guido Holzknecht, the famed Viennese proponent of fluoroscopy, wrote[25]:

> And it is clear to all of us that fluoroscopy affords to us in the very shortest time—so very easily—a virtually endless number of pictures, all of equally good quality, which very definitely are superior

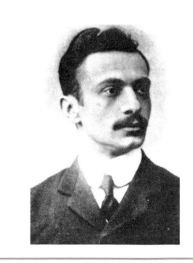

Guido Holzknecht (1872-1931).[1]

265

to the indistinct—and what can that which is dead tell us of the living?—distorted radiographs. We can also easily understand that, with the increasing quality and availability of fluoroscopic screens, the quality of whose images is constantly improving, radiography will be forced to yield a large area to fluoroscopy.

The fluoroscopic school was also the school of "symptom-complexes." Although often called the *Continental School,* it also had prominent protagonists in the United States, such as Russell Carman. This method of "indirect diagnosis" stressed the need for palpation of the opacified areas under fluoroscopic control. Accordingly, Holzknecht developed a wooden spoon ("distinctor") that enabled him to exert pressure on the abdomen without actually placing his hand in the irradiated field.[27]

The "symptom-complexes" method using indirect signs of gastro-intestinal disease appears to the modern reader as a form of radiological voodoo (see boxes on facing page).

By 1903, the development of improved power sources and intensifying screens reduced the exposure time for an abdominal film to 15 or 20 seconds. This enabled Rieder and his co-workers to rely primarily on a series of photographic plates of a moving organ (bioroentgenology) rather than on fluoroscopy.[23] As Bruwer[1] wrote, "It is perhaps not surprising that Rieder, the protagonist of roentgenography, avoided apparent damage from the rays, whereas Holzknecht, the prime protagonist of roentgenoscopy, died of roentgen-induced cancer."

The ability to detect *direct* evidence of disease processes, rather than relying on indirect signs, required the development of technical methods for demonstrating the gastric mucosa. John C. Hemmeter (1906)[28] showed that an experimentally produced "loss of substance in the gastric mucosa extending as far as the muscularis mucosae could be made visible

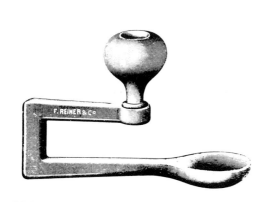

Holzknecht's "distinctor" (1911).[27]

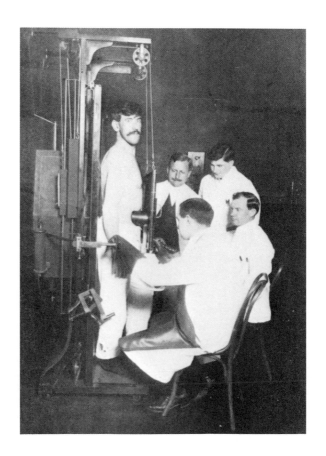

Group fluoroscopy (1915).[30]

266

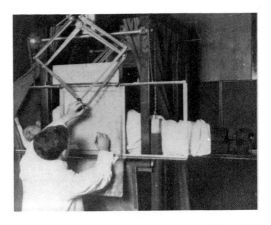

Use of fluoroscopic screen held vertically in front of a patient in the right lateral position (1915).[29]

by the bismuth method and that the bismuth adhered to the floor of the ulcer in sufficient quantities to prevent the passage of x-rays for 24 hours provided that no nourishment was given during this period." Turning his attention to three patients with confirmed gastric ulcers, Hemmeter showed that

> if a gastric ulcer is present, an experienced fluoroscopist can recognize a smaller, somewhat darker field in the generally dark region which corresponds to the stomach. The bismuth which covers the healthy part of the stomach disappears in 3 to 6 hours, provided that no food has been eaten. But in the field which corresponds to the gastric ulcer, the bismuth can still be demonstrated with x-rays 24-36 hours later, since gastric peristalsis can only remove it from there with great difficulty.

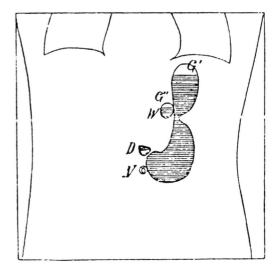

Interestingly, Hemmeter noted that "when the fluoroscope occasionally failed to disclose the presence and location of the ulcer, it still proved possible in two cases to discover the ulcer by making roentgenograms of the bismuth-coated stomach."

In 1910, Martin Haudek of Vienna first described the niche sign of gastric ulcer.[31] At that time, the appearance of an "hourglass stomach" was considered to represent a constriction from scar formation secondary to a gastric ulcer. After making this diagnosis on one patient who was later operated on, the surgeon haughtily chastised him saying, "Haudek, you have been wrong on two counts. You saw an hourglass stomach and there was none, you missed an ulcer which certainly was there." When Haudek reviewed the glass plates that had been preserved ("retrospectoscope"), he saw a projecting pocketlike irregularity just opposite the indentation, which he had called an hourglass deformity. Following similar observations on 25 additional cases, Haudek termed this protrusion an ulcer *nische*.[26]

Some authors considered that duodenal ulcers (unlike those in the stomach) were too small for radiographic delineation and based their diagnosis on the presence of duodenal deformity and secondary signs. However, Ake Akerlund[32] of Sweden (1917) was able to demonstrate tiny niches in a high percentage of surgically confirmed duodenal ulcers with the use of pressure devices and spot films. Akerlund also called attention to the radiographic diagnosis of hiatal hernia and gastric diverticula. The

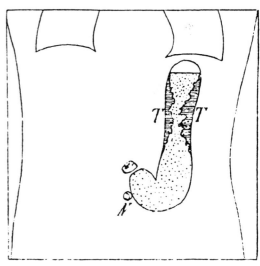

Gastric ulcer vs cancer (1910). *Top,* Penetrating ulcer with hourglass deformity. *Bottom,* Narrowing from carcinoma. *G',* Gas bubble in cardia; *G'',* gas in ulcer niche; *W,* contrast material in bottom of ulcer; *D,* duodenum; *N,* umbilicus; *T,* tumor.[31]

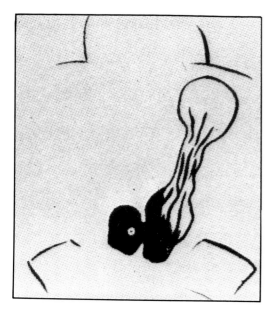

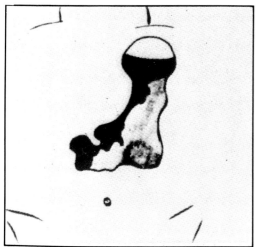

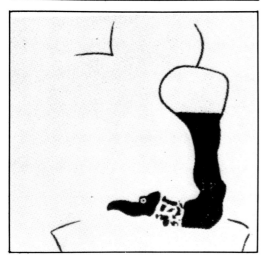

Drawings of mucosal fold pattern (1911) in a normal stomach (*top*) and in two patients with gastric carcinoma (*middle* and *bottom*).[33]

pressure and spot film technique was later perfected through the inventiveness of Hans Heinrich Berg of Hamburg, who developed such devices as rubber bags, cones, and belts for this purpose.[26]

The next major advance in gastrointestinal radiology was the development of techniques to demonstrate the mucosal fold pattern of the stomach. Gyula von Elischer[33] of Hungary (1911) used an emulsion of zirconium oxide to coat the entire inside of the stomach "so that a complete projection of the organ is made clearly visible, whereas bismuth rapidly sinks into the caudal pole and thus makes visible only one part of the stomach." Von Elischer showed several cases in which his method was "much richer in detail" and showed "much more delicate changes . . . The highly fluid zirconium emulsion, in spreading over the tumor, fills its irregularities and recesses very perfectly and in this way portrays the shape of a tumor or of a stenosis much more exactly than the bismuth meal which penetrates with much greater difficulty into such irregular surfaces." Therefore he asserted that his method would "make possible an earlier diagnosis of gastric carcinoma and pyloric stenosis."

Fritz Eisler and Robert Lenk (1921) presented an extensive study of the importance of what they termed the *fold pattern* of the stomach.[34] Contradicting previous studies indicating that "the occurrence of mucosal folds in the roentgenogram would always be a pathologic sign," Eisler and Lenk showed that by using a suitable technique "the mucosal folds can almost always . . . be visualized in at least a part of the stomach; and that they must therefore be regarded as a normal feature of the fluoroscopic and roentgenographic pictures obtained by this technique." In patients with gastric ulcer, they noted "in addition to the usual parallel shadow streaks there are single streaks which run diagonally, often almost transversely across the stomach and converge toward a point in the lesser curvature. In the region of this point they appear to be blunt-ended, broken off and pushed more closely together." This initial description of "radiating folds" made it possible to

confirm the diagnosis of an ulcer or of an ulcer scar. Usually one finds an ulcer niche at the apex of the triangle formed by the converging folds. Often one's attention first is called to this point by the very striking feature of the converging folds and on careful examination one then finds a thin layer of radiopaque material indicating a niche.

Gosta Forssell (1923), an anatomist who was the founding editor of *Acta Radiologica* and the major figure in Swedish radiology, produced a series of anatomical preparations and radiographs demonstrating the normal and abnormal appearances of the mucous membranes of the stomach and small bowel. Using a special fluoroscope he designed primarily for positioning the patient to obtain "focus roentgenograms" (spot films), Forssell noted that "the folds of the mucous membrane of the alimentary canal (are) formed by active movements of the mucous membrane itself."[35]

Richard Rendich (1923) stressed the appearance of the contour of the gastric rugal folds. He showed that in hypertrophic gastritis "the rugae are enlarged and of somewhat irregular formation, and tend to resist obliteration," whereas the atrophic type of gastritis was associated with "marked thinning of the mucosa and all coats of the stomach wall . . . (and) characterized by an absence of rugae formation."[36]

The ability of barium studies to show the lesion itself rather than only indirect signs brought to an end the era of the "symptom-complex" method. Nevertheless, some prominent physicians and surgeons contin-

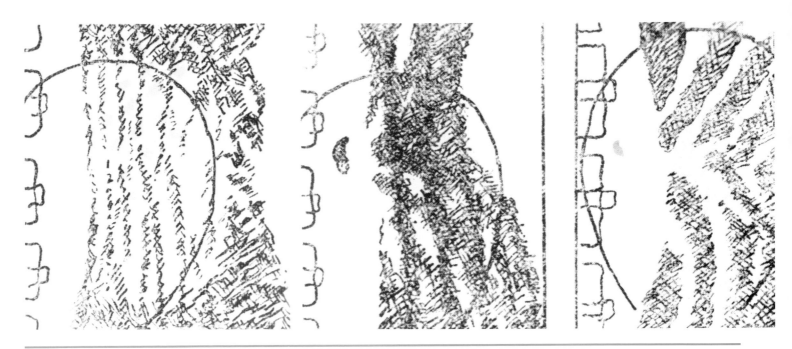

Gastric fold pattern (1921). *Left*, Normal pattern of folds. *Middle*, Ulcer niche with radiating folds. *Right*, Converging folds produced by an ulcer with no evidence of ulcer niche.[34]

ued to be skeptical. With regard to duodenal ulcers, one of the famed Mayo brothers was said to have sarcastically remarked "There are x-ray men who claim that they can see this little bit of a thing with the x-ray." After critical discussion following a paper he gave, the radiologist, Henry Hulst, complained "When you do work of this kind they will tell you that it is better not to do it because it will blunt your diagnostic abilities. You must not use a thermometer; you ought to be able to feel your patient's temperature. You must not use the stethoscope, because if you do, you will blunt your hearing."

At the 1914 meeting of both the Gastrointestinal Society and the

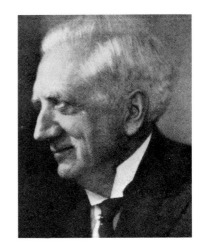

Gosta Forssell (1876-1950).

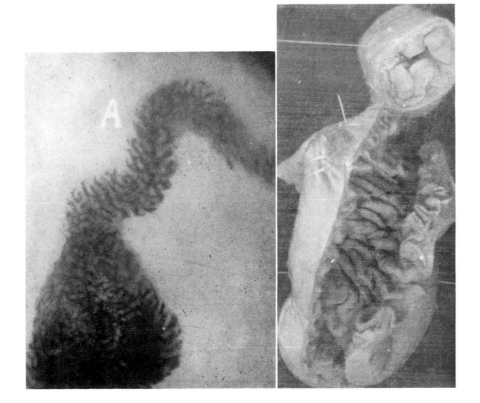

Mucous membrane of a proximal loop of jejunum (1923). *Left*, Radiograph in a live subject. *Right*, Anatomical preparation.[35]

269

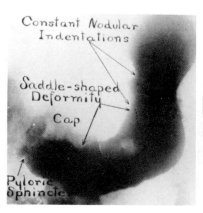

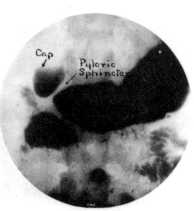

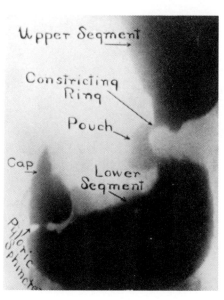

Brewer and Cole surgical challenge (1914). *Left,* Clinical diagnosis: gastric cancer. Roentgenologic diagnosis: extensive carcinoma, involving entire lesser curvature. Surgical findings: extensive carcinoma, involving most of lesser curvature. *Center,* Clinical diagnosis: definite ulcer of the cap. Roentgenologic diagnosis: normal stomach and cap. Surgical findings: normal stomach and cap. *Right,* Clinical diagnosis: gastric lesion of three months' duration. Roentgenologic diagnosis: hourglass stomach. Surgical findings: hourglass stomach.[37]

Medical Section of the American Medical Association, it was repeatedly asserted that the early diagnosis of gastric ulcer by x-rays was impossible. Even surgeons who agreed that a *positive* x-ray diagnosis of gastric ulcer could be relied on doubted the reliability of a *negative* diagnosis; they went right on operating, despite the negative x-ray findings, if clinical symptoms suggesting an ulcer were present.[9] Lewis Gregory Cole of New York, "a perfectionist and a maverick, not only willing but delighted to buck the opinions of his peers," bluntly insisted that his negative, as well as positive, diagnoses were reliable. If he saw no ulcer on his plates, none was present. To test Cole's claims, an objective study was arranged. A New York City surgeon, George Emerson Brewer (one of the doubters), sent Cole 27 patients. After radiographic examination, Cole sent Brewer a typewritten report "giving the exact findings and an opinion regarding the presence or absence of a gastric or duodenal lesion, its location, extent, and probable cause." Regardless of Cole's x-ray findings, Brewer then operated—and reported back to Cole the physical findings at operation.

In 11 cases (40%), there was no radiographic evidence of ulcer or cancer in the stomach or duodenal cap.[37] In all of these cases, the clinical findings seemed to Brewer strong enough to warrant an operation. But in not a single one of these cases, when the operation was performed, did Brewer find any surgical lesion of the stomach or cap! Cole's negative diagnoses were 100% correct. In another 11 cases, Cole made a positive diagnosis and was correct in nine. In the remaining five cases, Cole could only give Brewer an opinion rather than a firm diagnosis, "owing to incomplete observation, or unusual findings which could not be definitely interpreted." Still, Cole's opinion was right four times and wrong only once. Thus Cole's overall "batting average" for the series was 89%, an astounding result.

The stage was now set for one last battle between the advocates of fluoroscopy, led by Russell D. Carman, and the champions of plate radiography, led by Lewis Gregory Cole.

Russell D. Carman was head of the Section on Roentgenology at the Mayo Clinic and coauthor with Albert Miller of the influential textbook, *The Roentgen Diagnosis of Diseases of the Alimentary Canal.* Unlike Cole, who used the fluoroscope primarily to line up his tube and plate with the patient, to check the hardness of the rays, and to make a preliminary survey while relying on the plates for diagnosis, Carman relied primarily on the fluoroscope for diagnosis and only exposed a few plates per patient to clear up a doubtful point or to record some unusual feature which he might later want to show students or other physicians.[9]

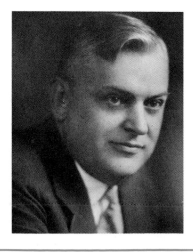

Russell D. Carman (1875-1926).[1]

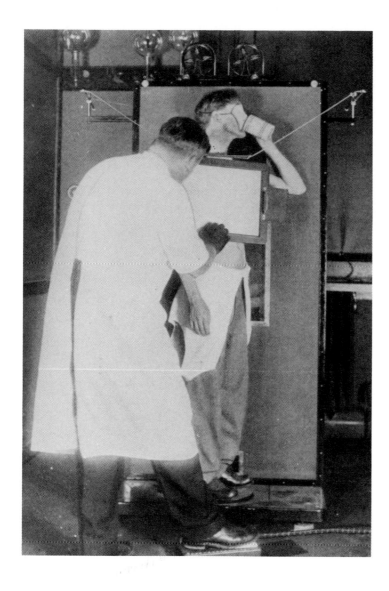

Carman at the fluoroscope (1917). Screen examination of the esophagus with the patient in a right anterior oblique position.[38]

As Carman and Miller wrote in their 1917 textbook[38]:

We believe that the advantages of the (fluoroscopic) screen in the examination of the digestive tract can hardly be too strongly emphasized. Only by its use can exact information be obtained as to mobility and flexibility, the phenomena of peristalsis and antiperistalsis, the nature and permanence of irregularities of contour, and the effects of palpation, respiratory movement and varying positions. All changes can be seen at every instant, in the order of their succession, at any desired angle, and in these respects a few minutes screening is equivalent to hundreds of plates.

The vast number of cases at the Mayo Clinic offered Carman many examples of virtually all pathological conditions. In 1919 alone, he and his staff performed more than 50,000 x-ray examinations. According to Carman, in determining whether a stomach was normal, "account must be taken of its length, breadth, capacity, contour, position, form, tonus, mobility, peristalsis, and motility." Carman stressed that "stomachs which are markedly dissimilar in their roentgenologic characteristics may each be appropriate for its possessor and function in a normal manner," although he added the proviso that "these variations have limits, even though wide, which can be determined in a general way."[38]

Carman found that his fluoroscopic observations were greatly enhanced by direct palpation of the abdomen. He recommended the use of a leaded protective apron and gloves and developed his fluoroscopic tech-

FLUOROSCOPIC SHEET.
MAYO CLINIC.

Case No. A ___ Sex ___ Age ___ Date ___

Name ___

	Total Acidity			Food remnants
Chemical	Free Hcl.		Microscopic	Oppler-Boas
	Comb. Acids			Yeasts
	Lactic Acid			Sarcines

Habitus N. E.
Residue 0. 1. 2. 3. 4.
Head 1. C. H. F. T. C. S. F. D. S.
Peristalsis Nor. Active Vigorous Not Seen
Bulb Seen Size 1 2 3 Reg. Irreg. Not Seen
Duod. Visualized Immediately Delayed Not Seen
Antrum Seen Regular Irregular Not Seen
Mobility Free Slightly Fixed Fixed
Filling Defects Card. Media. Pylorica GC. LC.
Incisura Card. Media. Pylorica Transient
Hour-Glass Stomach Organic Intermittent
Niche ___
Tender Point L. C. Duod. G. B. McB. Epig.
Diverticulum ___

Trouble—Esophagus, Stomach, Bowels, Duration ___ Increased Severity ___
Pain—Slight, severe, dull, gnawing, fullness, distress, where ___ radiates ___
continuous ___ intermittent ___ frequency ___ duration ___
after meals ___ night, time ___ any time ___
aggravated by food, quantity, solid, acid, fats, fibrous; relieved by food, soda, belching, vomiting.
Stomach feels better full, formerly, now; empty, formerly, now.
Vomits—Rarely, occasionally, often ___ blood, ___ mucus, bile, forced, delayed, tube.
Sour Stomach ___ Gas ___ Jaundice, sl., distinct ___ Cramps ___ Morph. ___
B. M.—Regular, constipation, diarrhoea, black, clay, blood, mucus. Typhoid ___ Alcohol ___
Weight—Increasing, stationary, off ___ lbs. in ___ Reduced diet ___
General Condition—Good, fair, poor, weakness, emaciation, pallor, appetite ___
Operations:

REPORT, X-RAY DIGESTIVE TRACT.

Case No. A 8.8.4.9.4. X-Ray No. 23298 Phy. Graham Murray Date 7-23-13
Name Henry Miller Sex male Age 58

STOMACH
Tonus Hypertonic
Filling defect None
Form S tee form
Position Oblique
Size (1, 2, 3, 4) 2 Peristalsis Vigorous
Incisura None
Residue in Stomach after 6 hrs. (0, 1, 2, 3, 4) 0
Pylorus Position Normal
Patency Free
Opening Immediate

DUODENUM
Duodenum Visualized Yes Dilated Obstructed Residue Yes
Cap Irregular Residue (0, 1, 2, 3, 4) 3

DIAGNOSIS:
Probable Duodenal Ulcer. Hypertrophic arthitis of spine.
Question of a filling defect in pars cardiaca.

Signed Carman

Left, Mayo Clinic checklist for gastro-intestinal procedures and *right*, an example of Cannon's report (1913).[38]

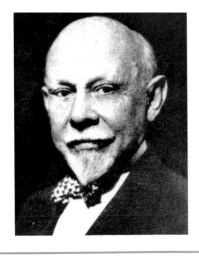

Lewis Gregory Cole (1874-1954).[42]

---

nique to the point where it would take an average of 5 minutes to adequately examine the stomach and duodenum. He did not rely on the reports of others to confirm his diagnosis or point out his mistakes but routinely followed his patients to the operating room to directly observe the surgical findings.[39]

Carman is perhaps best known for the sign of ulcerating gastric cancer that bears his name. As he described it in 1921[40]:

> When the ulcer is on the vertical portion of the lesser curvature or on the posterior wall near the lesser curvature, approximation of the walls of the stomach by palpation causes a dark, slightly crescentic shadow of the barium-filled crater to appear on the screen. In these situations, the convexity of the crescent is toward the gastric wall and the concavity toward the gastric lumen. The resemblance to a meniscus is so obvious that the word aptly applies to the sign.

Carman's most celebrated diagnosis was made in 1925. Returning from Europe as the newly elected president of the American Roentgen Ray Society, Carman suffered a severe gastric upset. As Albert Miller related,[41] Carman "stood gaily before the screen where thousands of patients had confronted him. In the darkness, the x-ray tube gave out its steady drone. No other sound was heard, for his associates were dumb as they gazed at a distorted gastric shadow." The image on the fluoroscopic screen was unequivocal.

> Finally they found voice. Spasm, they told Doctor Carman evasively. They would make some films.
> Carman returned to his office. It was a gray afternoon. On his desk was a rough draft of a new paper on cancer of the stomach. It had been the theme of the first paper he had published from Rochester. When the films were ready his assistants could not withhold them. Gravely they were laid before the Chief. Holding the films toward the window, Carman announced his diagnosis, just as he had done so many thousands of times before: "Cancer of the stomach and inoperable."

Lewis Gregory Cole, the spokesman for radiography, was described[26] as "an outspoken and contentious man . . . wont to debate every issue vigorously. He irritated many of his colleagues by his belligerent, sometimes almost abusive, remarks." Nevertheless, all acknowledged him a brilliant radiologist who coined the term *duodenal cap* when he observed that this portion of the duodenum sat like a stocking cap on the pyloric

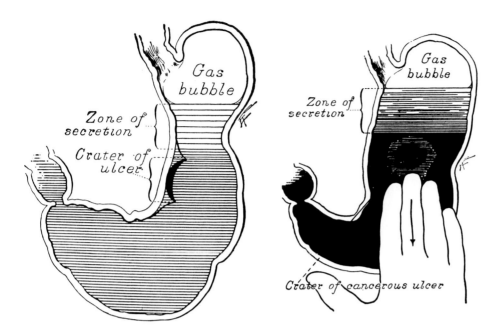

Carman's meniscus sign (1921). Drawings depicting (*left*) meniscus-like crater on the posterior wall of the stomach near the lesser curvature and (*right*) visualization of an ulcer crater on the posterior wall by stroking pressure of the hand.[40]

end of the stomach. Abandoning a reliance on fluoroscopy early in his career, Cole was known for the vast number of plates he made with patients in various positions and at different times. In 1908, Cole devised a special plate-changing table that allowed the changing of 18 to 25 plates in 5 minutes to show various phases of different gastric cycles.[43] When a patient came in for stomach radiography, Cole typically exposed 12 plates in rapid succession with the patient prone, 6 from the side, 2 from the rear, and 12 with the patient standing erect. After the patient ate a full meal mixed with barium, an additional 6 to 12 plates were made 2 hours later (two of them stereoscopic views of the entire gastrointestinal tract). He often made additional plates 4 to 6 hours after the meal. Thus 40 plates per stomach examination were a minimum in Doctor Cole's practice; 50 or 60 were common.

Cole termed this multiple-plate technique *serial radiography*.[44] Beneath his table was a fluoroscopic screen and the image was reflected onto an angled mirror so that the operator, peering at the mirror under the table, could move the patient into various positions while keeping the patient's stomach visible within the small opening in the leaded table top. Efforts at protection were made, but it is probable, especially considering the open bowl containing the tube above the table, that the operator received excessive radiation. In effect, it was an effort to simulate fluoroscopic observation but enabled study at leisure of the greater detail of

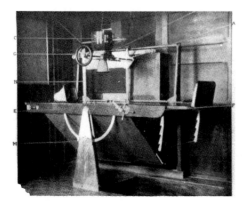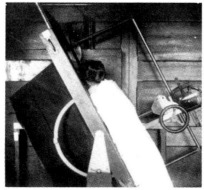

Cole's radiographic table in (*left*) supine and (*right*) upright positions (1908).[43]

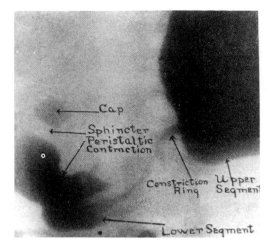

Serial radiography (1912).[44]

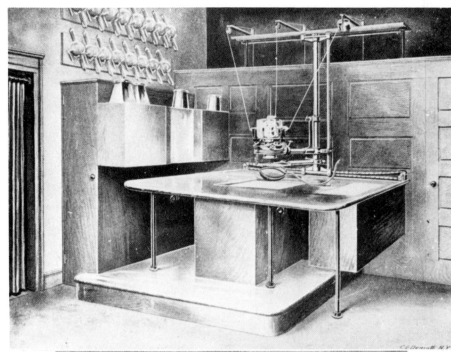

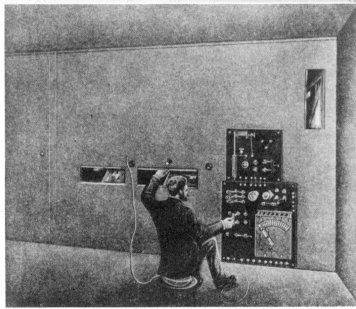

Top, X-ray table with ray-proof cabinet behind it (1912). *Bottom*, Interior of the ray-proof cabinet, showing the window through which the plates are manipulated and the compression bag on the operator's seat.[45]

the multiple radiographs. It also avoided the radiation hazard implicit in fluoroscopy.[26] Cole later designed an x-ray table associated with a ray-proof cabinet where the radiologist sat.[45] Compression of the patient was obtained using a rubber bag fastened to a celluloid diaphragm with a rubber tube leading from the bag to a similar one placed on the stool where the operator sat. By sitting down on the bag containing the air, he forced air through the tube into the bag placed on the patient. A variation of Cole's table, including a lead-lined protective cabinet, was developed by A. Howard Pirie of Montreal.[46] The wall of the cabinet contained an opening through which the operator could see the fluorescent screen reflected in a mirror.

To speed his technique, Cole replaced his glass plates with celluloid film bought in long rolls. He designed a special examining table, which in addition to many other complex and ingenious features contained a semiautomatic mechanism to advance the film each time a lever was

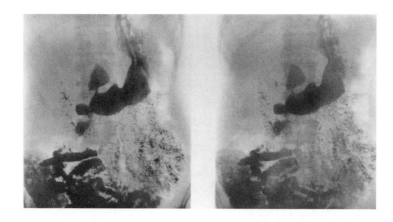

Stereoradiographs of the upper gastrointestinal tract (1915).[29]

pressed (much like the modern roll-film camera). Up to 50 exposures in succession could be made rapidly without reloading. By projecting the films in rapid succession (an early attempt at cineradiography), Cole could simulate the appearance of gastric motility.

Using his multiple-plate technique, Cole soon learned that when there was a constant defect in outline of the cap, a duodenal ulcer would invariably be found during surgical exploration. As he observed, "While there are many normal variations in the size, shape and position of the cap, a persistent deformity of outline is an accurate sign of the presence of a duodenal ulcer."[39]

As the Brechers questioned in their book[9]:

> Did Carman get better results with his primary emphasis on fluoroscopy, or Doctor Cole with his serial roentgenography? A radiologic tournament at which the two might pit their skills against each other was often discussed by other radiologists, and it has been said that Doctor Cole was actually invited to the Mayo Clinic to match his technique against Carman's, but no such confrontation actually occurred. Radiologists today, of course, draw upon both techniques; the complete gastrointestinal work-up now includes both a series of films and a thorough fluoroscopic examination.

DOUBLE-CONTRAST STUDIES OF UPPER GASTROINTESTINAL TRACT

Conventional single-contrast examinations had some limitations that could result in diagnostic error. To distend the organ under study, additional opaque barium had to be added. Although this permitted demonstration of lesions causing contour defects, those not imaged in profile might be obscured because of insufficient radiographic penetration. Single-contrast studies relied heavily on palpation and compression for detection of lesions. However, some parts of the anatomy such as the gastric fundus and cardia were not easily accessible to palpation. In addition, some patients had physical conditions such as obesity and recent surgery that precluded effective compression. Conventional single-contrast studies also emphasized diagnostic fluoroscopy, which even in the best of hands might miss small, subtle lesions. Reliance on fluoroscopic observation frequently made it difficult for anyone other than the fluoroscopist to adequately interpret the examination.

These potential problems were greatly alleviated by the double-contrast technique. Increasing the degree of distention was achieved by gas rather than barium. Thus the contour of the bowel could be seen without

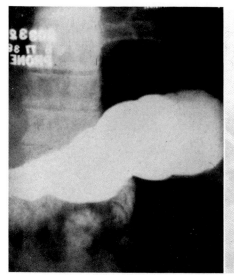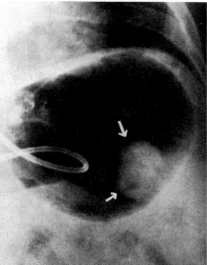

Tumor of the gastric cardia demonstrated by double-contrast technique (1944). *Left,* Prone radiograph of the barium-filled stomach shows no pathological condition of the cardia. *Right,* Radiograph of the cardia after air insufflation clearly shows a polypoid tumor projecting from the posterior wall into the gastric lumen.[52]

the loss of en face mucosal surface detail. Although still useful, compression was not as critical with the double-contrast technique, and areas such as the gastric fundus that were inaccessible to palpation could be well examined. In most double-contrast studies, fluoroscopy was used primarily to judge the correct volumes of barium and air and to allow for correct positioning and timing of spot films. The final diagnosis, however, relied on evidence documented on the permanent radiographs.

Igor Laufer, whose popular book[48] did much to encourage the use of the double-contrast technique, recommended that this examination was particularly valuable in the following situations[47]:

1. For the detection of superficial mucosal lesions
2. For the evaluation of areas not accessible to palpation or for the examination of patients in whom palpation is ineffective
3. In situations when someone other than the fluoroscopist must review and assist in the interpretation of the films

The combination of bismuth and gas (from effervescent agents) was first used by Holzknecht in 1906. Leonard (1913), in discussing the value of distending the stomach with gas, noted that "if a method of coating the mucosa uniformly with an opaque salt can be combined with this method of radiography, the lesser lesions of the mucosa might be revealed."[49] Limited double-contrast studies of the upper gastrointestinal tract using ingested air plus barium to demonstrate duodenal and gastric ulcers were reported by Hampton in 1937[50] and by Schatzki and Gary in 1958.[51] In 1937, Arens and Mesirow used barium and carbon dioxide liberated by Seidlitz powder for the demonstration of gastric mucosal relief patterns. The special value of double-contrast radiographs in the demonstration of tumors of the gastric cardia was described by Wasch and Epstein in 1944.[52] In the 1950s, Hikoo Shirakabe and other Japanese gastroenterologists used double-contrast techniques extensively for screening and the early diagnosis of gastric cancer, which has a very high incidence in that country.[53] This type of examination became standard in Japan during the 1960s and has been largely responsible for their superb results both in mass screening programs and in evaluating symptomatic patients. However, because of the low (and decreasing) incidence of gastric cancer in the West, these reports provoked relatively little interest in the United States and Europe. In the 1970s, Obata[54] and Gelfand[55] described important modifications of the Japanese technique. Soon afterwards, Laufer[56] and Poplack[57] applied the technique to the diagnosis of more preva-

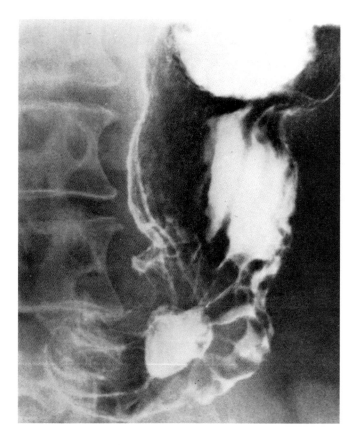

lent Western disorders such as erosive gastritis and peptic ulcer disease. This led to the development of improved barium suspensions and effervescent agents that now make it possible to routinely obtain high-quality, double-contrast studies of the upper gastrointestinal tract.

The use of the double-contrast technique was enhanced by the development of agents to produce intestinal atony and distention. Hypotonic duodenography was first described by Porcher (1944), who used morphine to relax the duodenum. For the next three decades, intestinal hypotonicity was generally achieved using parenteral anticholinergic drugs. However, these agents were associated with substantial side effects (tachycardia, blurring of vision, urinary retention, and dry mouth) and were contraindicated in patients with glaucoma, uncompensated cardiac disease, severe angina pectoris, and urinary retention. In 1974, Roscoe Miller reported the use of glucagon to produce intestinal hypotonicity. A polypeptide normally produced by the pancreas, glucagon was shorter acting, had substantially fewer side effects, and could be used in all patients except those few with suspected insulinoma or pheochromocytoma.[58]

STUDIES OF THE COLON

For more than 30 years prior to the discovery of x-rays, a variety of tubes had been inserted into the rectum and passed for varying distances into the colon. Turck is considered to have been the first to use x-rays to observe the position of metallic rectal tubes. The first radiographic observation of the colon was recorded by Walsh, who saw a faint outline in an abdominal radiograph of a patient receiving bismuth therapeutically. However, he and other investigators failed to pursue the possible value of this observation in making contrast studies of the large intestine.[26]

Most of the early examinations of the colon were performed as part of motility studies in which the distribution of opaque material was recorded at specific times following the ingestion of a bismuth meal. At times, air or oxygen was injected into the colon, either alone or in conjunction with an opaque material.

To effectively demonstrate pathology, it was necessary to directly inject opaque material into the colon. As early as 1901, Francis Williams[19] wrote in his classic text that "the large intestine may be injected with fluid containing an opaque substance like subnitrate of bismuth, and its outline and position studied." However, Williams apparently did not pursue this method. "I think, however, that we should remember that any liquid which is opaque to the rays must be heavy, and that the risk of putting into the large intestine such a weight as might be dangerous to its integrity should not be taken."

Schule (1904) is credited with performing the first opaque enema as a method for x-ray examination of the colon.[59] He published radiographs of patients who had received 300 to 400 ml of an oily suspension of bismuth subnitrate that was administered with the patient in the knee-chest position. The enemas were given before x-ray examination, without fluoroscopic control. However, the author cautioned that "for the average case one will, of course, be able to avoid the use of the somewhat complicated (unfortunately also expensive!) oil-bismuth method. But if it is desirable to visualize the course of the colon in an exact manner, then the best pictures can definitely be obtained with the above-described procedure."

In the same article, Schule described the appearance of radiopaque tubes introduced per rectum in an attempt to identify a site of obstruction. He noted that successful intubation of the descending colon "has up to the present time still not been achieved and on the basis of our present knowledge it will probably prove very difficult to achieve in the future." He considered this approach to detecting colon pathology to be inherently limited since

> the anatomical configuration of the structures involved makes it an impossibility to detect a stenosis or tumor above the rectum by means of a tube, since the numerous turns, folds, and protrusions of the normal large intestine already offer so many hindrances to the passage of the tube that in any given instance one can never be certain of the normality or abnormality of the obstruction which one has encountered.

A major contributor to contrast enemography was Georg Fedor Haenisch, who in 1910 described his technique for the fluoroscopic examination of the colon after the retrograde instillation of a mixture of bismuth carbonate, bolus alba, and water.[60] He made use of his own invention, the trochoscope, a horizontal table equipped with facilities for fluoroscopy that "enables me to follow the progress of the bismuth column on a small fluorescent screen." Haenisch stressed the importance of the fluoroscopic observation of the opaque material as it filled the colon to detect any interruption in flow that might be caused by a tumor (which might be missed if the stenosis were not sufficiently narrow to cause proximal dilatation).

> In my experience the only suitable method for this purpose is the contrast enema, and even this is only satisfactory when the advance of the fluid is observed and studied on the fluoroscopic screen from the moment of its entrance into the rectum until it has reached the cecum. Even with such a contrast enema, roentgenography alone is

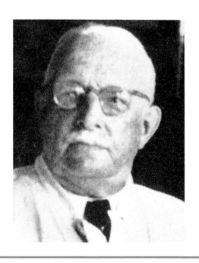

Georg Fedor Haenisch (1874-1952).[61]

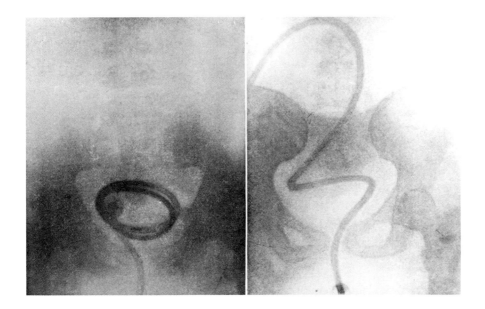

Use of radiopaque tubes inserted per rectum to identify a site of obstruction (1904). *Left*, Tube coiled within the rectum. *Right*, In another prone patient, the tip of the tube has extended into the left side of the colon.[59]

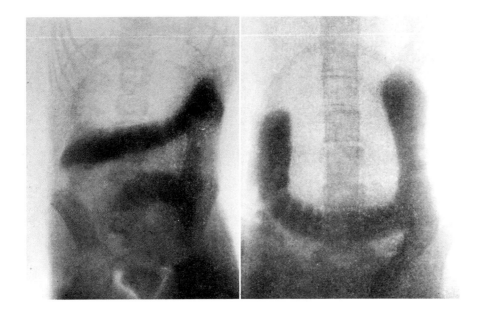

First published examples of opaque enemas (Schule, 1904). *Left*, Normal child. *Right*, Enteroptosis.[59]

completely inadequate and should only be used as an aid for the confirmation and permanent recording of important individual stages or unclear places in the fluoroscopic examination.

Haenisch strongly criticized the oral examination of the colon as "a very time-consuming and, in my opinion, a not very certain or reliable diagnostic procedure. An uninterrupted filling of the entire large intestine from the cecum to the ampulla of the rectum is rarely observed. To distinguish among the numerous breaks in the shadow, a truly pathologic interruption would be almost impossible."

Haenisch stressed the importance of cleansing the colon with cathartics and enemas, remarkably similar to that practiced today. After the examination was completed, he recommended that the bismuth mixture should be siphoned out under fluoroscopic observation for two reasons: "to avoid injury or discomfort to the patient from thickening and hardening of the injection, but also in order to observe for a second time on the screen passage of the bismuth through the stenosed portion of the bowel."

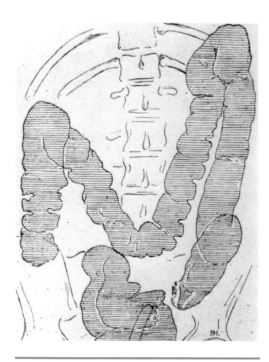

Stenotic carcinoma at the junction between the sigmoid and descending colon (1911).[60]

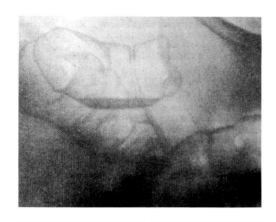

Double-contrast barium enema (1923). With the patient in a left-side down position, a cecal-filling defect with termination in a rounded contour was considered "strongly suggestive of tuberculosis."[63]

Although convinced of the validity of his method, Haenisch remained cautious:

If the fluoroscopic examination results in a definite or suspiciously pathologic finding which is confirmed in the developed roentgenograms, I have made it an absolute rule, before making any definitive diagnosis, to require an identically performed control examination several days later. Only when a second examination reveals the same findings do I believe myself justified in reservedly making a cautious diagnosis, in which, of course, the clinical symptoms are given the utmost consideration. By such a control examination, I believe that a high percentage of the sources of error can be avoided.

Haenisch clearly was concerned about the radiation exposure of his patients. "I do not let the (x-ray) tube go all the time. I have an assistant stationed at the switch to turn the current off and on, as I need it. Therefore, I do not burn the patient."[62]

Various clinical studies showed that the most reliable signs for carcinoma of the colon included obstruction of the retrograde flow of the opaque material, narrowing of the bowel lumen, and a persistent unilateral filling defect. Stierlin first pointed out the absence of the barium shadow of the cecum and ascending colon in tuberculosis, while Carman and Case showed that persistent narrowing of the bowel associated with diverticula usually represented diverticulitis. Carman noted that the so-called mucous and catarrhal colitis showed no abnormal x-ray findings, whereas the true chronic ulcerative colitis involving more than the rectum invariably produced lack of haustration, shortening of length, absence of flexures, stenoses, or granularity of the mucosa. During this period, polyposis and megacolon were correctly diagnosed by several radiologists, and Carman conclusively proved that the so-called incompetence of the ileocecal valve to the retrograde flow of contrast material was of no diagnostic or clinical significance.[39]

The next major achievement in radiographic studies of the colon was the report by A. W. Fischer (1923) of the "double-contrast" technique, which combined the contrast enema with the insufflation of air.[63] The artificial introduction of air into the colon had been used in pre-Roentgen days in the topical diagnosis of abdominal tumors by percussion and by several authors for the purpose of outlining the spleen, lower border of the liver, and gallbladder. Cole and Einhorn (1910) had suggested that air insufflation alone might permit detection of small mucosal lesions of the colon, although Schwarz considered that "what many authors would like to have recognized as tumor shadows belong in the realm of fantasy." Although Laurell and Odquist in Sweden (1921) were probably the first to use the double-contrast method, they insufflated air only after an opaque meal had arrived in the colon, rather than in conjunction with a contrast enema.[26]

As Fischer wrote[63]:

If one partially fills the intestine with the usual contrast material– barium sulfate-bolus suspension . . . and subsequently insufflates the intestine with the usual amount of air, then, after the peristaltic churning, a thin deposit of the contrast adheres to the mucosa which produces in the roentgen picture a sharp outline of the contours of the intestinal walls. . . . Depending on the circumstance of the individual case, after as much of the contrast fluid as possible has reached the cecum, one permits all, part or none of it to be evacuated . . . Next, one proceeds with the administration of air per anum by means of the usual double bellows, which is equipped with a rectal tube and a stopcock which only opens during the emptying of the two bellows and should thus protect the bellows from soiling with a backflow of the contrast material. The administration of the air is controlled by observation of the fluoroscopic screen with the patient lying on his right side or standing. . . . The contours and lumen of the intestine are very clearly recognizable, so that any stenosis or tumor is certain not to pass unnoticed.

By taking multiple radiographs with the patient in various positions, Fischer could visualize intraluminal tumors that might be obscured by a solid column of barium.

In the 1930s, Kirklin and Weber at the Mayo Clinic modified and improved Fischer's double-contrast examination of the colon to produce consistently excellent radiographs that could detect small intraluminal tumors. They also developed criteria for determining whether a colonic lesion was benign or malignant, a differentiation that had proved extremely difficult for earlier radiologists. Other innovations included the use of high-kilovoltage technique, the addition of tannic acid to promote colonic evacuation, and the intensive study of postevacuation films. Cook and Margulis even introduced the use of silicone foam for the examination of the rectum and sigmoid.[26]

The most recent development in contrast examinations of the colon has been the intensive effort to demonstrate small polypoid lesions that may contain cancerous tissue at an early, curable stage. Many refinements of the double-contrast technique were introduced by S. Welin in Malmö, Sweden (1967), who reported the detection of colonic polyps in about 13% of the patients he examined (about 25,000 in 13 years), a figure equivalent to the incidence of polyps in autopsy reports in that country.[64] The development and widespread use of colonoscopy employing the flexible fiberoptic colonoscope (mid-1970s) sparked an often bitter debate as to whether colonoscopy or the double-contrast barium enema should be the procedure of choice for detecting colonic polyps. Supporters of each technique gleefully reported cases in which the opposite approach failed to detect often sizable lesions. Many now consider colonoscopy and the double-contrast barium enema examination to be complementary rather than competitive procedures, with each having a major role to play in the detection of colonic pathology.

STUDIES OF THE SMALL BOWEL

The examination of the small intestine has always been a stepchild of roentgenology. In all other parts of the gastrointestinal tract the examination is performed by observing roentgenoscopically the actual filling of the organ in question and then by studying the partially or completely filled organ. If the usual roentgenological methods are used such an examination of the small intestine is not possible due to the obstacle which the pylorus causes in the continuous outflow of barium.[65]

For more than 50 years after the discovery of x-rays, only limited progress was made in the radiographic demonstration of diseases of the small bowel. Narrowing of the lumen with proximal dilatation and "long-lasting stagnation of the radiopaque material in the small intestine" could be demonstrated in patients with partial obstruction. Another sign of severe obstruction was "the enormous gas- and fluid-filled hollow spaces which only showed alterations in position, indicating a high degree of

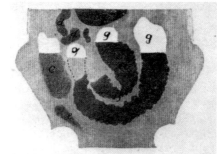
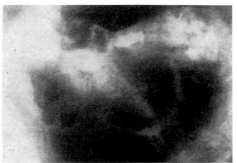

Small bowel obstruction (1911). *Left,* Direct sketch. *a,* Distended loops of small intestine; *g,* gas bubbles in loops of small intestine; *c,* ascending colon.[66] *Right,* radiograph of a patient with carcinoma of the cecum demonstrates obstructive masses with overlying gas bubbles in two distended loops of the small bowel which show a ribbed appearance.

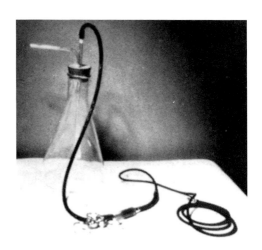

Barium enteroclysis (1939). Flask, transfusion syringe, and duodenal tube used during the procedure.[68]

stagnation of the shadow-producing masses."[66] Narrowing and spasm in the terminal ileum were noted in patients with tuberculous involvement. A similar appearance was seen in Crohn's disease.

Radiographic study of the small bowel was difficult to accomplish because of rapid peristalsis and overlapped bowel loops. A truly effective examination of the small bowel "would become possible if the barium were introduced through a duodenal tube. In this way, the filling of the small intestine would become similar to that of the colon through a rectal tube; it would in fact be an enema examination of the small intestine."[65]

Gilberto S. Pesquera in New York (1929) was apparently the first to recommend the use of a duodenal tube for continuous and controlled filling of the small intestine.[67] Ten years later (1939), Gershon-Cohen and Shay in Philadelphia first termed this technique *barium enteroclysis.*[68] In addition to a simple water suspension of barium sulfate, they injected air to produce a double-contrast effect. They stressed the "ease and rapidity with which the entire small intestinal tract may be visualized . . . The patient is spared repeated examinations of a progress meal and errors of diagnosis incident to incomplete filling of the intestines and the poor timing of the serial examinations of a progress meal are avoided."

Although the results of enteroclysis were far superior to those of routine oral examinations, its use was limited because of the need for intubation that was troublesome and time-consuming because a guidewire was not used. A major improvement was the development of an elongated Bilbao tube, which contained a stiff guidewire and was origi-

Stages of filling with barium enteroclysis (1939). "*Top left,* Duodenal tube in place; tip curled back in third duodenal segment. *Top middle,* At the end of 2 minutes with 200 cc injected, the duodenum and the first coils of the jejunum are filled. *Top right,* At the end of 5 minutes, 500 cc injected; jejunum is filled. *Bottom left,* At the end of 8 minutes, 800 cc injected and head of column is near ileocecal valve. *Bottom middle,* At the end of 10 minutes, air has been injected into jejunum and the head of the opaque column, already in the colon, has advanced to the splenic flexure. *Bottom right,* At the end of 12 minutes after the injection of more air. Note that the duodenal cap has remained full and that only a negligible reflux has occurred into the stomach, the pylorus having remained competent during the entire examination."[68]

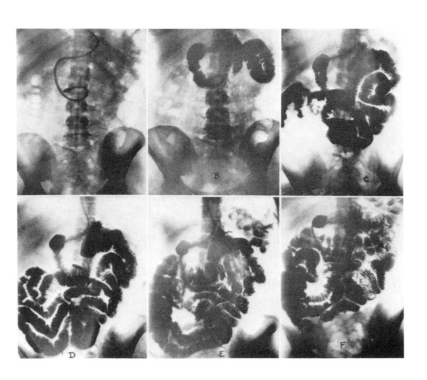

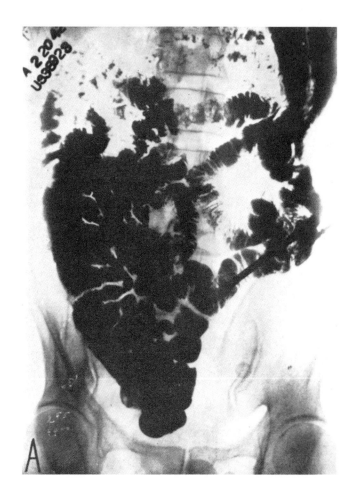

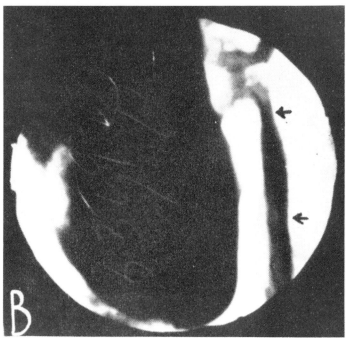

Small intestinal enema in a case of regional ileitis (1943). *Above left*, Overhead view. *Above right*, Spot film showing the narrow terminal ileum.[65]

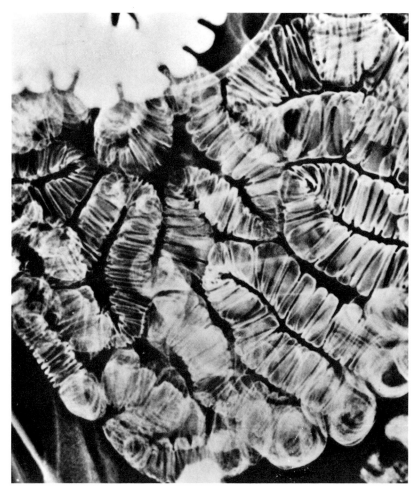

Modern enteroclysis.[71]

nally employed for hypotonic duodenography. Improved contrast material led to better coating of the small bowel. Trickey and co-workers (1963) found water to be an unsuitable double-contrast material because it produced an excessive dilution of barium. Searching for a fluid that would not readily mix with barium, they selected a 0.75% solution of hydroxymethylcellulose together with a wetting agent and used it to flush 80 ml of barium through the small bowel to produce a double-contrast effect.[69] The use of large volumes of barium combined with a 0.5% solution of methylcellulose in water was first described by Herlinger in 1978.[70] Up to 2 liters of this solution was introduced at a rate that produced distention and transradiancy of the small bowel without causing reflux into the stomach. Further improvements were suggested by Johan Sellink[71] and Dean Maglinte.

WATER-SOLUBLE CONTRAST

Although it was universally agreed that barium sulfate was the contrast material of choice for examination of the gastrointestinal tract, there were some situations in which the use of barium appeared to be contraindicated. Barium was known to incite a granulomatous reaction following leakage of the substance into body cavities or following retention within fistulous tracts. Therefore it was potentially dangerous to use barium in patients with suspected perforations, fistulas, and abscess cavities. In addition, many surgeons believed that if barium entered obstructed bowel or an abscess cavity from which it could not be removed, absorption of the suspending water could cause barium inspissation and the danger of partial or complete impaction.

To meet the radiographic needs in these specific situations, Wilma J. Canada (1955) introduced the use of water-soluble Urokon for gastrointestinal studies.[72] Already in use as a urographic contrast agent, Urokon "penetrates small tracts and cavities readily and does not become inspissated . . . Urokon disappeared rapidly from fistulas and abscess cavities, presumably by absorption or diffusion, thereby allowing subsequent contrast examinations, if required, without the confusion of residual opaque material." However, Canada noted that "Urokon is somewhat less dense (than barium) and mucosal coating is less adequate; therefore the examinations are less satisfactory for diagnostic purposes." Major disadvantages of Urokon were its high cost and "the extremely bitter taste of the material which makes the use of a tube obligatory for its introduction into the upper gastrointestinal tract."

After several enthusiastic articles, the use of water-soluble contrast in the gastrointestinal tract became controversial. It was shown that these agents often caused profuse diarrhea, acting like saline laxatives because of their hyperosmolarity.[73] Other authors noted that water-soluble contrast administered orally became rapidly diluted in the mid and distal small bowel. In the mid-1960s, two reports stressed the danger to dehydrated patients, especially infants, because of the use of water-soluble, iodine-containing contrast.[74] Consequently, these agents became unpopular and many radiologists stopped using them.

In 1959, Lessman and Lilienfield introduced Gastrografin as a water-soluble contrast for the study of the gastrointestinal tract. Gastrografin was a "palatable, lemon-flavored preparation identical, except for the added flavoring, with Renografin 76%" used for intravenous urography. Lessman and Lilienfield noted that "the filling of the small bowel distal to the second portion of the duodenum was not quite sufficient for detailed morphological study but adequate for detection of obstructive lesions and bowel fistulae."[75]

The hyperosmolarity of water-soluble contrast media draws interstitial fluid across the intestinal mucosa into the lumen. The increased volume of intestinal contents stimulates peristaltic activity, permitting rapid visualization of the small bowel, but also marked dilution of contrast that severely limits demonstration of mucosal detail. The ability of water-soluble contrast to accelerate interstitial transit time has led many radiologists to add 10 ml of Gastrografin to the barium mixture for small bowel follow-through examinations.[76]

After years of controversy, it has been generally agreed that water-soluble contrast is the agent of choice to demonstrate leakage from the gastrointestinal tract, as well as stab wounds, sinuses, and fistulas involving the peritoneal cavity. Because of its dilution effect, most radiologists prefer to evaluate possible small bowel obstruction with barium, except in patients with large bowel obstruction (to avoid the danger of barium inspissating proximal to the obstruction) and possibly in extremely ill patients in whom it is critical to make a rapid diagnosis.[77]

Although early articles recommended the use of water-soluble contrast in examinations of the esophagus where there was the possibility of aspiration, this technique is no longer performed because of the danger that the hypertonic contrast might draw large amounts of fluid into the tracheobronchial tree and produce severe pulmonary edema.

NEWER IMAGING MODALITIES

As in other areas of radiology, cross-sectional techniques (ultrasound, computed tomography [CT], and magnetic resonance [MR] imaging) have played an increasingly important role in the imaging of the gastrointestinal tract. In addition to demonstrating luminal and intramural lesions, these modalities can define the extent of an abnormality in various planes, assess the effect on adjacent organs, and detect disease at distant sites. Because of its nonionizing character and absence of known biolog-

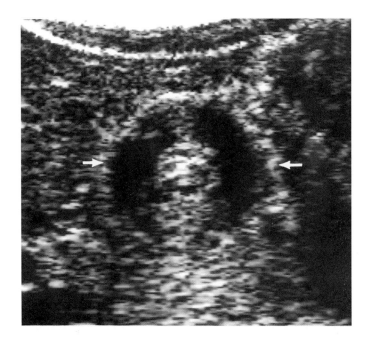

Ultrasound of pyloric stenosis. Characteristic doughnut lesion (*arrows*) consisting of a prominent anechoic rim of thickened muscle and an echogenic center of mucosa and submucosa.

CT staging of gastric carcinoma. There is narrowing of the antrum by the tumor (*arrows*) and adjacent lymph node metastases (*arrowheads*).

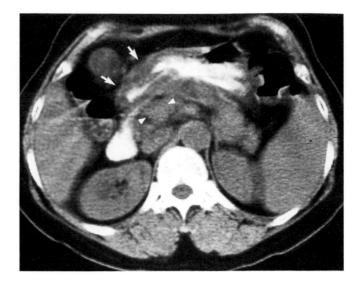

ical effects, ultrasound has become the primary screening modality for intraabdominal and pelvic pathology in children. It can detect gastrointestinal masses, such as pyloric stenosis and intussusception, and inflammatory disorders such as appendicitis. Esophageal and rectal transducers are being used to assess the extent of wall invasion in patients with malignant neoplasms in these areas. CT has become the imaging procedure of choice for staging cancers of the gastrointestinal tract and planning treatment, assessing tumor response to therapy, and detecting recurrent disease. With advances in respiratory gating, fast scanning, and new contrast agents, MR imaging will undoubtedly play a more important role in imaging the gastrointestinal tract because of its higher contrast resolution and its ability to directly image in sagittal and coronal, as well as axial, planes.

Bibliography

Bruwer AJ: Gastrointestinal tract. In Bruwer AJ (ed): Classic descriptions in diagnostic roentgenology. Springfield, Ill, Charles C Thomas, 1964.

Brecher R and Brecher E: The rays: A history of radiology in the United States and Canada. Baltimore, Williams & Wilkins, 1969.

References

1. Bruwer AJ: Gastrointestinal tract. In Bruwer AJ (ed): Classic descriptions in diagnostic roentgenology. Springfield, Ill, Charles C Thomas, 1964.
2. Hirsch SI: The roentgen ray study of the esophagus. Inter Med J 23:42-67, 1916.
3. Becher W: The use of Roentgen procedures in medicine. Deutsch Med Wschr 22:202-203, 1896.
4. Wegele C: A proposal for the use of Roentgen procedures in medicine. Deutsch Med Wschr 22:287, 1896.
5. Lindemann E: Demonstration of Roentgen pictures of the normal and distended stomach. Deutsch Med Wschr 23:266-267, 1897.
6. Einhorn M: Observations on radium. Medical Record 66:164-168, 1904.
7. Hemmeter JC: Photography of the human stomach by the Roentgen method: A suggestion. Boston Med Surg J 134:609-610, 1896.
8. Rumpel T: The clinical diagnosis of fusiform dilatation of the esophagus. Muenchen Med Wschr 44:420-421, 1897.
9. Brecher R and Brecher E: The rays: A history of radiology in the United States and Canada. Baltimore, Williams & Wilkins, 1969.
10. Skinner EH: American Roentgen Ray Society 1900-1950. Springfield, Ill, Charles C Thomas, 1950.
11. Leonard CL: The application of the roentgen rays to medical diagnosis. JAMA 29:1157-1159, 1897.
12. Walsh D: The roentgen rays in medical work. Baillière, Tindall and Cox, 1897.
13. Cannon W: Early use of the roentgen rays in the study of the alimentary canal. JAMA 62:1-3, 1914.
14. Cannon W: The movements of the stomach studied by means of the roentgen rays. Am J Physiol 1:359-382, 1898.
15. Barger AC: New technology for a new century: Walter B. Cannon and the invisible rays. AJR 136:187-193, 1981.
16. Cannon WB: Some reflections on the digestive process: Caldwell lecture. AJR 32:575-588, 1934.
17. Cannon WB and Moser A: The movements of food in the oesophagus. Amer J Physiol 1:435-444, 1898.
18. Roux JC and Balthazard V: A study of the contractions of the stomach in man through the use of Roentgen rays. C R Soc Biol (Paris) 10:785-787, 1897.
19. Williams FH: The roentgen rays in medicine and surgery, as an aid in diagnosis and as a therapeutic agent. New York, MacMillan, 1901.
20. Rieder H: Radiologic examination of the stomach and intestines in the living man. Muenchen Med Wschr 51:1548-1551, 1904.
21. Rieder H: Beitrage zur Topographie des Magendarm Kanales beim lebenden Menschen nebst Untersuchungen über den zeitlichen Ablauf der Verdauung. Fortschritte Roentgenstr 8:141-172, 1905.
22. Forssell G: Hermann Rieder: In memoriam. Acta Radiol 14:1-12, 1933.

23. Kestle C, Rieder H, and Rosenthal J: Cinematographically recorded roentgenograms (bioroentgenography) of the internal organs in man: A preliminary communication. Muenchen Med Wschr 56:280-282, 1909.

24. Bachem C and Gunther H: Barium sulfate as a shadow-forming contrast agent in roentgenologic examinations. Zeitschr für Rontgenkunde 12:369-376, 1910.

25. Holzknecht G and Brauner L: Die radiologische Untersuchung des Magens. Wien Klin Rundschau 19:273-276, 1905.

26. Rigler LG and Weiner M: History of radiology of the gastrointestinal tube. In Margulis AR and Burhenne HJ (eds): Alimentary tract roentgenology. St. Louis, CV Mosby, 1983.

27. Holzknecht G: Distinctor. Fortschr Rontgenstr 17:170, 1911.

28. Hemmeter JC: New methods for the diagnosis of gastric ulcer. Arch F Verdauungskrankh 12:357-363, 1906.

29. Case JT: Roentgen observations on the duodenum with special reference to lesions beyond the first portion. AJR 3:314-321, 1915.

30. Lippman CW: Cylinder with Bucky effect. AJR 3:452-453, 1915.

31. Haudek M: Die Rontgendiagnose des Kallosen (penetrierenden) Magengeschwurs und ihre Bedeutung. Muenchen Med Wschr 57:2463-2467, 1910.

32. Akerlund A: The roentgen diagnosis of ulcus duodeni with respect to local "directed" roentgen symptoms. Acta Radiol 2:14, 1928.

33. Von Elischer G: A new method for the roentgen examination of the stomach. Fortschr Rontgenstr 18:332-340, 1911.

34. Eisler F and Lenk R: The importance of the pattern of stomach folds in the diagnosis of gastric ulcer. Deutsch Med Wschr 1:1459-1461, 1921.

35. Forssell G: Studies of the mechanism of movement of the mucous membrane of the digestive tract. AJR 10:87-104, 1923.

36. Rendich RA: The roentgenographic study of the mucosa in normal and pathological states. AJR 10:526-537, 1923.

37. Brewer GE and Cole LG: The roentgenologic diagnosis of surgical lesions of the stomach and duodenum. Ann Surg 61:55-72, 1915.

38. Carman RD and Miller A: The roentgen diagnosis of diseases of the alimentary canal. Philadelphia, WB Saunders, 1917.

39. Stevenson CA: The development of gastrointestinal radiology. AJR 75:230-237, 1956.

40. Carman RD: A new roentgen-ray sign of ulcerating gastric cancer. JAMA 77:990-992, 1921.

41. Miller A: Carman. AJR 16:53-55, 1926.

42. Editorial. AJR 73:127, 1955.

43. Cole LG: A new radiographic table. Trans Amer Roent Ray Soc 174-276, 1908.

44. Cole LG: Serial radiography in the differential diagnosis of carcinoma of the stomach, gallbladder infection, and gastric or duodenal ulcer. Arch Roent Ray 17:172-181, 1912.

45. Cole LG: An x-ray table for serial and stereoscopic radiography and fluoroscopy. Arch Roent Ray 17:147-150, 1912.

46. Pirie AH: Cinematography of the antrum pylori, pylorus, and first part of the duodenum. Arch Roent Ray 17:163-172, 1912.

47. Laufer I: Double contrast examination of the gastrointestinal tract. In Margulis AR and Burhenne HJ (eds): Alimentary tract radiology. St. Louis, CV Mosby, 1989.

48. Laufer I: Double contrast gastrointestinal radiology with endoscopic correlation. Philadelphia, WB Saunders, 1979.

49. Leonard CL: The radiography of the stomach and intestines. AJR 1:1-42, 1913.

50. Hampton AO: A safe method for the roentgen demonstration of bleeding duodenal ulcers. AJR 38:565-570, 1937.

51. Schatzki R and Gary JE: Face-on demonstration of ulcers in the upper stomach in a dependent position. AJR 79:772-780, 1958.

52. Wasch MG and Epstein BS: The roentgen visualization of tumors of cardia. AJR 51:564-571, 1944.

53. Shirakabe H: Double contrast studies of the stomach. Stuttgart, Thieme-Verlag, 1972.

54. Obata WG: A double-contrast technique for examination of the stomach using barium sulfate with simethicone. AJR 115:275-280, 1972.

55. Gelfand DW: The Japanese-style double contrast examination of the stomach. Gastrointest Radiol 1:7-12, 1976.

56. Laufer I, Hamilton J, and Mullens JE: Demonstration of superficial gastric erosions by double contrast radiology. Gastroenterology 68:387-391, 1975.

57. Poplack W, Paul RE, Goldsmith M, et al: Linear and rod-shaped peptic ulcers. Radiology 122:317-319, 1977.

58. Miller R, Chernish SM, Skucas J, et al: Hypotonic roentgenography with glucagon. AJR 121:264-274, 1974.

59. Schule A: Intubation and radiography of the large intestine. Arch Verdauungskr 10:111-118, 1904.

60. Haenisch GF: Roentgenologic examination in narrowing of the large intestine: The early roentgenologic diagnosis of carcinoma of the large intestine. Muenchen Med Wschr 45:2331-2375, 1911.

61. Editorial. AJR 69:861, 1953.

62. Haenisch GF: The value of the roentgen ray in the early diagnosis of carcinoma of the bowel. Amer Quart Roentgenol 3:175-180, 1911.

63. Fischer AW: A new roentgenologic method for examination of the large intestine: A combination of the contrast material enema and insufflation with air. Klin Wschr 2:1595-1598, 1923.

64. Welin S: Results of the Malmo technique of colon examination. JAMA 199:369-372, 1967.

65. Schatzki R: Small intestinal enema. AJR 50:743-751, 1943.

66. Schwartz G: The roentgenologic detection of deeper stenoses of the small intestine. Wien Klin Wschr 40:1386-1390, 1911.

67. Pesquera GS: A method for the direct visualization of lesions in the small intestines. AJR 22:254-257, 1929.

68. Gershon-Cohen J and Shay H: Barium enteroclysis: A method for the direct immediate examination of the small intestine by single and double contrast techniques. AJR 42:456-458, 1939.

69. Trickey SE, Halls J, and Hobson CJ: A further development of the small bowel enema. Proc Roy Soc Med 56:1070-1073, 1963.

70. Herlinger H: A modified technique for the double-contrast small bowel enema. Gastrointest Radiol 3:201-207, 1978.

71. Sellink JL and Miller RE: Radiology of the small bowel: Modern enteroclysis technique and atlas. The Hague, Martinus Nijhoff, 1982.

72. Canada WJ: Use of Urokon in roentgen study of the gastrointestinal tract. Radiology 64:867-873, 1955.

73. Davis LA, Huang KC, and Pirkey EL: Water-soluble, nonabsorbable radiopaque media in gastrointestinal examination. JAMA 160:373-376, 1956.

74. Nelson SW, Christoforidis AJ, and Roenigk WJ: Dangers and fallibilities of iodinated radiopaque media in obstruction of the small bowel. Am J Surg 109:546-559, 1965.

75. Lessman FP and Lilienfield RM: Gastrografin as water soluble contrast medium in roentgen examination of the gastrointestinal tract. Acta Radiol 51:170-178, 1959.

76. Goldstein HM, et al: Comparison of methods for acceleration of small intestinal radiographic examination. Radiology 98:519-523, 1971.

77. Margulis AR: Water-soluble radiographic contrast agents in the gastrointestinal tract. In Miller RE and Skucas J (eds): Radiographic contrast agents. Baltimore, University Park Press, 1977.

CHAPTER 16

Gallbladder and Biliary Tree Radiology

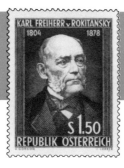

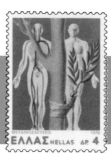

PLAIN RADIOGRAPHY

The first radiograph of a gallstone was published by Henry Cattell on February 15, 1896,[1] less than 3 months after the discovery of x-rays. Cattell placed a penny, a lead pencil, and a gallstone in a segment of small intestine that contained mucus and fecal material and was wrapped in three thicknesses of paper. After placing this preparation on a photographic plate and exposing it to x-rays, the penny was distinct and the lead of the pencil clearly visible (but not the surrounding wood); the shadow of the irregular gallstone could also be seen (although not as well as the other two objects). Gilbert and co-workers (1897) presented x-ray photographs of surgically removed gallstones, some composed of pure cholesterol and others of mixed material. They concluded that the degree of penetration by the x-ray depended on the chemical compositions of these stones, which often appeared as a central nidus surrounded by peripheral lamellation.[2] After placing several large mixed calculi underneath both the human thigh and lower thorax and failing to produce an identifiable shadow on the photographic plate even after a 15-minute x-ray exposure, they concluded that gallstones would be difficult to demonstrate in vivo because they would be obscured by human tissues.

George E. Pfahler (1900) reported strikingly clear radiographs of autopsy specimens of gallbladders filled with calculi.[3] Although he initially thought that respiratory motion would prevent gallstone detection in live patients, subsequent improvements in x-ray equipment allowing shorter exposure times permitted him in 1915 to report the successful detection of gallstones in vivo.[4]

The first preoperative radiographic diagnosis of gallstones with surgical confirmation was apparently made by Carl Beck in 1899.[5] To avoid the overlying soft-tissue shadow of the liver, Beck recommended that "the direction of the beam should be at an angle of 45° to the plate." When Beck presented two cases at the New York County Medical Society, many in the rather skeptical audience dubbed his interpretation "erroneous."

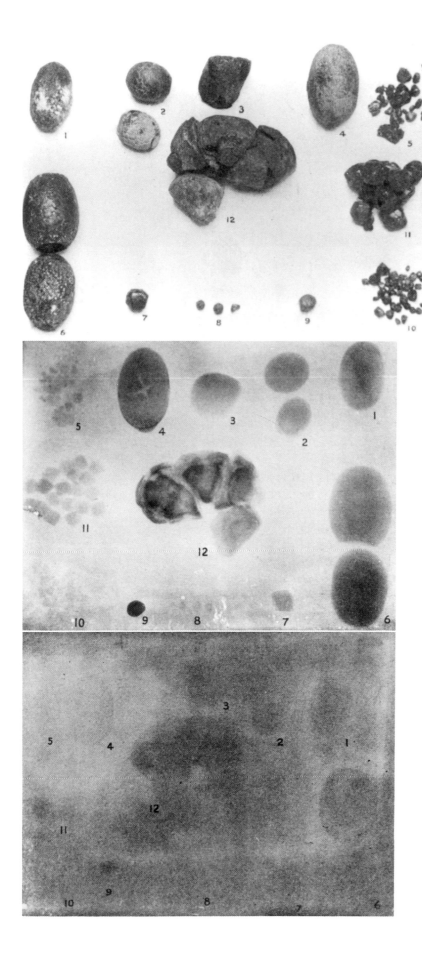

Translucency of gallstones (1900). *Top*, Plain photograph of twelve sets of calculi containing various chemical compositions. *Middle*, Radiograph of the same calculi. *Bottom*, Radiograph obtained when the calculi were placed under a living body.[5]

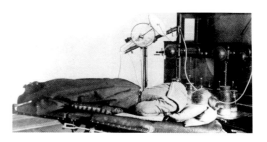

Method for gallstone radiography (1902). The tube access passes through the gallbladder at an angle of 60 degrees to avoid the liver. An exposure time of 50 seconds was used.[6]

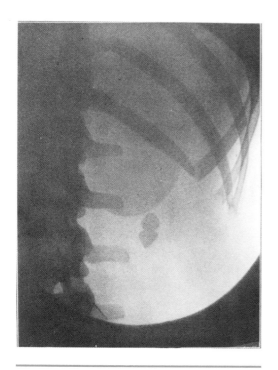

Two calcified gallstones (1913).[9]

A number of reports soon followed of the diagnosis of gallstones either as an incidental finding or in cases of suspected cholelithiasis. It was well recognized, however, that the radiographic demonstration of gallstones depended on their calcium content. Since the majority of calculi contained little, if any, calcium, it was clear that plain abdominal films would at best be able to detect only a minority of gallstones.[7]

In the mid-1910s, four reports documented the unequivocal radiographic detection of gallstones. James T. Case (1913) stressed the use of intensifying screens to provide more soft-tissue detail, as well as having the plate anterior to the patient (thus bringing the gallstones nearer the plate) rather than posteriorly as for the examination of urinary stones.[8] Thurston Holland (1913) noted that the calcification in gallstones typically was most pronounced on the exterior of the calculi, so that "the center of the stone is less opaque, whereas (it) is denser at the circumference."[9] Pfahler[4] (1914) emphasized the importance of oblique projections to exclude renal stones and calcified cartilage: "The patient is placed obliquely upon the right side. The cylinder is compressed strongly into the upper gastric region, so that the center of the cylinder is resting posterior to the right costal border. This will project the shadow of any gall-stones clearly to the outer side of the kidney." Lewis Gregory Cole (1914) concluded that "it is safe and sane to make a positive diagnosis of gall-stones when they are composed of calcium, or have a definite calcareous coating."[10] However, all agreed with Pfahler's earlier caveat that "if a calculus is not found it can by no means be interpreted as meaning that no stone is present."[3]

Enlargement of the gallbladder indicating underlying disease could be detected on contrast examinations of the upper gastrointestinal tract. As George and Leonard noted in their heavily illustrated book (1922), an enlarged gallbladder often produced pressure effects on the antrum of the stomach, as well as on the first and second portions of the duodenum.[11]

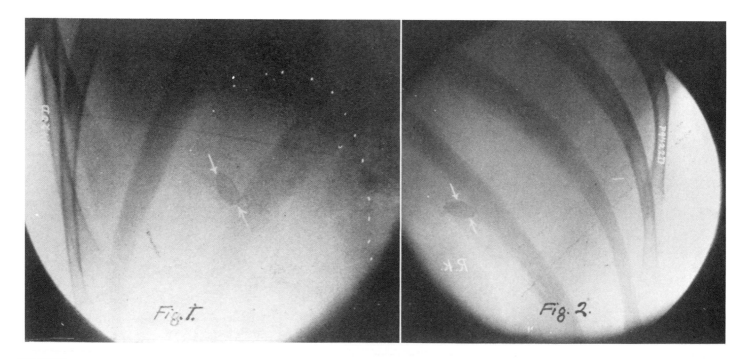

Value of oblique projections (1914). *Left,* Initial film shows the calcified gallstone lying within the shadow of the kidney. *Right,* Oblique projection clearly shows the gallstone projected outside the kidney shadow.[4]

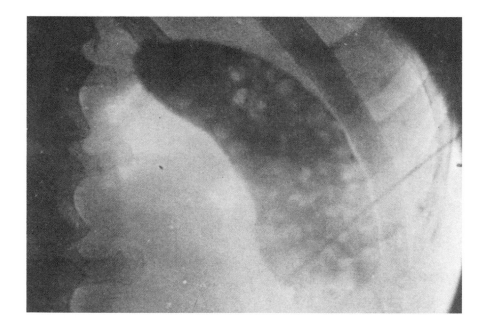

DIRECT GALLBLADDER PUNCTURE

In 1921, Burckhardt and Mueller inserted a needle into the gallbladder cavity by direct transhepatic puncture.[12] In studies on cadavers and subsequently in five patients, they injected a silver-containing contrast agent and air and clearly visualized the surface of the gallbladder and gallstones lying within it. Burckhardt and Mueller stressed that puncture of the gallbladder and other visceral organs was basically harmless as long as tiny needles (0.8 mm or smaller) were used. Although they "obtained incontrovertible evidence that gallstones can be visualized very beautifully in roentgenograms," Burckhardt and Mueller believed that "the chief value of the method was shown to lie not in the roentgenologic detection of gallstones, but in the possibilities which it afforded for obtaining bile and for injecting fluids for therapeutic purposes." They questioned whether some day by using this technique it might be possible

> by injection of a narcotic agent into the gallbladder to abort temporarily an acute attack of gallstone colic . . . to influence cholecystitis by direct injections into the gallbladder . . . by the injection of certain fluids into the gallbladder to dissolve gallstones or to reduce their size.

More than 60 years would pass before interventional techniques could answer these questions in the affirmative.

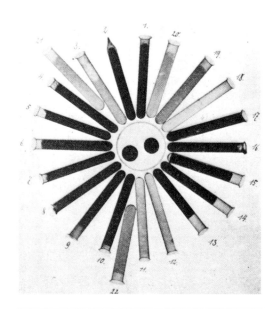

ORAL CHOLECYSTOGRAPHY

Cholecystography, the noninvasive technique for radiographic visualization of the gallbladder, was the culmination of an ingenious application of several basic pharmacological and physiological observations. In July, 1896, Ernst Sehrwald reported that the halogens (chlorine, bromine, and iodine) in pure liquid form were highly impermeable to x-rays.[13] In addition, he demonstrated that chemical compounds containing halogens had an impenetrability to x-rays that was proportional to the percentage of the halogen in the compound.

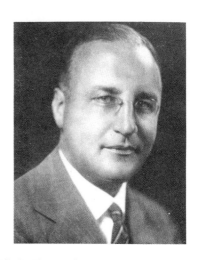

Evarts A. Graham (1883-1957).

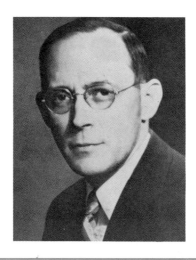

Warren H. Cole (1898-1990).

In 1909, Abel and Rowntree of Johns Hopkins Hospital conducted a series of experiments "on the pharmacological action of some phthaleins and their derivatives, with a special reference to their excretion, reabsorption, and purgative action."[14] One effective cathartic was phenoltetrachlorophthalein which, they noted, was almost entirely excreted by the liver into bile. By 1913, Rowntree, Horowitz, and Bloomfield reported on the use of this compound as a test for liver function.[15] They also found that phenolsulphonphthalein was excreted partly by the liver but mostly by the kidneys. Utilizing this information, Rosenthal and White (1925) developed the classic Bromsulphalein test for hepatic function.[16]

Another critical bit of basic information necessary for the development of cholecystography was the demonstration by Peyton Rous and Phillip Duryee McMaster (1921) that, by absorbing water, the normal gallbladder could concentrate bile eight to ten times.[17]

In the spring of 1923, Evarts A. Graham, Professor of Surgery at Washington University in St. Louis (and later the organizer and first Chairman of the American Board of Surgery), convinced Warren H. Cole, a first-year resident, to take a year off to work on the problem of visualizing the gallbladder. Graham theorized that an iodine or bromine derivative of phenolphthalein, because of the high atomic number of the halogen, might be radiographically visible in the gallbladder once it had been excreted by the liver and concentrated in the gallbladder. Cole recalled almost 40 years later,[18]

> I must have injected as many as 200 dogs and rabbits without obtaining a single gallbladder shadow. We knew that it would require six to ten hours after injection of the solution for the gallbladder to concentrate it to a maximal degree. Therefore, if we started our injections at 8:30 a.m. or 9:00 a.m. it would be undesirable to take roentgenograms much before 5:00 p.m. We had no x-ray equipment in our laboratory so we had to transport the animals across the street (via a tunnel) to the x-ray room at the hospital; this transportation fell to my lot since our laboratory assistants stopped work at 5:00 p.m. sharp.

After 4½ months of uninterrupted failure, in November, 1923, Graham and Cole achieved the first successful cholecystogram in a dog. "I called Dr. Graham, who was working late as usual. We stood there admiring the dripping film with a white blob in the center, as if we had found a treasure chest full of gold." But to their chagrin, other dogs injected in similar fashion that day and on succeeding days failed to demonstrate opacification of the gallbladder. Why did only one dog display a visualized gallbladder? As Cole recalled:

> Finally, in desperation, I called on Bill (the animal caretaker) and asked him if the treatment of that dog had been in any way different from the treatment of the other three dogs. Bill hesitated a bit, but stated he could think of nothing different in that dog. When I told him that this dog showed exactly the thing we were looking for, his expression of apprehension changed, and meekly stated, 'Well, Dr. Cole, there *was* one thing different. I forgot to feed that dog the morning he was injected.' I lunged at him, trying to slap him on the back, and grabbed his hand in appreciation at the same time. He hastily backed away, thinking no doubt that I was going to manhandle him. However, I was able to convince him I was very grateful for the entire incident, even though it represented an error of omission

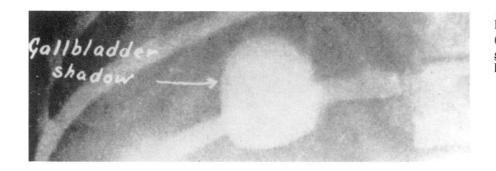

First successful cholecystogram in a dog (1923). The animal, weighing 5.25 kg, was given 1.5 gm of tetrabromophenolphthalein with 0.3 gm of calcium hydroxide.[18]

on his part. I recognized immediately that lack of food in the dog's stomach might readily be responsible for the great difference in behavior of the gallbladder, because I had read only a few days previously that Boyden had reported at the Annual Meeting of the American Society of Zoologists that feeding (especially fatty food) would cause emptying of the gallbladder in the cat. This would mean that with food in the stomach, the gallbladder would not be able to fill. I felt confident that eating was vital in filling and emptying of the gallbladder. Accordingly, the next day I gave three more dogs an injection but omitted their morning feeding. From that time on we were able to get good shadows. Having found a method of visualizing the gallbladder in animals, we moved rapidly to develop a technic which could be utilized in the human being.

Graham and Cole tested their new cholecystographic agent on fifteen patients without success. In retrospect, they realized that they had either given too small a dose (to check for toxic reactions) to permit visualization of the gallbladder or had given adequate doses to patients suffering from gallbladder disease that did not permit bile containing the compound to enter it (a major diagnostic sign). However, at the time, Graham and Cole could not be sure whether they were in fact demonstrating diseased gallbladders unable to take up bile or merely proving the worthlessness of contrast cholecystography. Moreover, some of the patients developed reactions to the injection, ranging from mild to quite severe.[19]

The sixteenth patient was a nurse from Cole's hospital who complained of right upper quadrant pain and had a questionable diagnosis of gallbladder disease.

> This was on February 21, 1924. I had already learned that rapid injection of this solution tended to increase the reaction. Accordingly, I gave the injection very slowly, hoping to avoid a reaction completely. However, my hopes were blasted . . . After injection of slightly over half of the solution the patient began complaining of nausea, followed shortly by pain in the back and elsewhere. I stopped the injection and waited ten minutes; the nausea disappeared so I renewed the injection.

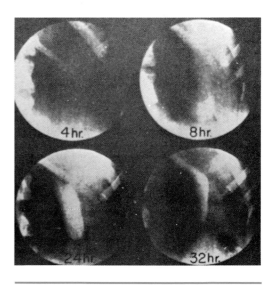

As Cole later declared, if the x-ray film in this case also had revealed no gallbladder shadow, "after seeing (her) in such misery with severe nausea, retching, and generalized pain, I doubt that I would have had the courage or the 'cruelty' to continue with injection of other patients."

The cumbersome technique consisted of an intravenous drip infusion of a mixture of 5 g to 6 g of tetrabromophenolphthalein and 1 g to 1.2 g of calcium hydroxide, dissolved in 3 to 5 ml of distilled water.

First successful cholecystogram in a human being (1924). Films taken at 4 (*upper left*), 8 (*upper right*), 24 (*lower left*), and 32 hours (*lower right*). No shadow is seen on the 4-hour film; on the 8-hour film the shadow is large and faint. A dense shadow is observed at 24 hours. Persistence of the shadow is attributed to the prolonged starvation.[20]

Cole's notebook recorded the results:

At 3¾ hours, gallbladder probably outlined, but exceedingly faintly.
At 7½ hours, gallbladder definitely outlined and distended . . .
At 24 hours, gallbladder spectacularly outlined . . .

Following the radiological diagnosis of "normal gallbladder," the nurse was saved from an unnecessary operation for gallbladder disease, and her symptoms were later traced to her kidney.[19]

The only problem with this technique was the patient's severe adverse reaction. This reaction and those of subsequent patients convinced Graham and Cole to switch from the calcium salt, which was poorly soluble and thus required a large and prolonged injection, to the more soluble sodium salt that could be given in smaller divided doses injected approximately 30 minutes apart. They designed an ingenious carrier for two syringes that made it possible to

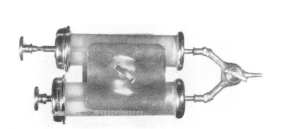

Carrier for two syringes made to allow alternate injections of physiologic saline solution and contrast material (1925).[18]

> allow alternate injections of physiologic saline solution and dye. This allowed us to stop the injections temporarily (and keep the needle open with saline) if a reaction was sustained. Often, early mild symptoms would disappear in a few minutes if the injections were stopped or the rate decreased.[18]

Nevertheless, the intravenous injection of cholecystographic contrast material continued to cause unpleasant side effects. This led to a search for an effective oral contrast agent. Merrill Sosman had observed that the gallbladder opacification from a "Graham-Cole test" that had disappeared after 24 hours had reappeared at 72 hours when he was performing a routine gastrointestinal series. He reasoned that some of the opaque salt excreted by the biliary system had been reabsorbed from the alimentary tract and, after circling through the liver again, must have reached the gallbladder a second time. This demonstration of the enterohepatic circulation meant that there was a good likelihood that an opaque agent administered orally would also be absorbed through the alimentary tract.[21]

In early 1925, two groups working independently reported the first successful oral cholecystography: Whitaker, Milliken, and Vogt[21] using sodium tetraiodophenolphthalein and Menees and Robinson[22] using sodium tetrabromophenolphthalein. The bromine compound was more toxic and soon abandoned. To avoid the nausea associated with the oral contrast agent, Whitaker and associates searched for a method "whereby the substance would pass through the stomach without coming in contact with the mucous membrane." They succeeded by producing "pills of the salt, double coated with salol in syrup of Tolu." Using these pills, "a cholecystogram after 6 hours showed a well outlined shadow of the gallbladder. At the 12 hour interval this shadow was more distinct." Nevertheless, the shadows produced by the oral method were less dense than those following intravenous injection of contrast material. As they noted,

> the roentgenographic technique must be exceptionally good and particular pains taken to eliminate respiratory movements which tend to erase the shadows. The patient should not be told to take a deep breath, but a moderate breath—one cannot hold the diaphragm perfectly still after filling his lungs to the limit. Furthermore, reliance should not be placed on a single exposure but several should be made at each interval. All this is important since the absence of a shadow, granted perfect technique, almost certainly indicates cholecystic disease.

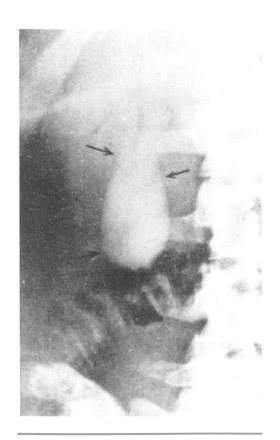

Oral cholecystography (1925). Twelve-hour film shows excellent visualization of the gallbladder.[21]

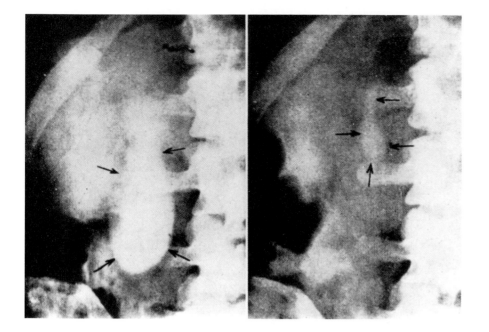

Effect of a fatty meal (1925). *Left,* Sixteen-hour film after oral administration of cholecystographic contrast shows excellent visualization of a normal gallbladder. *Right,* Tremendous reduction in size of the shadow about 2 hours after taking food rich in fat (egg yolks and cream).[22]

After reporting good-quality cholecystograms in 93% of normal subjects, Whitaker et al. recommended

> the use of the oral method first in cases suspected of gall-bladder disease, to be followed by the intravenous method in a few instances in which the result with the former is not conclusive. The advantages of the oral method are that it relieves many patients of the hospitalization necessary for the intravenous method, and that it causes them very little inconvenience and few unpleasant symptoms.

Some of the residual side effects of sodium tetraiodophenolphthalein (marketed as Iodeikon) were overcome with the development (1940) of a new class of compounds by Dohrn and Diedrich of Berlin.[23] The best of these, Priodax (iodoalphionic acid), was shown to be reasonably well tolerated and to produce improved images. Because it was primarily excreted by the urinary tract, Priodax was often associated with burning on urination. Nonvisualization of the gallbladder after oral administration of this contrast agent had a high correlation with the presence of gall-stones.

In 1951, Hoppe and Archer[24] developed iopanoic acid (Telepaque), a tri-iodo-alkanoic acid derivative. This compound was much safer than previously used agents and had a higher concentration in the bile, which produced increased gallbladder opacification. It also resulted in a substantial incidence of bile duct visualization.[7] Slight changes in the basic structure of this molecule produced other compounds (Cholebrine, Bilopaque, Oragrafin) that have been used for oral cholecystography.

In patients with severe vomiting, adynamic ileus, or inflammatory bowel disease, attempts were made to instill cholecystographic contrast material per rectum.

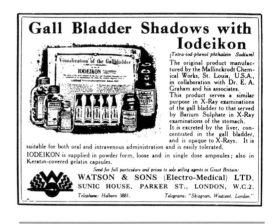

Advertisement for Iodeikon.

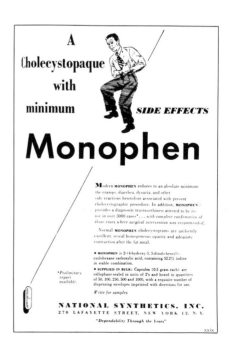

Amusing advertisement for Monophen (AJR, 1951). Note that the patient with biliary colic is clutching his *left* upper quadrant rather than his right.

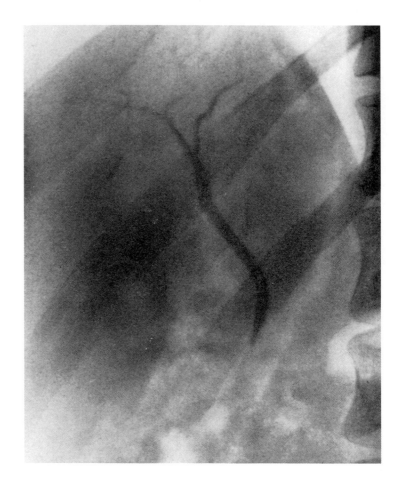

INTRAVENOUS CHOLANGIOGRAPHY

Intravenous cholangiography was used to obtain radiographic opacification of the bile ducts and to determine patency of the cystic duct. Therefore it required a contrast agent with physicochemical properties that allowed hepatic excretion of the compound in sufficient quantities and concentrations to permit direct radiographic visualization of the bile ducts. The first contrast agent for intravenous cholangiography was sodium iodipamide (Biligrafin), which was introduced in 1953.[26] Two years later (1955), this agent was replaced by the methylglucamine salt (Cholografin). The demonstration of the bile ducts using these intravenous agents usually required tomography for adequate visualization.

Iodipamide had six iodine atoms per molecule, and thus the concentration of iodine that was achieved when this material was excreted in bile was substantially higher than that with oral contrast agents, which were excreted at the same rate but had only three iodine atoms per molecule. Because radiographic opacification depends on the number of iodine atoms in the path of the x-ray beam, the concentration of iodine with iodipamide was adequate for opacification of the bile ducts directly, and further concentration of the contrast material by the gallbladder was unnecessary.[27]

The major developer of intravenous cholangiography was Robert E. Wise of the Lahey Clinic. He demonstrated the value of this technique in the diagnosis of acute cholecystitis, which was often associated with cystic duct obstruction that prevented gallbladder visualization on oral cholecystography. In addition, the nausea and vomiting that accompanied this condition interfered with the absorption of oral contrast agents, while the prolonged length of the oral examination was incompatible with the

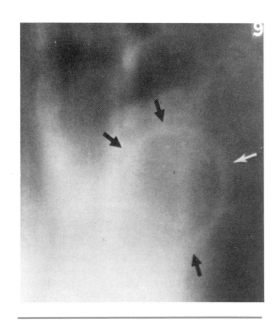

Infusion tomography of the gallbladder (1973). Distended gallbladder with a 4-mm thick wall in a patient with acute and chronic cholecystitis with gallstones. The gallbladder did not visualize on an oral study.[29]

frequent need for prompt surgical decision. Opacification of the common bile duct without opacification of the gallbladder during intravenous cholangiography was characteristic of obstruction of the cystic duct.[28]

Until the mid-1970s, intravenous cholangiography was the only preoperative method available for evaluating the bile ducts. Numerous combinations of dose and duration of infusion of Cholografin were studied in an attempt to improve opacification of the biliary tree and reduce the frequent and often severe toxic side effects. With the advent of ultrasound, computed tomography, cholescintigraphy, and transhepatic and endoscopic cholangiography to demonstrate the bile ducts, intravenous cholangiography has completely disappeared from the diagnostic scene.

Tomography of the gallbladder following the intravenous infusion of urographic contrast agents was suggested for direct demonstration of the thick, inflamed gallbladder wall in acute cholecystitis. Rabushka, Love, and Moncada (1973) showed that in patients with acute cholecystitis, the abnormal gallbladder wall could be opacified within a few minutes.[29] However, the use of infusion tomography was soon supplanted by the development of radionuclide biliary tract imaging.

RADIONUCLIDE IMAGING (CHOLESCINTIGRAPHY)

For many years, I-131 rose bengal was the only widely available radionuclide that was selectively taken up by liver cells and provided effective imaging of the hepatic parenchyma. However, a combination of technical problems, the high photon energy peak of I-131, and the significant patient exposure to particulate (beta) emission eventually contributed to its decline as a clinically useful imaging modality. Although rose bengal was excreted through the bile duct, imaging of these smaller structures had to await new radiopharmaceuticals and higher resolution gamma cameras.[30]

The successful labeling of a molecule of iminodiacetic acid (IDA) with Tc-99m, with its pure gamma energy, ideal 6-hour physical half-life, and 140 kev photon energy peak, represented a major breakthrough for hepatobiliary scintigraphy. Easily distributed commercially in kit form, IDA was readily taken up by the hepatocytes and excreted into the bile. The first IDA derivative successfully labelled with technetium was dimethyliminodiacetic acid (HIDA), a structural analog of lidocaine. In 1975, Harvey and co-workers showed that by using ^{99m}Tc-HIDA, the liver, bile ducts, gallbladder, and intestine could be rapidly visualized with serial gamma camera images.[31] Since that time, numerous other IDA molecules have been commercially produced that have an enhanced hepatobiliary excretion (with concomitant decrease in renal excretion) and provide better visualization of the common bile duct, even in patients with high bilirubin levels.

Persistent nonvisualization of the gallbladder (up to 4 hours) in a fasting patient who otherwise demonstrates normal liver cell uptake and excretion into the duodenum was shown to be dependable evidence for acute cholecystitis. With none of the undesirable side effects of Cholografin, these radiopharmaceuticals have established biliary scintigraphy as the preferred initial imaging modality when acute cholecystitis is suspected.[32]

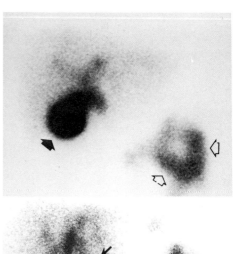

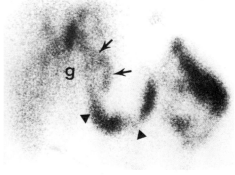

Acute cholecystitis demonstrated by radionuclide cholescintigraphy. *Top*, Normal scan demonstrates the bile ducts, the gallbladder (*black arrow*), and early excretion of radionuclide into the duodenum and proximal jejunum (*open arrows*). *Bottom*, In a patient with acute cholecystitis, the cholescintigram shows no visualization of the gallbladder (*g*) but good visualization of the common bile duct (*arrows*) and duodenum (*arrowheads*), indicating obstruction of the cystic duct.[33]

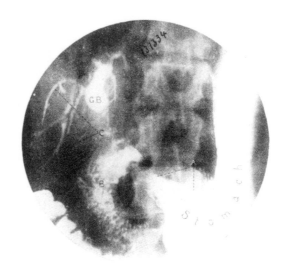

Filling of gallbladder and biliary tree during upper gastrointestinal examination (1915). *A*, Carcinoma, pyloric end of stomach; *B*, duodenum; *GB*, barium in gallbladder; *C*, barium in hepatic ducts.[34]

DIRECT CHOLANGIOGRAPHY AND INTERVENTIONAL TECHNIQUES

The injection of contrast material into the biliary tree began with two accidental observations. Russell D. Carman (1915) described a case of pathological communication between the gallbladder and duodenum in which barium was shown to fill the hepatic ducts during an upper gastrointestinal examination.[34] Three years later, Adolph Reich (1918) reported opacification of the bile ducts following injection of a cutaneous sinus tract with petrolatum and bismuth paste.[35] Reports of additional similar cases and the discovery (1921) of oil-based Lipiodol as an opaque contrast agent led to the development of a series of procedures to deliberately delineate the biliary tree. The first postoperative cholangiogram was performed in 1925 by G. Cotte of Lyon, who injected fistulas and post-surgical T-tubes in an intentional search for strictures and retained stones.[36] Six years later (1931), Mirizzi and Losada of Argentina extended the principle to operative cholangiography.[37] Mirizzi showed that operative cholangiography permitted a rapid and complete evaluation of the bile ducts and demonstrated the nature and extent of the pathological condition, often revealing findings that were not suspected preoperatively. He stressed that the diagnostic accuracy of operative cholangiography was far greater than that attained by surgical exploration alone. As Mirizzi noted, his aim was not only to discover overlooked stones before the abdominal wall was closed but to eliminate injuries to the ductal system.

> The bile in the peritoneum observed by surgeons, who believe its presence is due to slipping of the ligature, in most cases is a testimony that there is an anatomofunctional lesion of the hepatic and common bile ducts that has not been noted because of the inaccuracy, deceptiveness, and lack of precision in the methods of exploration used.

Unfortunately, the physical properties of Lipiodol limited its value as a contrast agent for operative cholangiography. Lipiodol was thick and did not flow freely, was poorly miscible, and produced considerable fragmentation. This problem was solved with the introduction of water-soluble contrast material. Improvements in instrumentation, refinements in technique, and the introduction of television monitoring into the operating room have greatly contributed to the advancement of operative cholangiography.[7]

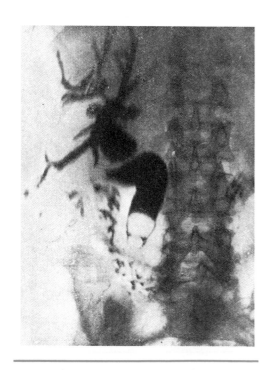

Lipiodol injection via a T-tube demonstrates retained stones impacted in the distal common duct (1925).[36]

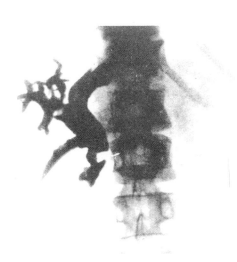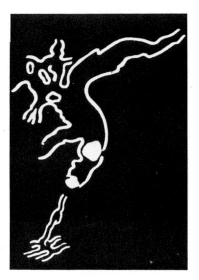

Nonsurgical transhepatic cholangiography probably originated in Indochina. In 1937, Huard and Do-Xuan-Hop[38] described radiographs obtained after the percutaneous transhepatic puncture of the biliary tree followed by the instillation of a Lipiodol in patients with biliary obstruction resulting from parasitic infestation. Fifteen years later, Carter and Saypol (1952) described a percutaneous method for prolonged drainage of an obstructed biliary tract.[39] However, the introduction of intravenous cholangiography the next year effectively ended for the time being the use of transhepatic cholangiography as the method of choice for nonsurgical visualization of the bile ducts.

Although intravenous cholangiography proved useful for demonstrating retained calculi after cholecystectomy, it was of no value in the heavily jaundiced patient in whom the distinction between bile duct obstruction and liver parenchymal disease was of crucial importance. The high surgical mortality in diagnostic explorations of these patients stimulated renewed interest in transhepatic cholangiography. A large series reported by Evans and co-workers[40] (1962) at New York Hospital established the usefulness and relative safety of the method:

> It carries two potentially serious complications: internal bleeding, due to perforation of a blood vessel, and bile peritonitis as a result of seepage of bile into the peritoneal cavity. These can be minimized by close collaboration between surgeon and radiologist both in the conduct of the examination and in the immediate post-examination.

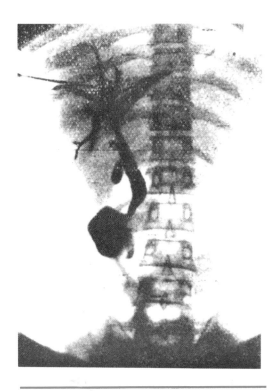

Transhepatic cholangiography (1937).[38]

The development of a catheter-sheathed needle added the important advantage of therapeutic drainage of the obstructed ducts after the procedure. This technique was first described in the surgical literature in 1964[41] and was modified by radiologists 10 years later.[42] Use of the transhepatic radiological approach could spare patients with advanced disease and limited life expectancy the need for major palliative surgery. Nevertheless, percutaneous transhepatic cholangiography was still infrequently performed except as an immediate preoperative maneuver in densely jaundiced patients, since the rigid needle could easily lacerate small hepatic vessels and create bile leaks. The major discovery transforming this procedure from "a greatly feared, dangerous technique into a widely accepted routine clinical procedure for direct bile duct opacification"[27] was the introduction in 1974 of the thin, flexible "Chiba" or

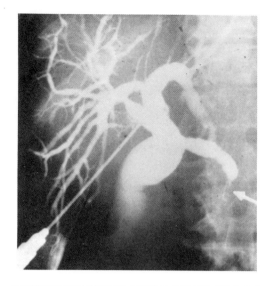

Percutaneous transhepatic cholangiography (1962). Recurrent carcinoma of the stomach obstructing the common duct. Note the small "rat-tail" deformity at the point of obstruction (*arrow*).[40]

"skinny" needle by Okuda and co-workers in Japan.[43] This technique had a low risk of bleeding and sepsis and could differentiate between the various causes of severe jaundice. By borrowing the catheter replacement principle from percutaneous angiography, stents could be placed across benign and malignant strictures to provide palliative treatment for patients who were not operative candidates.

The other direct approach to the biliary ductal system is retrograde cholangiography by endoscopic catheterization of the papilla of Vater. The first peroral cannulation of the duct was performed by two radiologists, Rabinov and Simon, who used a remotely manipulated catheter-cannula device under fluoroscopic guidance.[44] The major breakthrough in popularizing this technique was the development of the fiberoptic endoscope, which permitted nonsurgical visualization of the duodenal papilla. In 1968, McCune[45] reported a 25% success rate in duct cannulation; within 2 years, Oi and co-workers in Japan had achieved a 70% rate of successful cannulation.[46] Other major champions of this technique, called endoscopic retrograde cholangiopancreatography (ERCP) included Anacker in Germany and Vennes and Bilbao in the United States. Although ERCP has a 3% risk of complications (mainly sepsis induced in obstructed pancreatic and biliary ducts), it is a valuable technique for evaluating the patient with jaundice of undetermined etiology, for obtaining cytology and biopsy, and for therapeutic papillotomy and placement of biliary catheters and stents.[47]

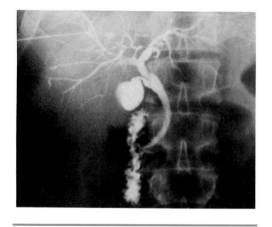

First normal cholangiogram reported using the "Chiba," or "skinny," needle technique (1974). The caliber of the entire biliary tract is normal in this patient with intrahepatic cholestasis.[43]

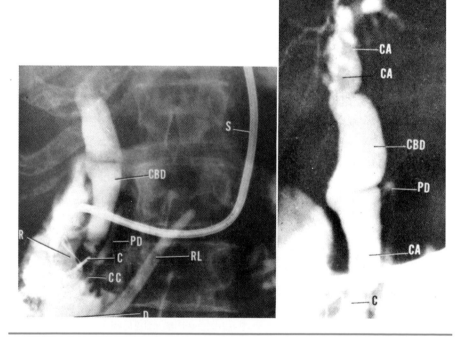

First peroral cannulation of the ampulla of Vater (1965). *Left,* Radiograph obtained early in the injection with the cannula in the ampulla partially opacifies the biliary and pancreatic ducts. *Right,* Film taken later during the injection with the patient in an erect position shows that the cannula has advanced slightly further into the common bile duct. The intrahepatic ducts are also delineated. Several calculi are noted in the biliary ducts. *C,* Cannula; *CA,* calculus; *CBD,* common bile duct; *CC,* common channel of biliary and pancreatic ducts; *D,* duodenum; *PD,* pancreatic duct; *R,* runners; *RL,* rubber leader; *S,* portion of instrument in stomach.[44]

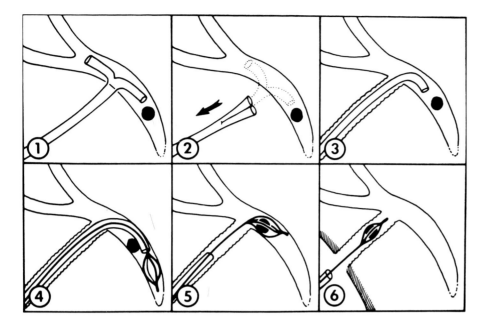

Technique for extraction of retained common duct stone (Burhenne, 1973). (*1*) Repeat T-tube cholangiogram is obtained on the day of stone extraction 4 to 5 weeks after choledochotomy. (*2*) After the location of the retained stone has been ascertained, the T-tube is withdrawn. (*3*) Using the sinus tract of the T-tube, the steerable catheter is guided into the bile duct, and its movable tip is advanced beyond the retained stone. (*4*) The basket is inserted through the steerable catheter, the catheter is withdrawn, and the basket is opened. (*5*) The open basket is withdrawn to engage the stone. The basket is only retracted, never advanced, outside the enclosure of the steerable catheter. (*6*) The stone is extracted through the drain tract.[48]

In patients with retained gallstones following cholecystectomy, surgical reexploration was associated with twice the operative mortality and morbidity of the initial operative procedure. As T-tube cholangiography became widely practiced, the possibility of removing retained calculi through the sinus tract was recognized. Mondet (1962) and Mazzarielo (1970) used forceps to extract biliary stones, while Lagrave and Plessis (1969) and Magarey (1969) used the Dormia ureteral stone basket.[27] Catheters and guidewires were used to dislodge obstructions in T-tubes and the common duct by encouraging the distal passage of stones and plugs. The major figure in nonsurgical stone extraction was H. Joachim Burhenne of Canada, who developed a remote-controlled catheter through which extraction baskets of several sizes could be introduced.[48] Using this technique, Burhenne has succeeded in removing 95% of retained calculi under fluoroscopic control.

In the 1980s, biochemical techniques for the dissolution of gallstones were developed. Initially, solvents such as ursodiol (named because it was a naturally occurring bile salt in bears) were administered orally. However, these agents, as well as those directly infused into the biliary system, had a slow rate of stone dissolution and often were associated with troublesome side effects. More rapid and predictable stone dissolution could be achieved after the percutaneous infusion into the biliary tree of monooctanoin[49] and the far more potent methyl tert-butyl ether (MTBE).[50] Both agents are effective against cholesterol stones. Although calcium bilirubinate stones or stones with a thick calcium rim cannot be completely dissolved, they may be reduced in size and "softened" sufficiently to be extracted with baskets or be destroyed by extracorporeal shock wave lithotripsy (ESWL). Because MTBE has substantial side effects if the agent escapes from the gallbladder into the duodenum, MTBE is preferred currently for dissolution of gallbladder stones while monooctanoin is used for common duct stones.[51]

Another noninvasive alternative to surgery in the treatment of gallstones is ESWL. Using high-energy shock waves, this technique produces alternating mechanical stresses on brittle substances such as gallstones, attempting to reduce them to sandlike particles that can pass through the cystic and common bile ducts.[52]

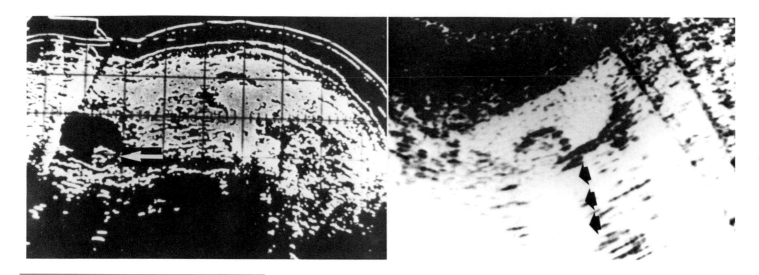

Ultrasound of gallstones. *Left*, Early
bistable B-mode ultrasound image of a
gallstone (1972). *Right*, Improvements in
resolution by gray-scale ultrasound allowed
detection of an acoustic shadow from a
gallstone (1974).

ULTRASOUND

In the early 1970s, several investigators (primarily Huvlitz and associates, Leopold and Sokoloff, and Doust and Makalad) recognized the potential to visualize the gallbladder with first B-mode and subsequently grey-scale sonography. This technique offers the ability to rapidly and noninvasively assess the gallbladder with an extremely high accuracy. The presence of an acoustic shadow posterior to an echodense intraluminal focus was shown to be virtually pathognomonic of a gallstone. Gallbladder size and wall thickness could be accurately measured, pericholecystic fluid collections could be detected, and the presence of sludge (low level echoes that move slowly with changes in patient position and do not cause acoustic shadowing) and polypoid lesions (cholesterolosis, adenomyosis, carcinoma) could be easily seen. In most centers, ultrasound has almost completely replaced oral cholecystography as the primary modality for evaluating the gallbladder. Ironically, oral cholecystography has begun to make a small comeback with the advent of ESWL, since the degree of gallbladder function and presence or absence of calcification within gallstones are critical factors in determining whether a patient is a candidate for this therapeutic procedure.

Advantages of ultrasound include the absence of side-effects from contrast material, the ability to perform the study in patients with various underlying conditions (e.g., liver disease, jaundice, malabsorption, or pregnancy), the rapid establishment of a diagnosis, and the absence of ionizing radiation.[53]

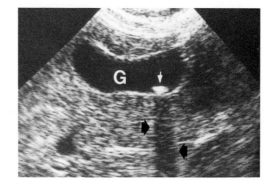

Modern sonogram (1991) showing a gallstone as an echogenic focus (*white arrow*)
in an otherwise sonolucent gallbladder (*G*).
Note the acoustic shadowing immediately
inferior to the stone (*black arrows*).

References

1. Cattell HW: Roentgen's discovery: Its application in medicine. Medical News 68:169-171, 1896.
2. Gilbert AC, Fournier A, and Oudin P: Photography of biliary calculi. Transactions of the Biology Society (Paris) 4:506, 1897.
3. Pfahler GE: Detection of gallstone by the roentgen ray. Amer Quart Roentgenol 3:23-33, 1911.
4. Pfahler GE: An improvement in the technique of gallbladder diagnosis. AJR 2:774-775, 1914.
5. Beck C: On the detection of calculi in the liver and gallbladder. NY Med J 71:73-77, 1900.
6. Monell HS: A system of instruction in x-ray methods and medical uses of light, hot-air, vibration and high-frequency currents. New York, Pelton, 1902.
7. Shehadi WH: Clinical radiology of the biliary tract. New York, McGraw-Hill, 1963.
8. Case JT: Roentgenoscopy of the liver and biliary passages with special reference to gallstones. JAMA 61:920-925, 1913.
9. Holland T: On gall-stones. Arch Roentgen Ray 17:374-377, 1913.
10. Cole LG: The detection of pure cholesterine gall-stones by the roentgen rays. AJR 2:640-651, 1914.
11. George AW and Leonard RD: The pathological gallbladder. New York, Hoeber, 1922.
12. Burckhardt H and Mueller W: Experiments on puncture of the gallbladder and its visualization with roentgen rays. Deutsch Ztschr Chirurgie 162:168-197, 1921.
13. Sehrwald E: The behavior of the halogens toward roentgen rays. Deutsch Med Wschr 30:477-480, 1896.
14. Abel JJ and Rowntree LG: On the pharmacological action of some phthaleins and their derivatives, with especial reference to their behavior as purgatives. J Pharmacol Exper Ther 1:231-264, 1909.
15. Rowntree LG, Hurwitz SH, and Bloomfield AL: Experimental and clinical study of the value of phenoltetrachlorphthalein as a test for liver function. Bull Johns Hopkins Hosp 24:327-342, 1913.
16. Rosenthal SM and White EC: Studies in hepatic function. J Pharmacol Exp Ther 24:265, 1925.
17. Rous P and McMaster PD: The concentration activity of the gall bladder. J Exper Med 24:47-73, 1921.
18. Cole WH: The story of cholecystography. Amer J Surg 99:206-221, 1960.
19. Brecher R and Brecher E: The rays: A history of radiology in the United States and Canada. Baltimore, Williams & Wilkins, 1969.
20. Graham E, Cole W, Copher G, and Moore S: Diseases of the gallbladder and bile ducts. Philadelphia, Lea & Febiger, 1928.
21. Whitaker LR, Milliken G, and Vogt EC: The oral administration of sodium tetraiodophenolphthalein for cholecystography. Surg Gynec Obstet 40:847-851, 1925.
22. Menees TO and Robinson HC: Oral administration of tetraiodophenolphthalein: Preliminary report. AJR 13:368-369, 1925.
23. Dohrn M and Diedrich P: Ein neues Rontgen Kontrastmittel der Gallenblase. Deutsche Med Wschr 66:1133-1134, 1940.
24. Hoppe JO and Archer S: Aryl-triiodo-alkanoic acid derivatives as cholecystographic media. Federation Proc 10:975-977, 1951.
25. Hornykiewytsch VT and Stender HS: Intravenose cholangiographie. Fortschr Roentgenstr 79:292-309, 1953.
26. Frummhold W: A new contrast agent for intravenous cholecystography. Fortschr Roentgenstr 79:283-291, 1953.
27. Berk RN, Ferrucci JT, and Leopold GR: Radiology of the gallbladder and bile ducts: Diagnosis and intervention. Philadelphia, WB Saunders, 1983.
28. Wise RE: Intravenous cholangiography. Springfield, Ill, Charles C Thomas, 1962.
29. Rabushka SE, Love L, and Moncada R: Infusion tomography of the gallbladder. Radiology 109:549-552, 1973.
30. Figley MM: History of radiology of appendage organs. In Margulis AR and Burhenne HJ (eds): Alimentary tract radiology, St. Louis, CV Mosby, 1988.
31. Harvey J, Loberg M, and Cooper M: Tc 99m-HIDA: A new radiopharmaceutical for hepatobiliary imaging (abstract). J Nucl Med 16:533, 1975.
32. Weissmann HS, Frank M, Bernstein LH, and Freeman LM: Rapid and accurate diagnosis of acute cholecystitis with ^{99m}Tc-HIDA cholescintigraphy. AJR 132:523-528, 1979.
33. Harned RE: Diseases of the gallbladder. In Eisenberg RL and Amberg JR (eds): Critical diagnostic pathways in radiology. Philadelphia, JB Lippincott, 1981.
34. Carman RD: Roentgen observation of the gallbladder and hepatic ducts after perforation into duodenum. JAMA 65:1812, 1915.
35. Reich A: Accidental injection of bile ducts with petrolatum and bismuth paste. JAMA 71:1555, 1918.
36. Cotte G: Exploration of the biliary ducts with lipiodol in a case of fistula. Bull Mem Soc Natl Chir (Paris) 23:759-767, 1925.
37. Mirizzi PL and Losada CQ: Exploration of the bile ducts during an operation. Proceedings of the Third Argentine Congress of Surgery 1:694-703, 1931.
38. Huard P and Do-Xuan-Hop: Transhepatic puncture of the bile ducts. Bull Soc Med-Chir Indochine 15:1090-1100, 1937.
39. Carter R and Saypol GM: Transabdominal cholangiography. JAMA 148:253-255, 1952.
40. Evans JA, Glenn F, Thorbjarnarson B, and Mujahed Z: Percutaneous transhepatic cholangiography. Radiology 78:362-370, 1962.
41. Wiechel KL: Percutaneous transhepatic cholangiography: Technique and application. Acta Chir Scand (suppl) 330:1, 1964.
42. Molnar W and Stockum AE: Relief of obstructive jaundice through percutaneous transhepatic catheter: A new therapeutic method. AJR 122:356-367, 1974.
43. Okuda K, Tanikawa K, Emura T, et al: Nonsurgical percutaneous transhepatic cholangiography: Diagnostic significance in medical problems of the liver. Am J Digest Dis 19:21-36, 1974.
44. Rabinov KR and Simon M: Peroral cannulation of the ampulla of Vater for direct cholangiography and pancreatography: Preliminary report of a new method. Radiology 85:693-697, 1965.
45. McCune WS, Short PE, and Moscovitz A: Endoscopic cannulation of the ampulla of Vater: Preliminary report. Ann Surg 167:752-757, 1968.
46. Oi I, Takemoto, and Kondo T: Fiberduodenoscope: Direct observation of the papilla of Vater. Endoscopy 3:101-105, 1969.
47. Stewart ET and Vennes JA: Endoscopic retrograde cholangiopancreatography. In Margulis AR and Burhenne HJ (eds): Alimentary tract radiology. St. Louis, CV Mosby, 1988.
48. Burhenne HJ: Nonoperative retained biliary tract stone extraction: A new roentgenologic technique. AJR 117:388-399, 1973.
49. Thistle JL, Carlson GL, Hofmann AF, et al: Monooctanoin, a dissolution agent for retained cholesterol bile duct stones. Gastroenterology 78:1016-1022, 1980.
50. Allen MJ, Borody TJ, Bugliosi TF, et al: Rapid dissolution of gallstones by methyl tert-butyl ether. N Engl J Med 312:217-220, 1985.
51. Van Sonnenberg E, D'Agostino HB, Casola G, et al: Interventional radiology in the gallbladder. Radiology 174:1-6, 1990.
52. Steinberg HV, Torres WE, and Nelson RC: Gallbladder lithotripsy. Radiology 172:7-11, 1989.
53. Jacobson HG and Stern WZ: The Graham-Cole "test" revisited: The oral cholecystogram today. JAMA 250:2977-2982, 1983.

CHAPTER 17

Uroradiology

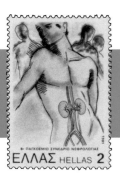

Urology can be said to owe its existence as a specialty to the inventive genius of Thomas Edison and Wilhelm Conrad Roentgen. The incandescent light made possible the development of the cystoscope which permitted precise examination of the urinary tract as well as endoscopic treatment of many conditions that had previously been accessible only by open surgical methods. And the Roentgen Ray provided a means whereby diagnostic studies of the entire urogenital tract could be carried out.

R.M. NESBITT, 1956[1]

At the time of the discovery of x-rays, renal, ureteral, and vesical stones and other causes of hematuria were diagnosed with "uncertainty." Error was frequent, and the location of a stone was often missed. Surgical explorations lacked precision and frequently, even among the most experienced, were fruitless. The extent of individual kidney function was unknown. Many deaths resulted from nephrectomy for tuberculosis because "contralateral renal function was unknowingly inadequate to sustain life."[2]

Although primitive cystoscopes were first devised in 1806, it was not until 1877 that Max Nitze developed a practical instrument with an improvised electric light source (using a platinum wire lamp) and lens system. After Edison's invention of the incandescent lamp was announced in 1880, Nitze immediately recognized the advantages of this light source for his work. However, it was not until 1887 that he was able to obtain a small bulb that could be adapted to his instrument.[3]

Urologists soon began passing catheters up both ureters through the cystoscope. In 1895, for example, Howard Kelley introduced the wax-tipped ureteral catheter. Scratches on the wax were diagnostic of calculi in the ureter. This was an extremely useful test and far more precise than early radiographs.[2]

The first preoperative radiographic diagnosis of a renal calculus was reported by John MacIntyre in July, 1896.[4] Two years later, "various American journals were dotted with case reports of plain film findings of renal and ureteral calculi."[5] The major advocate of plain radiography for the detection of renal and ureteral stones was Charles Leonard[6] of Philadelphia. "The diagnosis it affords is absolute both positively and negatively, and it has the advantages of mathematical accuracy." Unfortunately, Leonard was unaware of or refused to recognize a variety of problems that would void his results, such as nonopaque stones or technical difficulties. The low output of x-ray apparatus and the absence of intensifying screens required exposure times of 10 minutes or more, so that only large and dense calculi could be detected. Even when identified, the precise position of a stone within the kidney could not be localized, since the renal margins were rarely shown.[2]

Another unexpected problem was that some calcific densities in the pelvis did not represent ureteral calculi. To make this distinction, a French physician, Theodore Tuffier (1897), introduced a metal stylet into a ureteral catheter to make the latter radiopaque and thus outline the course of the ureter.[7]

Four years later (1901), three groups working independently reported similar methods of demonstrating the ureters radiographically. Lewis Ernst Schmidt and Gustav Kolischer of Chicago[12] used

> lead wire of various diameters as catheters. The central end of the lead wire is rounded by melting. While, on the one hand, lead wire is tough enough not to break off, on the other hand, it is so soft and flexible that injuries to the linings of the ureter or kidney are excluded, as is dislocation of the ureter . . . The diagnostic possibilities which this technique made possible are as follows:
> (a) The absolutely exact determination of the shape of the ureter.
> (b) The exact localization of a possible obstruction of a ureter.
> (c) The exact topographical localization of the renal pelvis.
> (d) The resolving of a possible differential-diagnostic difficulty in the differentiation between gall and kidney stones.
> (e) Information concerning the size of the renal pelvis.
> (f) Indications concerning the nature of a blockage of the ureter.

Loewenhardt equipped a catheter with a lead mandrin and advanced it into the renal pelvis. He noted that[13]

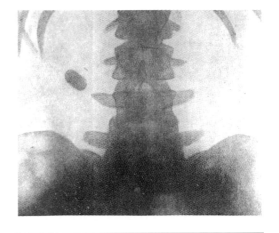

Kidney stone (1902).[9]

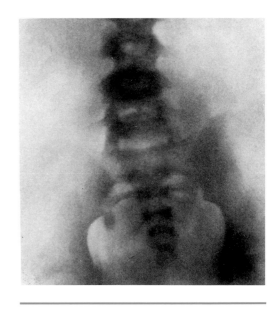

Ureteral stone (1904).[10]

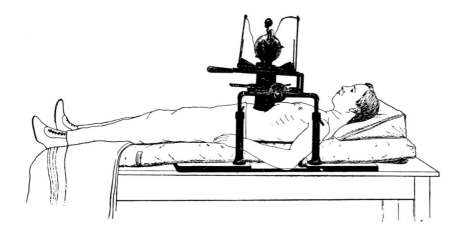

Skiagraphing renal calculus by using a compression device (1904).[11]

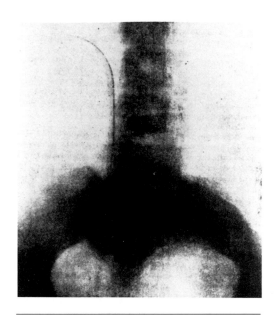

Course of the ureter in a living subject after retrograde placement of a catheter provided with a metal mandrin (1897).[7]

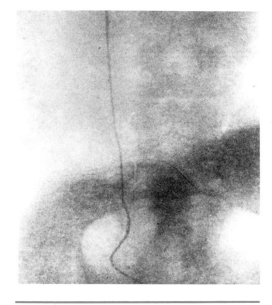

Lead wire catheter in the ureter (1901).[12]

Use of radiographic bougie in suspected ureteral calculus disease (1905). *Top*, Multiple opacities (*arrows*) in a patient with flank pain. *Bottom*, With the bougie in the ureter, the opacities are clearly seen to be outside the ureter. They represented calcified lymph nodes.[16]

the opening of the abdominal cavity and the palpation of the second kidney (to make certain that it was there!—author note) is still always necessary for a number of the surgical operations on one of these organs. In an effort to avoid whenever possible this diagnostic last resort through the use of other examination methods, the author sought to obtain information regarding the condition of the second kidney by the determination of the position of the ureter.

In Hungary, Illyes von Sofalva Geza (1901) preferred the use of a catheter rather than a lead wire alone. He suggested that instilling bismuth into the lumen of the catheter would make it more flexible, as well as radiopaque.[14] Three years later (1904), Bernhard Klose anticipated retrograde pyelography when he noted that he would have liked to fill the renal pelvis with contrast material by means of a ureteral catheter. He did not actually perform this procedure, because "one must consider whether the mucous membrane of the renal pelvis would not be too severely irritated by the bismuth powder."[15] E. Harry Fenwick (1905) introduced a "radiographic bougie," a ureteral catheter whose wall was impregnated with iron oxide and was described as "solid, aseptic, easily passed and proves very dense to x-rays."[16] It was not until 16 years later (1921) that Sgalitzer and Hryntschak recognized the value of oblique and lateral projections when it was unclear whether a calculus overlying the radiopaque ureteral catheter was actually in the ureter.[2]

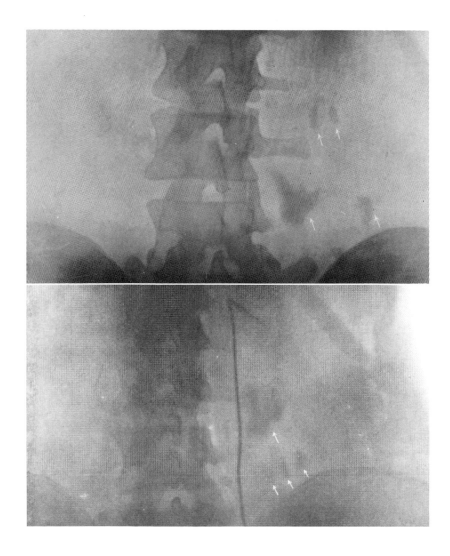

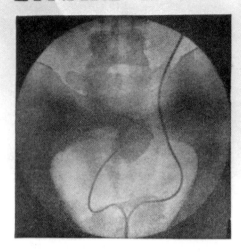
Advertisement for urological x-ray catheters (AJR, 1918).

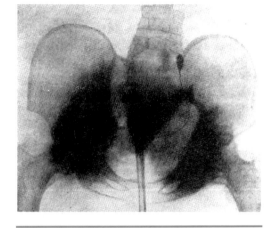

Catheter demonstration of ureteral obstruction (1901). Tip of the opaque catheter ends near the level of the iliac crest close to a dim shadow representing a stone wedged in the ureter.

CYSTOGRAPHY AND RETROGRADE PYELOGRAPHY

The first cystogram was reported by Wittek (1903), who filled a bladder with air to demonstrate a stone within it.[17] The next year, Wulff showed a bladder anomaly by opacifying the organ using a mixture of bismuth subnitrate, starch, and water.[18]

The possibility of demonstrating the upper urinary tract by an injection of contrast material was discovered fortuitously by Fritz Voelcker and Alexander von Lichtenberg (1905) while making radiographs of the bladder using Collargol (a colloidal silver preparation). One of their x-ray

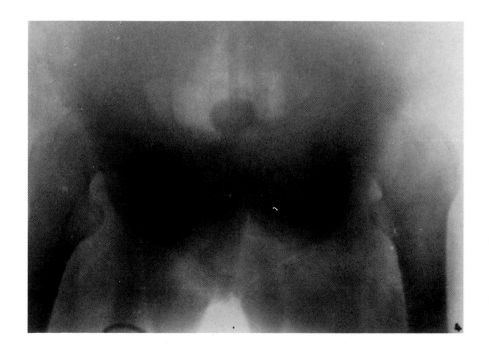

First cystogram (1903). After the introduction of 150 cc of air to fill the bladder, there is clear visualization of a stone within it. The tubular structure that is projected over the large calculus represents the catheter.[17]

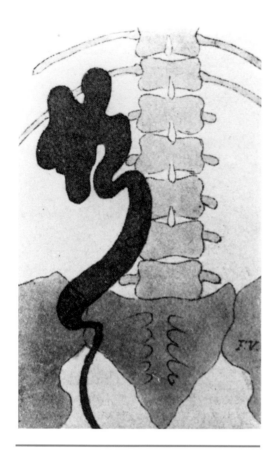

One of the first successful retrograde pyelograms (1906). Sharp kink of the ureter somewhat above the pelvic brim (from a left ovarian tumor) causes striking dilatation of the proximal ureter and renal pelvis.[19]

plates showed that the silver solution had entered the ureter and renal pelvis and outlined them on the radiograph.[1] The next year (1906), Voelcker and von Lichtenberg deliberately attempted to fill the renal pelvis by instilling a 5% solution of Collargol through ureteral catheters to produce the first successful retrograde pyelogram.[19] After completion of the procedure, the renal pelvis was rinsed out with a boric acid solution. Voelcker and von Lichtenberg noted that "since it is not possible even with the highest pressures to force a fluid from the bladder into the ureters and the renal pelvis, it is necessary to force a path into the renal pelvis by means of the insertion of a ureteral catheter." They emphasized the importance of pyelography "not only for the diagnosis of dilatation, kinking, and displacement of the renal pelvis and ureter, but also for malformations and possibly also for renal tumors."

A major advocate of retrograde pyelography was William Frederick Braasch, a prominent urologist at the Mayo Clinic, who was largely responsible for popularizing the technique in the United States. Using a 10% solution of Collargol, "we were able to outline the pelvis quite definitely."[20] He noted that

> moderate dilatation of the renal pelvis occurred in conditions other than hydronephrosis; furthermore, that the ureteral catheter could meet with obstruction in the pelvis without a stone being present . . . Most of the hypernephromata . . . showed on section marked deformity of the renal pelvis; either irregular dilatation of the pelvis, entire or in part, or encroachment upon the pelvic lumen by projections of the surrounding tumor substance. It occurred to me that a radiographic demonstration of these deformities could be of considerable aid in the diagnosis of hypernephromata, frequently so difficult to establish clinically.

With regard to localization of renal stones, Braasch recognized that "frequently a shadow is seen in the region of the kidney and its exact relation to the pelvis is in doubt. If the stone is within the pelvis its shadow will be either obliterated in a collargol plate, or it will appear dimmed by the surrounding collargol shadow. If the shadow is shown to be distinct from the pelvis . . . the stone must be without the pelvis." Braasch next turned to the problem of determining the site of origin of large abdominal tumors. He showed that "if a collargol radiograph is made, and the renal pelvis is found to be in the *normal position* and with a *normal outline*, the tumor is probably not renal." In his major text, Braasch[21] described and categorized a broad spectrum of renal structural lesions including neoplasms, chronic pyelonephritis, congenital abnormalities, and cystic diseases.

Retrograde pyelography (1910). Deformities of the renal pelvis caused by (*left*) tuberculosis and (*right*) renal neoplasm.[20]

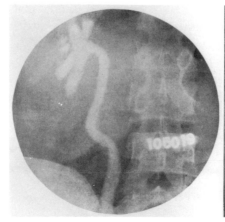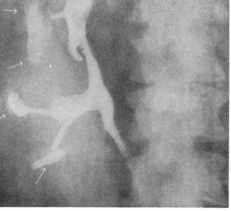

Uhle and Pfahler (1910), who recommended the use of silver oxide and later silver iodide as contrast media, described their technique for retrograde pyelography[22]:

> The injections are given by means of a syringe of 10 cc capacity and injected slowly so as not to cause sudden distension of the kidney pelvis, a condition which will provoke renal colic. To prevent over-distension, or the too rapid distension, we have devised the following technique: The buttocks of the patient are raised and warmed solution allowed to flow by gravity from a graduated burette which is held about two feet above the level of the patient. This method of examination determines the size of the kidney, pelvis, the amount of destruction of the kidney substance, and the position of the kidney in its relationship to other structures. It also determines the position and alterations in the size and shape of the ureter.

For more than 10 years, various silver preparations were used as the contrast material in retrograde pyelography. These compounds were difficult to handle and prepare, dirty to use, expensive, and often resulted in injury to the kidney. In these early days, injuries were caused by over-distention of the renal pelvis with resultant tearing and infiltration of the renal parenchyma and spread of contrast material into the local and general circulations. This led to large renal infarcts or small deposits of silver in the kidney or perirenal tissues, hemorrhage into the spleen or liver, and various lung changes such as emboli, hemorrhagic infarcts, pneumonia, or acute pulmonary edema. Collargol could be fatal as a result of urinary suppression or severe hemorrhage from the bowel, mouth and nose.[23] By 1916, Zindel[3] had collected from the literature a series of 35 cases of severe damage and 11 deaths after the use of silver complexes for retrograde pyelography.

To prevent rupture of the urinary tract by overzealous filling via syringe, Baker (1910) introduced a popular method for retrograde pyelography that included simultaneous filling of both ureters by means of a gravity device.[24]

Multiple other chemicals were tried for retrograde pyelography. In 1915, Burns recommended a 15% solution of thorium nitrate-citrate, which produced radiographs of good quality. Although this thorium compound irritated the urinary tract and resulted in occasional fatalities, for want of a better medium it remained the contrast agent of choice for 3 years.[25] The break from silver compounds was completed in 1918, when Cameron introduced potassium and sodium iodide for retrograde pyelography.[26] The potassium salt was soon excluded because of its depressant effect on the heart.

Oily contrast agents were also used for retrograde pyelography. These compounds were unsatisfactory because they were immiscible in urine and formed oily bubbles that led to errors in interpretation.

Oxygen, air, and carbon dioxide were tried for retrograde pyelography but all proved completely unsatisfactory. The gas formed bubbles that appeared as filling defects, leading to errors in diagnosis. It was difficult to maintain full distention of the pelvis and ureter with gas, which also could easily be confused with gas in the intestinal tract. Several cases of fatal air emboli were also reported.

Eventually, the iodinated contrast agents developed for excretory urography were also applied to cystography and retrograde pyelography. The sodium salts were found to be irritating to the bladder, and thus the meglumine salts of diatrizoate and iothalamate are now almost universally employed for cystography.[27]

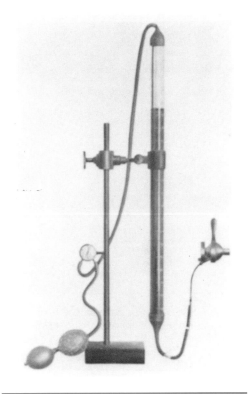

Device for measuring the capacity of the renal pelvis (1910).[24]

EXCRETORY UROGRAPHY
(INTRAVENOUS PYELOGRAPHY)

Although retrograde pyelography permitted accurate determination of some diseases of the urinary tract, the procedure required ureteral catheterization with the risk of developing a serious infection in this pre-antibiotic era. There was clearly the need for a simple, painless method for depicting the kidney, ureters, and bladder. In 1923, it occurred to Leonard G. Rowntree[28] that

> If, in roentgenography of the urinary tract, advantage could be taken of the fact that sodium iodid after its introduction into the body, is normally excreted in the urine, roentgenograms of the ureters and bladder might be secured without the need of catheterization. An ideal opportunity for the clinical testing of this idea presented itself in the section on dermatology and syphilology of the Mayo Clinic, where one of us (Earl D. Osborne) was utilizing intravenously from 50 to 250 cc of a 10% solution of sodium iodid in the study of the pharmacology and therapeutics of iodids. This circumstance made possible an immediate and direct clinical study, eliminating the necessity of carrying out time-consuming preliminary investigations on animals. The patients were informed of our interest in this problem, and many of them volunteered to undergo the roentgen-ray studies.

As they observed, "the striking lack of toxicity has long been known, but not fully appreciated. Enormous doses have been used clinically by syphilogists in the treatment of syphilis."

Following intravenous or oral administration of sodium iodide, visualization of the kidneys, ureters, and bladder was obtained. (However, oral ingestion of the salt produced local gastric irritation and upset, which precluded its further use.) As Osborne and co-workers wrote[28]:

> The method uniformly gives excellent and accurate shadows of the urinary bladder and renders reliable information relative to its size, shape, and location. It has been partially successful in depicting the renal pelves and the ureters in a limited number of cases. In a number of cases it assists in revealing the kidney itself through intensifying the renal shadow. It has been proved a success in revealing the existence of residual urine in the bladder and in furnishing approximate information of the amount, thus eliminating the necessity of catheterization and its attendant dangers of infection. Oral administration of the drug will prove satisfactory for routine use in making roentgenograms of the bladder, while for shadows of the ureters and kidneys intravenous injection of large doses of sodium iodid is desirable.

Larger doses of contrast material produced much better visualization, although they were also associated with a higher frequency of reactions. They also noted that the shadows of the kidneys and the lower margins of the liver and the spleen were sharply outlined after the administration of the sodium iodide. This probably was the first observation of the so-called nephrogram effect during excretory urography[29] (see p. 313).

Several other investigators experimented with a variety of compounds for excretory urography. However, these were either impractical because of poor opacification or too toxic because of the large amounts of iodine employed. A safe, efficient agent was still needed.

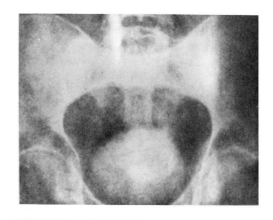

Excretory urography using sodium iodide (1923). Radiograph made 2 hours after the intravenous injection of 200 ml of a 10% solution of sodium iodide demonstrates "a perfect outline of the full bladder."[28]

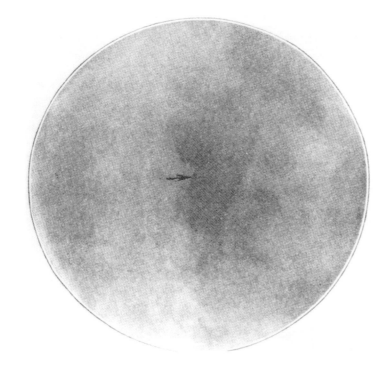

Throughout much of the 1920s, Arthur Binz and his assistant, C. Rath, biochemists in Berlin, synthesized a large number of pyridine compounds with components of arsenic and iodine. Their objective was a bacteriocidal agent against syphilis, a sort of "magic bullet" in the tradition of Ehrlich and his Salvarsan.[30] One of the compounds synthesized was called *Selectan-neutral*, an iodinated material that was considerably less toxic than simple iodide salts because its iodine was attached to a pyridine ring. Selectan-neutral was tried with some success against coccal infections of the gallbladder and urinary tract on the medical service of Leopold Lichtwitz in Hamburg. More importantly, it was shown that this compound was excreted primarily by the kidneys rather than by the liver. Could this iodine-containing compound be used as a contrast agent for radiography of the urinary tract?

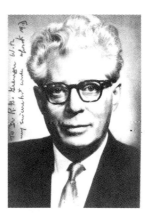

Arthur Binz (1868-1943).[31]

At this time, Emanuel Libman of the Mount Sinai Hospital in New York had just awarded a fellowship for foreign travel to one of his promising medical interns, Moses Swick. Swick was excited by the possibility of this new urinary contrast agent and accordingly went to work as Lichtwitz's assistant, changing the focus on the use of the drug from a potential therapeutic agent to one of possible diagnostic value.

As Swick wrote,[32]

> This led to the question whether selectan-neutral, whose tolerance has proved to be rather good considering the iodine content (54%), could not be used as a radiologic contrast substance in intravenous or oral administration. The first experiment on an animal did not show the gallbladder, but such a prominence of the kidney shadow resulted that the experiments were confined to the investigation of the kidneys and the urinary passages. In all cases, we obtained a good representation of the bladder. It seemed that also the kidney shadow was quite distinct.

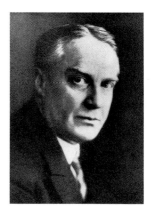

Moses Swick.

311

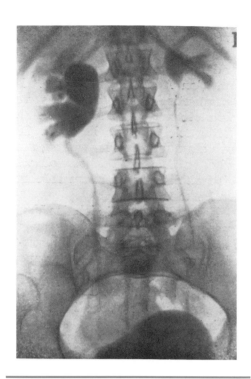

Early excretory urogram using uroselectan (1929). "Thirty-six-year-old female with obstructed right kidney at the moment of elimination. Complete urogram on left normal side."[32]

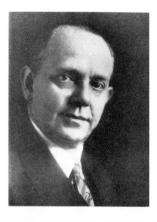

Alexander von Lichtenberg (1880-1949).[31]

However, the renal pelvis and ureter were poorly seen unless they had been ligated. "Some patients complained of headache, nausea, and vomiting. But in none of the cases were the reactions severe enough to interrupt further studies."

According to Swick, he suggested certain modifications of Selectan-neutral to Binz that would diminish the toxicity and increase both the solubility and the iodine content of the molecule. Meanwhile, Swick transferred to a large urological hospital in Berlin under the direction of the famed Alexander von Lichtenberg, which "afforded me close contact with Binz, who followed these investigations with great interest and was confident that the specifications could readily be fulfilled."[23]

Soon afterward, von Lichtenberg departed for urological meetings in the United States, where the German baron was enthusiastically received. About this time, Binz and Rath sent Swick a soluble, relatively nontoxic compound (Uroselectan) that was excreted in a high concentration in the urine. After several consecutive successes on patients, Swick (July, 1929) cabled the momentous news to his benefactor, Libman, with the request that von Lichtenberg be informed. Meanwhile, work continued, von Lichtenberg returned, and a presentation at the 1929 meeting in Munich of the German Urologic Society was planned.[30]

At this point, controversy and confusion come to the fore. According to Victor Marshall,[30] von Lichtenberg felt that he should be the principal author, since he was an internationally renowned urologist and director of the institution where the work had been performed. He thought that Swick should be relegated to a minor role in the presentation. However, due to the efforts of Lichtwitz, Swick's earlier mentor, a compromise was reached. The first presentation (1929), given y Swick alone, concerned the developmental work done on animals and humans, mostly in Hamburg. The second presentation on clinical applications was offered by von Lichtenberg and Swick.[33] Binz and Rath were credited as the actual makers of the compounds.

Swick was soon ushered into the background. In 1930, von Lichtenberg gave the first American lecture on intravenous pyelography. Referring to Swick just once: "Lichtwitz's assistant, Swick, from this standpoint, continued the work in my clinic under my direction." Although von Lichtenberg took most of the credit, it appears that his role was clearly secondary, providing Swick with the facilities to expand his continuing studies. Nevertheless, for the next 35 years, Swick did not get the recognition he deserved, even in his own country. Finally, after careful investigations by Victor Marshall of the Urology Section of the New York Academy of Medicine, Swick was awarded the distinguished Valentine Medal following introductory remarks referring to the many unkind years of headache and oblivion he had suffered.[39]

In association with Victor Wallingford, a chemist at Mallinckrodt, Swick succeeded in attaching iodine to a natural metabolite, hippuric acid, to produce Hippuran. Although this agent produced some systemic side effects, it was the forerunner of a valuable class of contrast agents including Urokon and the three major currently used hypertonic iodinated contrast media: Hypaque, Renografin, and Conray. In addition, Hippuran labelled with radioactive iodine played a major role in evaluating renal tubular function and effective renal plasma flow.

In 1929, Binz introduced Uroselectan B (Neo-Iopax), which was much less toxic than Uroselectan (Iopax). Three years later, Per-Abrodil (Diodrast) was produced. Over the next 20 years, Neo-iopax and Diodrast were the contrast agents used almost exclusively for excretory urography in the United States.

These iodides of the pyridine nucleus also proved excellent for retrograde pyelography. They produced no systemic toxicity or local irritation to the uroepithelium or renal parenchyma. These agents were miscible with urine; did not precipitate when mixed with urine, blood, or pus; and were of high viscosity, low capillarity, and high radiopacity.[2]

For more than 60 years, excretory urography has been used as a rough test of renal function and to demonstrate the renal parenchyma and pyeloureteral system. To estimate renal function, some early investigators determined the amount of iodine in the urine in a given time after injection. Others, observing the effect of diuresis that accompanies the injection of contrast material, correlated the amount of urine excreted after the injection with the specific gravity curve of the urine. A far simpler method of estimating renal function was to analyze the degree of visualization obtained. In general, opacification of good intensity indicated good renal function, although the converse was certainly not true. Poor opacification might be due to a number of technical or pathological findings such as poor preparation of the patient, inadequate dose or extravasation of contrast material, the development of hypotension during the injection, and a broad spectrum of pathological processes, especially an obstructing stone or tumor.[3]

The ability of the excretory urogram to assess morphological change in the renal parenchyma was increased with the appreciation of the "nephrogram" by Wesson and Fullmer in 1932.[34] This intensification of the renal shadow was first noted in radiographs taken many minutes or several hours after the intravenous injection of contrast material. These delayed nephrograms were in patients with acute ureteral obstruction, in whom renal function on the affected side was not yet markedly diminished. Recognition of the diagnostic value of opacification of the renal parenchyma encouraged some investigators to artificially obstruct the ureters with bougies to produce nephrograms,[35] but the many practical disadvantages of such a procedure soon led to its abandonment. It was not until organic compounds of high iodine concentration and low toxicity were developed that practical methods of visualizing the renal parenchyma became available. Steinberg and Robb (1938), during the course of their early studies on angiocardiography, noted that the rapid intravenous injection of a high concentration of iodinated contrast produced excellent visualization of the renal parenchyma.[36] However, it was not until more than a decade later (1950) that the first reports on intravenous nephrography appeared.[37,38]

Even with improved contrast media and excretory urography techniques, the diagnostic evaluation of renal masses continued to be performed primarily by urologists, who used retrograde pyelography to demonstrate changes in the collecting system rather than urographic alterations in the renal parenchyma and renal contour.[39] David Davis, a urologist, wrote in 1950 that retrograde pyelography was necessary to definitely exclude a renal tumor. "The intravenous urogram in practically every case represents a complete loss of time and money, and in my opinion may well be entirely abandoned as a step in the diagnostic investigation of renal tumors."[40]

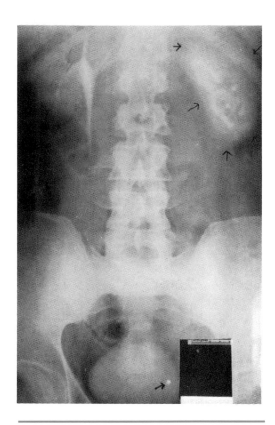

Obstructive nephrogram (1932). "After the intravenous injection of contrast material, the right kidney and ureter were normal. A stone 0.6 cm in diameter was seen in the lower left ureter (*arrows*). Note that the shadow of the left kidney is denser than that on the right, indicating that apparently none of the contrast material has been excreted on that side."[34]

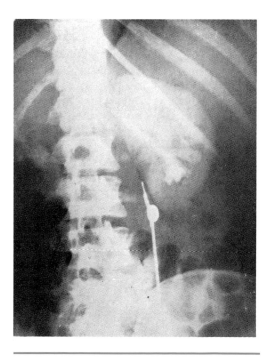

Obstruction of the ureter with a bougie to produce a good nephrogram of the left kidney (1947).[35]

313

NEPHROTOMOGRAPHY

As John Evans[41] and co-workers observed in 1954,

> Despite good opacification of functioning renal parenchyma by the intravenous technique, the clarity of the renal mass is compromised by the superimposition of intestinal contents and gas. Furthermore, small renal lesions imbedded in the substance of the kidney might easily be missed on plain nephrography because of being enveloped by functioning parenchyma. These difficulties are not of major importance if the procedure is to be used mainly as a test of differential renal function. However, if, as it would seem to us, the most important contribution of the method permits recognition of areas of nonfunctioning or malfunctioning renal parenchyma as occurs in cysts and neoplasms, then any impediment to complete delineation of the renal parenchyma would be of paramount importance. A technique which eliminates the adulteration of the nephrogram by extraneous abdominal contents and in addition visualizes the midcoronal plane of the kidney should then permit precise study of renal morphology. Body section roentgenography combined with intravenous nephrography we feel accomplishes this aim. This conjoint technique we have called "nephrotomography."

They noted that the possibility of nephrotomography was recognized in 1942 by Eugene Pendergrass,[42] who observed that "body section roentgenograms of the kidneys after the injection of a contrast medium may reveal changes that cannot be seen in the conventional examination."

Using a 12-gauge angiocardiographic needle inserted into an antecubital vein, Evans and associates rapidly injected 50 cc of Urokon after determining the precise time for obtaining the exposure by means of the arm-to-tongue Decholin circulation time. Good nephrotomograms were obtained in 15 of their 20 cases. Three years later, Evans reported a 93% adequate nephrogram rate using 90% Hypaque. Of major importance, this technique was reported to be 95% accurate in differentiating between renal cysts and neoplasms.[43]

Unfortunately, as Schenker and co-workers[44] observed, nephrotomography required "technical skill and experience for optimal results. Placement of a 12-gauge needle is frequently difficult and surgical exposure of a vein is often a necessity. Precise timing and rapid exposures are prerequisites for success. Repeat injection is often necessary and the

Nephrotomography (1954). *Left*, Retrograde pyelogram in a 54-year-old male with hypertension suggests the presence of a mass (cyst or neoplasm) in the upper pole of the right kidney. *Middle*, Nephrogram shows opacification of both kidneys, but the right kidney is obscured by overlying bowel. *Right*, Nephrotomogram demonstrates a clear cut, rounded radiolucency in the upper pole of the right kidney representing a large cyst.[39]

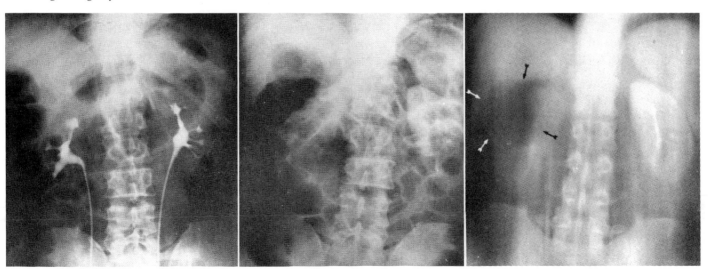

procedure, in most cases, demands an hour or more of the radiologist's time." Citing a report indicating that a nephrogram could be produced using a 2 minute injection through a 21-gauge needle,[45] Schenker and associates (1965) infused large volumes of dilute contrast material intravenously to produce striking pyelograms that lasted up to 45 minutes after infusion and combined this drip infusion technique with tomography to produce superb results.

RETROPERITONEAL AIR INSTILLATION

Retroperitoneal masses, especially involving the kidney and adrenal gland, can be brought into relief by the injection of air, oxygen, or carbon dioxide into this area. In 1902, Kelling of Dresden was the first to introduce large quantities of gas into the peritoneal cavity in an attempt to view the organs by means of the direct introduction of a cystoscope into the abdominal cavity.[46] He performed this "coelioscopy" several times without damage, but apparently never thought of radiographically examining the abdominal cavity after the insufflation of air. Twelve years later (1914), Rautenberg first described the radiographic findings in artificial pneumoperitoneum.[47] Using this technique, he "succeeded in gaining unsuspected views into the unopened peritoneal cavity, in determining adhesions and in studying all the abdominal organs in both healthy and diseased conditions with the help of x-rays."[48] Rautenberg stated that by using this nondangerous and simple method, the "representation of kidney tumors, kidney swellings, concretions and also of diminution of the kidneys is so far superior to previous results of radiological examination that this method of examination deserves general acceptance."[47]

In 1921, Rosenstein[48] and Carelli and Sordelli[49] independently published their accounts of the injection of air, oxygen, or carbon dioxide into the retroperitoneal perirenal space as a means for demonstrating the ipsilateral kidney and adrenal gland. To perform this "pneumoretroperitoneography," Rosenstein typically injected 500 cc to 1000 cc of oxygen through each flank. "In comparison with pneumoperitoneum, this process has exceptional advantages even if its effective area is more limited. It is absolutely safe, since no incidental injuries can occur . . . Finally, the technique and apparatus are so simple that anyone who is

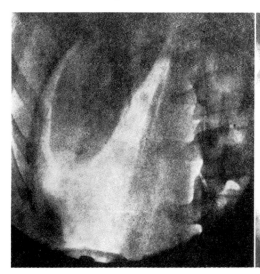 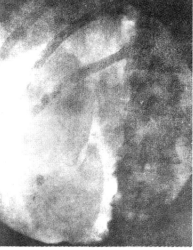

Retroperitoneal air insufflation (1921). "*Left,* Normally positioned right kidney. The uncatheterized ureter is clearly recognizable (from the kidney hilus, crossing diagonally toward the junction below the psoas muscle and the transverse process of the third lumbar vertebra). *Right,* Enlarged floating kidney, which has moved downward and turned (the lower kidney pole has approached the spinal column)."[46]

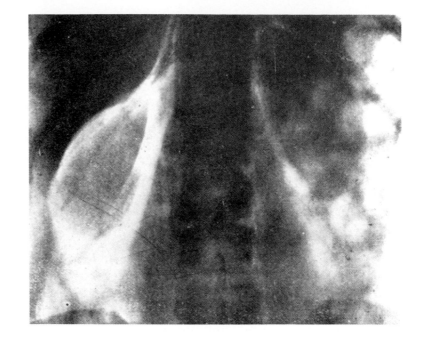

Pneumoretroperitoneography (1948). The contours of both kidneys and the psoas muscles are well seen. Note the visualization of the inferior border of the liver and its anatomical relation to the right kidney.[49]

aseptically trained can handle it."[48] Advantages of this technique included: "(1) in cases of doubt, whether both kidneys or only one is present; (2) determination of the size relationship of both kidneys; (3) clearer definition of renal stones; (4) demonstration of changes in shape and position of the kidney; and (5) demonstration of renal and perirenal tumors." Unfortunately, bilateral visualization required separate injections for both sides.

George Cahill (1935) first described the use of perirenal insufflation of air to outline suspected adrenal masses.[50] In 1948, Ruiz-Rivas described a new technique for pneumoretroperitoneography in which he injected oxygen presacrally or retrorectally.[51] Although he considered this technique safer than direct injection into the flank, deaths from gas embolism were reported with both methods.

With the availability of a successful technique for excretory urography, pneumoretroperitoneography disappeared from clinical practice (although it still was occasionally performed for evaluating enlargement or masses of the adrenal glands before cross-sectional imaging).

CYSTOURETHROGRAPHY

Cystourethrography in the male was first described by John H. Cunningham (1910), a well-known Boston urologist.[52] Cunningham introduced a silver colloid solution into his patient's urethra and produced a series of radiographs that clearly showed the presence of a stricture. In the introduction to his paper, Cunningham wrote, "It is not desired to convey the idea that this form of diagnosis is of any real practical importance, but rather to be an additional means of obtaining a clear interpretation of the character of the obstruction, whether single or multiple, annular or tortuous, etc." For more than 20 years, readers apparently took Cunningham's advice seriously. Although bismuth, barium, and Lipiodol were all tried as contrast materials, cystourethrography was rarely performed until it was revived and popularized by Rubin Flocks (1933), who injected a semisolid contrast medium into the urethra and filled the bladder with gas.[53] He demonstrated the value of this technique for defining urethral strictures and diverticula, as well as stenosis of the vesical neck.

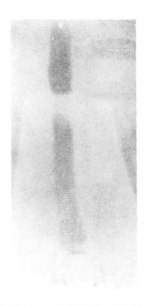

Urethral stricture (1910). Annular stricture at penoscrotal angle. "Note lightness of shadow at point of stricture dependent on small amount of fluid in the constricted area."[50]

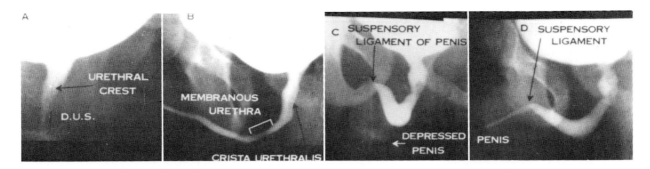

In 1945, Edling stressed the value of voiding cystourethrography (VCU), using the micturition method and performed under fluoroscopic control to adequately visualize the bladder and urethra in the adult male.[54] The value of this procedure in children was emphasized in monographs by Kjellberg, et al[55] and Burrows, et al,[56] as well as in a series of articles by Shopfner in the 1960s that popularized the technique of micturition cystourethrography.[57] Cinecystourethrography in children was popular in the late 1950s and early 1960s, but the cine film image was not as sharp as spot films and the dose to the gonads was much higher. Since that time, the use of 70-mm and later 105-mm cameras has replaced the spot film technique, greatly reducing the gonadal radiation dose while preserving excellent visualization of the bladder and urethra.[27]

In women, voiding cystourethrography is difficult because of the short urethra. A more valuable technique was the placement of a fine meshed chain in the female urethra followed by the exposure of radiographs in frontal and lateral positions to show the course and degree of angulation, especially in patients with stress incontinence.

RADIOGRAPHY OF THE SEMINAL VESICLES

Radiography of the seminal vesicles was first described by William T. Belfield in 1913: "Through an incision in the vas deferens just above the testicle (vasotomy), a solution of collargol or other metallic compound can be injected into vas and vesicle, and skiagrams made of these."[59] This technique was recommended for differentiating distended seminal vesicles from prostatic enlargement. Belfield warned that "if there be no occlusion of the seminal duct, collargol is passed with the urine for days following the injection, and the emitted semen is black—the latter phenomenon, inspired in one patient to fear that this future children might be Ethiopians."

INTERVENTIONAL PROCEDURES

In 1934, Dean performed the first percutaneous puncture of a renal mass and showed that it was possible to differentiate between cysts and renal cell carcinoma.[60] Dean also noticed that simple renal cysts often disappeared if the fluid was completely evacuated. Although the procedure was well tolerated with no substantial complications, renal puncture remained an uncommon practice until the method was revived a decade later by Lindblom of Sweden. Initially unaware of Dean's earlier work, Lindblom (1946) described a method of percutaneous puncture of the kidney using

Voiding cystourethrography in children (1970).[55]

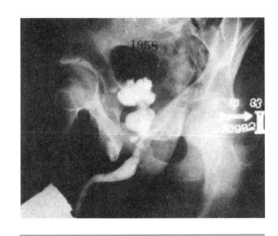

Cystourethrography (1933). Young man with a traumatic stricture of the urethra and a suprapubic cystostomy.[51]

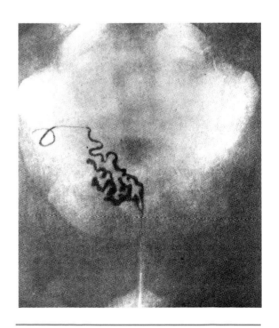

Radiography of the seminal ducts (1910). "Injection of a 15% Collargol solution through a vasotomy in a patient with chronic vesiculitis demonstrates tortuous vas deferens, seminal vesicle, and deflected ejaculatory duct."[59]

317

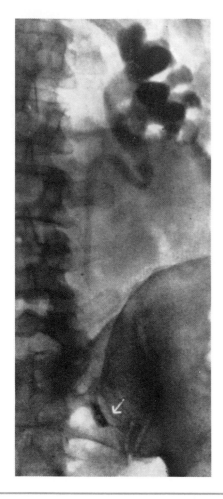

Antegrade pyelography (1954). After direct puncture of the left renal pelvis, contrast material demonstrates dilatation of the pelvis and upper part of the ureter. There is complete obstruction of the ureter at the pelvic inlet (*arrow*).[60]

fluoroscopic localization that permitted puncture of small lesions. After renal puncture and aspiration, contrast material injected through the needle was noted to diffuse into characteristic patterns permitting the differential diagnosis of renal cysts and tumors.[61] Extending this technique to the diagnosis of hydronephrosis, in 1954, Wickbom[62] and Weens and Florence[57] independently reported the technique of antegrade pyelography, in which contrast material was injected directly into the renal pelvis after percutaneous puncture. As Weens and Florence noted,[63]

> In the large majority of cases hydronephrosis may be adequately demonstrated by excretory or retrograde pyelography. In practice, however, circumstances occur in which a definitive diagnosis with conventional urographic procedures is not possible. This is usually the case if complete obstruction of the ureter is present preventing visualization of kidney, pelvis and calyces on radiologic examination.

In their patients, renal puncture permitted demonstration of the level of ureteral obstruction in patients with urethral or ureteral strictures in whom retrograde studies could not be performed.

In the next year (1955), Goodwin and associates[64] described the new therapeutic procedure of trocar nephrostomy, "performed by percutaneous lumbar tap of the renal pelvis with a large needle, followed by insertion of a plastic tubing for temporary urinary drainage in selected cases of hydronephrosis." They considered this procedure to be of greatest use

> in cases of large hydronephroses when a temporary diversion of the urinary stream, without open operation, is required before definitive surgery at a later date. The temporary diversion may be for the purpose of doing plastic work on the lower urinary tract, or it may be to allow return of function while working on the opposite side. It may also be used as a test of function in cases of hydronephrosis when it is uncertain whether or not the kidney is worth saving.

Percutaneous trocar nephrostomy (1955). "*Left*, Method and landmarks. The optimum site of puncture usually is about 5 finger breadths lateral to the midline and at a level where a thirteenth rib would be. *Right*, Cross-sectional anatomy of the left renal area (after Brodel). About 2 inches of tubing is allowed to coil in the hydronephrotic pelvis."[62]

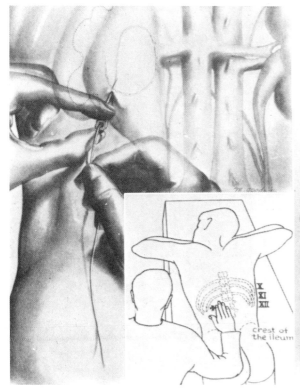

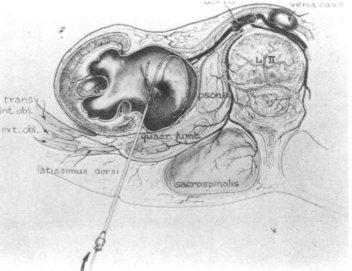

Ten years later (1965), Bartley and co-workers[65] introduced permanent percutaneous drainage of the renal pelvis by a modified Seldinger technique that could be carried out under local anesthesia and was especially valuable in patients with uremia "so advanced as to entail an appreciable operative risk." Nevertheless, urologists continued to perform open nephrostomies because of problems with the percutaneous technique. The arterial tubes inserted into the collecting system tended to slip out or become occluded. In 1973, Almgard and Fernstrom[66] introduced a self-retaining balloon catheter into the pelvis following a dilatation procedure. They concluded that percutaneous nephrostomy was so safe and successful that "operative nephrostomy should be resorted to only if the new method be unsuccessful."

Since that time, percutaneous nephrostomy became a routine procedure in many hospitals and open nephrostomies were performed much less frequently. In 1975, Fowler and associates[67] introduced the technique into the United States in a paper that rekindled the awareness of the vast possibilities inherent in percutaneous manipulation of the urinary tract.[68] A major new procedure was percutaneous pyelolithotomy, the extraction of kidney stones without an open operation, which was first reported in 1976 by Fernstrom and Johansson.[8] Initially, only small stones could be removed in this way, since they would have to pass through the relatively small track. With the development of flexible nephroscopes and a variety of snares and baskets, larger stones could be removed, and this procedure became extremely popular.

In 1980, after extensive testing in vitro and in animal models, the management of upper urinary tract stones was dramatically changed by the development of extracorporeal shock wave lithotripsy (ESWL). Non-invasive disintegration of human urinary stones by means of extracorporeally induced shock waves was based on the following principles: generating energy outside the body (shock wave), focusing the energy to a point distant from the energy source, coupling the energy into the body without damaging bodily tissues, and localizing and positioning the stone.[9] ESWL has become the treatment of choice for the majority of upper urinary tract calculi, and at the most experienced stone centers more than 95% of all patients are treated without resorting to open surgery. Although percutaneous stone removal has been supplanted by ESWL, ureteral strictures are frequently dilated using percutaneous techniques, and pyeloscopy has become an important procedure for the diagnosis of kidney disease.[68]

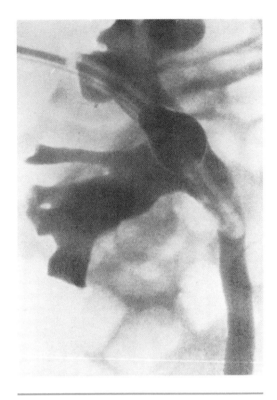

Balloon catheter for percutaneous nephrostomy (1974).[64]

Percutaneous pyelolithotomy (1976). *Left,* The stone before nephrostomy. *Middle,* The position of the nephrostomy tube and the stone. *Right,* Insertion of a narrow pair of stone-grasping forceps into the renal pelvis through the nephrostomy channel. Under fluoroscopic guidance, the stone could be grasped and extracted without any difficulty.[67]

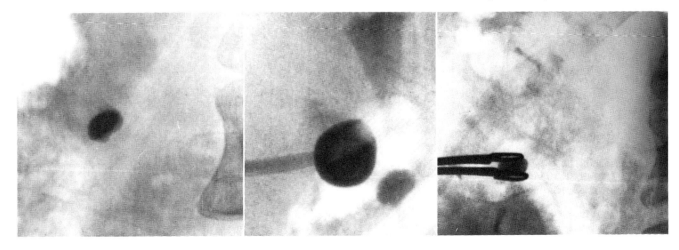

NEWER IMAGING MODALITIES

Cross-sectional techniques have become an essential component of the radiographic evaluation of urological disorders. In most institutions, ultrasound has become the most commonly performed examination for evaluating the urinary tract. Because an ultrasound study does not require contrast material and is not affected by renal function, this modality is routinely used in patients with renal failure to evaluate the kidneys and exclude hydronephrosis. Clots can be identified in the inferior vena cava or renal veins, and Doppler studies can assess renal blood flow. Ultrasound can detect renal and inflammatory masses, discriminate between fluid-filled cysts and solid tumors, and evaluate complications in renal transplant patients. The speed of ultrasound and the portability of the equipment make it an ideal guide for needle aspiration procedures either at the bedside or in the main radiology department.

Computed tomography (CT) combines an unsurpassed definition of the anatomy of the urinary tract and surrounding structures with the ability of contrast studies to differentiate normal functioning renal parenchyma from areas of infarction, inflammation, or tumor. Dynamic scanning can demonstrate vascular anatomy and lesion vascularity so well that angiography is now rarely needed to diagnose most surgical lesions in

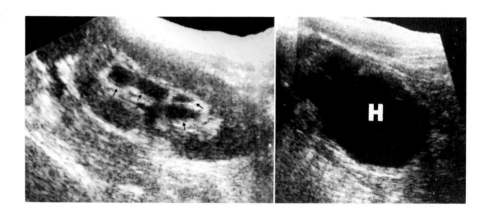

Ultrasound of hydronephrosis. *Left,* In a patient with moderately severe disease, the dilated calyces and pelvis appear as echo-free sacs (*arrows*) separated by septa of compressed tissue and vessels. *Right,* In a patient with severe hydronephrosis, the intervening septa have disappeared, leaving a large fluid-filled sac (*H*) with no evidence of internal structure and no normal parenchyma apparent at its margins.

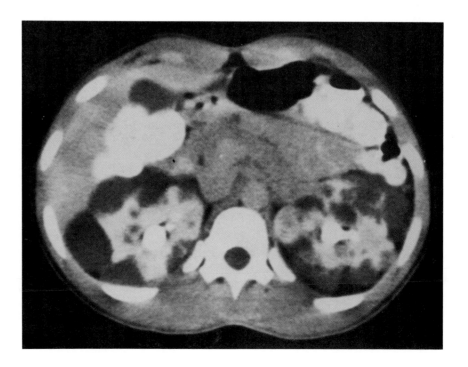

CT of multiple renal hamartomas. There are innumerable low-attenuation masses in both kidneys of this patient with tuberous sclerosis.

320

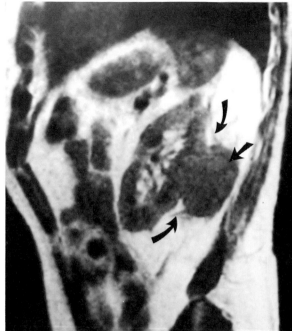 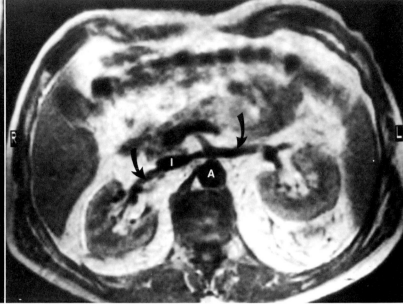

the kidney. CT is the modality of choice for evaluating retroperitoneal and pelvic trauma, as well as for staging malignancies of the urinary tract and detecting recurrences.

The precise role of magnetic resonance (MR) imaging in the assessment of urinary tract disorders is still unclear. The direct multiplanar imaging capability and absence of any need for intravenous contrast material to show vessel patency permits accurate preoperative staging of renal neoplasms. The extent of tumor, renal vein and caval thrombosis, and perihilar lymphadenopathy can be well demonstrated. A current problem is the lack of satisfactory tissue specificity in the differential diagnosis of solid renal masses and renal parenchymal disease, but this may be overcome by developments in pulse sequences and in vivo spectroscopy.

MR imaging of renal cell carcinoma. *Left*, Sagittal T1-weighted image shows the large tumor (*straight arrow*) arising from the posterior aspect of the kidney and displacing Gerota's fascia outward (*curved arrows*). *Right*, Transverse image at the level of the renal veins (*arrows*) and inferior vena cava (*I*) shows normal signal from flowing blood with no evidence of tumor thrombus.

References

1. Nesbitt RM: Radiology and its contribution to urology. AJR 75:995-996, 1956.
2. Maluf NSR: Role of roentgenology in the development of urology. AJR 75:847-854, 1956.
3. Tondreau RL: Roentgenography of the urinary tract. In Bruwer AJ (ed): Classic descriptions in diagnostic roentgenology. Springfield, Ill, Charles C Thomas, 1964.
4. MacIntyre J: Roentgen rays: Photography of renal calculus. Description of an adjustable modification in the focus tube. Lancet 2:118, 1896.
5. Cunningham JJ and Friedland GW: Early American uroradiology (1896-1933). Urolog Survey 22:226-228, 1972.
6. Leonard C: Roentgen ray diagnosis of renal calculus. Phila Med J 3:886-889, 1899.
7. Tuffier T: Sonde urétérale opaque. In Duplay et Reclus: Traite de chirurgie. Paris, Masson, 1897-1899, pp 412-413.

8. Fernstrom I and Johansson B: Percutaneous pyelolithotomy: A new extraction technique. Scand J Urol Nephrol 10:257-259, 1976.
9. Chaussy CG and Fuchs GJ: Extracorporeal shock wave lithotripsy for the treatment of urinary calculi. In Pollack HM (ed): Clinical urography. Philadelphia, WB Saunders, 1990.
10. Williams FH: The roentgen rays in medicine and surgery. New York, MacMillan, 1901.
11. Walsh D: The röntgen rays in medical work. New York, Wood, 1902.
12. Schmidt LE and Kolischer G: Radiography of catheterized ureters and kidneys. Mschr Urol 6:427-431, 1901.
13. Loewenhardt F: Determination of the position of the ureter before operation. Jahresbericht d. Schlesische Gesellsch f. Vaterl Kultur 79:136-137, 1901.
14. Von Illyes G: Ureteral catheterization and roentgenography. Orvosi Hetilap 45:659-662, 1901.

15. Klose B: Radiography of a case of complete ureter duplication diagnosed by cystoscopy. Deutsch Z Chir 72:613-617, 1904.
16. Fenwick EH: The value of the use of a shadowgraph ureteric bougie in the precise surgery of renal calculus. Brit Med J 1:1325-1327, 1905.
17. Wittek A: Technique for roentgen photography (lumbar spine, bladder stones). Fortschr Roentgenstr 7:26-27, 1903.
18. Wulff P: Applicability of x-rays in the diagnosis of bladder deformities. Fortschr Roentgenstr 8:193-194, 1904.
19. Voelcker F and von Lichtenberg A: Pyelography (roentgenography of the renal pelvis after filling with Kollargol). Muenchen Med Wschr 53:105-106, 1906.
20. Braasch WF: Deformities of the renal pelvis. Ann Surg 51:534-540, 1910.
21. Braasch WF: Pyelography. Philadelphia, WB Saunders, 1915.

22. Uhle AA, Pfahler GE, MacKinney WH, and Miller AG: Combined cystographic and rontgenographic examination of the kidneys and ureter. Ann Surg 51:546-551, 1910.

23. Swick M: Radiographic media in urology. Surg Clin North Am 58:977-994, 1978.

24. Baker HW: An improved method for measuring the capacity of the renal pelvis. Surg Gynec Obstet 10:536, 1910.

25. Burns JE: Thorium: A new agent for pyelography. JAMA 64:2126-2127, 1915.

26. Cameron DF: Aqueous solutions of potassium and sodium iodide as opaque mediums in roentgenography. Preliminary report. JAMA 70:754-755, 1918.

27. Hertz M: Cystourethrography. In Pollack HM (ed): Clinical urography. Philadelphia, WB Saunders, 1990.

28. Osborne ED, Sutherland CG, Scholl AJ, and Rowntree LG: Roentgenography of urinary tract during excretion of sodium iodid. JAMA 80:368-373, 1923.

29. Evans JA: Roentgenography of the urinary tract. JAMA 250:2854-2855, 1983.

30. Marshall VF: The controversial history of excretory urography. In Witten DM, Myers GH, and Utz DC (eds): Clinical urography. Philadelphia, WB Saunders, 1977.

31. Leonard CE: The results of the roentgen method in the diagnosis of renal calculus. Trans Amer Roentgen Ray Soc 56-68, 1904.

32. Swick M: Visualization of the kidney and urinary tract on roentgenograms by means of intravenous administration of a new contrast medium: uroselectan. Klin Wschr 8:2087-2089, 1929.

33. Von Lichtenberg A and Swick M: Clinical test of uroselectan. Klin Wschr 8:2089-2091, 1929.

34. Wesson MB and Fullmer CC: Influence of ureteral stones on intravenous urograms. AJR 28:27-33, 1932.

35. Weens HS and Florence TJ: Nephrography. AJR 57:338-341, 1947.

36. Steinberg I and Robb GP: Mediastinal and hilar angiography in pulmonary disease. Am Rev Tuberc 38:557-569, 1938.

37. Vesey J, Dotter CT, and Steinberg I: Nephrography: Simplified technic. Radiology 55:827-833, 1950.

38. Weens HS, Olnick HM, James DF, and Warren JV: Intravenous nephrography method of roentgen visualization of kidney. AJR 65:411-414, 1951.

39. Elkin M: Stages in the growth of uroradiology. Radiology 175:297-306, 1990.

40. Davis DM: Diagnosis of renal tumors in the adult. Radiology 54:639-645, 1950.

41. Evans JA, Dubilier W, and Monteith JC: Nephrotomography. A preliminary report. AJR 71:213-223, 1954.

42. Pendergrass EP: Excretory urography as a test of urinary tract function. Radiology 40:223-246, 1943.

43. Evans JA: Nephrotomography in the investigation of renal masses. Radiology 69:684-689, 1957.

44. Schencker B, Marcure RW, and Moody DC: Simplified nephrotomography: The drip infusion technique. AJR 95:283-290, 1965.

45. Lowman RM and DeLuca JT: Nephrotomography: Its role in routine urographic studies. J Urol 83:308-312, 1960.

46. Kelling G: Über Osophagoskopie, Gastroskopie, und Kolioscopie. Muenchen Med Wschr 49:21-27, 1902.

47. Rautenberg E: Rontgenphotographie der Leber, der Milz und des Zwerchfells. Deutsch Med Wschr 40:1205-1208, 1914.

48. Rosenstein P: "Pneumoradiology of kidney position." A new technique for the radiological representation of the kidneys and neighboring organs (suprarenal gland, spleen, liver). Z Urol 15:447-458, 1921.

49. Carelli HH and Sordelli E: A new procedure for examining the kidney. Rev Assoc Med Argent 34:18-19, 1921.

50. Cahill GF: Air injections to demonstrate the adrenals by x-ray. J Urol 34:238-243, 1935.

51. Ruiz-Rivas M: Diagnostic radiology: pneumokidney—original technique. Arch Espan Urol 4:228-233, 1948.

52. Cunningham JH: The diagnosis of stricture of the urethra by the roentgen rays. Trans Amer Assoc Genitour Surg 5:369-371, 1910.

53. Flocks RH: The roentgen visualization of the posterior urethra. J Urol 30:711-736, 1933.

54. Edling NPG: Urethrocystography in the male with special regard to micturition. Acta Radiol (Suppl) 58:56-96, 1945.

55. Kjellberg SR, Ericsson NO, and Rudhe U: The lower urinary tract in childhood. Chicago, Year Book, 1957.

56. Burrows EH: Urethral lesions in infancy and childhood: Studied by micturition cystourethrography. Springfield, Ill, Charles C Thomas, 1965.

57. Shopfner CE: Cystourethrography: Methodology, normal anatomy, and pathology. J Urol 103:92-103, 1970.

58. Beck C: Roentgen-ray diagnosis and therapy. New York, Appleton, 1904.

59. Belfield WT: Skiagraphy of the seminal ducts. JAMA 60:800-801, 1913.

60. Dean AL: Treatment of solitary cyst of kidney by aspiration. Trans Am Assoc Genitourin Surg 32:91-95, 1939.

61. Lindblom K: Percutaneous puncture of renal cysts and tumors. Acta Radiol 27:66-72, 1946.

62. Wickbom I: Pyelography after direct puncture of the renal pelvis. Acta Radiol 41:505-512, 1954.

63. Weens HS and Florence TJ: The diagnosis of hydronephrosis by percutaneous renal puncture. J Urol 72:589-595, 1954.

64. Goodwin WE, Casey WC, and Woolf W: Percutaneous trocar (needle) nephrostomy in hydronephrosis. JAMA 157:891-894, 1955.

65. Bartley O, Chidekel N, and Radberg C: Percutaneous drainage of the renal pelvis for uraemia due to obstructed urinary outflow. Acta Chir Scand 129:443-446, 1965.

66. Almgard LE and Fernstrom I: Percutaneous nephropyelostomy. Acta Radiol 15:288-294, 1974.

67. Fowler JE, Meares EE, and Goldin AR: Percutaneous nephrostomy: techniques, indications, and results. Urology 6:428-434, 1975.

68. Fernstrom I: Preface: Interventional procedures. In Pollack HM (ed): Clinical urography. Philadelphia, WB Saunders, 1990.

CHAPTER 18

Neuroradiology

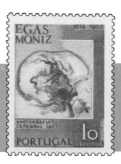
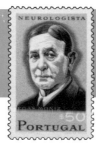
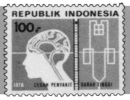
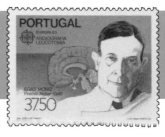

The story of neuroradiology begins with a celebrated failure. On February 5, 1896, Thomas A. Edison received a cable from William Randolph Hearst, the renowned publisher of the *New York Journal*. The cable read as follows[1]:

> WILL YOU AS AN ESPECIAL FAVOR TO THE JOURNAL
> UNDERTAKE TO MAKE CATHODOGRAPH OF HUMAN
> BRAIN KINDLY TELEGRAPH ANSWER AT OUR EXPENSE

As expected, Edison accepted the challenge. Three days later, it was reported that Edison would attempt that morning "to demonstrate the penetrating powers of the new light by an experiment in photographing a man's brain."[2] To prepare for this photographic experiment, Edison improved on the Crookes tube by making a tube out of a regular Edison incandescent light bulb. Later, he made longer, cylindrical tubes with the idea of placing these side-by-side so that the x-ray emitting electrodes of the set would form a surface that would be large enough in combination to emit parallel rays to cover the entire surface of the head.[3] Unfortunately, these tubes were unable to maintain the required degree of vacuum. As Edison's technical troubles mounted, there was grumbling among the army of reporters camped around his laboratory. Finally, on February 14, Edison gave up. In addition to his technical problems (breakage of tubes and difficulties in obtaining the appropriate vacuum), he placed part of the blame on the "insuperable obstacles" imposed by the skull itself.[4]

The initial value of x-rays in neurological diagnosis was the detection and localization of foreign bodies and fractures. In the United States, the first to use x-rays for the diagnosis of a patient with neurological disability (November 6, 1896) was Harvey Cushing, the father of modern neurological surgery.[5] Cushing was a house officer at Massachusetts General Hospital in Boston at the time of Roentgen's discovery. He arranged for an

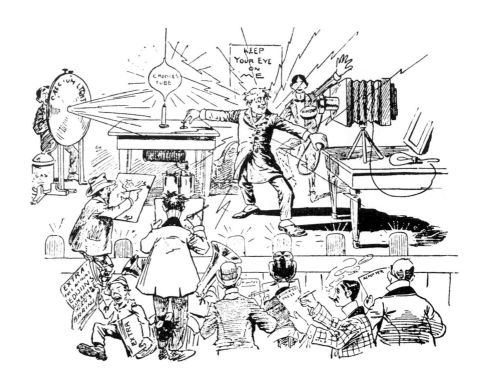

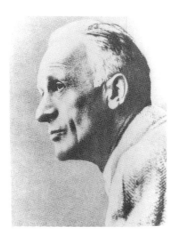

Harvey Cushing (1869-1939).

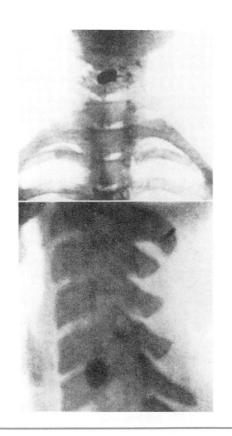

Top, AP. *Bottom*, Lateral projections of the cervical spine made by Harvey Cushing (November, 1896) revealing a bullet in the body of C6.[6]

x-ray tube to be acquired, but apparently received little support from his medical colleagues and was said to have taken the tube with him when he moved to the Johns Hopkins Hospital in Baltimore. Cushing's first radiographs were views of the cervical spine in a patient who was shot in the neck and subsequently developed the Brown-Séquard syndrome. The quality of the radiographs was superb, although the exposure time averaged 35 minutes and, as Cushing admitted, several plates of substantially poor quality were made "before plates were secured which were sufficiently good for reproduction."[6] Even in Baltimore, however, the application of x-rays to neurological problems was not an overwhelming success. As Cushing noted almost 30 years later,[7]

> I spent many weary hours for the next year or two in an improvised darkroom off from the old amphitheatre at the Johns Hopkins Hospital developing roentgen-ray plates in which no one at the time took any very great interest. Certainly no one of us could have had any possible conception of the increasingly important role the roentgen-ray was to play in clinical diagnosis and treatment.

For the next 20 years, neuroradiology was confined to plain film studies of the skull. The major figure of this era was Arthur Schüller, a Viennese physician who coined the term *Neuro-Roentgenologie* and has been called the "father of neuroradiology."[8] In 1912, Schüller published the first textbook on radiology of the skull,[9] which was translated into English in 1918 by an American, F. F. Stocking.[10] The foreword to the American translation was written by Ernest Sachs, a distinguished neurosurgeon, who stated "Since the roentgenologic technique has made such rapid strides in the past few years, it has become necessary to make a roentgenologic study of every case that may possibly have an intracranial lesion."[10] In his book, Schüller pointed out the value of observing the calcified pineal gland and noting how it became displaced by hemispheric tumors. Schüller also differentiated many types of normal and pathological intracranial calcifications. He wrote extensively on the changes in the sella turcica and stressed the difficulty of distinguishing intrasellar from extrasellar tumors by radiological means. Schüller's name is linked with Hand and Christian in the condition known as Hand-Schüller-Christian disease. He also was the first to describe osteoporosis

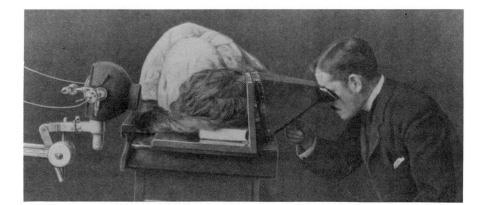

circumscripta and showed that it was a manifestation of Paget's disease. Schüller's more than 300 publications covered not only radiology of the skull but also various aspects of neurology, surgery, and psychiatry.[8]

The first case in which "a brain tumor has been clearly localized by means of the x-rays in the living subject" was reported by Church in 1899 on the basis of calcification within the tumor (a highly vascular glioma of the cerebellum).[14] Three years later, George Pfahler reported two additional cases and predicted that in addition to tumors, "other abnormalities and deficiency in brain tissue itself can be photographed, which will probably be of value in the diagnosis of cysts, softening and hemorrhages."[15,16] However, in virtually all these cases it was probably pure coincidence that some of these lesions were found at operation or postmortem, thanks to the diagnostic ability of astute clinicians rather than to the nebulous shadows on the x-rays.[5] Hematomas and tumors that were not calcified were virtually impossible to demonstrate radiographically since their density is approximately the same as that of normal cerebral tissue. Even Pfahler wrote that "I would never take the responsibility of an operation upon the brain *purely* upon skiagraphic evidence." Rather, the x-ray findings should be used for "confirming or adding to the clinical evidence."

A major advance in plain film radiography was the development of the "Sweet's method" for radiographically locating foreign bodies based on the triangulation of the planes of shadow of the body with the x-ray tube in two different positions. Measurements of the distance of the crossing of these planes from one or more points marked on the skin would indicate

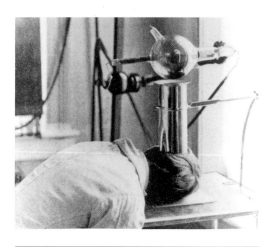

Early radiography of the skull. Note cylindrical cone but no radiation control about the tube.

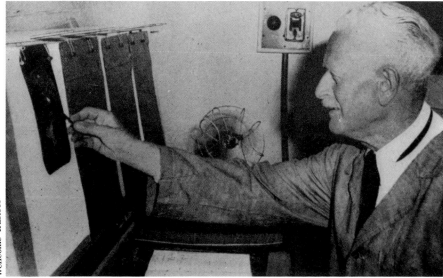

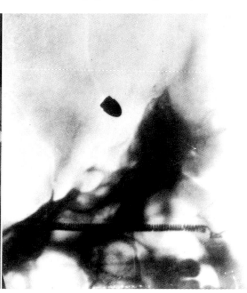

Left, Arthur Schüller (1874-1957).[8] *Right*, Radiograph of a bullet in the base of the brain, thought to be an experimental simulation to determine the required exposure factors for an examination of a young woman shot in the head by her husband (April or May, 1896).[13]

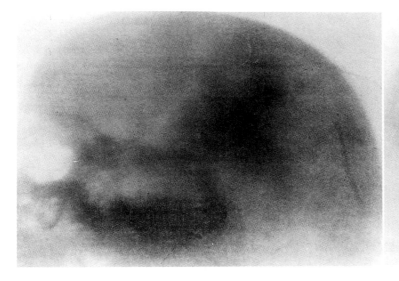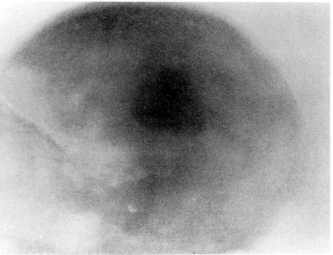

Brain tumor shown on skull radiographs (1902). *Left,* In a living subject, the shadow of the tumor is shown between the frontoparietal suture and the posterior meningeal artery. *Right,* Tumor inserted in the motor area of the unhardened brain of the cadaver.[15]

the precise position of the foreign body. Initially designed to identify the position of pieces of metal in the eyeball, Sweet expanded this procedure to localize foreign substances elsewhere in the head or in other portions of the body.[17]

The use of the pineal shift to localize brain tumors was popularized by Howard Naffziger (1924). He noted that

> When the pineal gland is calcified (in about 50 percent of all skulls), its position gives diagnostic information in cases *with intracranial pressure.* The shift has been found with brain tumors, brain abscess, and certain cases of brain swelling consequent upon a vascular block. A position of the pineal to the right of the mid-sagittal plane indicates a left sided lesion above the tentorium. A position of the pineal to the left of the mid-sagittal plane indicated a right sided lesion above the tentorium. A position of the pineal in the mid-sagittal plane in the presence of intracranial pressure indicates equal pressure on both sides.[18]

VENTRICULOGRAPHY/ENCEPHALOGRAPHY

The major early milestone in the development of neuroradiology was the introduction of ventriculography by Walter Dandy (1918). A protege of Cushing at Johns Hopkins Hospital, Dandy was bitterly disappointed when he was not invited to join Cushing's staff when the Professor returned to Boston. In collaboration with George Heuer, Dandy analyzed 100 consecutive brain tumors seen at Johns Hopkins.[19] They noted that "in only 6% of the cases did the tumor cast a shadow, and in these it was only the calcified areas that were differentiated by the roentgen-rays from the normal cerebral tissues." As Dandy later noted, "Although skull changes are shown by the roentgen-ray in 45% of our cases and are

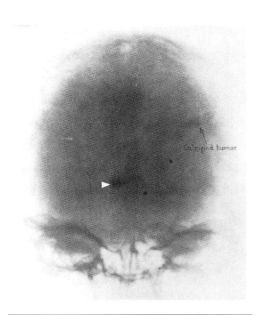

Pineal shift (1924). The calcified pineal (*arrowhead*) is displaced *away* from the side of the calcified tumor.[18]

frequently pathognomonic, on the whole they represent late stages of the disease." Consequently, Dandy[20] decided to test

> the possibility of filling the cerebral ventricles with a medium that will produce a shadow in the roentgenogram. If this could be done, an accurate outline of the cerebral ventricles could be photographed with roentgen-rays, and since most neoplasms either directly or indirectly modify the size or shape of the ventricles, we should then possess an early and accurate aid to the localization of intracranial affections.

Any substance injected into the ventricles, in addition to its ability to serve as a radiographic contrast, "must satisfy two very rigid exactions: (1) it must be absolutely non-irritating and non-toxic; (2) it must be readily absorbed and excreted." Dandy injected into the ventricles of dogs "various solutions and suspensions used in pyelography—thorium, potassium, iodide, collargol, argyrol, bismuth subnitrate and subcarbon-ate, all in various concentrations . . . but always with fatal results." He concluded that "it seems unlikely that any solution of roentgenographic value will be found which is sufficiently harmless to justify its injection into the central nervous system. Suspensions are precluded because they are not absorbed." The only possible solution to the problem was the "substitution of gas for cerebrospinal fluid."[20]

Dandy attributed the idea of using air as a contrast medium to his chief, William Halsted, who had noted the remarkable power of intestinal gases "to perforate bone." As Dandy[20] wrote,

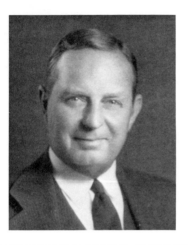

Walter Dandy (1886-1946).

> Striking gas shadows are present in all abdominal and thoracic roentgenograms. The stomach and intestines are often outlined by the contained air, even more sharply than when filled with bismuth. A small collection of gas in the intestines often obliterates the kidney outlines. A perforation of the intestines may be diagnosed by the shadow of the air that has accumulated under the diaphragm. Gas gangrene may be diagnosed by the air blebs . . . in the tissues. Pneumothorax is sharply outlined because the normal lung tissues

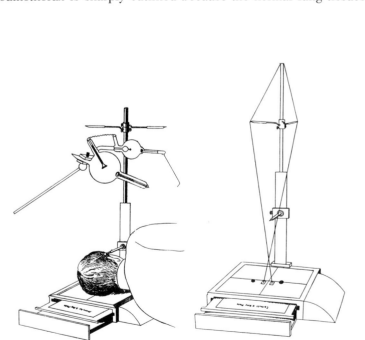

Sweet's method for radiographically locating foreign bodies (1903). "*Left,* Side view of the indicating apparatus, showing the position of the tube and indicator, as well as the receptacle for the photographic plates. *Right,* Planes of shadow, represented by threads, the point of crossing of which indicates the situation of the bullet."[17]

are eliminated. The paranasal sinuses and mastoid air cells show up in a thick skull by virtue of the air, and pathological conditions of the sinuses are evident because inflammatory or tumor tissue replaced the air. From these and many other normal and pathological clinical demonstrations of the roentgenographic properties of air it is but a step to the injection of gas into the cerebral ventricles—pneumoventriculography.

However, it is probable that Dandy was also influenced by an article in which Stewart radiographed a head injury case under the care of Luckett.[21] Initial radiographs demonstrated a fracture in the posterior wall of the frontal sinus. The patient was treated conservatively and discharged from the hospital but returned several weeks later after suffering a relapse. Repeat radiographs showed enormous dilatation of the ventricles by what was probably air or gas. At reoperation, one of the ventricles was tapped and air was released. Stewart noted that "it was subsequently learned that a severe pain in the head, with a free discharge of clear fluid from the nose followed a violent blowing of the nose, the logical deduction being that the patient had established a communication between the nose through the right frontal sinus and anterior lobe of the brain into the right lateral ventricle; that when he blew his nose he also blew up the ventricles of his brain." Perhaps this example of "spontaneous pneumoencephalography" was the inspiration for Dandy's revolutionary technique.

Ventriculography was easiest to perform in children before closure of the fontanels via a puncture through the interosseous defect. After union of the sutures, it was necessary to make a small opening in the bone. Dandy reported that the chief value of ventriculography was in the diagnosis of internal hydrocephalus in children, although he also noted that "tumors in either cerebral hemisphere may dislocate or compress the ventricle and in this way localize the neoplasm," while "tumors growing into the ventricles may show a corresponding defect in the ventricular shadow."

Within a year, Dandy introduced his second revolutionary neuroradiological procedure—encephalography. He had noted that on some ventriculograms gas had escaped into the subarachnoid space and concluded that the best way to outline these spaces would be via the lumbar route. Concerned about the danger of the injected air increasing pressure on the brainstem, he left his needle open to equalize the spinal pressure

Ventricular air following skull fracture (1913). *Left,* On the initial radiograph, two small arrows indicate the fracture of the outer table of the right frontal sinus. *Middle,* Lateral and (*right*) posteroanterior plates made three weeks later show the same fracture and the cerebral ventricles distended with air.[21]

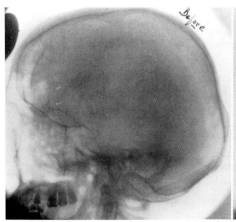
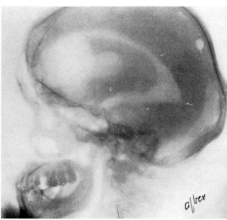
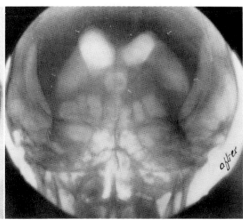

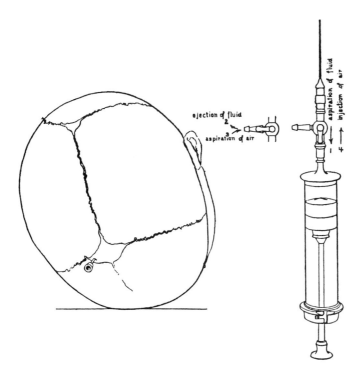

Ventriculography (1918). Diagram showing the oblique position of the head for aspiration of fluid and injection of air. The forehead is resting on the plate. Note the point of entrance of the needle into the anterior fontanel on the dependent side. The figure on the right shows the syringe and two-way valve attachment used for this purpose.[20]

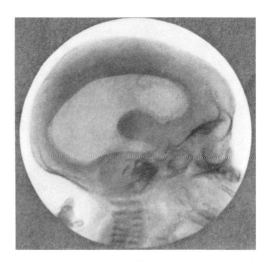

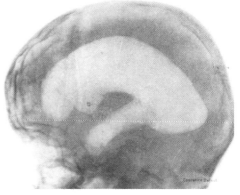

Ventriculography (1918). *Left*, Moderately distended ventricle in a case of communicating hydrocephalus. Note the diffuse posterior bulging of the posterior horn. *Right*, Hydrocephalus in a patient with large head and closed sutures. *III*, Third ventricle.

with that of the outside air. Dandy described how by maintaining the patient in a sitting position after introducing air via a lumbar puncture (after removal of an equivalent amount of cerebrospinal fluid) it was possible to outline the ventricles with air. He noted that this procedure filled all parts of the subarachnoid space and that, "the cisterns appear as large collections of air at the base of the brain; the cerebral sulci as a network of tortuous filaments of air. After an intraspinous injection, provided that the subarachnoid space is intact, the air will always fill the cerebral sulci. But if the cisterns are blocked at any point by a tumor or adhesions, the air will not be able to reach the cerebral sulci."[22] Somewhat over-optimistically, Dandy concluded that by using ventriculography and pneumoencephalography "it is difficult to see how intracranial tumors can escape localization."

Neurosurgeons now possessed two major diagnostic modalities. An excellent analysis of how to make the appropriate choice was offered by Leo M. Davidoff and Cornelius G. Dyke[23]:

> When air is injected directly into the ventricles, it is easily removed in case of untoward reaction later on, by reintroducing a brain cannula. Ventriculography is, therefore, the safer procedure in cases with increased intracranial pressure, whether due to tumor or some other cause. The disadvantages of ventriculography are that it is a relatively major surgical procedure, that it involves a certain amount of trauma to the brain, and that by the direct injection of air the ventricles alone are usually outlined. By means of the lumbar route, on the other hand, if no block exists, the air may enter into any region in the cranial cavity which is occupied by cerebrospinal fluid. Moreover, with a little experience the procedure can be carried out by anyone capable of performing a lumbar puncture. The interpretation of the resulting films, however, requires not only a familiarity with roentgenography generally and cranial roentgenography in particular, but a thorough knowledge of the anatomy of the brain and the physiology of the cerebrospinal fluid circulation.

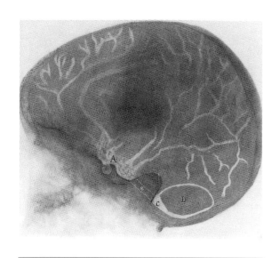

Encephalography (1919). A retouched photograph of a roentgenogram of the head after an intraspinous injection of air.[22]

We have, for these reasons, followed the simple rule of using ventriculography in patients with clinical signs of increased intracranial pressure, and encephalography in all other patients in need of such a test. Occasionally, when ventriculography fails to give adequate information for diagnosis, we use encephalography even in the presence of increased intracranial pressure. Under these circumstances, if alarming signs should occur following the air injection, the ventricles could be tapped directly through the trephine holes made for the ventriculography, but we have never had occasion to resort to this measure.

Ironically, several years passed before ventriculography was performed on Cushing's patients—and then only rarely. It is possible that the delayed use of ventriculography by Cushing may have been related to the poor personal relationship he had with Dandy.[5] The almost complete exclusion of encephalography from the Cushing practice was due to his fear that herniation of the cerebellar tonsils might occur and be fatal. Nevertheless, years later in retirement, Cushing admitted that he and his colleagues[24] were "altogether too slow to adopt the use of ventriculography for the identification or exclusion of brain tumors. Our conservatism . . . was, in retrospect, probably due to the insistence long laid in the clinic upon a thorough neurological examination in each case and the apprehension lest this be glossed over by the junior staff if a diagnosis in some instances could be more quickly arrived at in other ways."

Davidoff and Dyke[20] emphasized that

it is possible to obtain good encephalograms with much less air than is usually introduced and thereby to materially decrease the discomfort of the patient both during and after the procedure. The severity and duration of the symptoms occurring during and after lumbar air injection seem to depend upon the amount of air used, not, however, in absolute terms, but relative to the size of the ventricles. We have learned to determine the amount of air necessary in any given case by taking a film after 20 cc of air have been introduced, and immediately developing it. Inspection of this film shows whether the ventricular system is normal in size or whether it is dilated. If the size of the ventricles is within normal limits, 50 to 70 cc of air is sufficient for excellent encephalograms.

Davidoff and Dyke stressed the use of "stereoscopic roentgenograms from four sides with the head both vertical and horizontal," since they noted that "the practice of taking the films in only the vertical or horizontal position may lead to erroneous interpretations."

However, several published reports during the 1920s indicated a good deal of dissatisfaction with the accuracy of tumor localization by air studies. DeMartel considered that the injection of air into the ventricles was not a harmless procedure, since he had lost two patients. He preferred the injection of a dye such as methylene blue into one lateral ventricle.[25]

After 15 minutes, several milliliters of cerebrospinal fluid is extracted from the other ventricle. If the fluid is tinged blue, the conclusion is that there is ample communication between the lateral ventricles and the third ventricle. After another 15 minutes have elapsed, a puncture of the cisterna magna is done; if there is no dye in the fluid, it is reasonable to suspect two possibilities: a tumor of the posterior fossa which, pressing on the walls of the fourth ventricle, obstructs the aqueduct of Sylvius and interferes with the flow of fluid out of the third ventricle, or else a tumor in the vicinity of the third ventricle.

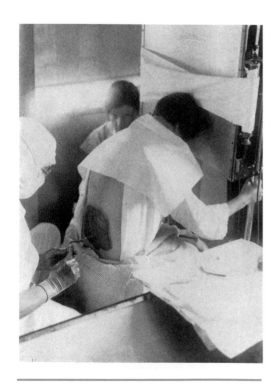

Position of the patient for encephalography (Davidoff and Dyke, 1932).[23]

At the first International Congress of Radiology in London (1925), Dandy's radiological colleague, J. W. Pierson,[8] admitted that ventriculography "is dangerous and complicated," but hastened to add that "in competent hands it should not be nearly so dangerous as an exploratory craniotomy and it frequently yields more information than the latter operation. Dandy reports but three deaths, which occurred very early in the series of at least 500 cases."

MYELOGRAPHY

The discoverer of air encephalography, Walter Dandy, also recognized the possibility of localizing spinal cord tumors by the lumbar injection of air. As he wrote in 1918[22]:

> It also seems probable that we shall be able to localize spinal cord tumors by means of intraspinous injections of air. In one of our cases the spinal cord and the surrounding air-filled spaces are sharply outlined. Should the spinal canal be obliterated, either by a tumor or possibly by an inflammatory process, it is conceivable that the air shadow will extend up to the level of the lesion. Its intensity will naturally be greatly reduced by the great density of the spine, and particularly of the bodies of the vertebrae. A lateral view of the spine, by eliminating the maximum amount of bone, will probably give the best results. If the spinal canal is not obliterated by the tumor, the injected air will pass freely into the intracranial subarachnoid space, none being left in the spinal canal. This happened in one of our cases in which a spinal cord tumor was suspected. The passage of air into the brain was difficult to explain at the time of the injection, as the symptoms had been present for four years and a tumor of such duration would certainly have blocked the spinal canal. At operation a chronic transverse myelitis was found. Instead of an enlargement of the spinal cord, there was a constriction, which readily explains the failure of air to stop at the suspected zone.

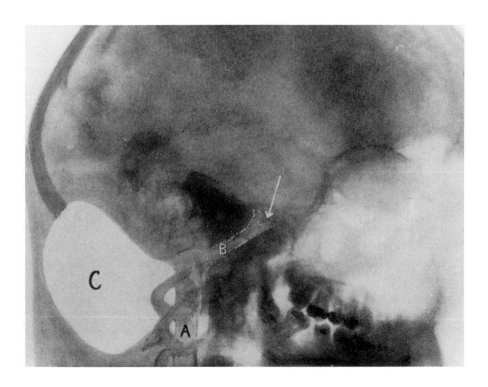

First air myelogram (1919). Retouched photograph of a roentgenogram of the head, after an intraspinous injection of air. The patient was suffering from the effects of an intracranial tumor that was localized only by the aid of the air injection and after a cerebellar exploration had revealed no growth. The enormous collection (C) of cerebrospinal fluid about the operative defect in the occipital bone corresponds to a greatly enlarged cisterna magna. The upper part of the spinal cord is visible because the spinal canal is filled with air (A). The cisternal block (*arrow*) represented a midbrain tumor. Note that none of the cerebral sulci contain air.[22]

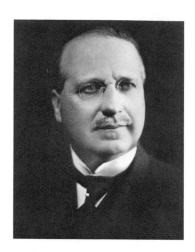

Jean-Athanase Sicard (1872-1929).

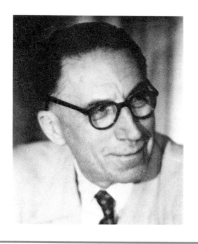

Jacques Forestier (1890-1978).

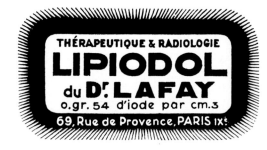

Advertisement for Lipiodol (1928).

Unfortunately, this first air myelogram was probably overlooked, since it had a minor place in the classic paper that first described pneumoencephalography. Dandy's first full paper on myelography did not appear until 1925.

The first deliberate air myelogram was apparently performed in 1919 by the Swedish internist, Jacobaeus. However, Jacobaeus was forced to conclude his paper by remarking that "the x-ray pictures, obtained by this method of examination, are however so difficult to read and so diffuse, that no successful and clear reproduction can be considered possible." Similar early results were also reported in 1921 by Wideroe and Bingel.[26]

The use of air myelography was supplanted by the development of positive contrast (Lipiodol) myelography by Jean-Athanase Sicard and Jacques Forestier in 1921.[27] The contrast material Lipiodol was originally prepared by the Frenchman, Lafay (1901), who was searching for an iodized oil that might have therapeutic properties. As Sicard and Forestier described, Lipiodol "is a dense, thick oil, of high density; it is colorless, not caustic and non-toxic, is well tolerated by tissues and has the remarkable quality of being very opaque to x-rays." It also appeared to have curative properties that were "indisputable in the pains of muscular rheumatism and particularly the sciaticas." Sicard and Forestier decided to try to inject Lipiodol into the epidural space, "a cavity of the body which up to now had escaped any such investigation." They had previously tried injection with Collargol, but this substance had been very painful, remained in place where injected, and produced poor radiographic images. Injection of air via the epidural sacrococcygeal route produced clearer pictures than the Collargol injection, but the intense pain it produced was a contraindication to the practical use of this procedure. With the patient tilted head-down in the Trendelenburg position, they noted that the heavy Lipiodol (following the law of gravity) slowly flowed to the upper regions of the dorsal and cervical spine. "After a day or two in this position, the Lipiodol is fixed within the epidural tissues. After two or three weeks the radiographic pictures appear practically unchanged." Sicard and Forestier stressed "the value of this examination for determining the permeability of the epidural space, to localize, for example, a tumor in this region, a compressing osteitis, etc." They noted that the inadvertent injection of oil into the cerebrospinal fluid should not be a cause for alarm, since "the cerebrospinal fluid tolerates Lipiodol remarkably well."

Reminiscing almost 40 years later, Forestier noted that ". . . the first injection of Lipiodol of the sub-arachnoid space was in fact accidental. Willing to inject Lipiodol into the epidural space through the lumbar route, I pushed my needle too far away; when we took the picture, we were confronted with the figure of a drop instead of blotches. To our great surprise there was no meningeal reaction. The drop was movable under the fluoroscope: the method of transit of Lipiodol was discovered."[26]

It was much easier to examine the subarachnoid space than the epidural cavity. Sicard and Forestier[28] noted that (after spinal puncture at the level of the fourth or fifth dorsal vertebra)

> in the normal subject, standing or seated, Lipiodol reaches the lower limit of the subarachnoid cul-de-sac in a few minutes after injection, accumulating in the vicinity of the second sacral vertebra in the form of an elongated ball or shortened caterpillar. Sometimes a little Lipiodol adheres like a fine, opaque thread along the roots of the cauda equina, outlining them by fine, opaque streaks.

However, "if the subarachnoid space is obstructed by a compressing process, serous meningitis, loculated or encysted, various neoplasms, etc., the Lipiodol will be retained or imprisoned in the canal and the reading of the radiographs will locate whatever point of the medullary axis corresponds to the site of the intra-arachnoid compression."

Sicard and Forestier preferred cisternal or cervical puncture, since they considered that the flow of Lipiodol would best be achieved "by injecting the iodized oil into the widest segments of the subarachnoid space." For lumbar puncture,[28] it was necessary that the patient be

> firmly tied to the table and the pelvis is raised higher than the head, to an inclination of from 45° to 60° or more. The slow progression of the lipiodol owing to gravity toward the cervical segment and the skull should be watched by fluoroscopy, and a film taken in this position when there is a stoppage. The drawback in this latter method lies in the fact that many patients cannot stand this declining position for more than 10 or 20 minutes; and if the lipiodol has shown a stoppage, it will not remain against the obstacle; but will fall down to the lumbosacral angle as soon as the patient gets up again.

Despite the emphasis on the postural advantages of cisternal injection of Lipiodol, it became apparent that the lumbar approach had great merit in diagnosing small nonobstructive intraspinal lesions, and that fluoroscopic observation together with spot radiographs was by far the superior method for myelography. This technique was facilitated by Camp's design of a tilt table that could be turned 90 degrees in either direction.[27]

Sicard and Forestier also developed a light version of Lipiodol by diluting the original contrast material in olive oil to produce a solution containing only 11% iodine. Less radiopaque than regular Lipiodol, light Lipiodol floated upwards (instead of sinking in the cerebrospinal fluid), and within about half an hour after injection into the subarachnoid space rose into the lateral ventricles. Sicard and Forestier ingeniously noted that "combined injections of ordinary Lipiodol (intracisternal injection) and light Lipiodol (lumbar injection) may outline the compressing tumor completely. The method is also advisable when multiple tumors are suspected; the stoppage, at long distances from one another, of the two kinds of Lipiodol would draw the physician's attention to the possibility of several tumors causing compression." Unfortunately, they found that light Lipiodol was "irritating and (it) was abandoned."[29]

Peiper and Klose showed that "a few drops of Lipiodol injected into the lateral ventricle glide down without symptoms through the foramen of Monroe, the aqueduct of Sylvius, the foramen of Magendie and Luschka to the terminal sac of the dural space."[26] This technique or the introduction of Lipiodol by lumbar injection could be used to differentiate the various forms of hydrocephalus and to outline brain tumors.

Initially, small amounts of Lipiodol (0.5 ml) were injected and only obstructing lesions could be identified. It was soon noted that fluoroscopic observation of the passage of Lipiodol in the spinal canal provided important information not obtainable from films alone and could lead to the detection of small intraspinal tumors.

In September, 1933, Mixter and Barr reported to the New England Surgical Society on the clinical significance of rupture of the intervertebral disks in the production of low back pain and sciatica. They immediately recognized the inadequacy of plain film examinations in identifying herniated disks and stressed the importance of myelography for detecting this lesion. "For this purpose the usual 1.5 to 2 ml of Lipiodol,

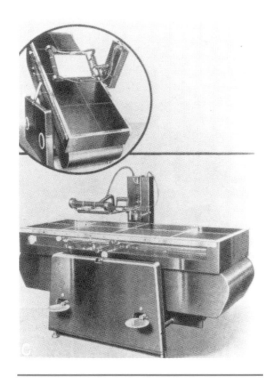

Camp's tilt table.

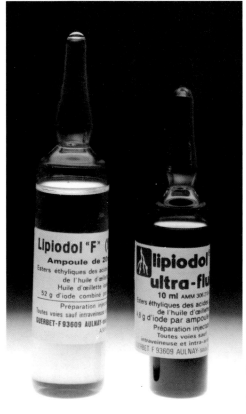

Ampules of Lipidol.

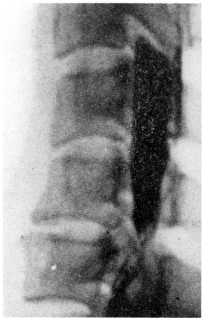

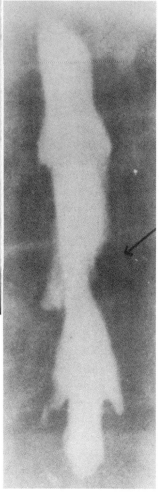

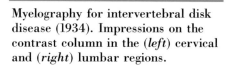

Myelography for intervertebral disk
disease (1934). Impressions on the
contrast column in the (*left*) cervical
and (*right*) lumbar regions.

sufficient to demonstrate a block, is not enough, and we now use 5 ml in order to nearly fill the lumbosacral canal . . . films taken with the patient sitting or standing and from various angles with the axis of the spine, usually localizes the lesion."[30] They also used Lipiodol myelography to identify herniated cervical disks. Although some authors strongly argued that clinical examination was more reliable in localizing intervertebral disk disease, many subsequent studies clearly showed the superiority of myelography.

Sicard and Forestier noted that the injection of Lipiodol into the subarachnoid fluid

> is well tolerated except for the fact that complete adaptation of the subarachnoid space to the presence of the lipiodol takes place only after a painful period of two to three days. It is thus necessary to warn the patient of the appearance during the initial stage, six to seven hours after the injection, of painful phenomena in the lower limbs. These consist of various paresthesias including tingling sensations, which are transitory and are markedly reduced by the usual doses of morphine.

They noted that the intensity of these reactions was dependent on the dosage and thus did not inject more than 0.5 ml. Using cervical or cisternal puncture, however, they reported no bad after effects such as headache, vomiting, malaise, or meningismus such as frequently followed lumbar puncture.

Untoward reactions to the subarachnoid instillation of Lipiodol were soon reported.[31] Ayer and Mixter noted marked cellular reaction in the cerebrospinal fluid in cats.[26] Mixter "hesitated to use it in the human subject . . . and . . . sought for some less toxic substance and for one that would move more freely and rapidly in the cerebrospinal space, but without success."[26]

Despite initial misgivings, contrast examinations of the spinal subarachnoid space became an acknowledged and valued neuroradiological diagnostic procedure. In 1923, the term *myelography* was first used by Berberich at a meeting of the Medical Society of Frankfurt.[26] Sicard and Forestier protested this term and wrote that "this word we consider to be a misnomer because no attempt is made at outlining the medulla itself. We prefer the original appellation of 'epereuve du lipiodol sous arachnoidien (the subarachnoid lipiodol test)'." By 1929, Globus and Strauss[32] reported their observations in 64 cases including not only spinal cord tumors but also various degenerative and inflammatory diseases. Lipiodol clearly was far better than conventional clinical methods in localizing the site of obstruction. Nevertheless, the problem of possible side effects persisted. In a discussion of the paper by Globus and Strauss, Elsberg remarked that "I have thoroughly believed that iodized oil is an irritant. I have seen, in a number of instances, fresh adhesions and marked congestion of the meninges and roots which are not ordinarily observed when the spinal cord is exposed during the course of a laminectomy, and have always explained this as a result of the irritating qualities of this foreign substance." However, it was only 12 years later (1941) that Marcovich, Walker, and Jessico[33] reported on the immediate and late effects of the intrathecal injection of iodized oil and clearly demonstrated its irritant properties.

That same year, Kubik and Hampton[34] reported a procedure for removing the iodized oil by simply aspirating it through a spinal puncture needle after myelography. As they stated,

> because of its irritating effects, there has been an increasing tendency to forego the use of iodized oil in myelography and to employ the less reliable procedure of pneumomyelography. If the oil can be removed shortly after its introduction, as may be done when it is accessible at operation, there is no serious objection to its use. One cannot always be certain, however, that a surgical condition is present, and the reluctance to use iodized oil under such circumstances is often responsible for prolonged disability of the patients who might be relieved by surgery . . . For some time we have been introducing the oil with the patient on the fluoroscopic table, leaving the needle in place during the examination, and removing the oil immediately afterward.

Ironically, 16 years previously Peiper and Klose remarked on the suggestion of Sicard and Forestier "to remove the oil from the lower lumbar sac by puncture in as much as it remains for a long time in that space.[26]

Many investigators searched for an improved intrathecal contrast agent. A variety of oil- and water-soluble substances were tried without success. In 1944, Ramsey and Strain described the use of Pantopaque (ethyl iodophenylundecylate) as a new contrast agent for myelography.[35] Pantopaque flowed more readily than Lipiodol, provided excellent contrast, and at first was considered to be absorbable. Although less toxic than Lipiodol, residual Pantopaque that was not removed after myelography did act as a meningeal irritant and in some cases produced arachnoiditis.

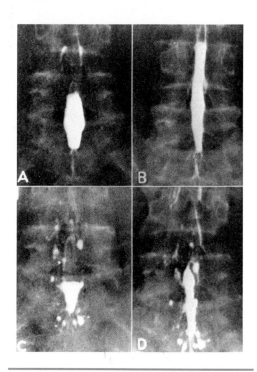

Long-term effects of intrathecal injection of iodized oil (1941). "Appearance of the caudal sac containing iodized oil, the day after its injection (*top left and right*) and four months after (*bottom left and right*). The iodized oil is movable at the latter, but the small globules fixed in the sheets of the lumbar and sacral roots are evident."[33]

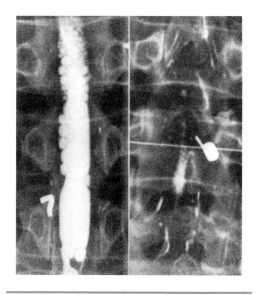

Radiographs before (*left*) and after (*right*) removal of iodized oil that had been injected into the lumbar subarachnoid space 4 days before removal (1941). Small amounts of oil remain in the cul-de-sac and in the sheaths of the nerve roots. The dense shadow represents the hilt of the lumbar-puncture needle, inserted between the third and fourth lumbar vertebrae; the heavy transverse line represents a needle on the surface used as a marker.[34]

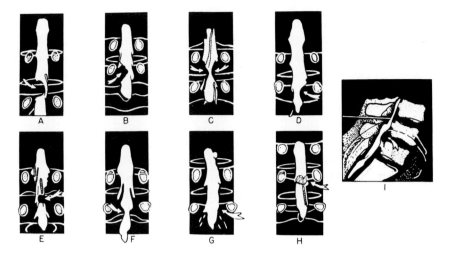

The first water-soluble agent for myelography was abrodil (Skiodan). Introduced in 1931 by Arnell and Lidstrom,[36] it never became popular outside Scandinavia because of its irritant effect on the spinal meninges. Almost four decades later, two other water-soluble contrast agents (Conray-60 and Dimer X) were developed, but they also were associated with unacceptable toxicity. During the late 1970s, the first successful nonionic, water-soluble contrast medium for myelography (metrizamide, Amipaque) was developed.[37,38] Unlike Pantopaque, metrizamide was miscible with cerebrospinal fluid and did not have to be removed, thus eliminating the need to reinsert the lumbar puncture needle to withdraw the solution. Its low density and viscosity permitted one to "see through" the contrast to better visualize the nerve roots. Metrizamide inadvertently injected outside the subarachnoid space was rapidly reabsorbed and thus had no permanent disturbing effect on image quality. Metrizamide myelography could be combined with computed tomography (CT). Perhaps of greatest importance, metrizamide was far safer than Pantopaque and much less likely to cause adhesive arachnoiditis. More recently, there has been the development of even less toxic nonionic agents such as iohexol (Omnipaque) and iopamidol (Isovue), which have essentially replaced metrizamide.[39]

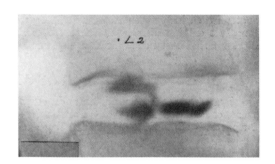

Diskography (1951). Incomplete anterior rupture.[40]

Epidural venography (1974). Venogram shows a block of the left anterior internal vertebral vein and radicular vein at L5-S1 (*single arrow*). Comparable veins on the right are shown with double arrows. Later phase of the venogram shows filling of the radicular vein and anterior internal vertebral vein superior to the block by collateral circulation via the external vertebral veins (*arrows*). The myelogram was interpreted as normal in this patient with a proven herniated disk.[41]

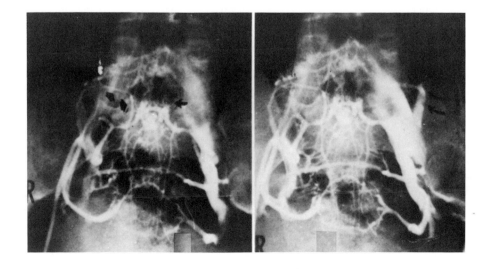

Mention should briefly be made of two other techniques for evaluating degenerative disk disease. In 1948, Lindblom[40] introduced *diskography*, in which a needle was introduced into the central portion of the intervertebral disk and a small amount of contrast material was injected. In a normal disk, the contrast material pooled centrally in the nucleus pulposus; in a degenerated disk, the contrast assumed a more irregular, distorted shape and dissected into more peripheral parts of the intervertebral disk.[39]

Another technique was *epidural venography*, which had a short period of popularity in the middle and late 1970s. Using a femoral venous approach, catheters were manipulated into one or both ascending lumbar veins and contrast material injected to outline the internal vertebral plexus. A herniated disk caused compression and lack of filling of veins in the ventral epidural space.[41] CT and magnetic resonance (MR) imaging have completely replaced both diskography and epidural venography.[39]

CAROTID ARTERIOGRAPHY

By the middle of the 1920s, the Portuguese neurologist, Egas Moniz, had found two major problems with the use of ventriculography: "the danger of injections of air and the lack of precision of diagnosis even in cases of ventricular deformity."[25] Moniz proposed to outline the brain radiographically with some positive contrast material, just as his Parisian friend, Sicard, had done with Lipiodol in the spinal subarachnoid space. Somewhat illogically he was inspired by the work of Graham and Cole in outlining the gallbladder following the intravenous injection of contrast material. His efforts to find a similar technique for the brain failed, since the brain possessed no parallel mechanism for the physiological concentration of contrast as existed in the biliary system.[8]

Moniz then turned to the concept of an intraarterial injection of some opaque material. He eliminated Lipiodol or other oily substances because they might produce harmful emboli. Moniz made a number of experiments on dogs and rabbits to assess the toxicity and opacity of such substances as the bromide and iodide salts of lithium, sodium, potassium, ammonium, and rubidium. He finally selected a 25% solution of sodium iodide.

After concluding his experiments on dogs, Moniz moved to the human cadaver to learn normal radiographic anatomy[25]:

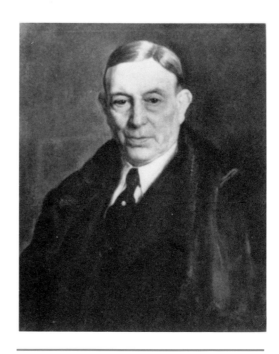

Egas Moniz (1874-1955).

> Once the arterial network was visualized, it was necessary to get acquainted with the normal pattern so that in cases of cerebral neoplasm appreciable changes could be recognized, at least in certain regions. We assume that, in the presence of a cerebral neoplasm, the arterial network would show appreciable changes in some localities that could define, if not the whole extent of the tumor, at least areas of distortion of small arterial branches. With highly vascular tumors, a visible shadow resulting from penetration of the opaque medium into the tumor should in all probability be evident.

Finally, Moniz was ready for his first patient. Since Moniz suffered severely from gout involving his hands, the actual arteriographic procedure was performed by his pupil and successor, Alemida Lima. However, following the percutaneous injection of contrast material in this and several additional cases, the radiograph showed no evidence of contrast material. Presuming that the contrast must have been injected outside the

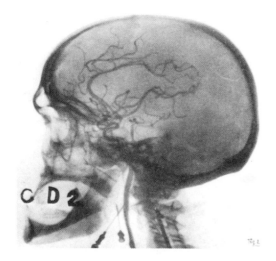

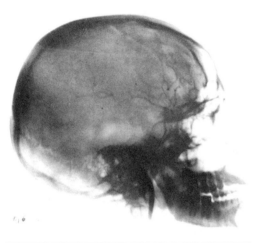

Cerebral arteriography (1927). *Top,* Internal carotid artery system. Injection of 30% NaI in a head preserved in formaline. *Bottom,* First arterial encephalography of the cerebral carotid system in a living man. In this patient with a large pituitary tumor, the carotid artery is pushed forward, although the origin of the middle cerebral artery is higher. There is displacement of the anterior cerebral artery, which is much reduced in volume.[25]

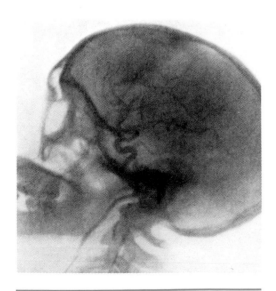

Direct percutaneous cerebral arteriography with thorotrast (1936). Note the needle in the internal carotid artery.[44]

artery, Moniz decided to make a surgical cutdown so that the internal carotid artery could be exposed for a precise puncture. The technique was a success, and in 1927 Moniz reported the first cerebral arteriogram.

Like Dandy's method of ventriculography, arteriography was accepted slowly, especially in the Anglo-Saxon countries. This may have been due in part to the fact that the procedure involved making two permanent scars, one on each side of the neck, unpleasant stigmata particularly for an attractive woman to carry for the rest of her life, especially if the investigation proved negative.[8]

In 1929, after much disappointment with the opacification and toxicity of sodium iodide, Moniz switched to a suspension of thorium dioxide as the contrast material for cerebral arteriography. He achieved spectacular success since thorium dioxide produced little acute intravascular toxicity (although it was locally harmful to the tissues of the neck if it extravasated), was almost painless on arterial injection, and was intensely radiopaque. These factors were beneficial and, indeed, essential to successful clinical arteriography because of the necessity for long radiographic exposure times because of slow film-screen combinations and the low output of the radiological equipment. Unfortunately, Moniz was completely unaware of the serious delayed effects produced by the radioactivity of thorium. Thorium is stored in the body in the reticuloendothelial system (liver, spleen, and lymph nodes). Since thorium is not excreted by the body and has an extremely long half-life (10^{10} years), the organs in which it is stored are continuously bombarded with dangerous alpha radiation that may produce malignant tumors 20 to 30 years later. Therefore thorium was abandoned as a diagnostic contrast agent a few years after its spectacular introduction.[42]

In 1931, Moniz published a book describing his first 90 cases (180 arteriograms). There were only two deaths in this group, both in arteriosclerotic patients.[43]

Moniz was awarded the Nobel prize for Medicine and Biology in 1949. Ironically, the award was given not for his extremely innovative and valuable work on carotid arteriography but for his many contributions to neurology and psychiatry, especially for the development of therapeutic prefrontal leukotomy for the treatment of mental diseases, a now largely discredited technique.[42]

In 1936, Loman and Myerson reported the feasibility of direct percutaneous carotid artery puncture for cerebral angiography.[44] As they wrote, "Because exposure and ligation of the carotid artery constitutes a formidable surgical technique which might cause clinicians to hesitate to utilize the procedure, we have developed a method by which thorotrast may be injected directly into the artery." To obtain sufficient concentration of contrast within the cerebral vessels, Loman and Myerson suggested two approaches: "(1) An assistant, standing opposite the operator, may compress the homolateral carotid at the root of the neck, preventing by this means the injected thorotrast from flowing through the cerebral vessels at too rapid a rate; or (2) you may slow down the outflow of blood from the cranial cavity by strongly compressing both internal jugulars over the sternomastoid muscles." They strongly recommended jugular compression, not only because it caused much less discomfort, but because of three disadvantages of carotid compression: "(1) It is apt by traction on the trachea to make the patient cough and as a result cause him to move his head while the roentgenogram is being taken; (2) it may displace the needle and thus cause an unsuccessful injection; and (3) it may produce an undesirable degree of cerebral anemia."

It is interesting to note that in this article Loman and Myerson mentioned that the Council of Pharmacy and Chemistry of the AMA "advise against the use of thorium dioxide because of its imperfect elimination from the body, its fairly high alpha-ray activity, and the possibility of its later radioactivity by the conversion of thorium dioxide into mesothorium and radiothorium, which may possibly render the tissues sensitive to roentgen rays." They were convinced that such possible complications would require far larger doses and pointed to an article by Robins and Goldberg who had injected 30 patients for visualization of the spleen and liver and "who were followed for from six weeks to four years (with) no apparent effects of the presence of the substance in the body."

In the succeeding 50 years, a variety of hypertonic and, more recently, isotonic contrast materials have been used for cerebral arteriography (see Chapter 25). Devices for obtaining rapid serial radiographs have been developed (see Chapter 25), the use of small catheters has been introduced, and digital subtraction techniques have been employed (see Chapter 25). These developments have transformed cerebral arteriography into a safe and widely performed procedure, which until the advent of CT and MR imaging was the single major imaging modality for neuroradiological diagnosis. Since the 1970s, the development of sophisticated interventional techniques has permitted dramatic therapeutic maneuvers in patients with cerebrovascular disease (see Chapter 31).

RADIONUCLIDE BRAIN SCANNING

George Moore, a young surgeon in training in Minneapolis, was attempting to design a method to more precisely define the margins of brain tumors at operation. Having known previously that fluorescein was taken up selectively by certain tumors of the eye and could be detected by applying ultraviolet light, Moore postulated that the same might apply to brain tumors.[45] In cases of suspected glioma, he injected a small quantity of fluorescein intravenously immediately before surgery. When the brain was exposed at surgery, a beam of ultraviolet light gave the glioma a yellowish color, while the surrounding normal brain appeared blue-gray. Well aware of the uptake of radioactive iodine by the thyroid, Moore wondered if the brain in similar fashion would selectively take up a radioactive compound. Would the skull block the emitted radiation or would it scatter it so much that precise localization would be impossible? In an attempt to answer these questions, Moore tried to tag a radioactive

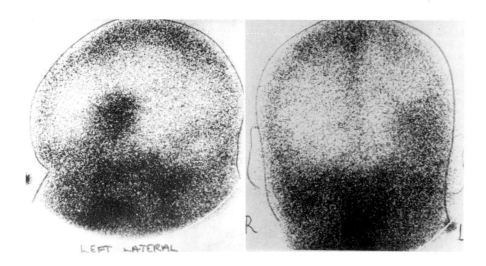

Radionuclide brain scan. *Left*, Left lateral and (*right*) anterior gamma-camera prints show a high concentration of the isotope (technetium) and the well-defined edges of a spherical mass extending superficially to the inner table of the skull in a patient with a meningioma.[8]

339

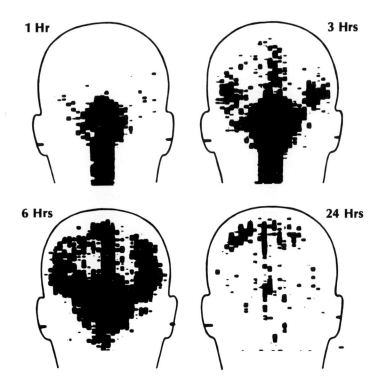

1 Hr   3 Hrs

6 Hrs   24 Hrs

Normal posterior radioisotope cisternograms. After the intrathecal injections of radioiodinated serum albumin, the cerebrospinal fluid flow is shown to be directional, rather than simply an ebb-and-flow phenomenon. Tracer is detected in the basal cisterns in about 1 hour, then ascends through the subarachnoid pathways to the hemispheric convexities, where most is resorbed.[47]

substance to fluorescein. He succeeded in preparing [131]diiodofluorescein, and injected this radioactive substance intravenously, exactly as he had simple fluorescein. Fortunately, the addition of iodine to the molecule did not endanger the benign quality of the drug. Moore used a Geiger counter to detect the radioactive emissions from the tumor and was immediately successful in localizing 12 out of 15 lesions.[45] Thus radionuclide brain scanning, or isotope encephalography, was born in 1948.

Since that time, dramatic improvements in equipment and isotopic agents (see Chapter 23) have greatly enhanced the efficiency and accuracy of radionuclide brain scanning. Because it could be readily performed on outpatients and was associated with no morbidity, radionuclide brain scanning revolutionized the approach to investigating patients with neurological disorders until it was supplanted by CT and MR imaging.

Other applications of isotopes in neuroradiology have included isotope cisternography and measurements of regional cerebral blood flow and metabolism. Isotope cisternography consists of the injection of a suitable radionuclide into the lumbar subarachnoid space and detecting its passage through the cerebrospinal fluid pathways. It is a useful confirmatory test in diagnosing communicating hydrocephalus and in detecting the site of leakage in patients with cerebrospinal fluid rhinorrhea.[46]

Cerebral blood flow was initially measured by the inhalation method of Kety and Schmidt (1948), in which the concentration of inspired nitrous oxide gas in blood taken from the jugular vein was used to estimate total cerebral blood flow.[48] Lassen and Ingvar (1961) introduced and developed the use of a radioactive inert gas ([85]K, ^{133}Xe) that permitted measurements to be made regionally by detectors outside the head.[49] The detectors measured the rate at which the radioactivity was removed by the cerebral blood flow. The accuracy of these regional estimates of blood flow were greatly improved when the inhalation technique was replaced by direct injection into the internal carotid artery. [133]Xe regional blood flow studies could show the proportionate differences in blood flow (1) between gray and white matter, (2) between one region of the brain and another, (3) in transitory and permanent vascular disturbances, and (4) in response to physiological stimuli such as altered arterial carbon dioxide tension and mental activity.[46]

For PET and SPECT scanning, see Chapter 23.

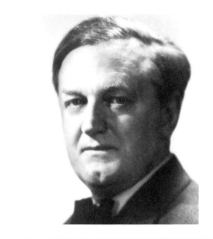

Erik Lysholm (1892-1947).

PRECISION RADIOLOGY AND OTHER ADVANCES

Precision radiology, in the nervous system and elsewhere, is a term associated with the Swede, Erik Lysholm. After first describing precision radiography of the petrous bone, a notoriously difficult structure to examine, Lysholm turned his attention to the entire skull. At the time, the x-ray tube was almost invariably set and fixed at right angles to the film and Potter-Bucky diaphragm. Lysholm developed his own head unit, based on the ingenious idea of moving the tube around a sphere with the central ray always directed to the center of the sphere. This required designing a new diaphragm that could be rotated so that the grid lines remained parallel to the x-ray beam. All movements of the tube were marked off in angles, as in a sextant. Lysholm related the angles to anthropological reference lines of the skull, particularly Reid's base line. He also incorporated a mirror system so that the underside of the patient's head (adjacent to the film) could be seen by the operator. This versatile device permitted the most difficult projections to be made precisely and, if necessary, reproduced exactly at a later date for comparative purposes. Another important facet of his head unit (designed in conjunction with the famed engineer, Georg Schonander) was the separation of the skull table from the patient's body, thus leaving the head free for precision radiography of the skull base. After much thought and experiment, Lysholm concluded that an adequate survey of the skull required at least four standard projections, each of which was logically worked out to display the maximum number of anatomical features.[8]

Lysholm also developed precision techniques for ventriculography. He stressed that the contrast material must always be placed up against the lesion. Consequently, Lysholm designed a systematic approach to filling the entire ventricular system and documenting the results by taking appropriate radiographs using his head unit. He suggested making two right-angle projections (and occasionally a third) without moving the patient's head, so that the position of air in the ventricles remained unchanged. The head was then moved into another position and the same procedure repeated. Both supine and prone positions were used. Lysholm recommended the use of a horizontal beam for the lateral projection, an unusual procedure for those days but one that was easy to perform with his skull table. Instead of using the traditional Potter-Bucky diaphragm, Lysholm designed an all-metal stationary grid for this projection.[8] After studying hundreds of cases confirmed by operation or autopsy, he demonstrated that tumors produced characteristic deformities of the ventricular system according to their site, and in 1935 and 1937 he published three classic papers on the ventricular system.

In all of his studies, Lysholm stressed that if only routine projections were taken, the diagnosis often could not be made. As he noted, "In addition to more standard projections, several special methods have been developed for the demonstration of various parts of the ventricular system. In this way routine radiography fell more and more into the background, and was replaced by methods of investigation designed for each individual case."

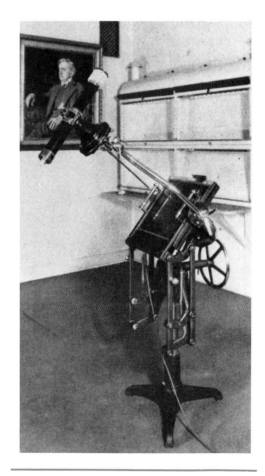

Original Lysholm-Schonander skull table (1931).[8]

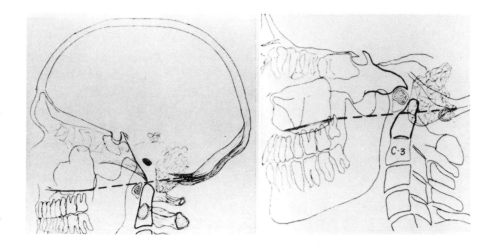

Chamberlain's line (1939). *Left,* Normal patient showing the tip of the odontoid below the line connecting the posterior margin of the hard palate to the back of the foramen magnum. *Right,* Cephalad displacement of the odontoid process above the line in a patient with basilar impression (platybasia).[53]

Among the noteworthy contributions to ventriculography and plain skull radiography during this period were the studies of Evans, Twining, and Chamberlain. Evans analyzed the ratio of the transverse diameter of the anterior horns to the internal diameter of the skull on air studies (AP projection, brow up) and determined that values above 0.30 indicated definite ventricular enlargement.[50] Twining measured the displacement of the third ventricle, aqueduct, and fourth ventricle by adjacent mass lesions[51] and introduced the line (between the tuberculum sellae and internal occipital protuberance) that still bears his name. Chamberlain was the true developer of the "Towne" projection,[52] as well as the line (posterior margin of hard palate to back of foramen magnum) used in the diagnosis of platybasia that bears his name.[53]

The introduction of somersaulting chairs combined with the development of autotomography greatly enhanced the technique of pneumoencephalography. Kurt Amplatz (1963) designed a mechanical chair capable of obtaining all radiographic positions "by tilting the patient in the chair rather than by positioning the patient's head alone." Although somersaulting techniques had been used for many years in some departments for children undergoing pneumoencephalography, the mechanical

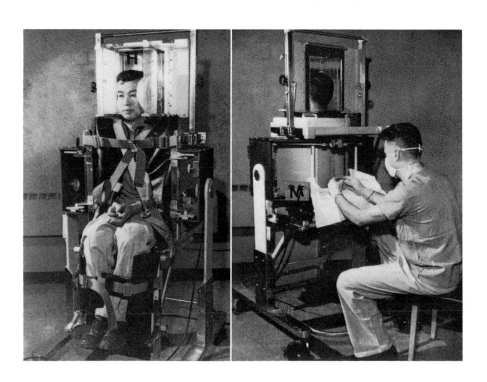

Amplatz chair for pneumoencephalography (1963). *Left,* The patient is firmly immobilized by seat belts, with the head firmly fixed by foam rubber cushions in the plastic head-holder (*H*). *Right,* Performance of spinal puncture.[54]

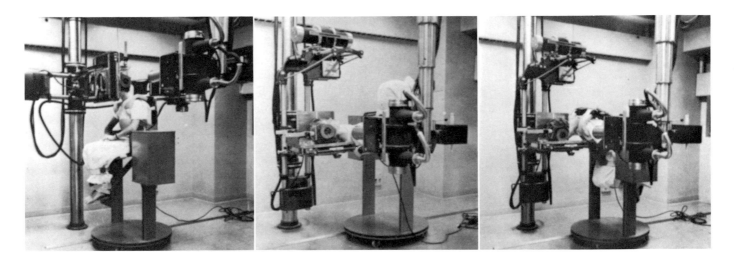

problems of somersaulting a heavy patient severely limited its use in
adults. Using the Amplatz chair or a subsequent device developed by
D. Gordon Potts and Juan M. Taveras (1964), which could be used in
conjunction with a Franklin or similar dedicated skull table, the patient
could be moved to a complete forward somersault and brought into the
supine position, thus filling and permitting accurate assessment of the
temporal horns of the lateral ventricles. Following this, the patient could
be brought into a sitting position to empty the temporal horns and then
manipulated through a slow backward somersault into the brow-down
position in which gas filled the posterior part of the third ventricle, the
aqueduct, and the fourth ventricle.[55] Another major improvement in the
pneumoencephalographic technique was the use of tomographic sections
in various planes to better demonstrate air in the cisterns and ventricles.
In 1949, Ziedses des Plantes[56] first suggested the use of autotomography
in pneumoencephalography, with the film and tube kept rigid while the
head was rotated. This method was rarely used until the concept was
revived 10 years later (1960) by Schechter and Jing.[57] They demonstrated
that this technique could provide good visualization of the third ventricle,
aqueduct, and fourth ventricle with obscuration of overlying bony structures.

In describing the glory days of pneumoencephalography, note should
also be made of Giovanni DiChiro, who developed a method for comput-
ing the volume of the sella turcica[58] and authored a classic atlas of
pneumoencephalographic anatomy.[59]

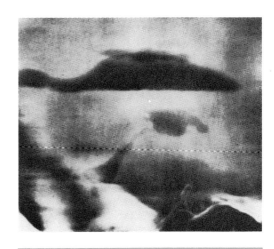

Lateral autotomogram (1963). Sharp
delineation of a normal aqueduct and
fourth ventricle.[54]

NEURORADIOLOGY AS A SUBSPECIALTY

For many years, neuroradiology was an unequal partnership in which the
various invasive procedures were performed by neurosurgeons while radiologists were relegated to taking appropriate exposures. The closest col-
laborations between radiologists and surgeons in the United States were at
the Peter Bent Brigham Hospital in Boston, where Harvey Cushing and
Merrill Sosman developed a close working relationship, and at the Mayo
Clinic, where John Camp teamed with Joseph Adson. Sosman's most
famous pupil, Cornelius Dyke, became the first full-time American
neuroradiologist when he joined the Neurological Institute of New York in
1929.[5] Dyke's fruitful collaboration with neurosurgeon Leo Davidoff resulted in many articles and a classic text on pneumoencephalography.[60]

With the introduction of ventriculography, which required surgical competence to incise the scalp and drill holes in the skull for inserting a needle to inject air, followed by suturing the incision, the surgeon became an essential participant in the examination. The neurosurgeon also took a dominant role in performing encephalography, myelography, and arteriography. These invasive procedures were financially valuable to the neurosurgeons, and thus the radiologists had to be content in merely providing the facilities and collaborating in the interpretation of the films.[5]

Radiologists had mixed feelings regarding this "turf battle." Most considered that the neuroradiologist should take complete command of the procedures, since his superior knowledge of the radiological possibilities for each particular examination allowed him to direct the study in such a way as to save time and avoid unnecessary procedures and discomfort to the patient while producing the information required for appropriate treatment. Nevertheless, radiologists in general hospitals were not properly qualified to supply maximum service in a field so specialized as neuroradiology.[5] The first "modern" American radiologist was Mannie M. Schechter, who developed a completely independent Neuroradiological Unit at St. Vincent's Hospital in New York. Schechter became the first radiologist in the United States to replace the surgeon for inserting the needles in neurodiagnostic procedures. Still, he always cooperated closely with neurologists and neurosurgeons and kept in contact with the patients he had studied by going to their operations and postmortem examinations.[5]

The first president of the American Society of Neuroradiology, Juan Taveras, reflecting on the development of his subspecialty in the United States on becoming the first editor of the *American Journal of Neuroradiology*, wrote in 1980[61]:

> An important problem affecting the education of individuals in this field related to the fact that training had to come after the completion of a residency and, given the great scarcity of radiologists prevailing during the decades of the 40's to the 60's, there was no hope that an individual would forego making a good living after the completion of his residency to obtain specialty training *for which there were no funds*. Consequently, only individuals who were appointed to the staff of departments and were assigned duty in the neurological area for a period of time had any opportunities to obtain postresidency experience.

In the absence of any formal training program, neuroradiology thus was performed by general radiologists with some interest in the field. This lack of training opportunity was recognized by the National Institute of Neurological Diseases and Blindness, which in 1960 decided to support training in neuroradiology that was to combine clinical and research training, similar to established training programs in neurology and neurosurgery. Two programs were established: one at the Albert Einstein College of Medicine under Schechter and the other at the Neurological Institute of Columbia-Presbyterian Medical Center under Taveras (who with Ernest Wood wrote the standard text, *Diagnostic Neuroradiology*). Interestingly, "almost immediately after the establishment of the fellowship programs, a significant number of individuals expressed a desire to obtain postresidency training in neuroradiology." In succeeding years, foundation support was no longer necessary "because the specialty of neuroradiology has been accepted and the needs recognized by the hospitals and universities."[54]

NEWER IMAGING MODALITIES

The development of CT in the 1970s revolutionized neuroradiology. The excellent spatial and contrast resolution of this modality permitted the rapid detection of brain parenchymal lesions, extraaxial tumors and collections of blood, and dilatation of the ventricular system without the need to resort to time-consuming, painful, and potentially dangerous arteriography and pneumoencephalography. The exquisite bony detail of the vertebral bodies and posterior elements provided by CT greatly improved the detection of spinal fractures, and the availability of axial sections permitted the diagnosis of herniation of intervertebral discs without the need for subarachnoid contrast material.

A decade later, the introduction of MR imaging again made a dramatic change in the approach to neuroradiological diagnosis. The multiplanar capability of this technique, coupled with its excellent contrast resolution and lack of need for intravenous contrast material, has led to MR imaging replacing CT in many clinical situations. MR imaging is especially valuable in assessing the posterior fossa and other areas that frequently have bone artifacts on CT. It has become the procedure of choice for imaging patients with suspected multiple sclerosis and other demyelinating disorders and is more sensitive than CT in demonstrating neoplastic and inflammatory processes and their precise relationship to adjacent structures. Impressions on the thecal sac and spinal cord can be easily demonstrated without the need for any intrathecal contrast material. Disadvantages of MR imaging include a lack of specificity, a slower scanning time (leading to image degradation from patient motion), the possibility of patient claustrophobia, and the contraindication to imaging patients with pacemakers or intracranial aneurysm clips. The role of MR imaging in acute head trauma is limited by problems in identifying acute hemorrhage, fractures, and displaced bone fragments, although it is more sensitive than CT in detecting nonhemorrhagic deep white-matter shear injuries that have important prognostic significance.

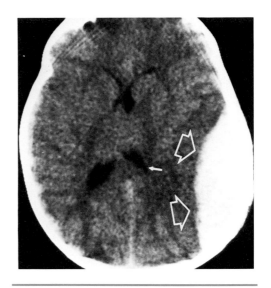

CT of acute epidural hematoma. Characteristic lens-shaped area of increased attenuation (*open arrows*). Substantial mass effect associated with the hematoma distorts the left lateral ventricle.

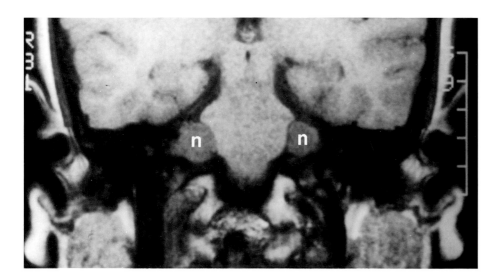

MR scan showing bilateral acoustic neurinomas (*n*) in a patient with neurofibromatosis.

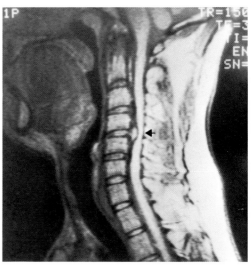

MRI of intervertebral disk herniation. There is an extradural impression on the cervical spinal canal (*arrow*).

References

1. Brecher R and Brecher E: The rays: A history of radiology in the United States and Canada. Baltimore, Williams & Wilkins, 1969.
2. New York Times, February 8, 1896, p 9.
3. Shephard DAE: Thomas Edison's attempts at radiology of the brain (1896). Mayo Clin Proc 49:59-61, 1974.
4. New York Daily Tribune, February 14, 1896, p 3.
5. Gutierrez C: The birth and growth of neuroradiology in the USA. Neuroradiology 21:227-237, 1981.
6. Cushing H: Haematomyelia from gunshot wound of the cervical spine. Bull Johns Hopkins Hosp 8:195-197, 1897.
7. Cushing H: Discussion. AJR 13:10-11, 1925.
8. Bull JWD: History of neuroradiology. Br J Radiol 34:69-84, 1961.
9. Schüller A: Röntgendiagnostik der Erkrankungen des Kopfes. Vienna, Holder, 1912.
10. Schüller A: Roentgen diagnosis of disease of head (translation F. F. Stocking). St. Louis, CV Mosby, 1918.
11. Tousey S: Medical electricity and röntgen rays. Philadelphia, WB Saunders, 1910.
12. Christie AC: A manual of x-ray technic. Philadelphia, JB Lippincott, 1913.
13. Mould RF: A history of x-rays and radium. London, 1980.
14. Church A: Cerebellar tumor: Recognized clinically, demonstrated by x-ray, proved by autopsy. Am J Med Sci 117:125-130, 1899.
15. Mills CK and Pfahler GE: Tumor of the brain localized clinically and by the roentgen rays: With some observations and investigations relating to the use of roentgen rays in diagnosis of lesions of the brain. Phila Med J 10:268-273, 1902.
16. Mills CK and Pfahler GE: An additional case of tumor of the brain localized clinically and by the Roentgen rays. Phila Med J 10:439-441, 1902.
17. Keen WW and Sweet WM: A case of gunshot wound of the brain in which the roentgen rays showed the presence of eight fragments of the bullet: Localization by Sweet's method made operation inadvisable. Am J Med Sci 126:1-10, 1903.
18. Naffziger HC: A method for the localization of brain tumors—the pineal shift. Surg Gynec Obstet 40:481-484, 1925.
19. Heuer G and Dandy W: Roentgenography in the localization of brain tumor, based upon a series of one hundred consecutive cases. Johns Hopkins Hosp Bull 27:311-319, 1916.
20. Dandy WE: Ventriculography following the injection of air into the cerebral ventricles. Ann Surg 68:5-11, 1918.
21. Luckett WH: Air in the ventricles of the brain following a fracture of the skull: Report of a case. Surg Gyn Obst 17:237-240, 1913.
22. Dandy WE: Roentgenography of the brain after the injection of air into the spinal canal. Ann Surg 70:397-403, 1919.

23. Davidoff LM and Dyke CG: An improved method of encephalography. Bull Neurol Inst NY 2:75-94, 1932.
24. Cushing H and Eisenhardt L: Meningiomas: Their classification, regional behavior, life history, and surgical end results. Springfield, Ill, Charles C Thomas, 1938.
25. Moniz E: Arterial encephalography: Importance in the localization of cerebral tumors. Rev Neurol (Paris) 34:72-90, 1927.
26. Epstein BS: Myelography. In Bruwer A (ed): Classic descriptions in diagnostic roentgenology. Springfield, Ill, Charles C Thomas, 1964.
27. Sicard JA and Forestier J: The radiographic method of examining the epidural space by means of lipiodol. Rev Neurol (Paris) 37:1264-1266, 1921.
28. Sicard JA and Forestier J: Clinical use of iodized oil: Therapeutic and diagnostic applications. Bull Soc Med Hop Paris 47:309-314, 1923.
29. Sicard JA and Forestier J: Roentgenologic exploration of the central nervous system with iodized oil (lipiodol). Arch Neurol Psychiat 16:420-434, 1929.
30. Mixter WJ and Ayer JG: Rupture of the intervertebral disc with involvement of the spinal canal. N Engl J Med 211:210-215, 1934.
31. DeMartel MT: The operative treatment of tumors of the spinal cord and its coverings. Rev Neurol (Paris) 1:701-707, 1923.
32. Globus JH and Strauss I: Intraspinal iodolography. Arch Neurol Psychiat 21:1331-1386, 1929.
33. Marcovich AW, Walker AE, and Jessico CM: Immediate and late effects of intrathecal injection of iodized oil. JAMA 116:2247-2254, 1941.
34. Kubik CS and Hampton AO: Removal of iodized oil by lumbar puncture. N Engl J Med 224:455-457, 1941.
35. Ramsey GHS and Strain WH: Pantopaque: A new contrast medium for myelography. Radiogr Clin Photog 20:25-33, 1944.
36. Arnell S and Lidstrom F: Myelography with Skiodan (abrodil). Acta Radiol 12:287-289, 1931.
37. Almen T: Contrast agent design. Some aspects on the synthesis of water-soluble contrast agents of low osmolality. J Theoret Biol 24:216-226, 1969.
38. Lindgren E (ed): Metrizamide-amipaque: The non-ionic water-soluble contrast medium: Further clinical experience in neuroradiology. Acta Radiol (suppl 355) 1-432, 1977.
39. Hesselink JR: Spine imaging: History, achievements, remaining frontiers. AJR 150:1223-1229, 1988.
40. Lindblom K: Discography of dissecting transosseous rupture of disks in lumbar region. Acta Radiol 36:12-16, 1951.
41. Gargano FP, Meyer JD, and Sheldon JJ: Transfemoral ascending lumbar catheterization of the epidural veins in lumbar disk disease. Radiology 111:329-336, 1974.

42. Grainger RG: Intravascular contrast media: The past, the present and the future. Brit J Radiol 55:1-18, 1982.
43. Moniz E: Cerebral angiography. Paris, Masson, 1931.
44. Loman J and Myerson A: Visualization of the cerebral vessels by direct intracarotid injection of thorium dioxide (thorotrast). AJR 35:188-193, 1936.
45. Moore GE: Use of radioactive diiodofluorescein in the diagnosis and localization of brain tumors. Science 107:56-57, 1948.
46. Bull JWD: Neurology's debt to Becquerel. Br J Radiol 45:881-890, 1972.
47. Wagner HN: Nuclear medicine. New York, HP Publishers, 1975.
48. Kety SS and Schmidt CF: The nitrous oxide method for the quantitative determination of cerebral blood flow in man: theory, procedure and normal values. J Clin Invest 27:476-483, 1948.
49. Lassen NA and Ingvar DH: The blood flow of the cerebral cortex determined by radioactive krypton. Experimentia 17:42-43, 1961.
50. Evans WA: An encephalographic ratio for estimating ventricular enlargement and cerebral atrophy. Arch Neurol Psychiat 47:931-937, 1942.
51. Twining EW: Radiology of the third and fourth ventricles. Br J Radiol 12:385-418, 569-598, 1939.
52. Towne EB: Erosion of the petrous bone by acoustic nerve tumor. Demonstration by roentgen ray. Arch Otolaryngol 4:515-519, 1926.
53. Chamberlain WE: Basilar impression (platybasia): A bizarre developmental anomaly of the occipital bone and upper cervical spine with striking and misleading neurologic manifestations. Yale J Biol Med 11:487-496, 1939.
54. Amplatz K: An improved chair for pneumoencephalography and autotomography. AJR 90:184-188, 1963.
55. Potts DG and Taveras JM: A new somersaulting chair for cerebral pneumography. AJR 91:1144-1149, 1964.
56. Ziedses des Plantes BG: Examination of the third and fourth ventricles using small amounts of air. Acta Radiol 34:399-407, 1950.
57. Schechter MM and Jing BS: Improved visualization of the ventricular system with the technic of autotomography. Radiology 74:593-598, 1960.
58. DiChiro G and Nelson KB: The volume of the sella turcica. AJR 87:989-996, 1962.
59. DiChiro G: An atlas of detailed normal pneumoencephalographic anatomy. Springfield, Ill, Charles C Thomas, 1961.
60. Davidoff LM and Dyke CG: The normal encephalogram. Philadelphia, Lea & Febiger, 1937.
61. Taveras JM: The development of neuroradiology in the United States. AJNR 1:1-2, 1980.

CHAPTER 19

Obstetrical and Gynecological Radiology

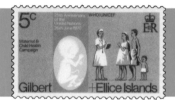
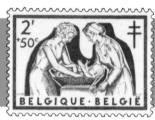
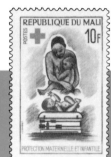

> Obstetricians will readily receive the immense value of ability to *see* the fetus in utero after ossification of its bones has occurred. The representation of deformed pelves in the living subject . . . all this opens up a tempting and promising field for practical research.
>
> HENRY W. CATTELL, 1896

Among the first to take up the challenge was Edward Parker Davis, Professor of Obstetrics at Jefferson Medical College, who attempted to image an unborn fetus inside the maternal uterus. Assisted by electricians and photographers, his first step was to radiograph (1½-hour exposure) a fetal skull placed within a female pelvis taken from a cadaver. The success of this experiment and one on a living 3-day-old baby encouraged Davis to try his equipment on a pregnant woman.[2] The almost-term woman was stretched out comfortably on a clinical table and a photographic plate was placed against her abdomen. As Davis[3] wrote,

> It was interesting to observe that the proximity of the electrical apparatus seemed to have no disturbing effect on the patient. She was informed that an effort would be made to ascertain the position of the child by the use of the electric light; she readily consented to the attempt, and aside from the slight fatigue from remaining quiet in one position, she seemed to be soothed by the constant sound of the apparatus, her pulse not varying through the entire time.

The first exposure lasted 1 hour and failed. After a second attempt lasting 1¼ hours,

> the faint outline of the trunk of her fetus could be recognized, the darker shadow of its pelvis occupying the upper right-hand portion of the plate, while projecting downward at about the center were irregular white masses showing the situation of the fetal limbs. The head of the child was so hidden by the mother's pelvis that no indication of its presence was obtained. While this experiment failed to outline distinctly the skeleton of the fetus, it offers information which may be of value in further attempts.

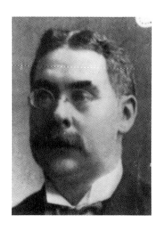

Edward Parker Davis.

Radiograph of fetal skull placed within the pelvis of a female cadaver (1896). Exposure time of 1½ hours.[3]

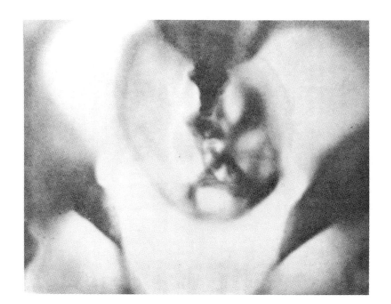

After examining ten patients, Davis reported that x-rays might be of value in obstetrics "to determine the position and attitude of the fetus; to determine the outlines of a contracted pelvis; to diagnose an abnormal condition of the fetus, such as a tumor; to reveal an accumulation of fluid within a cavity of the fetal body, as shown by the abnormal contour of the fetal tissues; to reveal the presence of more than one fetus in the uterus."

Davis concluded by stating that "the attempt to obtain information by this method is certainly a justifiable one, as it requires no exposure of the patient, no vaginal manipulation, and puts her to no essential discomfort. There has not been the slightest evidence that the passage of the rays through the uterus has affected either mother or child."

Left, Phototype print of the film obtained from the passage of x-rays through the uterus after 3½ months of pregnancy (1896). *Right*, Sagittal anatomical section (right half) of the same gravid uterus, natural size.[4]

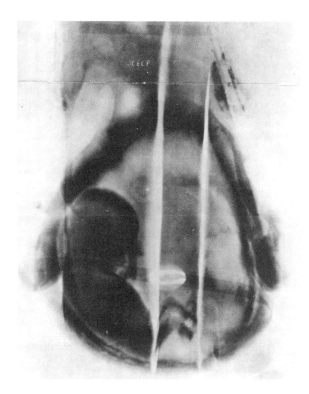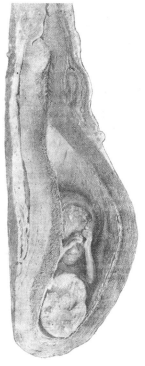

Soon afterward, Henri Varnier and co-workers[4] reported the radiography of "a gravid uterus which had been removed in December 1894 and had been preserved since then in alcohol." They could easily see the profile of the head, the trunk, and "in the visible upper extremity one can note two black bands parallel to the axis of the form and separated by a brighter space . . . the radius and the ulna . . . Extending from the buttocks in semiflexion one can see the two lower extremities, one of which is especially easy to recognize. In it one can distinguish the lower third of the thigh, the knee, and the foreleg. In the thigh the femur appears as a black band."

PELVIMETRY

For the next decade, early workers in obstetrical radiology devoted themselves to the demonstration of the pelvic inlet and its accurate measurement.[1] At an international congress in Moscow in August, 1897, Varnier presented the radiographs that he and Adolphe Pinard had obtained of the female pelvis in nonpregnant women and in women who were less than 6 months pregnant.[5] The living bony pelvis could be visualized "as if one were looking at a skeleton through a slightly dusty piece of glass and plate." They recommended an exposure time of "2 minutes per centimeter of body thickness at the region under examination, which would be 30 minutes for 15 centimeters thickness. Thus with this method the exposure time varies from 30 to 40 minutes." Radiography of pregnant women in the second half of pregnancy was of limited value because "the thickness of tissues to be traversed is too great for the sources of x-rays which are at present available." However, "in non-pregnant women and in women who have been pregnant for less than six months we have been able to make successful pelviographies." In each case, the resulting radiographs could show "a distinct and detailed silhouette of the pelvis and its femoral and vertebral articulations, a silhouette which permits us to gain as precise a general picture as we would gain by a direct view of the skeleton from a distance of several meters." Varnier and Pinard coined the term *pelvimetry* for the various measurements they could make (within 2 to 3 mm) of "the distance between the posterior superior iliac spines, the size of the sacrum, the distance between the spinous lumbosacral crest and the posterior superior iliac spines, and the distance from the middle region of the promontory to the sacroiliac symphyses." They stressed that "for those who are familiar with the difficulty that one experiences in external or internal exploratory examinations for making these measurements, which are so essential for the clinical study of oval, oblique, asymmetrical pelvises, this constitutes a great advance."

Levy and Thumim[6] in Berlin noted that

It is probably indisputably correct that a method which would make unnecessary an internal examination, or the usual, very complicated, and for both physician and patient very annoying methods which have been used up to the present time (1897), would have a great advantage over all others. We therefore set ourselves the problem of determining whether it would be possible by means of a few roentgenograms, to obtain the measurements of the conjugata vera of the pelvic inlet and of the transverse diameters of the pelvic inlet and outlet, as well as the picture of the whole pelvis.

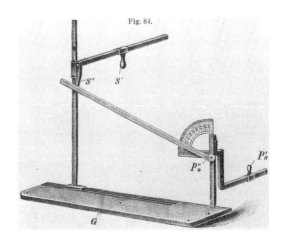

Pelvimetry device of Levy and Thumim (1897).[6]

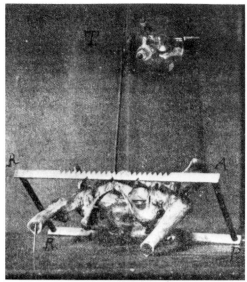

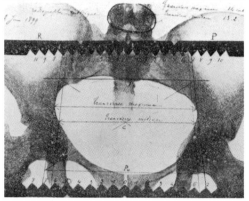

Pelvimetry technique of Fochier (1899). *Left,* Apparatus used to obtain measurable radiographs. *Right,* Radiograph of a dry pelvis preparation using this device. *RA,* Anterior metal strip; *T,* Crookes tube; *RP,* posterior metal strip; *Pu,* pubis; *Pr,* promontory; *C,* center of the pelvis. The maximum transverse distance is 14 cm, and the midtransverse distance is 13.2 cm.[7]

Utilizing a simple anteroposterior projection with the tube placed directly above the symphysis at a distance of 50 cm from the plate, they reported that "even at an advanced stage of pregnancy, we can now get a clear picture of the whole pelvis with an exposure time of 2 to 5 minutes. This picture shows the above-described dimensions, but with a distortion of perspective." By solving several reasonably simple equations, one could arrive at more precise measurements.

An ingenious method of pelvimetric measurement developed by Jean Fabre was reported in 1899 by Louis-Alphonse Fochier.

> The method consists essentially of placing around the person to be radiographed metal strips with serrations with 1 cm gaps between them, or some wooden strips in which metal nails are placed at 1 cm intervals, or screens made of metal wires spaced 1 cm apart. These strips or screens will undergo the same distortion as the region examined, but the interval between the wires, the serrations or the nails will always correspond to centimeters whatever may be the actual length of these intervals in the roentgenographic print.

The results obtained using this notched metal frame provided "very approximate" measurements of the diameter of the pelvic inlet. This technique also could be used to "obtain the transverse dimensions of the heart or the position of a foreign body."

In the same year (1899), Walter Albert performed pelvimetry with the spinous process of the fifth lumbar vertebra and the upper border of the symphysis pubis of the patient at a level so that the plane of the pelvic inlet was parallel to the surface of the photographic plate.[8] The measurements made on the radiograph were corrected by the principle of similar triangles in relation to the target-plate distance and the distance of the upper border of the symphysis.[1]

During the second decade of the twentieth century, measurements of the pelvis became more complex with the introduction of stereoradiography to pelvimetry.[9-11] One of these articles contained the following advice[9]:

> Roentgen ray pelvimetry should not be resorted to in the early months of pregnancy, because of remote possibility of harm to the embryo. After the third month, however, no ill results should follow the short exposures necessary for this method of measurement. In fact, we believe that unhealthy conditions during gestation might be improved by moderate roentgenization. During the last two months of pregnancy it becomes more difficult if the patient is of the short and thick type, but at this time the added information of position of the fetus, the presence of single or twin pregnancy, and at least one diameter of the fetal head may be gained.

During the 1920s, there was an appreciation of the importance of pelvic shape and contour, rather than mere linear measurements in affecting the course of labor. For example, Caldwell and Moloy (1932) studied variations in pelvic shape and classified them into gynecoid, android, anthropoid, and platypelloid.[12] Although stressing that these variations in the female pelvis "are not associated with or caused by pathologic processes," they could have an adverse effect on delivery. The most dangerous form of pelvis was the android type, which resembled that of a human male. This could lead to "midpelvic arrest . . . where forceps are difficult to apply, and version and breech extraction is equally dangerous. If the extreme forms are identified before the onset of labor, elective cesarean section can be sanely advised." During this era, the early preoccupation with the pelvic inlet yielded to the realization that the size and shape of the midplane and also the pelvic outlet must be taken into consideration.[1]

In the mid-1930s, the importance of measurements of the fetal skull was recognized. Ball worked out a system of measuring the cubic volume of the pelvis and fetal skull in an attempt to quantitate cephalopelvic disproportion.[1] With Marchbanks, Ball developed an instrument called the *pelvicephalometer* and a circular chart to correct the various measurements for size of the object and film-object distance.[13] They considered the mean circumference of the fetal cranium to be more accurate than a simple measurement of its diameter in calculating the volume of the fetal skull. Clifford (1934) introduced a technique of stereoradiography in which the biparietal fetal head diameter could be accurately predicted in utero to within 0.3 cm.[14]

The standard pelvimetry technique that is still included in positioning textbooks was introduced in 1944 by Colcher and Sussman.[15] They divided the true pelvis into three levels (actual inlet, mid-pelvis, outlet) with intersecting anteroposterior and lateral diameters that included all the major bony landmarks of the pelvis. They included a ruler that could be elevated, lowered, and rotated so that it was always parallel with the tabletop and film and thus gave the same degree of distortion as the pelvis itself. The ruler also permitted direct centimeter measurements on each

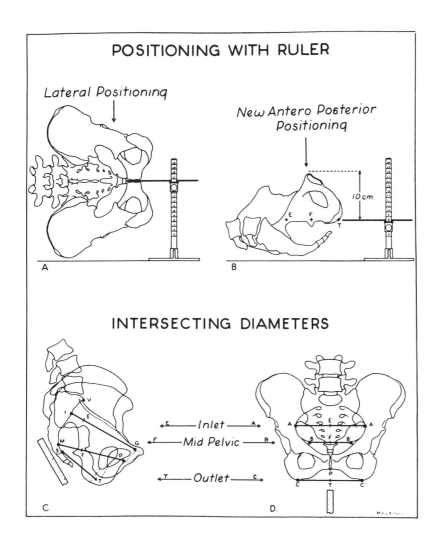

Colcher and Sussman technique for pelvimetry (1944). "*Top left and right*, Diagrams showing lateral and anteroposterior positions with ruler. *Bottom left and right*, Diagrams of the three pelvic levels with intersecting diameters. Inlet, Actual anteroposterior diameter of inlet line *G-I* crosses through inlet transverse diameter *A-A'*. Mid-pelvis, Anteroposterior diameter *P-M* crosses transverse diameter *B-B'*. Outlet, Anteroposterior diameter of outlet *T-S* bisects midpoint of transverse diameter line *C-C'*."[15]

351

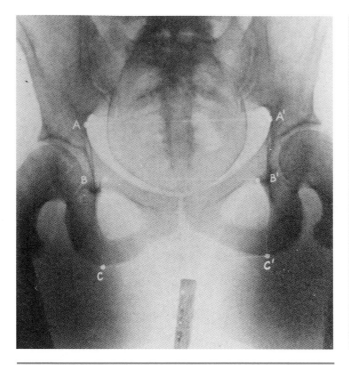

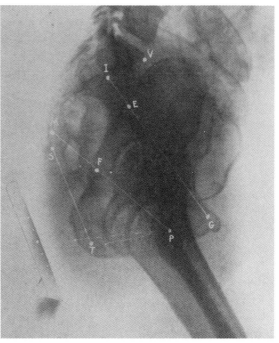

Anteroposterior pelvimetry radiograph (as in diagram of previous illustration). *A-A'*, Transverse diameter of the inlet; *B-B'*, transverse diameter of the mid-pelvis at the level of the ischial spines; *C-C'*, transverse diameter of outlet at level of tuberosities of the ischium. Centimeter ruler markings on radiograph used for measurements.[15]

Lateral pelvimetry radiograph. Line *G-V* is textbook true conjugate; *G-I*, anteroposterior diameter of actual inlet; *P-M*, anteroposterior diameter of mid-pelvis; *T-S*, anteroposterior diameter of outlet. Centimeter ruler markings on radiograph used for measurements.[15]

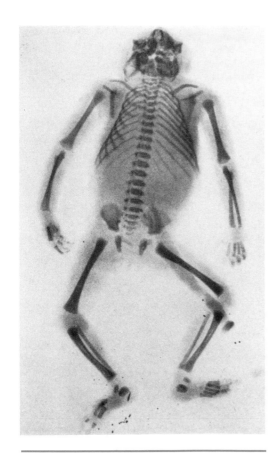

Anencephaly on a postpartum radiograph (1917).[19]

film without need for correction tables. Only two exposures were required, an anteroposterior and lateral view. They could be taken at any distance since any magnification could be corrected by the ruler. When presenting in the midline, the fetal head could be measured in both the lateral and anteroposterior projections.

RADIOGRAPHIC STUDIES OF THE FETUS

As early as 1898, Imbert performed an x-ray examination on a case of extrauterine pregnancy.[16] Edling (1911) reported a series of abnormalities in pregnancy studied radiographically. He showed several cases of twins and one of triplets and was able to decide whether a pelvic mass was due to tumor or pregnancy.[17] Marshall[18] reported a lithopedion, Case (1917)[19] successfully diagnosed anencephaly before birth, and Hess (1917)[20] analyzed the appearance of ossification centers to radiographically determine fetal age. In the 1940s, Jenkinson and co-workers were able to recognize achondroplasia fetalis in utero[21] and to diagnose osteopetrosis prenatally.[22]

Matthews (1930) stated that "we feel sure that no pregnancy, regardless of its stage of development, is damaged by diagnostic roentgenology properly carried out."[23] He noted that the fetal skeleton could be radiographically demonstrated as early as the fourteenth to fifteenth week. Matthews stressed the value of radiographs in making a positive diagnosis of pregnancy complicating fibroids of the uterus and in differentiating between pregnancy and other pelvic tumors such as fibroids and ovarian cysts. "Today the surgeon or gynecologist who removes a fibroid uterus that contains a four or five months' pregnancy may well feel chagrined and indeed not be surprised if suit is instituted against him for malpractice." In his series, "the diagnosis of anencephalic monster was made five times before delivery was accomplished, thereby enabling the obstetrician to fortify himself against criticism by informing the family (never the patient!) of the presence of a fetal monster." Matthews also reported two instances in which a preoperative radiograph demonstrating hydrocephaly or anencephaly could have spared the patient a cesarean section. Therefore he urged that "every patient who is a candidate for cesarean section should have a roentgenogram taken to determine the normalcy of the child."

A difficult clinical dilemma was the question of fetal death. In 1922, Spalding[24] and Horner[25] in independent studies noted that overlapping of the cranial bones before the onset of labor was a sign of intrauterine death. It was later shown that a minimal degree of overlapping could develop in a living fetus. Szello[26] and Kehrer[27], also working independently in 1931, noted that marked bending or angulation of the spinal column was an early sign of fetal demise. Thoms[28] reported that lack of change in the position of the fetal bones of the extremities on serial radiographs was evidence of intrauterine death. The presence of gas in the fetal circulatory system, best seen on lateral projection, was reported as a sign of fetal death by Roberts in 1944.[29] Other less precise signs of fetal demise included a fetal bone size that did not correspond to the duration of pregnancy and a vague haziness of pelvic landmarks and contours, which represented a late case of fetal death in which the skeletal structures degenerated, the bones decalcified, and the soft tissue detail became blurred.[1]

PLACENTOGRAPHY

The radiographic demonstration of the site of placental attachment to the uterus permitted a diagnosis of placenta previa. In 1930, Menees and coworkers[30] described the technique of *amniography,* in which injection of a strontium iodide solution into the amniotic fluid outlined the fetus and placenta. After injection, they advised "to wait half an hour to an hour before taking the films, to permit an even diffusion through the amniotic cavity. During this time the patient changes position frequently to assist in the mixing." The placenta appeared as "a filling defect or a flattened area, best seen when caught in profile." In certain instances, it was possible to identify the sex of the fetus by noting the outline of the scrotum and to show the umbilical cord encircling the fetal neck. Menees and associates[30] also reported "a shadow in the region of the left costal margin of the fetus . . . has been interpreted as strontium solution in the fetal stomach, indicating that the swallowing of amniotic fluid must be of frequent occurrence." Although they reported "no injurious or toxic effects" to the mother or fetus in normal pregnancies, subsequent studies indicated that strontium iodide was quite toxic and tended to precipitate premature delivery. The injection of Uroselectan B into the amniotic sac was somewhat less toxic to the fetus but still tended to initiate premature delivery; for this reason contrast opacification of amniotic fluid never became a popular procedure because of the inherent danger to the fetus.

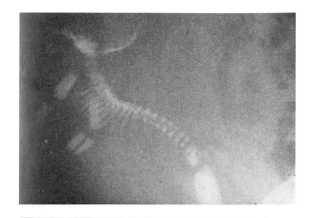

Prenatal diagnosis of osteopetrosis (1943). Lateral projection of maternal abdomen shows a fetus in utero with dense, widened, thickened bones.[22]

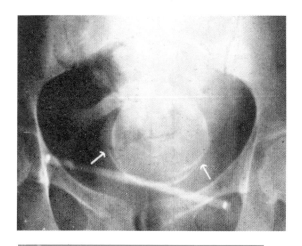

Spalding sign of fetal death (1922). Marked overlapping of the fetal skull bones (*arrows*) with some disproportion between the surface of the skull bones and the skull contents.[24]

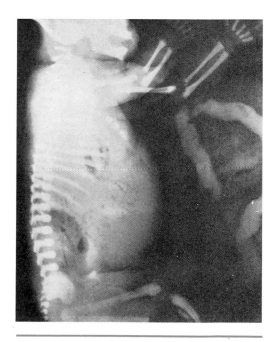

Roberts sign of fetal death (1944). Gas within the fetal circulatory system.[29]

Amniography (1930). *Left*, Posteroanterior radiograph and (*right*) tracing show the fetal small parts well outlined. Several loops of cord are visible. The breech shows no projecting shadow of a scrotum, justifying the diagnosis of a female fetus. The fetal stomach contains strontium iodide.[30]

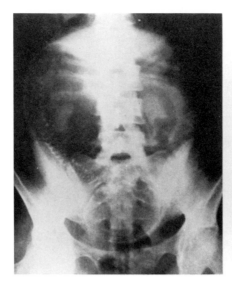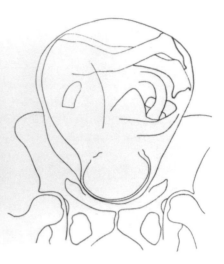

By partially filling the urinary bladder with radiopaque contrast, Ude and co-workers (1934) noted that in cases with placenta previa there was an increased distance between the opacified bladder and fetal head.[31] That same year, Snow[32] emphasized the value of studying the soft tissue pattern of the uterine wall, which was considerably thickened at the site where the placenta was attached. Ball and Golden (1941) noted that normally the "fetal head will dip into the pelvic inlet and occupy the mid-coronal and mid-sagittal planes of the superior strait when the mother is standing."[33] In placenta previa, there typically was some upward displacement of the fetal head since the interposed placenta did not permit the fetal head to completely descend. They cautioned that

> any pelvic tumor mass of sufficient size can displace the fetal head from the mid coronal or mid sagittal plane or prevent it from dipping below the level of the brim of the inlet. Such a mass might be a uterine fibroid, an ovarian cyst, an overdistended bladder or rectum, or the placenta implanted low in the uterus. All except the latter can be ruled out by the usual methods of examination.

Placenta previa (1934). *Left*, Radiograph and *right*, diagram show upward displacement of the fetal head by the pelvic mass lying between it and the upper margin of the bladder.[31]

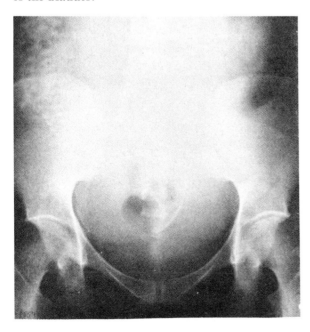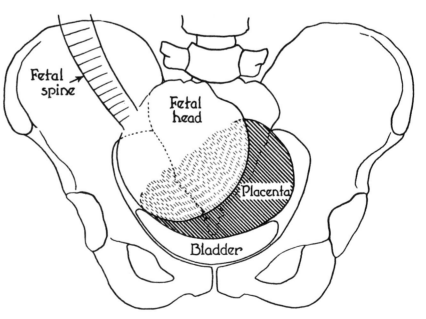

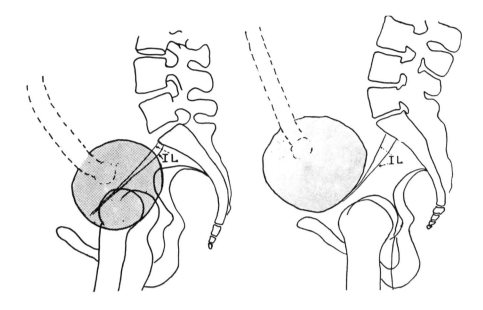

An invasive technique for diagnosing placenta previa was reported by Hartnett (1948), who injected opaque contrast material into the internal iliac artery via the femoral artery.[34] Although opacification of the placental vessels provided definite evidence of the site of placental attachment, this method was far too difficult and dangerous for general use.

ULTRASOUND

Because it does not use ionizing radiation and thus gives no x-ray exposure to the fetus, ultrasound has rapidly become the diagnostic modality of choice for imaging the pregnant woman. The initial application of ultrasound as a diagnostic study in obstetrics and gynecology was the work of Ian Donald and colleagues from the University of Glasgow's Department of Midwifery in the early 1950s. Ironically, Donald's work was initially slowed by fears at grant-giving institutions that ultrasound might possibly have toxic effects on the fetus and mother.[35]

In his initial experiment, Donald utilized an ultrasonic metal flaw detector to identify echo patterns from excised uterine fibroids and ovarian tumors. However, for clinical work his detector could only operate successfully through a water-filled tank at some distance from the patient's skin. The difficulties caused by this arrangement led to his consideration of various alternatives and ultimately to the development of the contact scanner. By 1957, Donald and an engineer, Tom Brown, had designed and constructed a prototype hand-operated, 2-dimensional contact scanner. The primary advantage of contact scanning (now universally used clinically for ultrasound imaging of the pelvis and abdomen) was the elimination of the inconvenience related to the sound-transmitting water tank. The transducer probe could be placed in direct contact with the patient's skin and acoustic coupling achieved by the use of an oil or jelly.[37]

Donald and co-workers had their earliest successes in gynecology (1956). Using A-mode equipment they distinguished between ascites, ovarian cysts, and fibroid tumors on the basis of their echo patterns. In obstetrics, the A-mode equipment initially was used to measure fetal

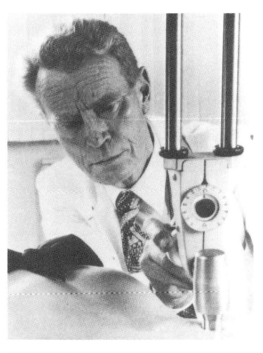

Ian Donald performing an ultrasound scan using a contact compound scanner of his design.[36]

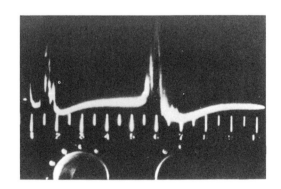

A-mode sonogram (1955) produced by Donald using his flaw-detection equipment. The sonogram shows two spike echoes separated by a clear sonolucent area, which was the recognized A-mode echo display of an ovarian cyst.[36]

355

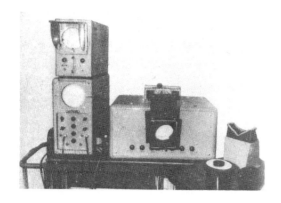

Ultrasound recording apparatus showing three cathode-ray tubes with camera folded back over the cathode-ray tube on the right (1958).[38]

biparietal diameter, which essentially represented in utero echoencephalography because of the nonreflective quality of the fluid-filled uterus and the thin skull of the fetus. This technique allowed obstetrical personnel to evaluate the rate of fetal growth, to estimate fetal weight at the time of measurement, to screen for certain abnormalities such as hydrocephaly, and to assess fetal head size close to delivery to determine possible fit through the birth canal.[36] However, the unidimensional method of recording was severely limited, since it was not possible to determine the exact origin of the recorded echoes. In 1958, Donald and co-workers reported the application of 2-dimensional ultrasound (in conjunction with compound contact scanning) to obstetrics and gynecology.[38] They also established sonographic criteria for the diagnosis of hydatidiform mole[39] and contributed greatly to the development of fetal cephalometry and the study of the "blighted ovum."[37] Although they realized that "ultrasonic diagnosis is still very crude and the preoperative diagnosis of histological structure is still far off, such a possibility in the future is an exciting prospect."

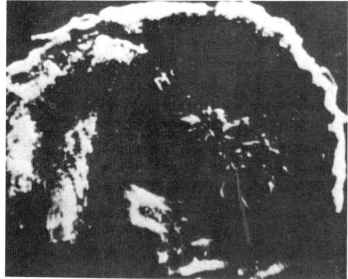

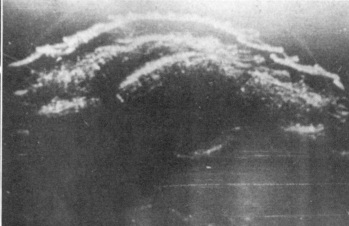

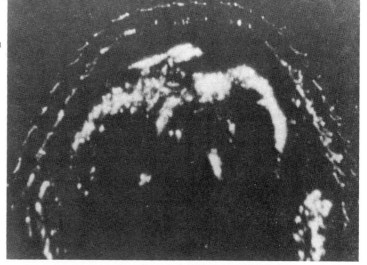

Early ultrasound scans (1958). *Top*, Very large complex ovarian cystadenoma. *Top right*, Outline of fetal skull at 34 weeks' gestation (suprapubic scan). *Right*, Twins, both in breech position (scanning across fundus of uterus).[38]

Donald and his colleagues[40] were the first to describe the "full bladder technique," whereby the distended urinary bladder displaces bowel loops out of the pelvis and becomes a "sonolucent" window to the uterus and ovaries. This simplified the examination and permitted better ultrasound images of the pelvic organs.[41] Following the successes of Donald's group, several other researchers worldwide began applying ultrasonic diagnosis in obstetrics and gynecology. In the United States, a compound contact scanner to replace the previous water bath was constructed in 1962 by a group at the University of Colorado. Because of its compact design, flexibility, and ease of use at the bedside, this instrument made an immediate commercial impact. Utilizing this scanner, extensive obstetric and gynecological studies were initiated by Horace Thompson and Kenneth Gottesfeld, working in the clinical ultrasound program under Joseph Holmes. In addition to being among the earliest investigators to visualize and describe the echo pattern of the placenta,[42] Thompson and Gottesfeld applied both A-mode and B-mode techniques to a wide range of clinical problems, including the evaluation of abdominal cysts and tumors, determination of the presence of twins and placenta previa, measurement of fetal biparietal diameter, and the detection of abnormal fetal growth patterns.[43]

Since those early days, ultrasound has become the major technique for evaluating fetal age, congenital anomalies, and complications of pregnancy. Because the traditional parameters used by obstetricians to assess gestational age (e.g., date of last menstrual period, size of the uterus, quickening, first fetal heart tones) are frequently unavailable or impre-

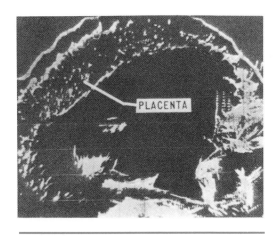

Placental scan (1963), showing the echo pattern of the anteriorly placed placenta in the upper left.[36]

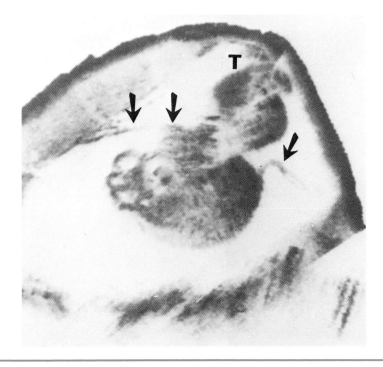

Omphalocele. Transverse sonogram shows a small fetal trunk (*T*) and herniated bowel and viscera within a covering membrane (*arrows*). Note that the covering membrane is distended by ascites.[50]

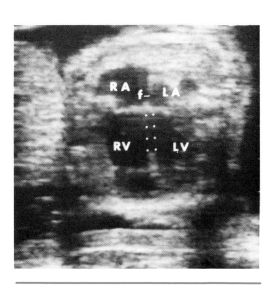

Ventricular septal defect (*white dots*) in a fetus with tetralogy of Fallot. *RA*, Right atrium; *LA*, left atrium; *RV*, right ventricle; *LV*, left ventricle; *f*, foramen ovale.[51]

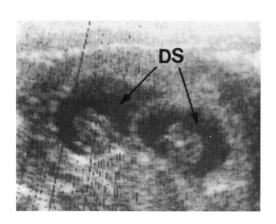

Ultrasound of twin pregnancy. *DS,*
Decidual sacs.

cise, ultrasound has become the major modality for estimating fetal age. Ultrasound can directly visualize the fetus, thus allowing the measurement of anatomical structures that reflect fetal growth and permitting comparison of these measurements with reference standards observed during normal pregnancies.[44,46] The first sonographic parameter used to assess gestational age was the longest biparietal diameter, usually measured at the level of the thalami. Subsequently, it was shown that the crown-rump length measurement was much more accurate in assessing gestational age in early pregnancy (less than 11 weeks). Ultrasound also has been used to diagnose multiple pregnancies, to detect abnormalities in the volume of amniotic fluid (often associated with underlying fetal anomalies), and assessing intrauterine growth retardation.[47] Because clinically significant errors of morphological development occur in up to 5% of all children, the ability of ultrasound to detect these anomalies in utero may permit in utero medical or surgical therapy, provide an indication for termination of the pregnancy, or influence the mode of delivery. Among the abnormalities that can be detected and often treated in utero are osseous and neural anomalies of the fetal cranium and spine, gastrointestinal atresias and developmental cysts, cystic and obstructive lesions of the genitourinary tract, congenital cardiac lesions, and short-limbed dwarfism syndromes.[48]

Ultrasound has become the major imaging modality for diagnosing ectopic pregnancy. In addition to showing an enlarged uterus that does not contain a gestational sac and is associated with an irregular adnexal mass and "ectopic fetal head," or fluid in the cul-de-sac indicating ectopic pregnancy, ultrasound can effectively exclude this diagnosis by the unequivocal demonstration of an intrauterine pregnancy (double decidual sac, small fetal pole, or the presence of movement or cardiac activity), since the incidence of coexisting ectopic and intrauterine pregnancies is only 1 in 30,000.[49] It also can well demonstrate the spectrum of pregnancy disorders ranging from benign hydatidiform mole to the more malignant and frequently metastatic choriocarcinomas.

GYNECOLOGICAL RADIOLOGY

The development of gynecological radiography can be divided into three phases. Before 1912, no contrast material was available and radiographic diagnosis was limited to detection of abnormalities that were inherently either more opaque or lucent than normal tissues. The second phase used gas as a contrast medium, while the third used opaque contrast agents.[1]

In the early days of radiography, a variety of metallic foreign bodies were detected in the bladder, uterus, and vagina. Calcified dermoid cysts and uterine fibroids were visualized, and a didelphic uterus and vagina were demonstrated by means of metal sounds.

The detailed vascular anatomy of the female genital tract was shown radiographically by several experimenters who injected opaque contrast material into specimens and cadavers during the first decade of the twentieth century. Perhaps the first invasive procedure in a live patient was performed by Schick,[35] who bravely injected bismuth salts into an abscess cavity that complicated the removal of a parametrial cyst. The abscess was drained and healed promptly.

Pneumoperitoneum

> The radiological examination of a bladder filled with oxygen, where the stone, as well as the hypertrophied prostate, appeared quite clearly on the picture (cystoscopic control) caused the thought to occur to me . . . that the introduction of sterile, inactive oxygen or air into the abdominal cavity could possibly make visible many organs, tumors and abdominal cavity areas which until now had not been accessible to radiological examination, or if so, with difficulty or by means of devious methods.

So began Eugen Weber (1913)[52] in an article describing his experimental studies with diagnostic pneumoperitoneum. One year later, E. Rautenberg (1914) described pneumoperitoneum in living humans.[53] Although neither of these articles specifically dealt with gynecological problems, it was clear that gas introduced into the peritoneal cavity could outline the peritoneal surfaces of the pelvic organs. The first specific applications of pneumoperitoneum to pelvic radiography were by Otto Goetze (1918) and by Arthur Stein and William Stewart (1919). Goetze[54] noted that

> the pelvic organs can, of course, only be differentiated by means of the introduction of gas into the peritoneal cavity through the simultaneous use of a highly elevated position of the pelvis combined with a great variety of lateral positions. Even in the knee-elbow position all of the movable parts drop out of the true pelvis. At first I needed the aid of other procedures to visualize the uterus, viz., inflation of the rectum with a rubber balloon and elevation away from the vagina of the very difficultly movable uterus either digitally or by tamponade. But it is now a very easy matter for me to visualize any uterus and usually also the ovaries fluoroscopically or roentgenographically, simply by a correct positioning of the patient without any such additional procedures.

Stein and Stewart[55] were able to "demonstrate not only the normal uterus with its round ligaments, small cystic ovaries and normal bladder but also myomatous tumors of the uterus, which, as is well known, have not

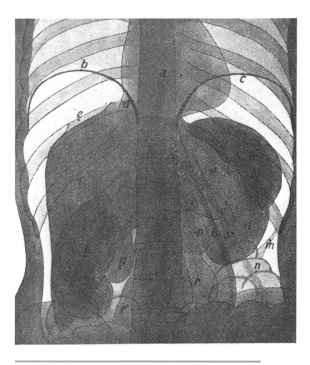

Diagnostic pneumoperitoneum (1918). *a,* Heart; *b,c,* hemidiaphragms; *d,* inferior vena cava; *e,* coronary ligament; *f,* right lobe of liver; *g,* gallbladder; *h,i,* kidneys; *k,* spleen; *l,* left lobe of liver; *m,* left colic ligament; *n,* splenic flexure of colon; *o,* greater curvature of stomach; *p,* pancreas; *r,* loop of small intestine.[54]

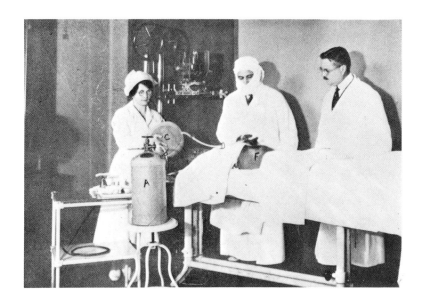

Technique of inflation of the peritoneal cavity with gas (1919). "*A,* Gas tank; *B,* section of rubber tubing connecting tank with inlet of bag; *C,* rubber bag distended with gas. Gentle pressure being made by nurse forcing gas into peritoneal cavity. *D,* Section of rubber tubing connecting outlet of bag with needle; *E,* needle during inflation. Note the angle. *F,* Peritoneal cavity becoming distended with gas."[55]

359

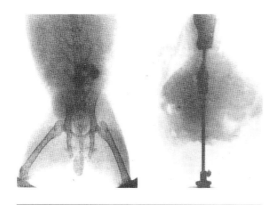

Collargol studies of the uterine cavity (1914).[57]

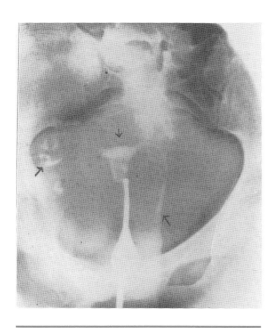

Collargol study of the uterus and fallopian tubes (1916). Elevation of the left tube and downward displacement of the tube on the right. The right tube was closed at the fimbriated end, while the left was patent and permitted a small amount of contrast to escape into the peritoneal cavity.[60]

heretofore been rontgenographically demonstrated." Using a tilting table (15 degrees Trendelenburg) with sandbags under the pelvis of the laterally positioned patient, "the intestines drop out of the pelvis and are replaced by oxygen, which surrounds the fixed organs."

Although some early workers used pelvic pneumoperitoneography with considerable success, the theoretical danger of gas emboli substantially limited its popular acceptance. The use of quickly absorbable gases, such as carbon dioxide and nitrous oxide, eliminated much of the danger from gas embolization.[1]

Hysterosalpingography

The introduction of contrast material into the uterine cavity was first performed by Walter Rindfleisch, who injected a liquid paste of bismuth via a long uterine syringe.[56] Four years later (1914), I. C. Rubin filled the uterine cavity with Collargol to demonstrate such abnormalities as "myomas, corpus carcinomas, uterine polyps, uterus bicornis, etc."[57] Ironically, Rubin stressed the need to exercise care lest the opaque material pass through the fallopian tubes and into the peritoneal space. "In cases of infected uterine contents (suppurative endometritis and infected carcinoma) the danger of ascending infection should not be overlooked, and this diagnostic method is not recommended in such cases." The use of Collargol was soon abandoned because it produced severe irritation of the peritoneal cavity and was reported to produce mucosal irritation of the fallopian tubes and even obstructive inspissation of a tube that had previously been patent. A variety of silver, thorium, and iodine solutions also proved to be too irritating to use safely.

In the same year, working independently, William H. Cary of New York used Collargol in a deliberate attempt to demonstrate tubal pregnancy.[58] As he wrote, "The principle is simple. If the tube be patent the shadow (of opaque contrast) extends throughout its length and irregularly into the lateral pelvis. The obstructed tube shows a shortened shadow."

Finally, in 1920, Rubin reported his method of using the intrauterine insufflation of oxygen to determine patency of the fallopian tubes[59]:

> If the gas injected into the uterus under certain measurable pressure would pass into the fallopian tubes, it ought to reach the general peritoneal cavity. In patients with patent fallopian tubes the gas would establish an artificial pneumoperitoneum identical with that produced when injected by direct abdominal puncture. In patients with occluded tubes no such result could be obtained.

If the tubes were patent, the pelvic organs could be studied radiographically. "The method has practically the value of an exploratory laparotomy for purposes of determining the continuity of the lumen of the fallopian tubes."

The Rubin test became widely accepted in the diagnosis of sterility from tubal obstruction. Although Rubin noted that "the two possible dangers, namely, embolism and infection, are more theoretical than actual," the original test was later modified by Alvarez, who showed that carbon dioxide was more quickly absorbed and theoretically less dangerous.[1]

In 1925, Williams and Reynolds[61] experimented with barium sulfate as a contrast agent for hysterosalpingography. Unfortunately, this opaque material caused peritoneal granulomas and adhesions and was quickly discarded.

The next major advance in hysterosalpingography was the use of Lipiodol by Carlos Heuser in 1921.[62] Heuser initially used the oil-based contrast for the early diagnosis of pregnancy and claimed that Lipiodol did not produce abortions. "Hitherto we have had no means of trustworthy diagnosis of pregnancy in the first months. The problem is a serious one, for in all maternity homes there are records of cases of early pregnancy which have been operated on for fibroma." Heuser also noted that "the radiographs may thus allow us to diagnose sterility due to obstruction of the tubes; for it may be observed that they do not fill or fill up badly. In cases of pyosalpingitis and old salpingitis a radiograph of the tubes can be obtained and the diagnosis confirmed." He noted that "during the injection the eyes of the patient must be observed, for the pupil is dilated when the liquid enters the tubes. The pupillary reaction is characteristic. When the injection enters the tube it produces a little colic, and first there is a dilatation and afterwards a contraction of the pupils. If the woman has had salpingitis, this reaction is much stronger, but the passing of the liquid through the tube does not cause any pain."

Later authors demonstrated uterine anomalies, ectopic pregnancy, and uterine carcinoma by Lipiodol hysterosalpingography. A combination of pneumoperitoneum and hysterosalpingography[63,64] produced superb radiographs that outlined the serosal coverings and lumens of the uterus and tubes, as well as the peritoneal surfaces of the ovaries.

In 1942, Kjellberg reported a new method of hysterosalpingography using the newer and less toxic water-soluble contrast agents used for urography.[65] An injection of contrast through the uterus and fallopian tubes and into the peritoneal cavity could outline both the lumens and peritoneal surfaces of the genital tract. In addition, the ovaries, pouch of Douglas, and small bowel loops in the pelvis could be seen.

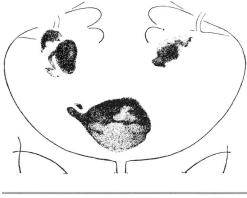

Williams and Reynolds (1925) method for determining patency of the fallopian tubes. Following insufflation of barium sulfate into the cervix of a normal woman, contrast material is found in the uterine cavity and distal portions of the tubes and their fimbriated extremities.[61]

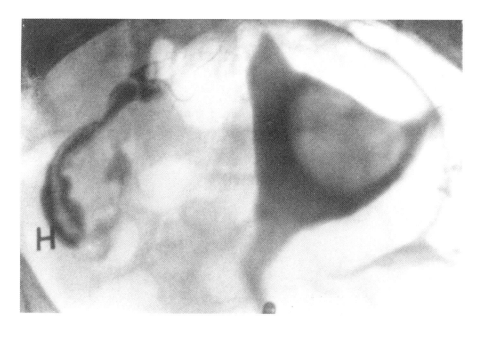

Hysterosalpingography with water-soluble contrast (1942). Large submucous myoma in an enlarged uterus. Free tubal passage on both sides. The right tube is slightly dilated within the ampullary port (*H*) and the longitudinal fold formation is distinctly shown.[65]

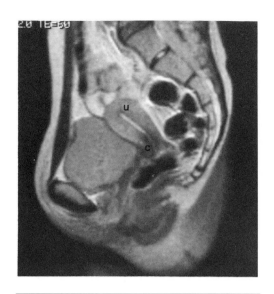

NEWER IMAGING MODALITIES

Both computed tomography (CT) and magnetic resonance (MR) imaging have had substantial impact on the evaluation of gynecological disease. In most centers, CT has become the modality of choice for staging gynecological malignancy. In addition to showing tumor invasion of the parametrium, CT can directly delineate the tumor mass and thus assist in the design of radiation treatment ports. Although MR imaging can more clearly demonstrate the primary neoplasm and is better than CT in determining the depth of myometrial invasion in endometrial cancer, it has not replaced CT for staging because it is less sensitive to extrauterine metastases, is more expensive, and requires a longer examination time. MR imaging appears to be of special value in determining the origin of large pelvic masses.

MR demonstration of normal pelvic anatomy. Sagittal image well demonstrates the uterus (u) and cervix (c). The uterine stroma appears as an intermediate-intensity signal. The endometrium is seen as a high-intensity signal area surrounded by the well-vascularized low-density signal region of the junctional zone.[67]

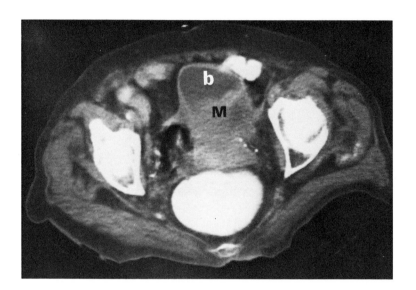

CT showing bladder invasion by endometrial carcinoma. The mass (M) obliterates the fat planes between the bladder (b) and uterus. Urine within the bladder outlines the irregular thickening of the posterior wall.[66]

References

1. Gould DM: Pioneer descriptions in obstetrical and gynecological roentgenology. In Bruwer AJ (ed): Classic descriptions in diagnostic roentgenology. Springfield, Ill, Charles C Thomas, 1964.

2. Brecher E and Brecher R: The rays: A history of radiology in the United States and Canada. Baltimore, Williams & Wilkins, 1969.

3. Davis EP: The application of the Röntgen rays. III. The study of the infant's body and of the pregnant womb by the Röntgen rays. Amer J Med Sci 3:263-269, 1896.

4. Varnier H, Chappuis J, Chauvel, and Funck-Brentano: A first encouraging result of intrauterine photography by x-rays. Annales de Gynécologie 45:185-190, March 1896.

5. Varnier H: Pelviography and pelvimetry by means of x-rays. Report to XIIth International Medical Congress in Moscow on August 23, 1897. (Cited in Bruwer, 1964.)

6. Levy M and Thumim L: A contribution to the evaluation of roentgen rays in obstetrics. Deutsch Med Wschr 23:507-509, 1897.

7. Fochier LA: An apparatus permitting precise measurements in radiographic experiments. Province Med Lyons 14:290-292, 1899.

8. Albert W: Concerning the value of roentgen rays in childbirth (with demonstration of roentgenograms). Centralbl für Gynäkologie 23:418-419, 1899.

9. Manges WF: Roentgenographic pelvimetry. Amer J Obstet Gynec 65:622-623, 1912.

10. Van Allen HW: Easy and accurate pelvimetry by roentgen ray. AJR 3:367-368, 1916.

11. Chamberlain WE and Newell RR: Pelvimetry by means of roentgen ray. AJR 8:272-276, 1921.

12. Caldwell WE and Moloy HC: Anatomical variations in the female pelvis and their effect in labor with a suggested classification. Amer J Obstet Gynec 26:479-505, 1933.

13. Ball RP and Marchbanks SS: Roentgen pelvimetry and fetal cephalometry: A new technic. Radiology 24:77-84, 1935.

14. Clifford SH: The x-ray measurement of the fetal head diameter in utero. Surg Gynec Obstet 58:727-736, 1934.

15. Colcher AE and Sussman W: A practical technique for roentgen pelvimetry with a new positioning. AJR 51:207-214, 1944.

16. Imbert MA: Radiographies d'artères et radiographie de grossesse extra-utérine. Comptes Rendus Soc Biol (Paris) 5:649, 1898.

17. Edling L: Über die Anwendung des Rontgenverfahrens bei der Diagnose der Schwangerschaft. Fortschr Rontgenstr 17:345-355, 1911.

18. Marshall E: Zur Diagnose eines Folles von Lithopadion mit Hilfe des Skiagrams. Fortsch Rontgenstr 4:115-116, 1900-1901.

19. Case JT: Anencephaly successfully diagnosed before birth. Surg Gynec Obstet 24:312-317, 1917.

20. Hess JH: The diagnosis of the age of the fetus by use of roentgenograms. Amer J Dis Child 14:397-423, 1917.

21. Jenkinson EL and Kinzer RE: Achondroplasia foetalis (chondrodystrophia foetalis). Radiology 37:581-587, 1941.

22. Jenkinson EL, Pfisterer WH, Lattier KK, and Martin M: A prenatal diagnosis of osteopetrosis. AJR 49:455-462, 1943.

23. Matthews HB: The roentgen ray as an adjunct in obstetric diagnosis. Amer J Obstet Gynec 20:612-632, 1930.

24. Spalding AB: A pathognomonic sign of intra-uterine death. Surg Gynec Obstet 34:754-757, 1922.

25. Horner DA: Roentgenography in obstetrics. Surg Gynec Obstet 35:67-71, 1922.

26. Szello F: Die Diagnose des intrauterinen Fruchttodes mit Hilfe der Röntgenphotographie. Arch Gynak 145:495-511, 1931.

27. Kehrer E: Zur Röntgendiagnose des intrauterinen Fruchttodes. Zbl Gynaek 55:2530-2540, 1931.

28. Thoms H: Observations on roentgenological evidence of fetal death. Surg Gynec Obstet 71:169-171, 1940.

29. Roberts JB: Gas in the fetal circulatory system as a sign of intrauterine fetal death. AJR 51:631-634, 1944.

30. Menees TO, Miller JD, and Holly LE: Amniography: Preliminary report. AJR 24:363-366, 1930.

31. Ude WH, Weum TW, and Urner JA: Roentgenologic diagnosis of placenta previa. AJR 31:230-233, 1934.

32. Snow W and Powell CB: Roentgen visualization of the placenta. AJR 31:37-40, 1934.

33. Ball RP and Golden R: A roentgenologic sign for the detection of placenta previa. Amer J Obstet Gynec 42:530-533, 1941.

34. Hartnett LJ: The possible significance of arterial visualization in the diagnosis of placenta previa. Amer J Obstet Gynec 55:940-952, 1948.

35. Schick R: Radiologische Untersuchungen einer der zweigten postoperativ entstandenen Abszesshöhlen. Zbl Gynaek 33:629-632, 1909.

36. Goldberg BB and Kimmelman BA: Medical diagnostic ultrasound: A retrospective on its fortieth anniversary. Eastman Kodak, 1988.

37. Holmes JH: Diagnostic ultrasound: Historical perspective. In King DL (ed): Diagnostic ultrasound. St. Louis, CV Mosby, 1984.

38. Donald I, MacVicar J, and Brown TG: Investigation of abdominal masses by pulsed ultrasound. Lancet 1:1188-1194, 1958.

39. MacVicar J and Donald I: Sonar in the diagnosis of early pregnancy and its complications. J Obstet Gynaecol Brit Commonw 70:387-395, 1963.

40. Donald I and Brown TG: Demonstration of tissue interfaces within the body by ultrasonic echo sounding. Brit J Radiol 34:539-543, 1961.

41. Azimi F, Bryan PJ, and Marangola JP: Ultrasonography in obstetrics and gynecology: Historical notes, basic principles, safety considerations, and clinical applications. CRC Crit Rev Clin Radiol Nucl Med 8:153-253, 1976.

42. Gottesfeld KR, Thompson HE, Holmes JH, and Taylor ES: Ultrasonic placentography: A new method for placenta localization. Amer J Obstet Gynecol 96:538-547, 1966.

43. Thompson HE, Holmes JH, Gottesfeld KR, and Taylor ES: Fetal development as determined by ultrasound pulse echo techniques. Amer J Obstet Gynecol 92:44-48, 1965.

44. Jeanty P and Romero R: Estimation of the gestational age. Semin Ultrasound CT MR 5:121-129, 1984.

45. Kurtz AB and Goldberg BB: Obstetrical measurements in ultrasound. Chicago, Year Book, 1988.

46. Sabbagha RE, Tamura RK, and Dal Compo S: Fetal dating by ultrasound. Semin Roentgenol 17:190-197, 1982.

47. Romero R and Jeanty P: The detection of fetal growth disorders. Semin Ultrasound CT MR 5:139-143, 1984.

48. Romero R, Pilu G, Jeanty P, Ghidini A, and Hobbins JC: Prenatal diagnosis of congenital anomalies. Norwalk, Conn, Appleton & Lange, 1988.

49. Callen PW: Ultrasonography in obstetrics and gynecology. Philadelphia, WB Saunders, 1983.

50. Mukuno DH, Lee TG, Hornsberger HR, et al: Sonography of the fetal gastrointestinal system. Semin Ultrasound CT MR 5:194-209, 1984.

51. DeVore GR: Fetal echocardiography. Semin Ultrasound CT MR 5:229-248, 1984.

52. Weber E: Concerning the significance of the introduction of oxygen or air into the abdominal cavity for experimental and diagnostic radiology. Fortschr Rontgenstr 20:453-455, 1913.

53. Rautenberg E: Radiography of liver, the spleen and the diaphragm. Verhandl d Deutschen Kongresses f innere Medizin, Wiesbaden 31:305-307, 1914.

54. Goetze O: Roentgen diagnosis in the gas-filled abdominal cavity: A new method. Muenchen Med Wschr 65:1275-1280, 1918.

55. Stein A and Stewart WH: Roentgen examination of the abdominal organs following oxygen inflation of the peritoneal cavity. Ann Surg 70:95-100, 1919.

56. Rindfleisch W: Representation of the uterine cavity. Berl Klin Wschr 17:780-781, 1910.

57. Rubin IC: X-ray diagnosis of tumors of the uterus by means of intrauterine collargol injections: Preliminary communication. Zbl Gynaek 38:658-660, 1914.

58. Cary WH: Note on determination of patency of fallopian tubes by the use of collargol and x-ray shadow. Amer J Obstet Dis Wom 69:462-464, 1914.

59. Rubin IC: Nonoperative determination of patency of fallopian tubes in sterility. Intrauterine inflation with oxygen, and production of an artificial pneumoperitoneum: Preliminary report. JAMA 74:1017, 1920.

60. Gottleib C and Rubin I: Collargol injection of the uterus and tubes. AJR 3:257-260, 1916.

61. Williams E and Reynolds RJ: Method of determining the patency of the fallopian tubes by x-rays. Brit Med J 1:691-692, 1925.

62. Heuser C: Lipiodol in the diagnosis of pregnancy. Lancet 2:1111-1112, 1925.

63. Carelli HH, Gandulfo R, and Ocampo A: The radiographic examination in gynecology. Semana Med 32:85-88, 1925.

64. Stein IF and Arens RA: Iodized oil and pneumoperitoneum combined in gynecologic diagnosis: Preliminary report. JAMA 87:1299, 1926.

65. Kjellberg SR: Acta Radiol (Suppl) 43:1-179, 1942.

66. Gross BH and Callen PW: Ultrasound of the uterus. In Callen PW (ed): Ultrasonography in obstetrics and gynecology. Philadelphia, WB Saunders, 1990.

67. Thoeni RF and Margulis AR: Introduction. In Eisenberg RL (ed): Diagnostic imaging: An algorithmic approach. Philadelphia, JB Lippincott, 1988.

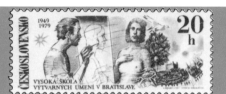

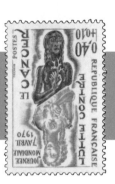

CHAPTER 20

Breast Radiology

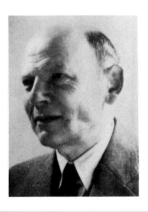

Albert Salomon.

The first report of radiography of the breast was made in 1913 by Albert Salomon, a German surgeon. He studied approximately 3,000 mastectomy specimens in an attempt to correlate the radiographic picture with the gross and microscopic anatomy of breast tumors. Salomon's primary concern was to study the extent and mode of spread of breast cancer so that a more adequate biopsy specimen could be removed at the time of surgery.[1]

Salomon's most important observation was the recognition that an x-ray film gave a true picture of the margins and extent of a tumor. He described the radiographic appearance of the most common forms of breast cancer, clearly differentiating the scirrhous or infiltrating type from the circumscribed or nodular form. Salomon identified the punctate calcifications characteristic of ductal carcinoma, although this was not recognized as a separate pathological entity until many years later. Salomon also reported the first "clinically occult" breast cancer found by radiographic examination. In this case the breast had been removed because of a large palpable cyst. Histological sections taken from the obvious lesion were reported as benign by the pathologist. However, the specimen radiograph not only showed the large, rounded, sharply defined cyst but also a tiny, dense, spiculated tumor with the typical appearance of a scirrhous carcinoma. Unfortunately, the gross specimen in this case was lost or discarded before the films became available for study so that no real confirmation could be made.[1]

For more than a decade, there were no references to breast radiography in the medical literature. There were two major reasons for this lack of clinical interest. First, radiography of the breast was technically difficult, and the quality of the resulting radiographs was poor. Perhaps more important, Halstead (1898) and Steinthal (1905) had reported markedly improved survival rates after radical mastectomy and axillary lymph node resection for breast cancer. Because it was generally accepted that every palpable nodule must be removed surgically and examined histologically, there was little interest in further diagnostic methods.[2]

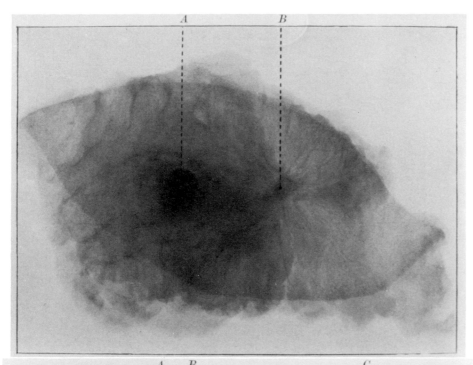

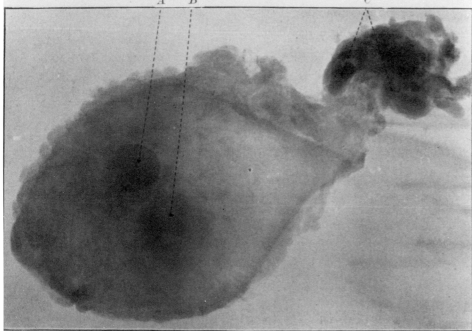

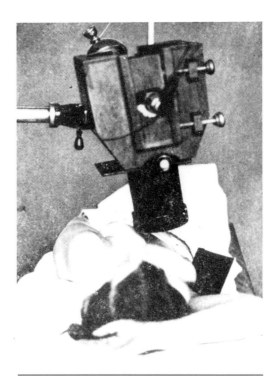

Mammography apparatus of Vogel (1932).[4]

Earliest radiography of the breast (1913). *Top*, "Chronic mastitis and carcinoma solidum. Radiating extensions between the nipple (*A*) and a carcinoma the size of a hazel nut (*B*), and extending beyond the nipple, cystadenomatous proliferation. Together with the small carcinoma, this constitutes the tumor that clinically is the size of an egg." *Bottom*, "Movable tumor. *A*, Nipple; *B*, sharply delimited tumor with a process extending to the nipple; *C*, carcinomatous axillary glands."[1]

In the 1920s, several independent groups began investigating clinical radiography of the breast. The earliest report by Otto Kleinschmidt (1927) came from the surgical clinic at the University of Leipzig under the directorship of Erwin Payr.[3] Another member of the Leipzig group was Walter Vogel, who in 1932 proposed a radiographic classification of various benign lesions and discussed their differential diagnosis from carcinoma.[4] The other major paper from this clinic, by Finsterbusch and Gross (1934), described an unusual type of ductal calcification that was later shown to represent secretory disease.[5]

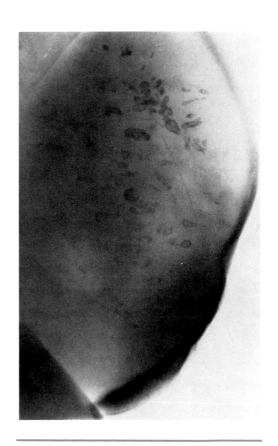

X-ray of the left breast with tumor shadows and calcification (1934).[5]

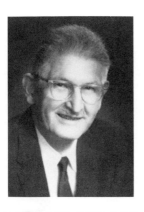

Stafford L. Warren.

In the United States, the pioneering work in breast imaging was performed by Stafford L. Warren, a radiologist in Rochester, N.Y. While trying to standardize the techniques in his new x-ray department for the interpretation and measurements of the thoracic aorta, Warren noted that the breast was silhouetted on the 6-foot oblique views of the chest. When fluoroscoping the chest, he began examining the breasts at various angles and found that by putting the arm over the head, an oblique anteroposterior exposure would clearly show the breast and the axillary fossa. After multiple trials, Warren decided that the optimal technique was to make stereoscopic films of each breast. A steady position for these two stereoscopic radiographs could be achieved by placing the patient in the recumbent semi-oblique position on a wooden table with sandbags under the opposite shoulder and with the patient retracting the opposite breast from the x-ray beam.[6]

Warren made extensive studies of surgical pathological specimens and cadavers by radiography and correlated them with gross dissection and histopathological study. He contributed some excellent descriptions of the normal gland at rest and during pregnancy and differentiated the normal radiographic appearance from that of the surprisingly common dysplastic gland. Warren used sequential x-ray films to study breast changes over a prolonged period and stressed the need for radiographing both breasts, with the opposite side being taken for comparison.

Initially, Warren's surgical colleagues did not take his work seriously until he made some astounding diagnoses of small tumors. In his initial publication (1930), Warren reported 119 patients, of whom 58 had histopathological evidence of malignancy. Only 8 cases (4 of which were malignant) were misdiagnosed, resulting in an incredible accuracy rate of almost 93%.[7]

Warren's report on breast radiography stirred considerable interest in the procedure. Numerous articles by radiologists and surgeons in the United States and Europe appeared in the literature in the early 1930s. Among the most important were Paul S. Seabold and Ira H. Lockwood. Seabold[8] stressed that

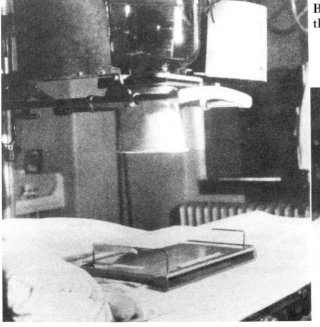

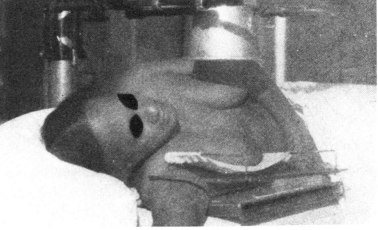

Breast radiography (1933). *Left*, General setup. *Below*, Position of the patient.[8]

it is not always possible to diagnose lesions of the breast by physical examination with the degree of accuracy necessary for a definite, therapeutic decision, particularly in the heavy, massive breast. A study of the breast by a roentgenographic method will demonstrate changes in the internal architecture of the organ not only in the normal, but also the pathological breast during the cycles of menstruation and pregnancy, and in tumors.

Lockwood[9] noted that

> the roentgen examination offers a diagnostic method in the study of diseases of the breast that is comparable to the gross examination of excised tissue. The pathological state responsible for any of the cardinal presenting breast symptoms, tumor, pain or discharge from the nipple, can often be recognized without exploratory section. The need for biopsy can be reduced in many tumors that are clinically only suspicious, but proved to be roentgenologically characteristic.

Nevertheless, Lockwood acknowledged several limitations of the radiographic method "shared by any method of gross observation: The inability to recognize, (a) microscopic areas of cancer, (b) early malignant degeneration in benign tumors and (c) early carcinoma associated with chronic cystic mastitis."

In general, most articles noted the potential value of breast radiography but reported rather erratic and discouraging results that usually were due to the inferior quality of the radiographs. Disregarding Warren's advice, many workers apparently paid little attention to the basic principles of technically good radiography of the breast and concentrated instead on various gadgets, positions, and injection techniques.[6] An important diagnostic sign—punctate calcifications found in 30% of all cancer cases—went unrecognized in series after series. The calcific deposits were not visualized on the films or, if seen, were confused with artifacts.[7] Another major problem was Warren's own high accuracy rate. Although he admitted that his patient population was highly selected and contained a large number of advanced cancers, subsequent workers became discouraged when their results in unselected series were far poorer.

In view of the technical difficulties in obtaining high-quality radiographs of the breast, various invasive techniques were proposed. Emil Ries (1930) succeeded in demonstrating a tumor of the lactiferous ducts by injecting Lipiodol.[10] Unfortunately, "seven weeks after the injection, the woman began to have pain in the nontumorous breast" related to abscess formation. N. Frederick Hicken (1937) fully developed this method by introducing thorotrast directly into the milk ducts.[11] This procedure, which gave "an accurate roentgenographic pattern of the ductal and secretory system of the mammary gland," he termed *mammography*. Hicken noted that

> tumors originating in the periductal tissues or sequestrated cysts which do not have a patent communication with the estuaries of the nipple cannot be visualized by injecting the milk ducts. In such instances, an exploring needle is plunged directly into the tumor mass and if cystic, its contents are aspirated and replaced by air or other contrast media. When air is used, the "aeromammograms" clearly depict the limiting walls of the cysts, denoting whether they are single, multilocular, or papillomatous.

Several years later, numerous reports warned of the dangerous sequelae of injecting radiopaque substances into the ductal system of the breast. Initial complications were mastitis and abscess; subsequently, cancers were reported years after the use of thorotrast.[12]

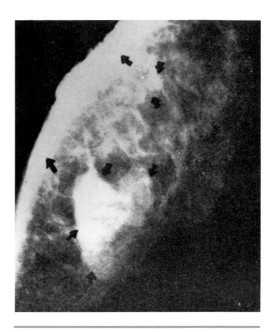

Radiograph of a section of the right breast through site of nipple showing infiltration of skin by tumor (1930). Tumor masses of all sizes are visible within the breast substance.[7]

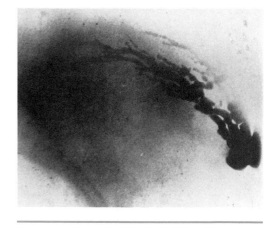

Initial study of the entire milk ductal system after Lipiodol injection (1930).[10]

Mammography (1936).[11] *Left*, Cannulization of milk ducts with a blunt no. 25-gauge needle using aseptic technique. *Right*, Injection of thorotrast into a bleeding duct shows two definite filling defects in the ductal lumen representing pedunculated papillomas.

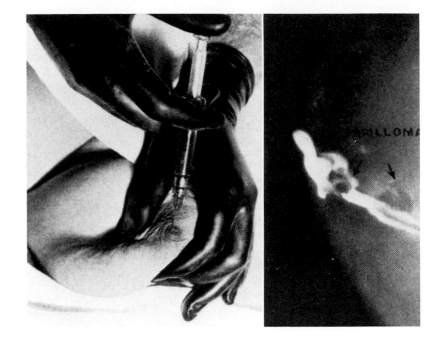

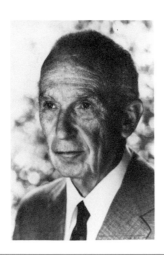

Raul Leborgne.

Mammography technique (1951). Position of the patient for obtaining a craniocaudal film (*below*) and a lateral view (*below right*). Note the cone and the compression pad interposed between it and the breast below. The film, enclosed in a black paper envelope, is in contact with the breast.[14]

Pneumomammography, the injection of air into the retromammary space in an attempt to obtain better visualization of lesions in the breast, was reported by Baraldi of Argentina in 1933.[13]

The next major contribution to radiography of the breast was by Raul Leborgne of Uruguay, who in 1951 published his discovery that microcalcifications were demonstrable in 30% of breast cancers.[14] He described the calcifications as "innumerable, punctate or slightly elongated, resembling grains of salt, and arranged in clusters." They could occur inside or outside the tumor shadow, or in the absence of a tumor shadow. Because these calcifications developed mainly in cancers of the intraductal type, which occur more frequently in dysplastic breasts, this sign provided an opportunity for tumor detection in a type of breast that had previously been the most difficult to examine both clinically and radiographically. In addition, since these neoplasms grew slowly, spread intraductally, and were typically asymptomatic, the ability of x-ray examinations to discover these tumors at an early stage made clinicians and surgeons realize more fully the diagnostic value of the method. As with other successful pioneers in breast imaging, Leborgne[14,15] stressed that "due to the complex pathology of the breast and to the small difference of opacity between normal and pathologic tissues, the roentgen study demands a perfect technique."

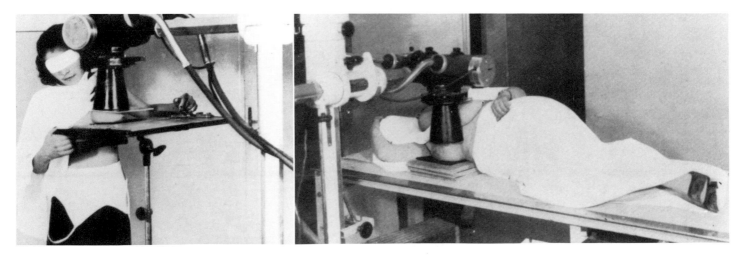

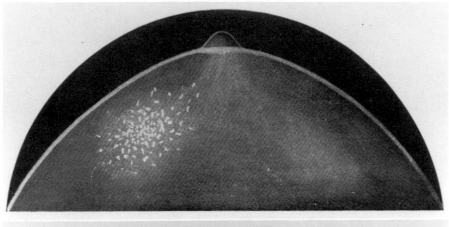

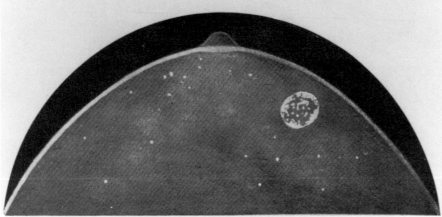

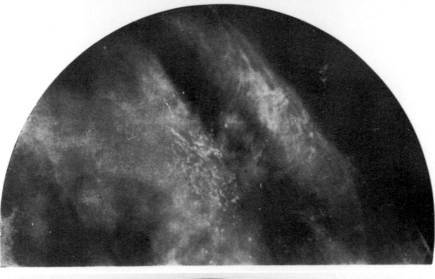

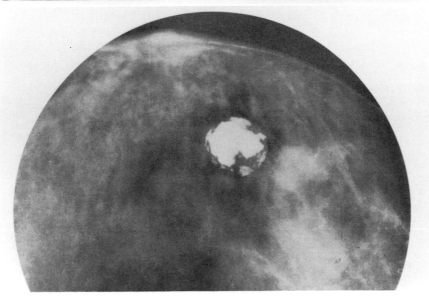

Diagrams of breast calcifications and coned compression views of the breast (1953). *Top*, Diagram of calcifications in carcinoma that appear as "scattering of countless, punctiform, or elongated calcifications, very closely grouped, particularly in center." *Middle*, Diagram of calcifications in fibrocystic disease appearing as "small calcifications in a circumscribed area, predominantly in the periphery (calcifications in cyst); and tiny, punctiform, rounded calcifications scattered throughout the breast in ductal desquamation." *Middle below*, Coned compression view shows calcifications in a carcinoma. *Bottom*, Plain radiograph shows a fibroadenoma as a rounded nodule with central calcification and a narrow peripheral calcified rim.[15]

369

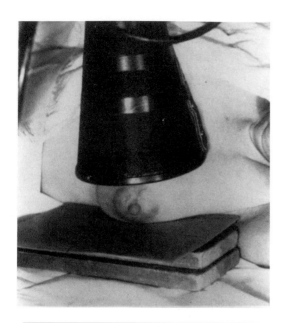

Mammographic technique (1958). Lateral radiograph of the breast is obtained with the patient in the lateral decubitus position, lying on the side to be examined. The breast is extended on the cassette or disposable film packet. Note the special cone designed by the author, which contained a flattened inferior surface for closer approximation to the chest wall.[17]

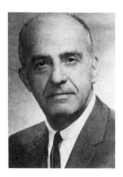

Jacob Gershon-Cohen.

Except for a few centers in the United States and Europe (especially Gros and Sigrist in Strasbourg), the use of mammography for clinical purposes remained limited. Victor Kremens wrote in 1958,[17]

roentgenography of the breast has been little used in this country up to the present time. This is explained, at least in part, by the difficulties encountered from a technical standpoint in obtaining roentgenograms of high diagnostic quality. More important, however, is the difficulty in roentgen interpretation. Considerable time and application must be expended by the radiologist before sufficient facility is developed to warrant a reasonable confidence in his ability to properly interpret and diagnose breast pathology . . . The question has been asked, "Why should we burden ourselves with the problems of roentgenographic examination of the female breast when proper management of the patient in most cases will lead to biopsy anyway?" This question may be answered by repeating the dictum that there are no shortcuts in medicine. Any diagnostic information which may be obtained by additional study without detriment to the patient should be sought without stint or reservation. There is no thought of omitting roentgen study of the chest in an individual with hemoptysis and a positive sputum. There similarly should be no hesitation to obtain whatever additional information may be made available by a roentgen breast examination despite the clarity of the clinical picture. Completely unsuspected pathology may be uncovered in either the breast under observation or, as has occurred in many instances in our experience, in the contralateral breast. One of the great values of the roentgen examination has been the opportunity it has afforded in detecting a disease process *before* it is clinically manifest.

Perhaps to allay one fear of the surgeons regarding the use of mammography, Kremens noted that "it is not intended that biopsy be supplanted by roentgen examination. Increased use of breast roentgenography may well lead to an increased number of biopsy examinations as a result of detection of previously unsuspected abnormalities."[17]

Most clinicians, however, were not impressed. For example, Haagensen[18] in his 1956 textbook emphatically stated that radiography had no place in the diagnosis of breast diseases.

In the United States, virtually the only major advocate of mammography was Jacob Gershon-Cohen. As early as 1938, Gershon-Cohen (in collaboration with Albert Strickler) published an article on the radiographic examination of the normal breast in which he stated that a precise knowledge of the normal breast at all ages and stages of activity was a prerequisite to recognizing pathological conditions that might arise.

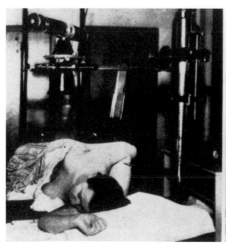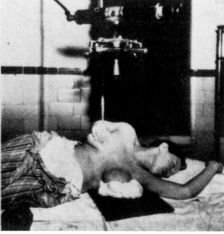

Technique of mammographic examination (1938). "The patient is placed in the lateral recumbent position, the breast to be examined on the film, the other retracted with the homolateral hand."[19]

If the roentgen examination of the breast is to be of real aid to the clinician, it must reveal the presence of pathological changes in their earliest stages—before they can be detected by clinical methods; but even if it can only confirm the nature of clinically detected abnormalities of the breast, it would still be a very helpful diagnostic aid.[19]

In the early 1950s, Gershon-Cohen began his rewarding collaboration with the renowned pathologist, Helen Ingleby. In an attempt to base mammography on a sound anatomical basis, they stressed the close correlation of breast lesions on radiographs with the gross and microscopic specimens. This eventually permitted recognition on the films of shadows that had previously appeared unimportant. With increasing experience, Gershon-Cohen and Ingleby could correlate radiographic and pathological findings with a variety of specific clinical entities.[20]

Gershon-Cohen emphasized the importance of high-contrast images obtained without screens and with collimation and compression. To overcome the difficulty in obtaining adequate exposure of both the thinner peripheral and thicker juxtathoracic tissues, he recommended the simultaneous exposure of two films without intensifying screens, interposing between them a layer of aluminum 0.5 mm thick. The upper film revealed contrast of the thicker, posterior portion of the breast, and the film covered by the aluminum foil revealed contrast of the anterior portion.[16]

A major stimulus to the widespread use of mammography was the 1960 report by Robert L. Egan[21] of 1,000 studies from the M. D. Anderson Hospital and Tumor Institute in Houston. After extensive experimentation with variations in technical factors, photographic emulsions, and processing, Egan selected a high milliamperage–low kilovoltage technique using industrial film that resulted in dependable high-quality diagnostic images that were easily reproducible. He wrote that

> the palpatory method of detection and diagnosis of breast lesions is inaccurate even in an institution where a limited number of clinicians evaluate all patients attending the breast clinic . . . Soft-tissue roentgenography of the breast can reduce the error of preoperative diagnosis and reveal a number of unsuspected lesions. In addition, it can obviate a significant number of general anesthesias now administered for diagnostic purposes.

Using his technique, Egan and co-workers achieved the astounding accuracy of an error rate of "less than 1% in malignant disease."

Egan also addressed the question of what to call this radiographic procedure. He considered "roentgenography of the breast" too non-specific, whereas "mastography" was an unwieldy term (the prefix *mastos*

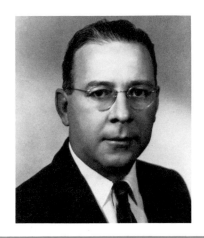

Robert L. Egan (1920-   ).

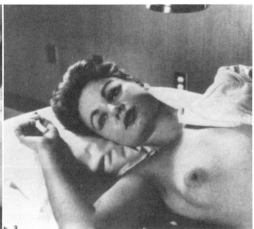

Mammography technique of Egan (1960). *Left*, Positioning for the cranial-caudad view. Identification marker is kept on the axillary side of the breast for localization of the mammary quadrant. *Middle*, Oblique or lateral position. The cardboard film-holder is supported on a small wood block. *Right*, Axillary view. The central beam is centered to the apex of the axilla and also parallel to the retromammary space. This arm position provided maximum visualization of the axilla as it reduced the number of skin folds without superimposition of the scapula.[21]

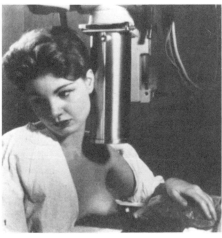

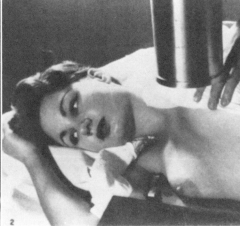

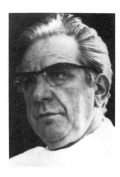

Charles M. Gros (1910-1984)[16]

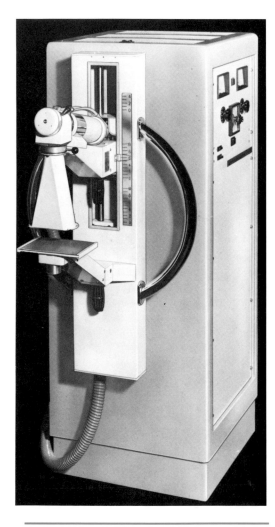

First production model of the CGR
Senographe (1966).[16]

had been used sparingly in reference to the breast and was easily confused with similar sounding terms). The term *mammography* had been first used by Hicken to describe the injection of contrast material into the milk ducts.[11] Nevertheless, Egan selected *mammography* as his term for breast radiography since it was "concise, short, and followed more closely the usual system of radiologic nomenclature and was the most frequently used combining form for the mammary gland."[6]

In the mid-1960s, Charles M. Gros[22] of France introduced two major innovations in mammographic technique. He substituted a molybdenum target for tungsten, which increased the contrast between low-density breast structures (fat, parenchymal tissue, and calcifications) because of the greater photoelectric effect of molybdenum at low energies (26 to 28 kVp). Gros also introduced vigorous compression of the breast during exposures to eliminate motion artifacts, diminish scattered radiation, and separate structures within the breast. However, the improved image quality was obtained at the expense of increased surface exposure (8 rad) compared to the Egan technique (4 rad).

In 1965, the CGR Company introduced the Senographe, the first mass-produced, "dedicated" mammography unit. The 0.7-mm molybdenum focal spot provided improved contrast, whereas the built-in compression device decreased scattered radiation and motion and separated breast structures.[23]

Until 1973, acceptable diagnostic quality in mammograms required hand development or the use of a slow mechanical processor. This problem was eliminated when the DuPont Company, stimulated by the investigation of Ostrum, Becker, and Isard, marketed a combined single-emulsion film/high-definition intensifying screen for mammography.[24] The intimate contact required between the film and the screen was initially accomplished by enclosing the envelope in a sealed, air-evacuated polyethylene bag. Subsequently, the bag was replaced with single-screen cassettes. With improvements in the speed of the single-emulsion film, this system permitted not only rapid automatic processing but also shorter exposures that reduced the surface exposure to about 1 rad.[23]

Other technical advances included fine moving grids, which greatly reduced the scattered radiation and improved mammographic contrast,[25] and microfocal spot tubes that allowed magnification techniques and improved diagnostic accuracy in distinguishing malignant from benign lesions. Indeed, most modern dedicated mammography units have two focal spots—one for standard surveys and a smaller one for magnification images of specific regions of interest.[26]

The most recent technological advances in mammography have been directed to reducing radiation exposure while preserving image quality. Geometric unsharpness of the image has been decreased by the development of smaller molybdenum focal spots, as well as by the utilization of a greater distance between the target and film (source-to-image distance). These improvements have allowed the development of faster film-screen combinations (e.g., rare-earth screens coupled with faster films), permitting significant reduction in radiation dose without degradation of the image.[23]

XEROMAMMOGRAPHY

A completely new technology for breast imaging was xeroradiography, which was first reported by Gould and co-workers in 1960[27] but not generally utilized by the medical community until the many technical refinements introduced by John Wolfe during the late 1960s.[28] Originally developed during the late 1930s, xeroradiography employed a photoconductive plate of selenium-coated aluminum instead of x-ray film as an image receptor (see Chapter 6). The plate was charged with positive ions and, with the breast superimposed, was exposed to x-rays. The resulting latent electrostatic image on the plate corresponded to differing densities within the interposed breast. Using xerographic processing equipment, the latent image was transformed into a permanent blue and white image on paper.

The resulting images were of high quality that was largely due to an edge enhancement phenomenon that accentuated high-density structures, particularly calcifications. Unlike film-screen mammography, xeromammography required a tungsten tube and higher-energy x-rays (40 to 50 kVp) and only moderate breast compression.[23]

Initially, xeromammograms were produced in the positive mode with pathological and anatomical densities appearing blue. With increasing concern over radiation dosage in mammography, Xerox shifted its emphasis from technological development to the reduction of dose. By combining added aluminum filtration of the tungsten x-ray beam with internal modifications of the system, the surface exposure was reduced from 3 to 1 rad per image; however, the quality of the images decreased because of diminished contrast (visual "flattening" of images). By reversing xeromammograms from the positive to the negative mode where densities were white on a blue background, the dose could be further decreased by about 30%.[23] The development of a black liquid toner to replace the original blue particles resulted in improved image quality with less radiation dose.[20]

For the past 20 years, an often-heated controversy has flared between proponents of film-screen mammography and xeromammography. Advocates of film-screen mammography pointed to the higher contrast images that facilitate identification of poorly defined masses, considerably lower radiation dose per exposure, decreased cost, and less maintenance. Champions of xeromammography stressed the ease of interpretation, increased latitude because of its diminished contrast, and convenience (no darkroom required). They also pointed to improved demonstration of microcalcifications resulting from the edge-enhancement phenomenon, although current film-screen mammography performed with dedicated equipment can depict calcifications especially well. A practical benefit of

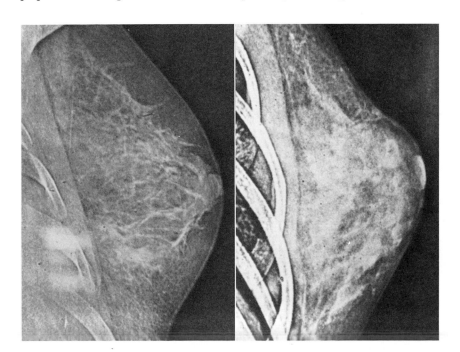

First xeroradiography of the breast (1960). "*Far left*, Enlarged view of the left breast of a 29-year-old nulligravida shows sharp detail in the subcutaneous tissues, the parenchyma, and behind the breast itself. *Left*, Enlarged view of the right breast of an 18-year-old multipara who was 45-days postpartum. Individual glands and ducts can be made out with difficulty, although the detail is much sharper than with conventional roentgenography in this type of breast."[27]

xeromammography has been the ability to perform high-quality examinations with standard ceiling-mounted, general purpose x-ray units, whereas good film-screen mammography requires specially designed x-ray equipment.

In general, the past several years have seen a swing from xeromammography, which was extremely popular during the 1970s—especially in high volume centers—to film-screen mammography.[2,29]

SCREENING MAMMOGRAPHY

Despite improvements in therapeutic methods, there was little change in mortality rates from breast cancer during the first 60 years of the twentieth century. From clinical experience, it became clear that the more extensive a tumor of a specific type at the onset of treatment, the worse the prognosis. Therefore the best way in which to reduce mortality from breast cancer was to diagnose the disease at an early stage before it had developed sufficiently to become incurable.[30] Gershon-Cohen and Gros pointed out the potential of mammography as a screening device for detecting breast disease in asymptomatic women. In a 1962 article describing 2,000 consecutive mammographic examinations, Egan reported 53 cases of "occult carcinoma," which he defined as "one which remains totally unsuspected following examination by the usual methods used to diagnose breast cancer, including an examination of the breast by an experienced and competent physician. To qualify for this definition, no symptoms or signs should be present."[31]

The first prospective, randomized, controlled diagnostic trial scientifically designed to determine the value of screening for breast cancer was performed from 1963 to 1969 under the auspices of the Health Insurance Plan (HIP) of New York. Organized by Philip Strax, Louis Venet, and Sam Shapiro, the purpose of the study was to determine whether periodic screening with film mammography and physical examination could decrease the mortality rate of breast cancer. Sixty-two thousand subjects were equally divided between study and control groups. Screening consisted of 4 annual mammograms and physical examinations over a 3-year period. Although not all of the women completed the 5-year study, there was a 30% to 40% decrease in mortality in the screened, randomly selected group when compared with the control group.[32,33] This was especially impressive considering that the mammograms performed in the study were of a quality far inferior to those currently obtainable. The only disturbing finding in the HIP study was that the reduction in mortality was limited to women over the age of 50. This probably related to the fact that the technically inferior mammograms performed at that time were not as effective in younger women with dense breasts as they were in older women.

The success of the HIP study led the National Cancer Institute and the American Cancer Society to co-sponsor the Breast Cancer Detection Demonstration Project (BCDDP) at 27 sites throughout the United States. These projects, which began in 1973, were not set up as controlled scientific studies but were designed to demonstrate to the medical profession and the public the application of periodic screening (physical examination, thermography, mammography) of essentially asymptomatic women for the detection of early breast cancer.[29] Almost one-third of cancers detected by the centers were either noninfiltrating or small infiltrating cancers less than 1 cm in size; more than 80% of all cancers

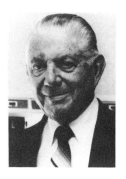

Philip Strax.

374

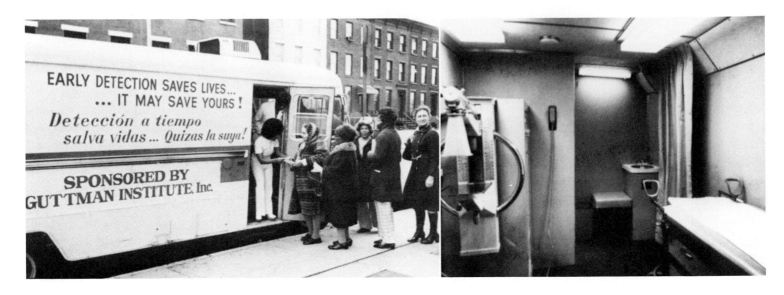

showed no evidence of nodal involvement. Physical examination and mammography were the important diagnostic modalities in all of the centers. Mammography demonstrated almost 90% of the cancers. Indeed, in almost 42% of cancers, mammography demonstrated a lesion in the absence of physical findings; conversely, physical examination alone (in the absence of positive mammographic findings) was positive in only 9% of the cancer patients.

A larger study of mammographic screening was done in Sweden under the leadership of Laszlo Tabar.[30] More than 130,000 women aged 40 to 74 were enrolled in a randomized study in which the only screening method used was a single, oblique-view mammogram. The results showed a 31% reduction in mortality from breast cancer in the study group and a 25% decrease in the absolute rate of more advanced cancers.[30]

The American and Swedish studies clearly indicated the value of screening women for breast cancer by regular physical examinations and mammography. However, during the late 1970s a bitter debate within the medical community over the relative value of mammography caused many women to avoid this most sensitive technique to detect breast cancer.[34] The controversy revolved around two points: the lack of a proved benefit of screening women under age 50 and the potential carcinogenic risk of mammography.[29] Although the results of the HIP study showed a substantial reduction in mortality in the screened population, this benefit was initially restricted to women over age 50. Later analyses also showed a 20% mortality reduction in women under 50. The BCDDP study showed a high detection rate of minimal cancers, especially in women under 50.[35] Many centers reported a detection rate of minimal cancers 10 or more times greater than that reported in the HIP study.

The carcinogenic effect of low-level radiation is unknown. However, if there is a risk it is immeasurably small, especially in women over age 30.[36] Large doses of radiation (1,000 times greater than that used in current film-screen techniques) have been shown to cause an increased number of breast cancers, but this increase is confined mainly to women under age 30. Today, although the controversial debate has subsided, the fear of radiation is still cited as one of the chief reasons women do not avail themselves of mammography.

The most recent American Cancer Society guidelines for mammography include a baseline study between ages 35 and 39, followed by examinations every 1 or 2 years between ages 40 and 49, and yearly examinations after age 50.

A major impediment to the widespread use of mammographic screening has been the relatively high price of the examination. To overcome this problem, several groups began offering low-cost screening to asymp-

Self-contained mobile mammographic unit used by Strax in the late 1960s. *Above left*, Mammograms could be obtained in 70 women per day. *Above*, The unit contained facilities for obtaining a medical history and performing physical examination, mammography, and thermography.[16]

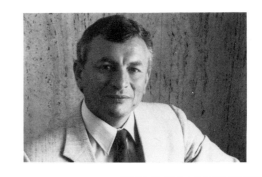

Laszlo Tabar.

tomatic women. This required an approach different from that appropriate for solving the more complex diagnostic dilemmas presented by symptomatic patients. Since the goal of screening was to detect unsuspected abnormalities, rather than to characterize them fully, operational procedures were streamlined to maximize patient throughput and achieve substantial cost savings. Income lost from asymptomatic patients paying lower fees was more than offset by the income generated by additional problem-solving mammograms needed to fully characterize screening-detected abnormalities and by the increased use of needle localization procedures to guide biopsy.[37]

In the late 1960s, Strax was the first person to develop and successfully operate a self-contained mobile unit for breast cancer screening with mammography.[16] Mobile vans for mammographic screening have been used in Sweden since the mid-1970s. This concept has been popularized in the United States by Edward A. Sickles, who observed that

> although start-up costs are somewhat higher than needed to remodel and equip an office, the operating expenses are considerably less, primarily because no rent is paid . . . We constructed our four-room mobile van by customizing the shell of a 34-foot recreational vehicle. The van is staffed by three mammographic radiologists who share (and rotate) the jobs of patient reception, imaging plus physical examination, and making appointments. They also share the driving of the van. All the equipment, including heating and cooling systems, is powered by gasoline generators . . . By situating the van near large downtown office buildings or at supermarkets, both working and nonworking women can undergo screening rapidly, typically in 10-15 minutes during a lunch hour, coffee break, or just before grocery shopping.[37]

OTHER MODALITIES FOR BREAST IMAGING

In 1929, Max Cutler introduced the technique of transillumination of the breast.[38] This method, also called light scanning or diaphanography, consisted of the passage of red and near-infrared light through the breast. Proponents believed that breast cancers absorbed these wavelengths from the increased amounts of blood in their neovascular network. Most systems attempted to evaluate the total light transmission through regions of the breast, as well as to compare the ratio of infrared/red light transmitted.[39]

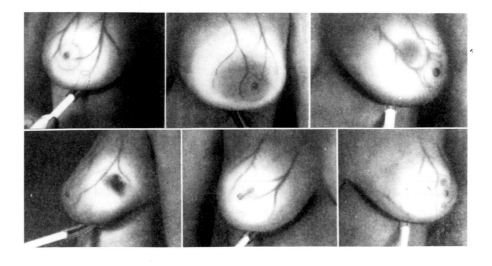

Transillumination of breast lesions (1929). "*Top left,* Normal breast demonstrating position of light during examination. *Top middle,* Diffuse opacity of breast with 'chronic mastitis.' *Top right,* Solid breast tumor. Character of opacity is same in benign and malignant tumor. *Bottom left,* Traumatic haematoma of breast. Opacity is intense, uneven, and irregular in outline. *Bottom middle,* Intracystic papilloma and dilated duct filled with blood in case of bleeding nipple. *Bottom right,* Multiple papillomata. Straight line represents site of local removal of one lesion which failed to stop bloody discharge."[38]

The examination is made in a totally dark room with the patient sitting in a revolving chair opposite the examiner. The lamp is placed against the undersurface of the breast and gradually moved as different areas in the breast are inspected successively, the object being to place the particular portion in question directly between the light and the examiner's eye. By means of gentle pressure on the upper surface, thus compressing the organ between the hand above and the light beneath, the degree of translucence may be increased. The tail of the breast is best transilluminated by placing the small curved lamp underneath the axillary fold, directing the light anteriorly. Both breasts are examined routinely, the normal sized being transilluminated first to serve as a standard for comparison.

Although Cutler reported characteristic appearances of solid tumors, cysts, traumatic hematomas, and ductal lesions causing bleeding from the nipple, subsequent studies clearly showed that this procedure was far inferior to screen-film mammography for detecting breast cancer. The broad, diffuse light source produced intense scatter that reduced resolution similar to the effect of scatter radiation and geometric unsharpness in x-ray imaging. Transillumination had poor depth resolution, making it impossible to detect a lesion at a depth greater than twice its diameter.[40]

Several investigators have recommended the use of ultrasound to detect and categorize benign and malignant lesions.[41,42] However, subsequent studies have shown a broad overlap between the supposedly typical sonographic characteristics of benign and malignant lesions.[43] Another study showed that whole-breast ultrasound could detect barely more than half of all biopsy-proven cancers and an even smaller percentage of cancers that had not yet spread to the axillary nodes.[44] Therefore it is clear that ultrasound is of little value in screening asymptomatic women to detect cancer. The major role of this modality is to differentiate cystic from solid breast lesions, especially nonpalpable masses detected by mammography.

Another technique used for diagnosing breast cancer was thermography, a noninvasive procedure designed to detect subtle differences in temperature between malignant tumors and normal breast. In 1956, Lawson[45] noted that the skin overlying malignant lesions in the breast was 1° to 3° F warmer than other areas of breast parenchyma. Although subsequent studies initially confirmed his findings, later reports demonstrated thermography as insensitive in detecting breast cancer and that no specific thermographic criteria for breast cancer could be developed.[46]

LOCALIZATION OF OCCULT BREAST LESIONS

When small masses, clustered microcalcifications, areas of architectural distortion, or asymmetry are detected by mammographic screening in asymptomatic patients, a surgical biopsy is recommended. Because a relatively large percentage of these biopsies will yield benign histology, the goal of surgery is to resect the smallest amount of tissue to include the suspected lesion while sacrificing a minimal volume of the breast.[47]

The simplest method for localizing nonpalpable breast lesions was quadrant localization.[48] However, this technique resulted in unnecessary sacrifice of large volumes of breast tissue and did not guarantee that the suspected lesion had been removed, since the mobility of deep lesions relative to the skin, anatomical coordinates, or radiopaque markers placed mammographically on the skin surface did not ensure accurate localization.

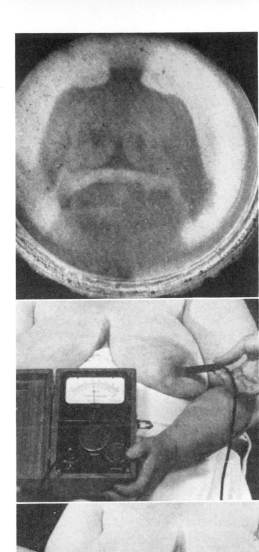

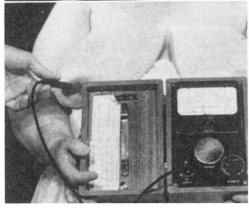

Thermography (1956). *Top,* Evaporograph image of patient with carcinoma of right breast. *Middle,* Carcinoma of left breast in another patient. *Bottom,* Note the lower temperature in the normal right breast.[45]

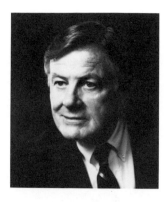

Gerald D. Dodd.

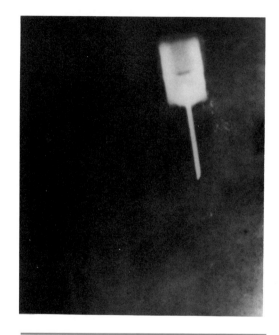

Needle localization (1965). Mammogram showing the position of the needle in the region of a cluster of carcinoma calcifications in an asymptomatic breast.[16]

Localization of nonpalpable breast lesion (1985). *Right,* Mammogram shows localization of a suspicious cluster of calcifications. After satisfactory positioning of the curved end of the wire with the pseudoelastic metal alloy end, the needle can be withdrawn or left in place, as shown, to stiffen the wire and permit easier palpation by the surgeon. *Far right,* Radiograph of the tissue specimen.[16]

The most accurate method of localizing an occult breast lesion required positioning a needle close to it. The first person to perform needle localization of nonpalpable, mammographically visible lesions before biopsy was probably Gerald Dodd in Philadelphia in 1963.[49] Numerous techniques of needle localization have been described subsequently, including the placement of single or multiple needles,[50,51] dye and contrast injections in the region of the suspected abnormality,[52,53] and needle-placed hook wires.[54] In this last technique, the marker was anchored in place by its hooked tip, and this self-retaining feature avoided displacement of the marker during subsequent mammography and preparations for operation. Dye injection methods were often much less accurate, especially in the fatty breast, because of possible diffusion of the dye into an undesirably large volume of breast tissue. Subsequent improvements in the needle–hookwire technique included the ability to repeatedly withdraw the wire back into the needle so that it could be repositioned as many times as necessary until the tip was positioned optimally and confirmed in two mammographic positions[55] and the development of a wire made from a pseudoelastic alloy that was tough enough to resist inadvertent transection by surgical scissors.[56]

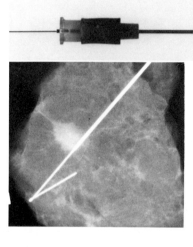

Localization of nonpalpable breast lesion (1980). *Above,* When the 20-gauge needle is pulled back over the spring hookwire, the hook is released and springs open. *Left,* Radiograph of a tissue specimen reveals an infiltrating ductal carcinoma.[16]

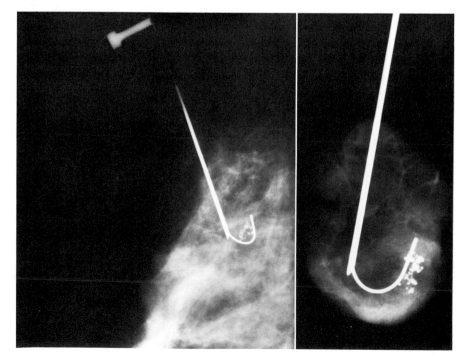

Bibliography

Gershon-Cohen J: Breast roentgenography. In Bruwer AJ (ed): Classic descriptions in diagnostic roentgenology. Springfield, Ill, Charles C Thomas, 1964.

References

1. Salomon A: Contributions to the pathology and clinical picture of carcinoma of the breast. Arch Klin Chir 101:573-668, 1913.
2. Hoeffken W and Lanyi M: Mammography: Technique, diagnosis, differential diagnosis, results. Stuttgart, Thieme, 1977.
3. Kleinschmidt O: Brustdruse. In Zweifel P, Payr E, and Hirzel S (eds): Die Klinik der bösartigen Geschwülste. Leipzig, 1927.
4. Vogel W: The roentgen visualization of mammary tumors. Arch Klin Chir 171:618-626, 1932.
5. Finsterbusch R and Gross F: Kalkablagerungen in den Milch und Ausführungsgängen beider Brustdrüsen. Röntgenpraxis 6: 172-174, 1934.
6. Egan RL: Mammography. Springfield, Ill, Charles C Thomas, 1972.
7. Warren SL: A roentgenologic study of the breast. AJR 24:113-124, 1930.
8. Seabold PS: Procedure in the roentgen study of the breast. AJR 29:850-851, 1933.
9. Lockwood IH: The roentgen-ray evaluation of breast symptoms. AJR 29:145-155, 1933.
10. Ries E: Diagnostic Lipiodol injection into milk-ducts followed by abscess formation. Amer J Obstet Gynec 20:414-416, 1930.
11. Hicken NF: Mammography: The roentgenographic diagnosis of breast tumors by means of contrast media. Surg Gynec Obstet 64: 593-603, 1937.
12. Brody H and Cullen M: Carcinoma of the breast seventeen years after mammography with Thorotrast. Surgery 42:600-602, 1957.
13. Baraldi A: Roentgeno-neumo-mastia. Rev Med Del Rosario 25:1536, 1935.
14. Leborgne R: Diagnosis of tumors of the breast by simple roentgenography: Calcifications in carcinomas. AJR 65:1-11, 1951.
15. Leborgne R: The breast in roentgen diagnosis. Montevideo, Uruguay, Impresora, 1953.
16. Gold RH, Bassett LW, and Widoff BE: Highlights from the history of mammography. RadioGraphics 10:1111-1131, 1990.
17. Kremens V: Roentgenography of the breast. AJR 80:1005-1013, 1958.
18. Haagensen CD: Diseases of the breast. Philadelphia, WB Saunders, 1956.
19. Gershon-Cohen J and Strickler A: Roentgenologic examination of the normal breast: Its evaluation in demonstrating early neoplastic changes. AJR 40:189-201, 1938.
20. Ingleby H and Gershon-Cohen J: Comparative anatomy, pathology and roentgenology of the breast. Philadelphia, University of Pennsylvania Press, 1960.
21. Egan RL: Experience with mammography in a tumor institution: Evaluation of 1,000 studies. Radiology 75:894-900, 1960.
22. Gros CM: Méthodologie. Symposium sur le sein. J Radiol Electrol 48:638-655, 1967.
23. Gold RH and Bassett LW: Mammography: History and state of the art. In Feig SA and McClelland R (eds): Breast carcinoma: Current diagnosis and therapy. New York, Masson, 1983.
24. Ostrum BJ, Becker W, and Isard HJ: Low-dose mammography. Radiology 109:323-326, 1973.
25. McSweeney MB, Sprawls P, and Egan RL: Mammographic grids. In Feig SA and McClelland R (eds): Breast carcinoma: Current diagnosis and therapy. New York, Masson, 1983.
26. Sickles EA, Doi K, and Genant HK: Magnification film mammography. Radiology 125: 69-76, 1977.
27. Gould HR, Ruzicka FF, Sanchez-Ubeda R, and Perez J: Xeroradiography of the breast. AJR 84:220-223, 1960.
28. Wolfe JN: Xerography of the breast. Radiology 91:231-240, 1968.
29. Milbrath J: Mammography. In Porrath S (ed): A multimodality approach to breast imaging. Rockville, Md, Aspen, 1986.
30. Tabar L and Dean PB: The control of breast cancer through mammographic screening: What is the evidence? Radiol Clin North Am 25:993-1005, 1987.
31. Egan R: Fifty-three cases of carcinoma of the breast, occult until mammography. AJR 88:1095-1101, 1962.
32. Strax P, Venet L, and Shapiro S: Value of mammography in reduction of mortality from breast cancer in mass screening. AJR 117: 686-689, 1973.
33. Strax P: Results of mass screening for breast cancer in 50,000 examinations. Cancer 37: 30-35, 1976.
34. Bailar JC: Mammography: A contrary view. Ann Intern Med 84:77-84, 1976.
35. Baker LH: Breast cancer detection demonstration project: Five-year summary report. Cancer 32:194-225, 1982.
36. Feig SA: Assessment of the hypothetical risk from mammography and evaluation of the potential benefit. Radiol Clin North Am 21:173-191, 1983.
37. Sickles EA, Weber WN, Galvin HB, et al: Mammographic screening: How to operate successfully at low cost. Radiology 160:95-97, 1986.
38. Cutler M: Transillumination as an aid in the diagnosis of breast lesions. Surg Gynecol Obstet 48:721-729, 1929.
39. Kopans DB: Nonmammographic breast imaging techniques: Current status and future developments. Radiol Clin North Am 25: 961-971, 1987.
40. Drexler B, Davis JL, and Scholfield G: Diaphanography in the diagnosis of breast cancer. Radiology 157:41-44, 1985.
41. Kobayshi T, Takatani O, and Hattori N: Differential diagnosis of breast tumors: The sensitivity graded method of ultrasonotomography and clinical evaluation of its diagnostic accuracy. Cancer 33:940-951, 1974.
42. Jellins J, Kossoff G, and Reeve TS: Detection and classification of liquid-filled masses in the breast by gray scale echography. Radiology 125:205-212, 1977.
43. Kopans DB, Meyer JE, and Lindfors KK: Whole-breast ultrasound imaging: Four-year follow-up. Radiology 157:505-507, 1985.
44. Sickles EA, Filly RA, and Callen PW: Breast cancer detection with sonography and mammography: Comparison using state-of-the-art equipment. AJR 140:843-845, 1983.
45. Lawson RN: Implications of surface temperatures in the diagnosis of breast cancer. Can Med Assoc J 75:309-310, 1956.
46. Martin JE: Breast imaging techniques. Radiol Clin North Am 21:149-153, 1983.
47. Kopans DB and Meyer JE: Localization of occult breast lesions. In Athanasoulis CA, Pfister RC, Greene RE, and Roberson GH (eds): Interventional radiology. Philadelphia, WB Saunders, 1982.
48. Berger SM, Curcio BM, Gershon-Cohen J, et al: Mammographic localization of unsuspected breast cancer. AJR 96:1046-1052, 1966.
49. Threatt B, Appelman H, Dow R, et al: Percutaneous needle localization of clustered mammary microcalcifications prior to biopsy. AJR 121:839, 1974.
50. Dodd GD, Fry K, and Delany W: Pre-op localization of occult carcinoma of the breast. In Nealon TF (ed): Management of the patient with breast cancer. Philadelphia, WB Saunders, 1965.
51. Curcio BM: Technique for radiographic localization of nonpalpable breast tumors. Radiol Technol 42:155, 1970-1971.
52. Simon N, Lesnick GJ, Lerer WN, et al: Roentgenographic localization of small lesions of the breast by the spot method. Surg Gynecol Obstet 134:572-574, 1972.
53. Horns JW and Arndt RD: Percutaneous spot localization of nonpalpable breast lesions. AJR 127:253-257, 1976.
54. Frank HA, Hall FM, and Steer ML: Preoperative localizations of nonpalpable breast lesions demonstrated by mammography. N Engl J Med 295:259-260, 1976.
55. Kopans DB and DeLuca S: A modified needle-hookwire technique to simplify preoperative localization of occult breast lesions. Radiology 134:781, 1980.
56. Homer MJ: Nonpalpable breast lesion localization using a curved-end retractable wire. Radiology 157:259-260, 1985.
57. Bruwer AJ (ed): Classic descriptions in diagnostic roentgenology. Springfield, Ill, Charles C Thomas, 1964.

CHAPTER 21

Dental Radiology

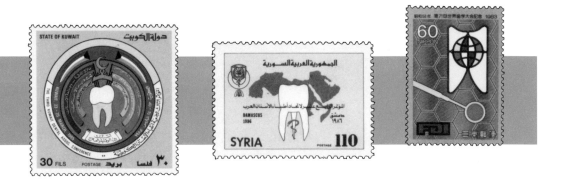

Within 2 weeks of Roentgen's discovery, Otto Walkhoff, a German dentist, made the first intraoral radiograph. Using a glass photographic plate wrapped in black paper and covered with thin rubber sheeting, this radiograph of his own teeth was a cross between present-day bite-wing and periapical projections and required an exposure of 25 minutes! The images consisted essentially of the gross outlines of the bicuspid and molar teeth but were useless for diagnostic purposes.[1] Three months later, Wilhelm Koenig of Frankfurt made dental radiographs that were more useful diagnostically and required only 9 minutes' exposure.[2] Soon afterward, an English dentist, Frank Harrison, constructed a special vacuum tube for dental use and " . . . was gratified to see the first image of roots of the teeth gradually develop in the negative." Although his exposure times initially were similar to those of Walkhoff, Harrison later succeeded in reducing them to 10 minutes.[2]

In the United States, the first dental radiograph was made in April, 1896, by William J. Morton, a New York physician. At a meeting of the New York Odontological Society, Morton reported that the density of the teeth was greater than that of the bone surrounding them. He stated that radiography offered[3]

> a wondrous field for investigation and study in diagnosis. Each errant fang is distinctly placed, however deeply embedded within its alveolar socket; teeth before their eruption stand forth in plain view; an unsuspected exostosis is revealed; a pocket of necrosis, of suppuration, or of tuberculosis is revealed in its exact outlines; the extent in area and location of metallic fillings are sharply delineated, whether above or below the alveolar line. Most interesting is the fact that the pulp-chamber is beautifully outlined, and that erosions and enlargements may be readily detected . . . Already painless dentistry is within your grasp by aid of electricity and simple anesthetics, and now the x-ray more than rivals your exploring mirror, your probe, your most delicate sense of touch, and your keenest powers of hypothetical diagnosis.

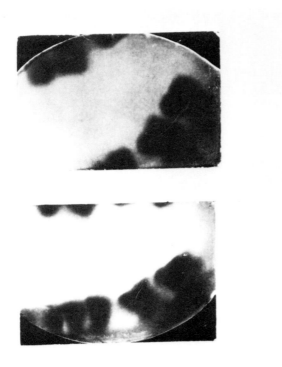

Erste Zahnaufnahme vom Lebenden angefertigt 14 Tage nach der Veröffentlichung Röntgens im December 1895 auf einer zu geschnittenen photographischen Glasplatte von D⁻ Walkhoff Zahnarzt in Braunschweig.

First dental radiograph (Walkhoff, December, 1895).

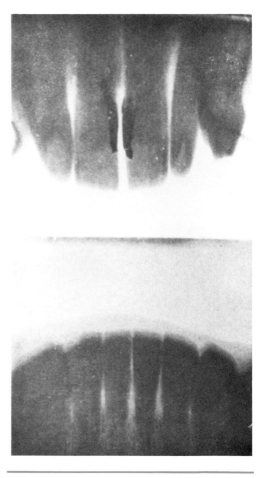

Early dental radiograph (Koenig, 1896).[1]

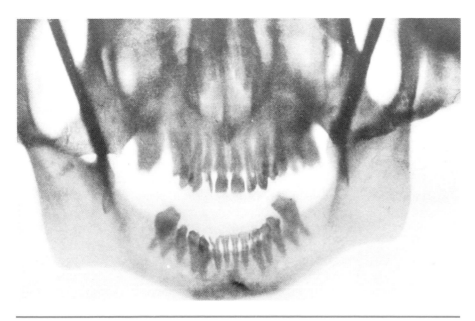

First dental radiograph made in the United States (1896). "Skiagraph of front of skull, showing the dentures, pulp, chambers of incisors, etc."[3]

381

The major figure in American radiodontics and a roentgen martyr was C. Edmund Kells, a New Orleans dentist who established the first radiographic dental clinic in the United States (July, 1896). Kells[4] described how he made his first dental radiograph:

> The patient, one of my assistants, was then seated in a chair, with the film holder in position. With the teeth held together and the mouth closed, she could swallow without causing a movement of the film. With the face leaning against a firmly fixed thin board, in order to steady her, the tube was placed on the other side of the board. Thus, I unknowingly used a filter, which possibly prevented my patient from being burned during the long exposure.
>
> Thus was my first dental radiogram taken. Picture the poor girl sitting there with her face against the board, for 15 long minutes.

Kells looked forward with enthusiasm to demonstrating his finding to a professional audience. Accordingly, he decided to attend the annual summer meeting of the Southern Dental Association in Asheville, North Carolina. Kells had to bring his own equipment (since nothing similar was available in North Carolina), a hand-held fluoroscope, and an assistant with an individual film holder. Unfortunately, the meeting was held during daylight hours at the Battery Park Hotel, which was supplied with electric current in the evenings only. As fate would have it, at the precise time allocated for his clinic, the hotel also scheduled a society ball.

> When it was noised about that there was an x-ray machine "going," those attending the ball, as well as others in the hotel, swarmed into our clinic rooms—there was no stopping them. Everyone wanted to see the bones in her hand. I say *her* hand, because the women predominated. The current was to be cut off at midnight, and the spectators would not allow me to take a picture and then take the time to develop it. The marvelous fluoroscope was all they wanted to see. I had gone to the expense of bringing a subject all the way from New Orleans and arranging a temporary darkroom for the developing of the film, and then did not get a chance to do it. However, we all had a wonderful time and our members and their wives did finally get a "look in" before the current was shut off.[4]

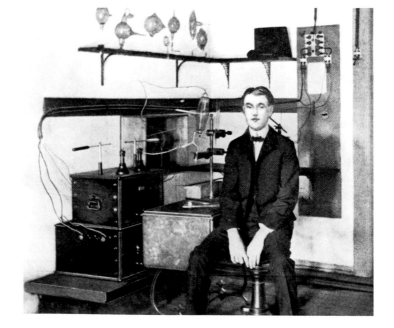

C. Edmund Kells' x-ray laboratory (1896). Patient with a film in his mouth positioned for a radiograph. The grounded aluminum screen shows faintly between the face and the tube. The patient could also be posed in a regular dental chair, which afforded a steady head-rest with an easy semirecumbent position. Note the variety of tubes in the rack above the apparatus. These were required because of the poor reliability of the tubes as a result of the variability of their vacuums.[5]

As more investigators learned to use the new x-rays for clinical purposes, it became apparent that there were many more applications of dental radiography than were at first envisioned. As an early editorial stated[6]:

> it is evident that for the diagnosis of impacted or unerupted teeth, locating the position of broken instruments in canals, detecting projection of portions of fillings beyond the apical foramen, the diagnosis of inflammatory lesions in the jaws, necrotic bone, etc., there is a wide field of utility in dentistry for the x-ray.

This statement indicates that in the early days no attempt was made to do routine radiodontic examination. The x-rays were employed only rarely, when there seemed to be a specific application for their use. [7]

Kells[4] was also the first dentist to use radiography in root canal therapy. As he later described the circumstances that occurred on May 10, 1899:

> I was attempting to fill the root canal of an upper and central incisor for a little boy. It occurred to me to place a lead wire in the root canal and then take a radiogram to see whether it extended to the end of the root or not. I carried out this inspiration, for an inspiration it surely was, and the result was all that was anticipated. The lead wire was shown very plainly in the root canal . . .

In the next year (1900), Weston A. Price[8] called attention to the ability of radiographs to disclose incomplete root canal fillings. Arthur Merritt (1916)[9] proposed the use of three radiographs: a pretreatment film, one after "cleaning and sterilizing" with a wire in place, and a postoperative film. He felt that ". . . without the aid of the Roentgen Ray, it is impossible in any given case to be certain that the operation has been properly performed."[9] Today, root canal therapy is absolutely dependent on preoperative, operative, and postoperative radiodontic evaluation.

The other dentist who was a major x-ray pioneer was William H. Rollins of Boston (see Chapter 4). He designed "an oral camera for röntgen photography," which consisted essentially of the familiar dentist's mirror mounted at the end of a rod but with a small film holder where the mirror would ordinarily be. To use the instrument, Rollins directed, "cut disks from a Kodak film and place six or more over each other with thin disks of aluminum between, enclosing them water and light tight in the camera. Give full exposure to the first film. As each film has less exposure than the one in front of it, the appearances vary and one is sure to give the information sought."[10]

Rollins also invented an x-ray tube arm and bracket for use in the dental office. Although this undoubtedly was the first dental x-ray apparatus described in the literature, it was never commercially manufactured.

Rollins was one of the first to recognize the potential of radiation injury and to advise caution with the use of x-rays. He recommended the use of radiopaque glasses, enclosure of the x-ray tube in a lead housing, and protection of the patient by covering those body areas not being clinically examined.[11] For the most part his advice went unheeded.

The first use of radiographs in the diagnosis of "pyorrhea alveolaris" was reported by Rollins in 1896.[12] Although today it is universally accepted that periodontal disease can be detected by means of radiography before it can be discovered by direct ocular examination, the diagnostic value of radiographs was challenged by Kells. He stated (1920) that "in periodontia alone, it (the radiograph) can have but little value. The

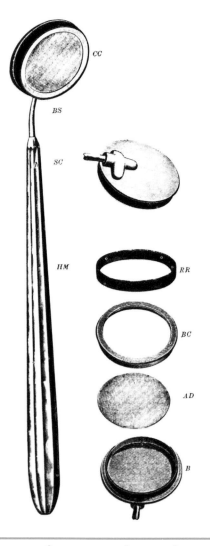

Oral camera for roentgen photography (Rollins, 1896). The instrument consists of a hollow metal handle (*HM*); a flexible sliding brass rod (*BS*), fastened by the screw (*SC*), and supporting the camera (*CC*). *B* is a brass cell ⅛-inch deep; the front is closed by the aluminum disk (*AD*), which is held in position by the ring (*BC*) over which is stretched the soft rubber ring (*RR*) to prevent painful pressure on the gum.[10]

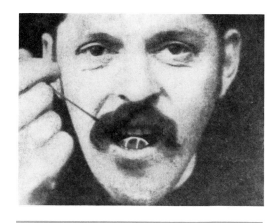

Dental fluoroscope in use (1910).[17]

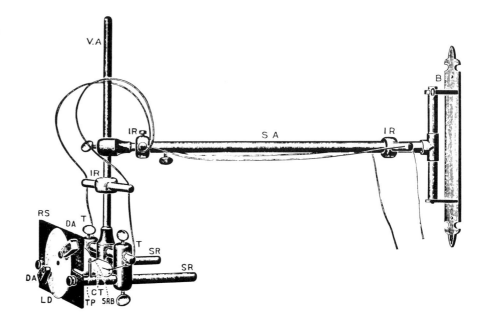

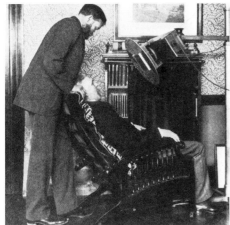

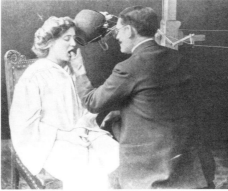

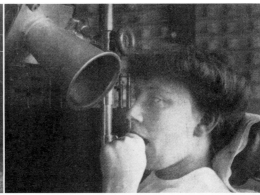

Radiographing the upper front teeth. *Left*, Williams (1904). *Middle*, Note the Friedlander shield and that the dentist is holding the film (1910).[19] *Right*, The patient is holding the film in position against the upper teeth by exerting slight pressure with the thumb (1916).[14]

Patient seated and apparatus arranged for making a radiograph of the left side (1916). "Patients seated comfortably find it easy to remain perfectly quiet."[14]

pyorrhea specialist, who cannot diagnose pyorrhea and sufficiently gauge its extent without the aid of the ray, had undoubtedly better engage in some other specialty."[13]

It was not until some years after the discovery of x-rays that it was thought necessary to examine all the teeth. When this need was finally recognized, eight or nine periapical radiographs were deemed sufficient. Later, 16- or 18-film examinations were used to preclude the possibility of overlooking oral pathology.[7] These extensive screening procedures have now been largely replaced by pantomography (see Chapter 24).

In succeeding years, the value of radiography in prosthetics, orthodontics, and oral surgery has been well established.[15]

The story of dental x-ray plates and film closely parallels the progress of its medical counterpart from the earliest days of radiography. Special emulsions, various plate or film sizes, and a practical packet were problems that had to be met to satisfy the needs of the dental profession.[15,16]

Early dental radiographs were made on photographic plates, films, and bromide papers. Glass plates proved satisfactory for the anterior region of the mouth, where the curved surfaces did not cause undue distortion of the image. However, distortion was a problem in the posterior region. Another difficulty was the need for cutting large glass plates to the sizes needed for dental radiography. Therefore film presented many advantages, particularly its thinness and flexibility, which made it easy to place in the mouth.

About 1900, Price[16] designed a celluloid-based dental film that was said to be thick enough to prevent curling but sufficiently flexible to be introduced into the mouth. In an attempt to obtain a greater degree of contrast between the tooth structures and the surrounding alveolar process, three emulsion layers instead of one were coated on the support. This product was made and marketed by the Seed Dry Plate Company. The films were cut to size from large sheets and wrapped in black unvulcanized rubber sheeting.

Placing the x-ray film in the mouth could prove to be a vexing problem. As Morton[3] described in 1896:

> The way I devised was to cut a pattern in gutta-percha or cardboard or anything that the patient could wear in the mouth without gagging too much. If they gag too much, I use the cocaine spray. Having cut this pattern, I took it to the darkroom and cut the film in the same shape and folded it into three folds of paper, and then wrapped it into a pocket of gutta-percha tissue and adjusted it to the roof of the mouth.

Kells' system was similar, except that instead of designing a pattern in the mouth he took an impression of the patient's upper and lower teeth and made a vulcanized plate with a pocket to act as the film holder.[4] In Germany, Hunstadbraten mentioned the use of "bite-guides," horseshoe-shaped mouthpieces with an inner part of rubber that could be inflated to press the film against the upper jaw when the patient closed his mouth. Although many pioneer dentists simply used their own fingers to hold the x-ray films in place, reports of malignancies made this an untenable solution. Protective gloves were recommended but were not considered practical. An alternative offered by Tousey[15] in 1908 was a horizontal occlusal film that would be retained when the patient closed down. Specially designed occlusal film was introduced in 1917 and remains in use today.

There was a critical need for a specially wrapped packet containing dental films. One of the earliest and most successful wrappings consisted of a black and orange or ruby paper and a black rubber sheeting. Later, the ruby paper wrapping contained a thin, external coating of paraffin. Kells was probably the first to suggest and use two dental films in a packet so that duplicate radiographs were available in case one was lost or sent to a referring physician. Each exposure in those early days required from 20 to 90 seconds.[16]

In 1913, a red, waxed, moisture-proof, hand-wrapped paper packet was introduced by Kodak. It contained two single-coated periapical films enclosed in black paper. These packets were superseded in 1921 by machine-made packets containing single-coated film. These packets were more sanitary, easier to place, and much more comfortable for the patient.[16]

In 1918, a dental film packet consisting of a lead-foil external backing was introduced. This packet was rigid and reduced the amount of secondary radiation reaching the film from surrounding tissues. Since that time, all dental film packets have contained lead-foil backings.

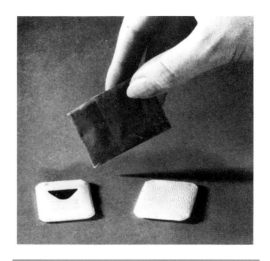

Dental x-ray film. Early hand-wrapped dental x-ray film packet (*above*), which was quite crude when compared with the sleek modern machine-made packet (*below*).[16]

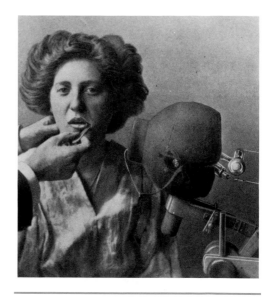

Vertical dental film carrier inserted in the mouth (1910). Note the prominent Friedlander shield.[17]

Kodak (1915) was the first to introduce dental x-ray films coated on both sides of the support with a fine-grain, high-contrast emulsion ("radiatized") that greatly aided visualization of detail. These films were enclosed in neatly designed machine-made packets. To detect caries in the interproximal surface of the teeth, an area inaccessible to clinical evaluation, the first "bite-wing" film packet was designed by Howard Raper (1924). These packets initially contained single-coated film, which was later changed to the radiatized type.[16] A severe critic of the bite-wing film was Kells, who stated[4]:

> The Bite-Wing packet [is] principally designed for the purpose of detecting cavities in the tooth, but I believe that if an operator cannot find cavities on the crowns of the teeth without the use of the ray, what he needs is a competent dental assistant to make his examination for him and not a roentgen-ray machine.

The first bite-wing technique called for a five- to seven-film series, which included the anterior teeth. Raper recommended these radiographs be taken once a year for patients under 30 years of age, and every 18 to 24 months for patients over 30.[15]

Like all medical films of that period, the early dental films were coated on a basis of cellulose nitrate. In 1929, however, the use of cellulose acetate (safety) base was begun. About the same time, the color of the packet was also changed from black to white. A smaller dental film packet designed for radiography of children's teeth was introduced by Kodak in 1930. Since that time, extremely fast, "rapid-processing" dental films have been introduced that permit a reduction in the x-ray dose to the patient, which is desirable in a complete dental examination.[16]

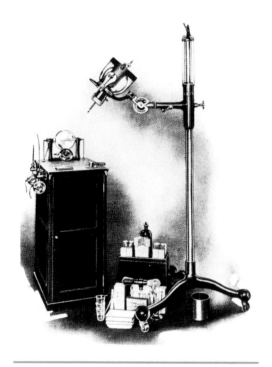

First American commercially manufactured x-ray machine made especially for the dentist (American X-ray Equipment Company). Note the lead glass tube shield on this 1917 model, which sold for $320.[21]

First European commercially manufactured x-ray outfit (1905). Called the *Record*, it was manufactured by Reiniger-Gebbert and Schall of Germany (predecessors of Siemens Corporation). The gas-filled x-ray tube was partially lead-shielded for protection against radiation; however, note the exposed high-voltage wires. The device included a collimator for intra-oral radiographs.[21]

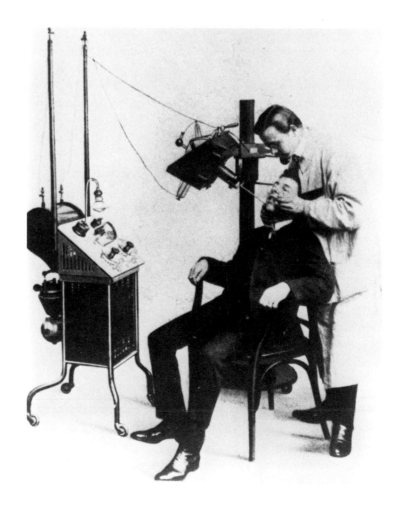

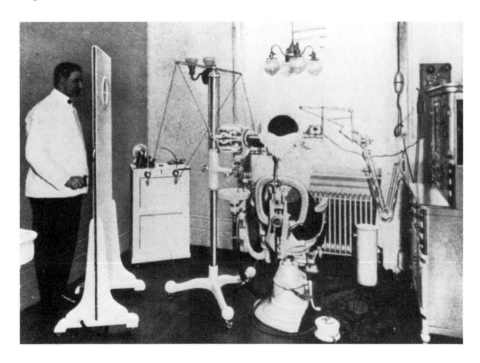

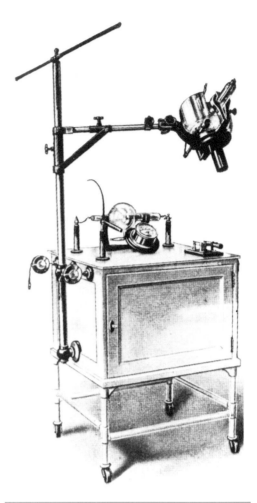

Compact early dental x-ray unit, which consisted of an induction coil x-ray machine with the tube holder mounted on the cabinet. It sold for $75.[21]

Although commercially manufactured dental x-ray outfits had been produced in Europe since 1905, before 1913 there were no American dental x-ray machines on the market. Medical equipment was adapted for dental purposes by using dental x-ray tube stands or wall-bracket or x-ray tube holders. The first American commercially manufactured x-ray machine made especially for the dentist was produced in 1913 by the American X-ray Equipment Company of Mount Vernon, New York. It was an induction coil machine, used with an x-ray tube stand for a "complete outfit." Either alternating or direct current could be used. Soon the need for a more compact outfit was realized, and smaller and less expensive units were produced. As with medical x-ray machines, early dental units often had a dangerously exposed high-tension wire that caused several serious accidents and a few fatal ones. As one example, a dentist was about to expose a film when his patient excitedly pointed out the window to a runaway horse. At that instant, the dentist pressed a button, touched the high-tension wire, and was thrown across the room into a solid wall, sustaining a fractured skull. In 1923, the Coolidge shock-proof oil-immersed dental unit was introduced by the Victor Corporation a few years before it became the General Electric X-ray Corporation. This safe, small unit, with a capacity of 85 kV at 10 mA, had an extension wall bracket or floor stand to lessen the required floor space.[1]

Prospective radiodontists were seriously handicapped by the lack of training in interpreting dental radiographs in the dental school curriculum. In 1910, Howard Riley Raper introduced dental radiography into the curriculum of the Indiana Dental School. Three years later (1913) he wrote *Elementary and Dental Radiology*, the first textbook in the field. At that time 15 colleges were offering a special course in radiography, and others incorporated the subject in other classes. However, dentists most often took private courses, and many of those who did not have x-ray

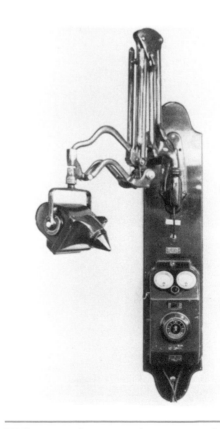

Wall-mounted version of an advanced model of the CDX x-ray unit (1933).[21]

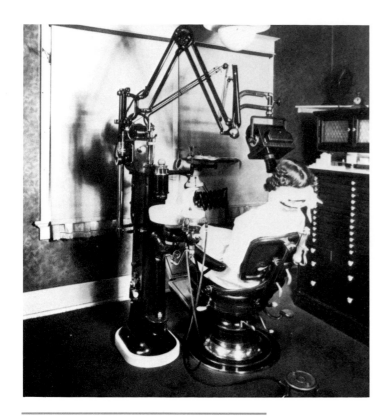

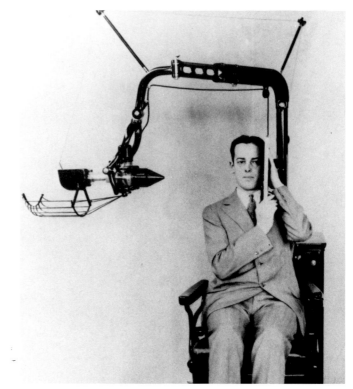

Left, Coolidge "shock proof" oil-immersed CDX x-ray unit in use.[21]

Right, Ritter x-ray unit (1928). A large Coolidge tube was used in this unit, which had an exposed high-tension wire and may have surprised the dentist with an occasional shock. Open-tube machines with exposed high-tension wires were manufactured into the 1930s.[21]

machines sent their patients to laboratories to have radiographs made. As late as 1929, Kodak offered an intensive course in x-ray technique for dentists and assistants. As the years went on, the teaching of radiodontics was taken over completely by the dental schools.[7]

As with other early x-ray workers, some of the pioneers of dental radiograph fell victim to radiation injury. As early as July 14, 1896, Harrison reported that his assistant, following several 10- to 14-minute exposures over a 4-week period, complained of itching, stinging, and red areas on his face. After several days, desquamation of the skin occurred, and some hair fell out.[18] In 1907, Kells enumerated the various injuries that could result from radiation exposure and the subsequent treatment of these injuries. Ironically, Kells was foreshadowing his own bleak future.[19] After numerous debridement and grafting operations and amputations, Kells was no longer able to practice his profession. In excruciating pain, he shot himself to death in his dental office.[20]

References

1. Glenner RA: 80 years of dental radiography. JADA 90:549-563, 1975.
2. Franke OC: Wilhelm Conrad Roentgen and other x-ray pioneers. Bull Hist Dent 31:11-17, 1983.
3. Morton WJ: The x-ray and its application in dentistry. Dental Cosmos 38:478-486, 1896.
4. Kells CE: Thirty years' experience in the field of radiography. JADA 13:693-711, 1926.
5. Kells CE: Dental skiagraphy. In Monell SH: A system of instruction in x-ray methods and medical uses of light, hot-air, vibration, and high-frequency currents. New York, Pelton, 1902.
6. Kirk EC: Editorial. Dental Cosmos 38:529-530, 1896.
7. Sweet APS: Some historical aspects of radiodontics. Dental Radiogr Photogr 15:9-11, 1942.
8. Price WA: The roentgen rays with associated phenomena, and their applications to dentistry. Dental Cosmos 42:117-129, 1900.
9. Merritt AH: The roentgen ray in dental practice. AJR 3:264-268, 1916.
10. Rollins W: An oral camera for Roentgen photography. Boston Med Surg J 134:90, 1896.
11. Kathren RL: William H. Rollins: Pioneer in reducing radiation hazard. J Hist Med 19:287-294, 1964.
12. Rollins W: Radiography in pyorrhea alveolaris. Int Dental J 18:140, 1897.
13. Kells CE: The x-ray in dental practice. JADA 7:241-272, 1920.
14. McCoy TR: Dental and oral radiography. St. Louis, CV Mosby, 1916.
15. Bober-Moken I and Perez RS: Historic insights on dental radiography. Bull Hist Dent 34:13-27, 1986.
16. Fuchs AW: Evolution of roentgen film. AJR 75:30-48, 1956.
17. Tousey S: Medical electricity and röntgen rays. Philadelphia, WB Saunders, 1910.
18. Bird PD: The development of dental radiology: The realization of a scientific dream. Br Dent J 151:28-32, 1981.
19. Kells CE: Roentgen-ray burns. JADA 14:235, 1927.
20. Gardiner JF: C. Edmund Kells: New Orleans' gift to dentistry. Bull Hist Dent 29:2-7, 1981.
21. Glenner RA: The dental office: A pictorial history. Missoula, Mont, Pictorial Histories, 1984.

CHAPTER 22

Military Radiology

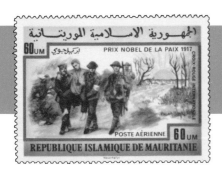
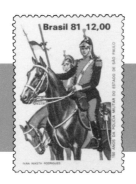
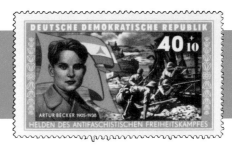

Doctors in the armed services of the major powers quickly grasped the importance of x-rays in military surgery. In Germany, the Royal Prussian Army almost immediately established a training school for radiographers and army doctors in Berlin and opened a laboratory for practical work in one of the military hospitals there. The British Army acquired its first x-ray set at the Royal Victoria Hospital, Netley, and clinical radiographs were produced by November, 1896.[1]

The first military use of x-rays came approximately 6 months after Roentgen's discovery. In May, 1896, Lieutenant Colonel Giuseppe Alvaro performed x-ray examinations on soldiers returning from the ill-fated Ethiopian campaign, in which the Italian Army suffered a crushing defeat by the Ethiopians at Adowa. In two patients, Alvaro was successful in localizing bullets with x-rays and subsequently removing them after initial probing had proved fruitless. These examinations were performed at the Military Hospital in Naples, Italy, thousands of miles from the front and more than 2 months after the battle had taken place.[2]

GRECO-TURKISH WAR (1897)

When war again broke out in the Balkans in the spring of 1897, the great European powers took sides. England, France, and Russia supported the Greeks, and Germany aided the Turks. This conflict was the first opportunity for evaluating the usefulness of radiography close to the firing line.[1] The German Red Cross sent a hospital unit to Constantinople. It contained a roentgen apparatus operated by Hermann Kuttner, who reported after the war that the x-rays were of great help in establishing the position of embedded bullets and facilitating their removal.[3] Radiography was especially valuable in cases of osteomyelitis or draining wounds in determining the extent of the fractures and the presence or absence of bullets

389

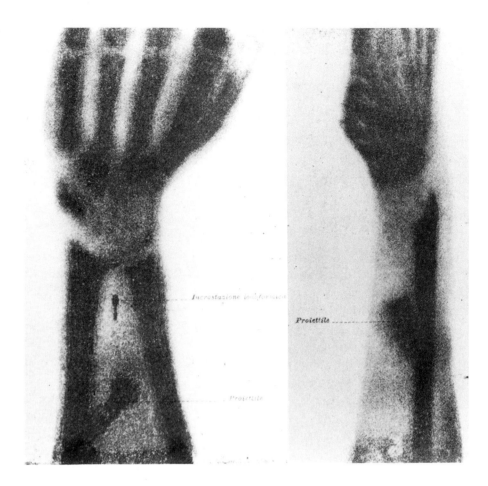

First military use of x-rays (1896). *Left,* Frontal and *right,* lateral projections successfully localizing a bullet (Proiettile).[2]

or fragments of lead or clothing. Kuttner stressed the importance of radiography in estimating injuries to the nervous system, especially in patients with severe paralysis, in whom the x-rays could determine whether the paralysis was a result of compression of the spinal cord from dislocated bone fragments or bullet injuries, thereby determining whether surgical intervention might be successful. Unfortunately, Kuttner's machine was extremely bulky, and he concluded that x-rays could only be employed in reserve or base hospitals and not in field or evacuation facilities.[4]

British x-ray units under the direction of Francis C. Abbott and Sir Robert F. Symons were sent to hospitals in Greece.[5] As much as possible, the British used a fluorescent screen to the exclusion of the photographic method, "as the position of the bullet or the seat of the injury may be viewed in many positions rapidly, and the time required to develop a dry plate constitutes a serious delay to a busy surgeon." The major technical difficulties included the heavy weight of the coil and secondary battery, the fragility of the Crookes tubes and glass plates, the danger of carrying strong sulfuric acid, and the general delicacy and temperamental nature of the apparatus. An amusing difficulty in Greece was the superstition of the people who viewed the x-ray apparatus and its use as the work of the devil. It was difficult, Symons complained, to take a skiagram when the subject was constantly crossing himself to ward off evil spirits.[1]

The most serious obstacle to field radiography was the lack of a reliable source of electrical power. The British were required to recharge their wet batteries on the H.M.S. Rodney, a warship of the Royal Navy, whereas the Germans had to discard their storage batteries and took their power directly from the hospital lighting plant.

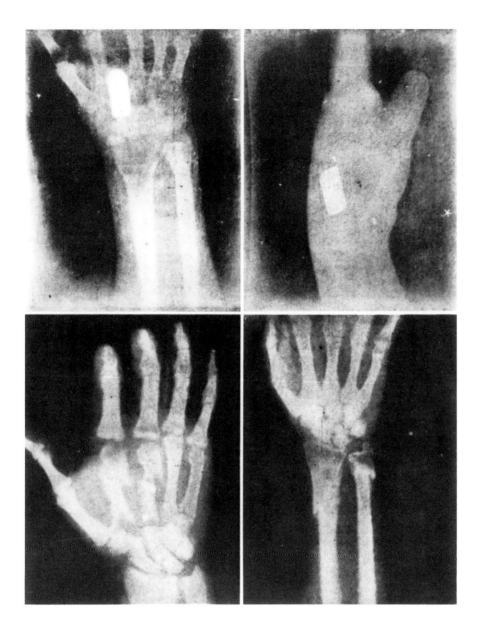

Greco-Turkish War (1897). *Top left*, Frontal and *top right*, lateral views showing a bullet wound of the right wrist. *Bottom left*, Fractures of the second and third metacarpals from a penetrating bullet wound of the hand. *Bottom right*, Fracture of the distal shafts of the radius and ulna due to a penetrating bullet wound of the forearm.[5]

It was the impression of the British surgeons and radiographers that the x-ray apparatus would prove to be of no use in the field because of the size and bulk of the machinery. In addition, Abbott advised the War Office that the use of x-rays at the front might be an incentive to surgeons to perform premature operations in poor surroundings. The new rifles used during the Greco-Turkish war fired a high-velocity steel-jacket bullet that tended to make a small entrance wound and frequently passed through the body. The gaping entrance wounds formerly seen, which were enlarged and infected by pieces of clothing being driven into the tissues, had almost completely passed into history. Thus the bullet was "practically aseptic" and there was no urgency for removal until the patient could be moved to a hospital far behind the lines.[1]

THE TIRAH CAMPAIGN (1897–1898)

The support of the English for the Greeks against the Moslem Turks led to a revolt of their co-religionists in Tirah and Malakand, districts on the Indian border with Afghanistan. The insurrectionists seized the forts in the Khyber Pass, closing it to travellers and to military transports. The

British-Indian government, realizing the importance of the Khyber Pass itself and the menace of the revolt among the natives, sent an expedition (Tirah Campaign) to quell the uprising.[4]

The wild, entirely roadless country in which the military operations were conducted made it extremely difficult to transport the wounded to base hospitals. Therefore for the first time x-rays were used on the field of battle. Walter C. Beevor, a well-to-do career army surgeon, purchased an x-ray apparatus at his own expense and shipped it to India. Transporting the x-ray apparatus posed a novel challenge in army logistics. After experiments with ox-carts, mule transport, and pack-bearers, Beevor chose to employ two *dhoolies* (Indian bearers) to carry each 100-pound box of equipment suspended from a pole. After a 200-mile journey along a route of breathtaking beauty but containing precipitous paths, icy mountain rivers with rapid torrents, and hostile tribesmen, the equipment arrived at its destination without incurring any damage.[1]

As in previous military experiences, the greatest problem involved in operating the x-ray apparatus was the generation of electricity. The only means Beevor had at Tirah was a heavy and cumbersome primary battery worked by a mixture of bichromate of potash and sulfuric acid. The latter was too dangerous for military transport unless accompanied by someone especially to look after it. Therefore Beevor condemned this form of battery for field work and recommended the employment of a hand dynamo and portable accumulator. This combination could stand rough transport and, if one malfunctioned, the other could be substituted. Despite the danger of their breakage in transport, glass plates were found to be more satisfactory than x-ray papers, whose emulsion tended to melt in hot weather.[4]

Tirah Campaign (1898). *Top left,* Bullet lodged in front of the elbow joint. *Top right,* Two bullets in the region of the hip joint. *Bottom,* Retained bullet in the leg of General Wodehouse lying in the calf muscles and framed by the leg bones (fibula above, tibia below). Note the safety pin in the bandage.[6]

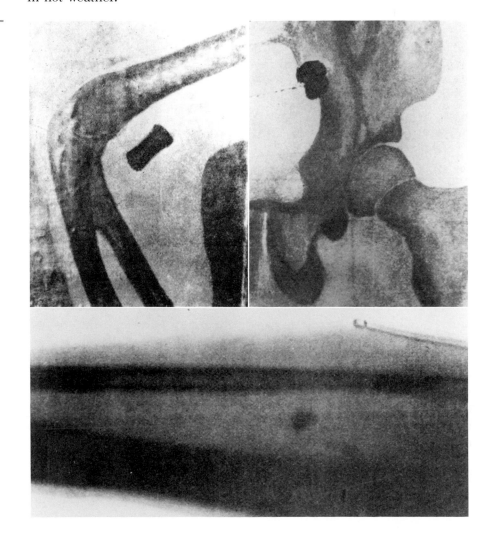

Beevor's exploits excited the curiosity of the British nation.[6] He had taken his x-rays in the midst of a battle in some far-off place, and two of his patients were public figures: General Wodehouse and General Sir Ian Hamilton. Wodehouse's stoicism as he had a bullet wound in his leg probed while under intense enemy fire was widely reported in the popular press. The wound failed to heal, and Beevor's subsequent radiograph dramatically revealed a retained bullet fragment as the cause of the suppuration. General Hamilton shattered the bones of his leg in a fall from his horse. The radiograph made after manipulation showed that the fracture had been perfectly reduced, "and there will be no need now for his proceeding home."[1]

As a result of his experience in the Tirah Campaign, Beevor recommended that all apparatus constructed for military work be "get-at-able," thus enabling one to repair the inevitable defects of wear and tear. He declared that "I maintain it is now the duty of every civilized nation to supply its wounded in war with an x-ray apparatus, not only at base hospitals, but close at hand, wherever they may be fighting and exposing themselves to injury."[6]

THE RIVER WAR (1896–1898)

Britain finally established control over the valley of the Nile in a 2-year campaign in which an army dispatched from Cairo liberated the Sudan from an Islamic fundamentalist group, the Mahdists. Among the many thousands of items dispatched to the expedition was an x-ray unit under the control of an army surgeon, Major John C. Battersby. Battersby recognized that his major adversary was the incredible heat and dust of the Sudan. To protect his equipment during the 100-mile river voyage and the long overland trek to the Sudan, Battersby surrounded the outer boxes containing coils and storage batteries with thick felt covers, which he kept constantly wet by applications of water every 2 hours. Though exposed to air temperatures up to 122° F in the shade, the apparatus reached its destination at Abadieh without mishap.[1]

As in other military campaigns, one of the most serious difficulties was the generation of the primary electrical current for charging the storage batteries or for directly working the coil. Battersby's solution was to produce electricity by charging wet batteries with a dynamo rigged up to the rear wheel of a tandem bicycle. This required two cyclists, pedalling as hard as they could to overcome the resistance, since the high temperature and humidity prevented Battersby's volunteers from "cycling" for more than 30 minutes at a time.[7]

The fierce sandstorms and the hot sun were more difficult to combat. Dust was everywhere, and all sensitive equipment had to be wrapped up. The glass plates were particularly vulnerable, since the wooden holders were not impervious, and each was kept in a cloth bag. The intense sunlight was impossible to "black out" and penetrated under the fluoroscopic hood and into the development room. Consequently, Battersby used the fluoroscopic screen only at night, and all the developing work was performed at 3:00 a.m., the darkest hour. This hour was also the coolest, when the temperature in the mud-hut darkroom fell to only 90° to 110° F, so that photographic development was no longer instantaneous.[1]

In 21 cases in which conventional surgical probing failed to find the bullet or to prove its absence, an accurate diagnosis was obtained using x-rays in all but one (a man with a chest wound who was too ill to

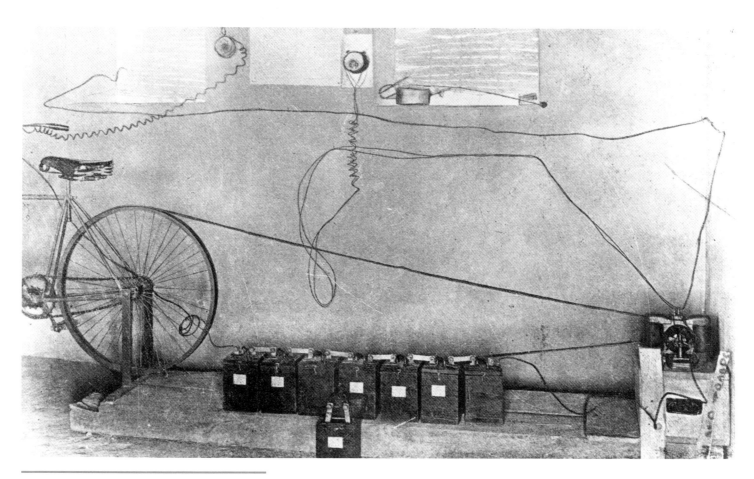

River War (1899). Method for generating electricity for charging storage batteries.[7]

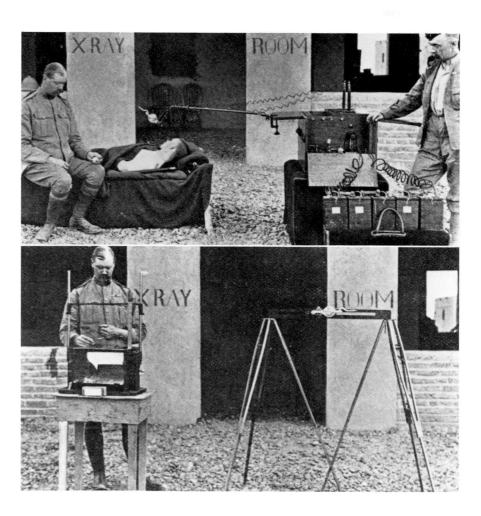

River War (1899). *Top*, Major Battersby and his orderly taking a radiograph. *Bottom*, Localizing apparatus.[7]

examine). As Battersby remarked, "I have shown you how probing for an uncertain bullet, with its subsequent pain, is now a thing of the past in military surgery."[7]

THE BOER WAR (1899)

The Boer War was a bitter struggle for ownership of the mineral wealth of South Africa that pitted the British Army against the Boers, the descendants of the Dutch immigrants who had settled the country almost 250 years before. During this conflict, the siege of Ladysmith was the first occasion in which radiography was performed for a substantial period under shell fire. The radiographer in Ladysmith was Lieutenant Forbes Bruce, who had served in the Sudan with Battersby and had become convinced of the futility of using bicycle power to generate electricity for the coils and storage batteries. The problem of recharging the batteries was ingeniously solved when Bruce discovered a flour mill nearby and gained permission from the manager to drive the dynamo from the mill shaft by means of a pulley. This arrangement proved so successful that Bruce even could provide the surgeon with an electric light for the operating room at night.[8]

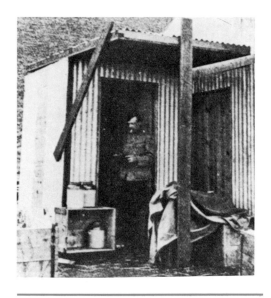

Boer War (1899). Temporary darkroom at Delfontein, with John Hall-Edwards standing in the doorway.[1]

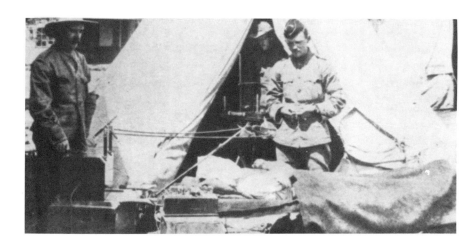

Boer War. Tented x-ray department outside Ladysmith during the siege of 1899. Quartermaster Forbes Bruce assisted by a Colonial scout x-rays the wrist of a soldier.[1]

Boer War (1899). *Left*, Gunshot wound to the right thigh shattering the upper third of the femur. This officer in the Imperial Light Horse received no amputation and returned to duty. *Right*, Gunshot wound causing a fracture of the head of the radius and lower end of the humerus.[8]

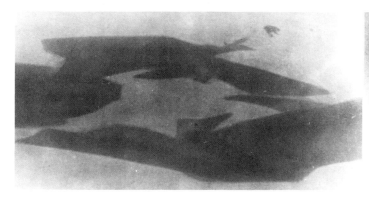
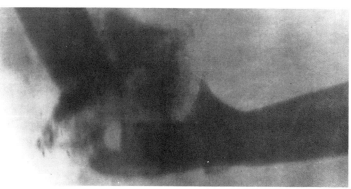

For a week the Boers besieged Ladysmith, and shells dropped continually near the town hall, where the x-ray apparatus was set up. As Bruce later wrote, "Great caution had to be used in photographing the patients when shells were heard in the immediate vicinity, as they (the patients) were sure to start, thinking the building would be hit. Exposures under these conditions had to be short." Bruce posted a lookout to report on the firing of the guns, and this resulted in far fewer radiographic failures.[8]

SPANISH-AMERICAN WAR (1898)

The United States Army first used x-rays in the Spanish-American War. However, x-rays were not used extensively, resulting from both the type of warfare and the fact that the Medical Corps was primarily occupied in caring for the large number of soldiers ill with typhoid fever. Nevertheless, the more important general hospitals and the three hospital ships (Relief, Missouri, Bay State) were supplied with x-ray apparatus. Two soldiers suffered x-ray burns from prolonged and frequently repeated exposure, probably the first incidents reported in military radiography.[9]

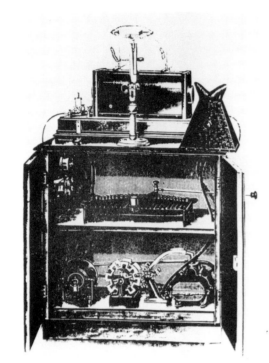

Spanish-American War (1898). Edison portable x-ray outfit representing the first x-ray installation in the U.S. Navy, placed into service on the hospital ship "Solace."

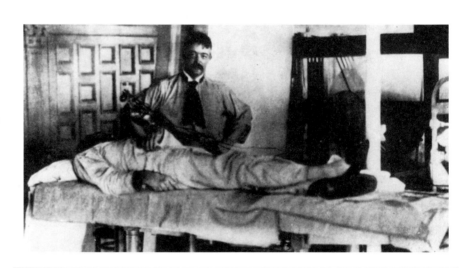

Spanish-American War (1898). Taking x-ray photograph on the hospital ship RELIEF at Siboney, Cuba.[9]

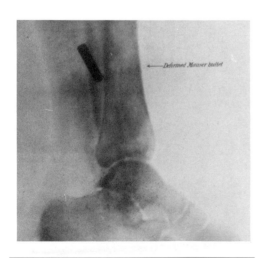

Spanish-American War (1898). Radiograph demonstrating an opaque Mauser bullet in the left leg of an American infantryman.[9]

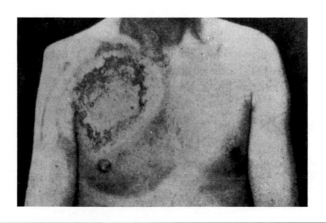

Spanish-American War (1898). Roentgen-ray burn of right breast following three unsuccessful prolonged exposures of the shoulder.[9]

WORLD WAR I

World War I was the bloodiest conflict yet recorded in terms of human life and suffering. Out of approximately 65 million men mobilized for war, it was estimated that 36 million were killed or injured. Space limitations preclude an examination of the role of radiology in the armies of all the combatants. Thus the following discussion deals only with the experiences of the United States Army in World War I.

The Division of Roentgenology was initially established from the Division of Supply and later became a section under the Division of Surgery. Its major objective, under Colonel Arthur C. Christie, was the procurement of x-ray supplies and equipment. Christie had been an efficient regular army officer before entering civil practice and thus was familiar with army regulations, knew how to procure supplies, and quickly earned the confidence of the heads of other army departments and the Surgeon General.[11]

A special Standard U.S. Army x-ray table with two removable tops was developed. In addition to being used in the x-ray room, the table top was used as a stretcher for carrying patients and could be employed as a

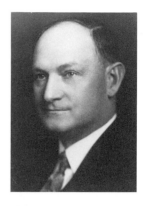

Colonel Arthur C. Christie (1879-1956), Director of Division of Roentgenology in World War I.

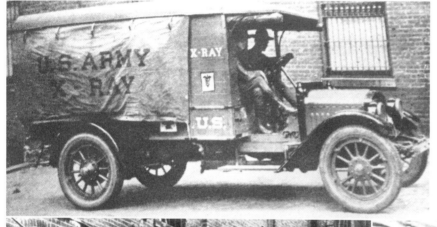

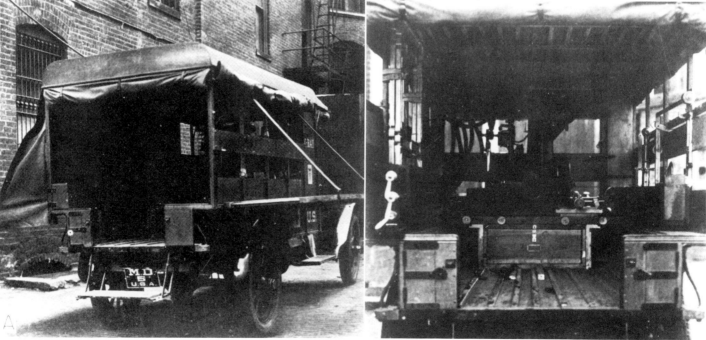

Mobile x-ray unit used in World War I. *Left*, X-ray truck. *Middle*, Exterior table tops used for beds.[12] *Right*, Interior of vehicle with packaged x-ray equipment.[12]

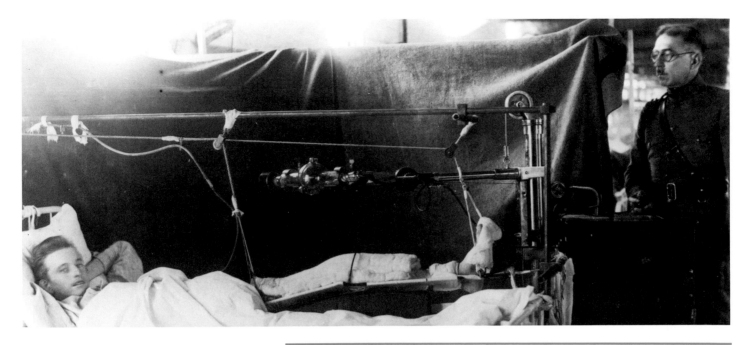

World War I. One of the earliest mobile bedside x-ray units at Base Hospital 69 in France.

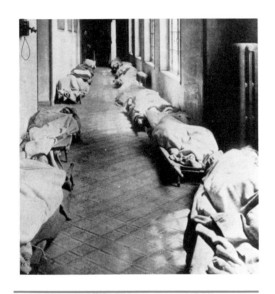

En route to the x-ray room. Corridor of a French castle transformed into an Army Hospital during World I. (AJR, 1918.)

surgical operating table, since its Bakelite covering was impervious to antiseptic solutions. A remarkably efficient and silent portable x-ray field unit was developed by William D. Coolidge. The current used in the transformer of this portable outfit was obtained from a generator driven by a single-cylinder, air-cooled gasoline engine. The voltage depended on the speed of the engine, which was easily controlled. This portable equipment had no moving parts (except in the engine and generator) and could be disassembled for transportation within 3 minutes. Because the unit employed alternating rather than direct current, the absence of rectifying switch or interrupter meant that there were fewer devices to get out of order. Using Coolidge's new hot cathode tube with its capacity for continuous efficient operation, this unit was one that could serve in regular hospital situations, as well as portable work.[11]

By the end of the war, 719 x-ray units were shipped overseas: 150 complete sets for base hospitals, 250 bedside machines, 55 x-ray ambulances, 264 portable machines, and hundreds of accessory items.[12]

Once the logistics were under way, the major problem was to obtain a sufficient number of radiologists. The results of a questionnaire sent to members of the American Roentgen Ray Society made it clear that "the

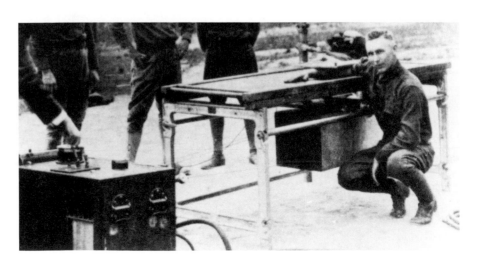

World War I. Portable x-ray field unit used by the U.S. Army Medical Department that could be disassembled for transportation within 3 minutes.

number of qualified roentgenologists in the United States was comparatively small and that some plan would need to be devised to train men for this work." The solution was to implement short and intense radiology training programs for active duty and reserve medical officers. Beginning in July, 1917, schools were established in various parts of the country in hospitals where there were ample facilities and materials for teaching. Medical officers were assigned to these civilian schools in groups of 10 for 2 weeks of x-ray training before some were shipped overseas. Within 6 months, about 200 men had been trained to serve as radiologists.[11]

The basic textbook was the *United States Army X-ray Manual*, one of the earliest (if not *the* earliest) formalized standard-setting works on medical radiography to be published in North America. With 506 pages and 219 illustrations, the *Manual* served both radiologists and technologists.[13]

In December, 1917, the civilian schools (except the one in New York) were closed, and two others were established at the Medical Officers' Training Camps at Camp Greenleaf, Georgia, and Fort Riley, Kansas. The purpose of these two schools was to select those incoming officers who would be suitable for x-ray work and to give them a preliminary course of training in radiology while they were being instructed in the rules and regulations of the Army. After a brief course in the Camp schools, the men were sent to New York for final instruction in the installation, care, and repair of apparatus and in the methods of localization of foreign bodies. Later, the Kansas school was closed, and the equipment at the New York school was shipped to Camp Greenleaf, where all instruction of military radiology was placed under the sponsorship of the United States Army Medical School under the command of Lieutenant Colonel William Manges.[11]

In addition to the training of radiologists, enlisted men were given an intensive 1-month course of training to become "manipulators." Many of these individuals had been technicians in radiology before entering the Army or had worked in factories where x-ray apparatus was made. Still others were electricians or photographers. All were thoroughly drilled in "trouble hunting" and repair work on apparatus, as well as in the care, handling, and filing of developing room material (films and plates).[11]

The curriculum of the Camp Greenleaf School of Roentgenology was based on the idea that its students were being trained to practice radiology under war conditions anywhere from the battlefront to base hospitals. It was considered critical that both the officers and enlisted men be able to work any kind of apparatus and keep it operating under all conditions possible, as well as to be able to install it, dismantle it, and pack it properly for transport. While medical officers concentrated on x-ray diagnosis, enlisted personnel spent time on proper positioning of patients for radiographic examinations. British, French, German, and American x-ray equipment were studied so that officers and enlisted radiological personnel would be prepared for whatever they might encounter overseas.[12]

In September, 1918, the demand for trained radiologists was so great that larger classes had to be taken into the school and the length of the course had to be decreased. Originally designed for 25 radiologists and 50 manipulators per month, by this time twice as many personnel had to be accommodated. The course of instruction for radiologists had to be reduced from 3 to 2 months; the more advanced clinical instruction was sacrificed in favor of studies in localization of foreign bodies, the care and operation of apparatus, and practical fluoroscopic and radiographic work.

UNITED STATES ARMY
X-RAY MANUAL

AUTHORIZED BY THE SURGEON-GENERAL OF THE ARMY

*Prepared under the Direction of the
Division of Roentgenology*

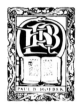

[219 ILLUSTRATIONS]

NEW YORK
PAUL B. HOEBER
67-69 EAST 59TH STREET
1918

World War I *United States Army X-ray Manual* (1918).

399

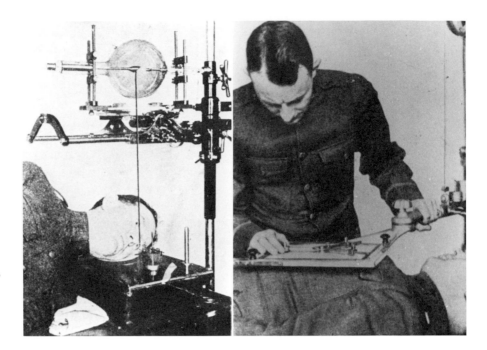

World War I. Techniques for foreign body localization in the eye. *Left*, Radiographic. *Right*, Fluoroscopic screen method.[12]

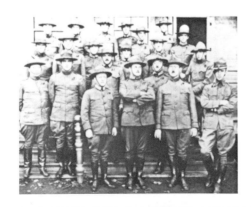

World War I. Staff of instructors at Camp Greenleaf School of Roentgenology.

Probably the most important clinical subject in both lecture and laboratory courses was the localization of foreign bodies. With the aid of manikins and other objects in which foreign bodies were placed, the student officers were taught the various methods of foreign body localization that had the approval of the Surgeon General's Office. The standard army table was provided with parts necessary to carry out the method of localization proposed by Professor Strohl of the French Roentgenological Service. This method was based on the construction of a triangle, with the foreign body as the apex and the base a measured distance on the fluorescent screen that represented the shift of the foreign body shadow during the localization. Other techniques that were taught included the parallax method, by which the depth of the foreign body could be determined from three different points on the skin surface; the nearest point method, a rapid technique involving palpating the soft tissues in the region of the foreign body with a rod having a metallic end and determining the point on the surface where the least amount of pressure would move the foreign body (this being the point on the surface nearest to the foreign body); stereoscopic radiographs (for use in hospitals at some distance from the front, where surgical work was more deliberately and carefully planned); and the Bowden modification of the Sweet Eye Localizer used for foreign bodies in the eyeball or near it.[11]

In the war zone itself, x-rays were used less in the field hospital, an emergency hospital for the battlefield 3 to 8 miles from the front, than in the evacuation hospital, the major surgical center to the rear of the battle area. In the field hospital, the radiographic unit was located close to the surgical room. The demands on radiologists were overwhelming, and x-ray teams often were forced to work constantly with little sleep for days on end. Few permanent radiographic plates were made, since the rapid and accurate fluoroscopic method was used almost exclusively.

Because of the tremendous number and types of wounds generated in battle and the possibility of their infection from less than optimum aseptic and sterile conditions, the x-ray localization procedures had to be simple, direct, and quick. "Surgeons were often tempted to perform the x-ray localization procedures themselves. However, this responsibility belonged to the roentgenologist. Surgeons not familiar with the x-ray localization procedure subjected themselves, coworkers, and patients to considerable x-ray overexposure."[14]

WORLD WAR II

During World War II, radiology played an important role in military medicine, both at home and in the war zone. The x-ray examination of the chest was an important phase of the physical examination of candidates for service in the U.S. Army. Photoroentgenograms, using 4 × 5 films for frontal and lateral projections, were obtained routinely before acceptance and again before discharge. The purpose of this procedure was "(1) to eliminate those whose physical condition would not withstand the rigors of army life; (2) to avoid dissemination of tuberculosis because of the close contact incident to groupings of large numbers as required in the service; and (3) to maintain graphic records of chest conditions in order to provide for proper adjustment of any claims which might be made against the Government."[15]

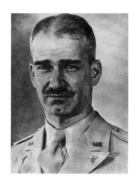

Colonel Alfred A. de Lorimer (1901-1960), Commandant of the Army School of Roentgenology in World War II.

World War II. Picker basic field unit packed for transportation. *A,* Tube unit and high-tension cables. Note the spring suspension provided for the tube and the device to keep the chest upright. *B,* Support mechanism. *C,* Controls of unit, with compartments for accessories. *D,* Localization and fluoroscopic attachments. *E,* Transformer component.

World War II. Field packing chest developed at the Army School of Roentgenology. *A,* Exterior of chest. *B,* Dryer, fixed by straps, packed in the lower section of the chest. *C,* Loading bin, fixed by straps, packed in the lower section of the chest. *D,* Lower section of the chest used as a table. *E,* Top section of the chest used as a desk. *F,* Top section of the chest converted into a reserve auxiliary wash tank. Any bulging of the sides caused by large volumes of water could be corrected by using the fixation straps for reinforcement.

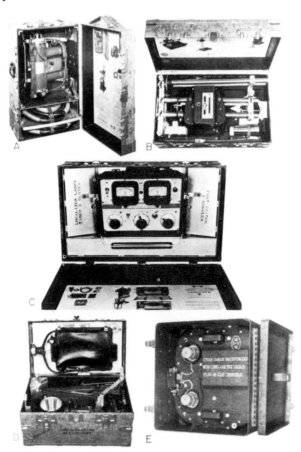

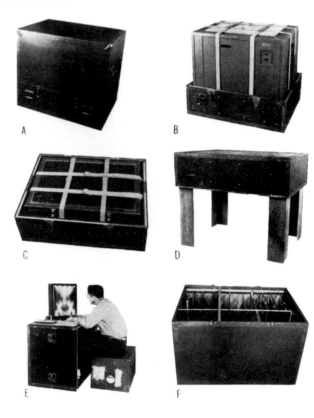

World War II. Auxiliary mobile x-ray unit set up in the field for daylight use.[18]

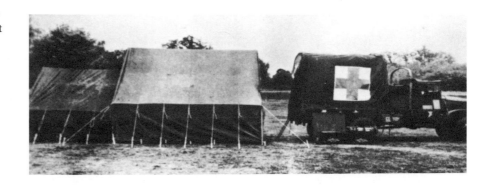

World War II. Radiography with the field table of a Picker Army X-ray Unit. This unit was widely used both in the front line, as well as in rear echelon military medical installations. Picker was the sole supplier of the Army Field X-ray Unit, although it should be noted that James Picker, then president of the company, donated all the profits the company made during the war to the United States Treasury.[16]

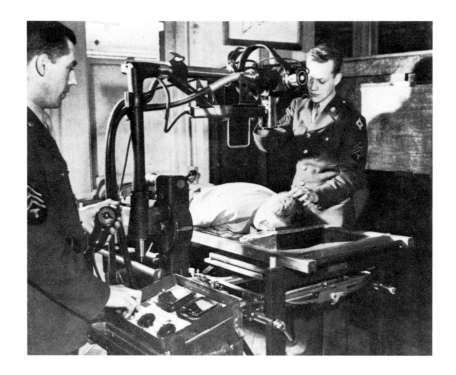

World War II. Actual Army radiography field operations. *Left*, 15th Base Evacuation Hospital, Anzio, shows inadequate radiation protection. *Right*, 95th Evacuation Hospital, Capua Sector, shows use of an improvised table with a mobile Picker x-ray unit.[18]

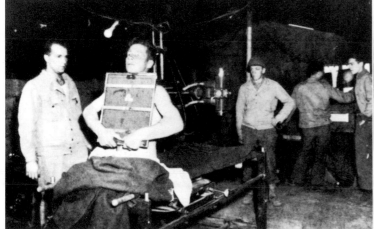

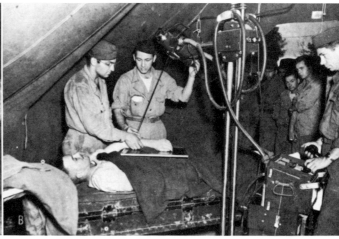

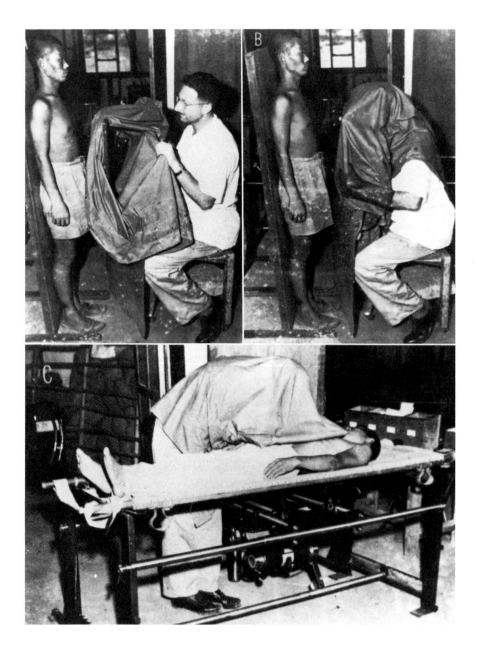

World War II. Improvised fluoroscopic technique used at the 20th General Hospital. *Top left*, In preparation for the examination, a fluoroscopist holds a pup tent with which he will secure sufficient darkness for the examination. *Top right*, Examination of an ambulatory patient. *Bottom*, Examination of a litter patient. Note the protective sandbags at the upper left.[18]

For the "theater of operations," the designing of equipment was governed by three axiomatic principles:

> (1) versatility of adaptation to the extent that each piece of equipment will function not merely for a single purpose, but for several requirements and installations; (2) portability to the extent that disassemblage of each item can be easily accomplished and that the component parts can be easily carried, the weight of any one part not exceeding 200 pounds; and (3) practicality in design to the extent that the equipment can serve the requirements of function in peacetime installations as well as in zones of combat.

It was considered beneficial to supply the Army with x-ray units that radiologists had already been using in their regular practices. In addition, the equipment could incorporate improvements made during peace time so that it would not be necessary "on mobilization day suddenly to develop new designs in order to incorporate new principles that may be discovered." Two other advantages of designing war-time equipment that was also practical for use in peace-time installations were:

(1) a war reserve stock of supplies is provided so that, in case of a sudden emergency, equipment will be available for moving into the field without awaiting supplies from manufacturers; (2) because of steady purchases, the manufacturers will be informed as to just what the army will need in large quantities, and they will therefore have set up the necessary jigs, dies, and other tools necessary for uniform and large-scale constructions.[15]

Applying these principles, the combination x-ray table unit, x-ray machine unit, and mobile x-ray chassis were designed to provide for a nine-way adaptation. These units offered:

(1) horizontal fluoroscopy; (2) foreign body localization by means of a rapid fluoroscopic method; (3) sitting fluoroscopy, the design of the x-ray tube and screen supports providing for easy and quick shifting for the study of a patient supported to a sitting position on the litter; (4) standing fluoroscopy, to the extent of accommodating routine chest studies and also gastro-intestinal studies; (5) horizontal roentgenography, with conventional focal-film distances from 25 to 40 inches; (6) six-foot vertical chest study; (7) six-foot horizontal chest studies, the patient lying on a litter, upon the floor; (8) ordinary bedside work in the wards, by means of mounting the component parts of the x-ray machine upon a mobile chassis; and (9) superficial roentgen therapy, to the extent of milliamperage capacities of 4 and kilovoltage potentials up to 100.[15,19]

The military also designed a light-proof tent that could be erected outdoors, within an ordinary corridor or war tent, or within a room, cellar, or dugout. As with all equipment, it was designed for a two-way adaptation, either as a fluoroscopic compartment or, with another arrangement, as a film-processing "darkroom."

The radiology requirements in the theater of operations were precisely organized. Nevertheless, it was realized that "because of the character of present-day warfare—the rapidity of movement and the frequent change in the battlefront with alterations of offensive and defensive tactics— medical installations can be considered merely in a relative manner. We cannot think of well identified and established situations."[20]

No radiographic assistance was provided for the front-line forces. The most advanced installation in which x-ray services could be utilized effectively was the *mobile surgical hospital*. This was an Army unit that moved forward to the vicinity of the "clearing station" of the medical battalion as casualties accumulated there. Its purpose was to provide the first real surgical care for those of the wounded who because of their condition could not be evacuated further to the rear (i.e., the evacuation hospital). Before this care became available, treatment consisted merely of first-aid dressings or the application of a tourniquet. Casualties typically reached the mobile surgical hospital (about 5 to 7 miles to the rear of the front lines) within 4 to 15 hours and were scheduled to be transported farther to the rear as soon as possible (usually within 1 to 4 days). Each mobile surgical hospital had two radiologists and three x-ray technicians. As in World War I, most of its x-ray activities were fluoroscopic, including localization of foreign bodies.[20]

Farther to the rear, about 15 to 70 miles from the front line and usually located at a railhead, was the *evacuation hospital*, which was allotted two radiologists and as many as 10 x-ray technicians. Casualties generally reached the evacuation hospital from 4 to 48 hours after injury, either directly from the clearing station or from the mobile surgical hospital as soon as they were in condition to permit further transportation.

With accommodations for as many as 750 patients, the evacuation hospital was set up in a temporary building or in some building taken over for the purpose and was more substantial than the tents of the mobile surgical hospital. Again, most of the x-ray procedures were performed under fluoroscopy; radiography was considered to be practical in only about 10% of cases.[20]

General hospitals were permanent or semipermanent structures designed to provide special and prolonged treatment. The radiological requirements were similar to those expected for any large institution in civilian practice. In comparison with the mobile surgical and evacuation hospitals, the equipment in a general hospital was substantially larger and of conventional commercial design. Three radiologists and nine x-ray technicians were allotted for each 1,000 patients.[21]

Two other types of hospitals required the services of a radiologist. *Convalescent hospitals* accommodating as many as 3,000 tended to treat more chronic problems, and only one radiologist and five technicians were deemed necessary. *Station hospitals,* which provided for medical and surgical care of personnel connected with units not usually engaged in conflict, often were allotted a single, well-qualified radiologist and several technicians.[20]

The critical role of x-ray studies in military medicine meant that proportionally more radiologists were needed than for general civilian care. As in World War I, there was a severe shortage of radiologists (and radiologic technologists), which had to be met by special training programs. Of the 1,000 radiologists needed, about half had to be comprehensively trained specialists. For certain assignments, however, it was considered that limited training in basic fundamentals would be sufficient. An "Intensive Basic Course in Roentgenology" was instituted, which consisted of 4 weeks of didactic lectures, conferences, and special problem investigations given 8 hours a day for 6 days a week. Enlisted personnel training as x-ray technicians received a 2- or 3-month course.[20]

References

1. Burrows EH: X-rays on the battlefield. In Pioneers and early years: A history of British radiology. Channel Islands, England, Colophon, 1986.
2. Alvaro G: The practical benefits to surgery of Röntgen's discovery: Diagnostic results in the location of bullets in wounded soldiers from Africa. Giornale Medico del Regio Esercito 44:383-394, 1896.
3. Kuttner H: The importance of Roentgen rays in war surgery based on experience in the Greco-Turkish war of 1897. Beit Klin Chir 20:167-230, 1898.
4. Reynolds L: The history of the use of the roentgen ray in warfare. AJR 54:649-672, 1945.
5. Abbott FC: Surgery in the Graeco-Turkish war. Lancet 1:80-83, 1899.
6. Beevor WC: The working of the roentgen ray in warfare. J Roy United Service Institution 42:1152-1170, 1898.
7. Battersby J: The present position of the roentgen rays in military surgery. Arch Roentg Ray 3:74-80, 1899.
8. Bruce F: Experiences of x-ray work during the siege of Ladysmith. Arch Roentg Ray 5:69-74, 1901.
9. Borden WC: The use of the Röntgen ray by the Medical Department of the United States Army in War with Spain (1898). Washington, DC, US Government Printing Office, 1900.
10. Matignon JJ: L'appareil à rayons X de l'armée Japonaise en campagne. Arch Electr Med 14:455-457, 1906.
11. Manges WF: Military roentgenology. In Glasser O (ed): The science of radiology. Springfield, Ill, Charles C Thomas, 1933.
12. Lauer OG: Radiography in the United States Army during World War I. Radiol Technol 56:400-408, 1985.
13. United States Army X-ray Manual. New York, Hoeber, 1918.
14. Case JT: Localization and extraction of foreign bodies under x-ray control. In Weed FW (ed): The Medical Department of the United States Army in the World War, Vol XI, Surgery. Washington, D.C., U.S. Government Printing Office, 1927.
15. De Lorimer AA: Wartime military roentgenology. Radiology 36:391-403, 1941.
16. Krohmer JS: Radiography and fluoroscopy, 1920 to the present. RadioGraphics 9:1129-1153, 1989.
17. Lauer OG: Radiography in the United States Army during World War II. 1. Radiologic Technology 58:123-133, 1987.
18. Lauer OG: Radiography in the United States Army during World War II. 2. Radiologic Technology 58:215-224, 1987.
19. De Lorimer AA and Dauer M: The Army roentgen-ray equipment problem. AJR 54:673-687, 1945.
20. De Lorimer AA: Requirements for roentgenological services in the field of combat. Radiology 38:590-598, 1942.
21. Bell JC and Heublein GW: Diagnostic roentgenology in an Army General Hospital during the present war. AJR 43:425-485, 1944.

THE EMERGENCE OF IMAGING MODALITIES

WE WANT TO KNOW

If the Roentgen rays, that are way ahead,
    Will show us in simple note,
How, when we ask our best girl to wed,
    That lump will look in our throat.

If the cathode rays, that we hear all about,
    When the burglar threatens to shoot,
Will they show us the picture without any doubt,
    Of the heart that we feel in our boot.

If the new x-rays, that the papers do laud,
    When the ghosts do walk at night,
Will show 'neath our hat to the world abroad
    How our hair stands on end in our fright.

If the wonderful, new, electric rays,
    Will do all the people have said,
And show us quite plainly, before many days,
    Those wheels that we have in our head.

If the Roentgen, cathode, electric, x-light,
    Invisible! Think of that!
Can ever be turned on the Congressman bright
    And show him just where he is at.

Oh, if these rays should strike you and me,
    Going through us without any pain,
Oh, what a fright they would give us to see
    The mess which our stomachs contain!

Homer C Bennett, *American X-ray Journal*, 1897

CHAPTER 23

Nuclear Medicine

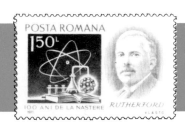
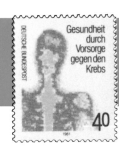
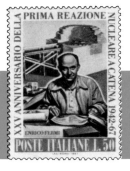
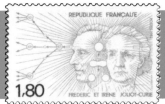

The use of radioactive materials in medical and biological studies was limited before 1932 because the only radioactive isotopes available were the naturally occurring forms that normally are present only in minute quantities in biological systems. Although important preliminary investigations were performed, it was necessary to develop a reliable source of relatively large amounts of reasonably stable artificial radio-isotopes (radionuclides).

A major landmark in the development of nuclear science was the classic experiment of Ernest Rutherford (1919) at the Cavendish Laboratory in Cambridge, England. Rutherford placed a small amount of radium in a container filled with oxygen and mounted a zinc sulfide screen nearby. Alpha particles emitted by the radium struck the zinc sulfide screen and produced on its surface pinpoints of light called *scintillations*, which could be observed and even counted by watching the screen through a microscope. Next, Rutherford placed enough silver foil between the container and the zinc sulfide screen to block the alpha particles so that the scintillations ceased. Finally, he substituted nitrogen for the oxygen in the container. Despite the continuing presence of the silver-foil barrier, scintillations reappeared on the zinc sulfide screen. Something different was now being emitted from the nitrogen-filled container—something capable of penetrating a barrier impervious to alpha particles. By studying the behavior of this material in electric and magnetic fields, Rutherford showed that they were not x-rays but rather positively charged nuclear particles, or protons.

Rutherford and an associate, James Chadwick, deduced the underlying process that must have been occurring inside the container. When an alpha particle emitted by the radium struck a nitrogen nucleus containing seven protons, one proton was ejected. The remainder of the nitrogen atom and the alpha particle joined together to form a new atom with eight protons—an oxygen atom. Rutherford had thus achieved the goal of the

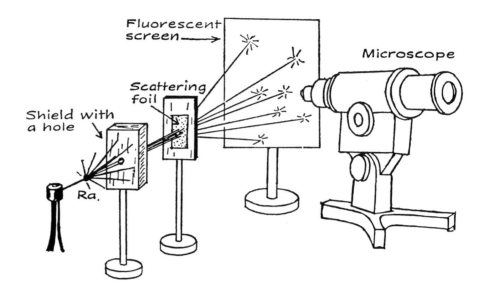

Radiumography (1907). *Top,* Experimental design for radiographing a block of granite with 60 mg of radium bromide using an exposure time of 3 days. *Bottom,* Resulting radiograph.[2]

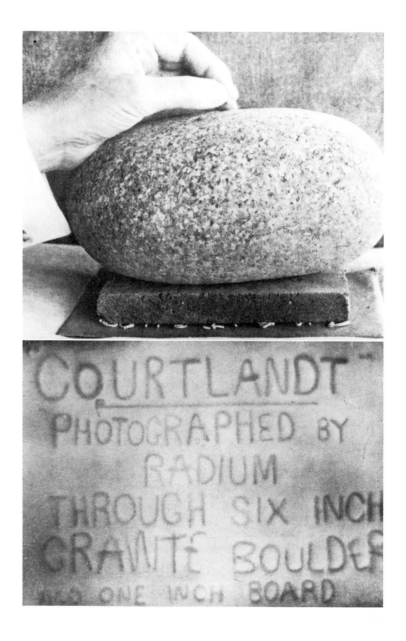

410

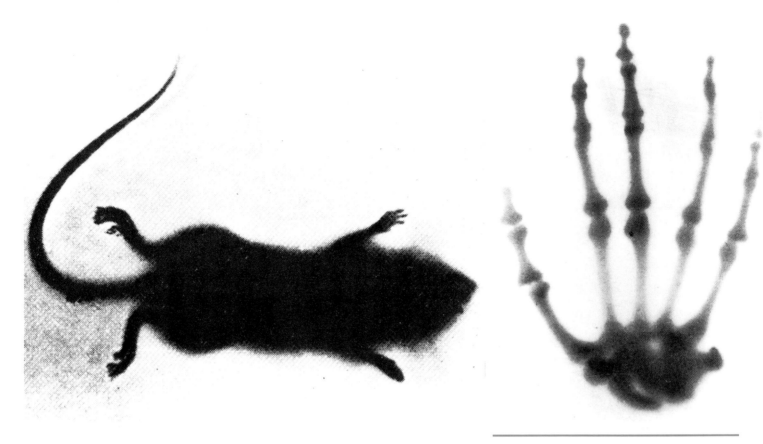

Radiumgraphs (1904). *Left*, Image of a mouse after 24 hours exposure.[3] *Right*, Image of a hand following 6 hours exposure.[4] "While there is considerable permeation, the contrasts are poor and another disadvantage is that it takes hours to represent an image."

medieval alchemist: the transmutation of elements. A critically important by-product of this artificial transformation of an atomic nucleus was the leftover proton, which was ejected at high energy.

Not only was it possible to convert one familiar element like nitrogen into another like oxygen, but bombardment also produced previously unknown species of matter. These isotopes of common elements had the same number of protons and electrons but different atomic weights.

Rutherford and other investigators soon realized the inherent limitations of using radium and other radioactive elements as sources of bombarding particles. Only the alpha particles from radium were effective in nuclear transformation. However, the emission of an alpha particle by an atom of radium is a relatively rare event, and the energy and penetration of these particles are severely limited.[5] To learn more about the nucleus and to produce the fascinating new isotopes on a useful scale, a far richer source of high-energy bombarding particles was urgently needed.

For the next decade, laboratories in many countries engaged in a scientific race to be the first to develop "particle accelerators" or "atom-smashers" capable of speeding up subatomic particles to the energies required for effective nuclear bombardment. Initially, they employed the one type of particle accelerator already familiar to physicists—the x-ray tube itself. Increasingly more powerful "supervoltage" x-ray tubes were constructed (see Chapter 7). Eventually, John D. Cockroft and Ernest T.S. Walton in England (1932) built a high-voltage transformer-type of accelerator capable of producing protons with sufficient energy to bring about a

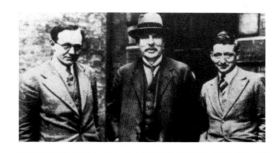

Ernest T.S. Walton, Ernest Rutherford, and John D. Cockroft.

nuclear transformation. The lithium nucleus, which contains three protons, captured a fourth from the beam to become a beryllium nucleus; this beryllium nucleus then split into two helium nuclei containing two protons each.

In the United States, Ernest O. Lawrence (1931), at the University of California Radiation Laboratory, developed the cyclotron, the first of the circular accelerators. Instead of using a high voltage for the initial acceleration of charged particles, the cyclotron employed a magnetic field and a series of accelerations to achieve high-energy particles with lower voltages. Lawrence and his co-workers were able to demonstrate nuclear transformation using the cyclotron almost immediately following the Cockroft and Walton report. Meanwhile, an American chemist, Harold C. Urey, discovered deuterium, or heavy hydrogen. In addition to permitting the labelling of hydrogen so that it could be used as a tracer in living systems, the nuclei of deuterium (deuterons) provided a new source of subatomic projectiles. By the end of 1933, a cyclotron had been developed that could produce a 3,000,000 electron volt beam of deuterons with a radiation intensity equivalent to enormous quantities of radium. This cyclotron was able to accelerate protons, deuterons, and alpha particles.[6]

The discovery of two new subatomic particles—the neutron (1932) and the positron, or positively charged electron (1933)—gave new impetus to the empirical studies of the effects of alpha particles emitted from radium on a variety of elements. At the Radium Institute in Paris, the pivotal experiments were conducted by Irene Curie, the daughter of Pierre and Marie Curie, and her husband, Frédéric Joliot. Their methods differed from Rutherford's of 15 years earlier only in that they were looking for positrons, as well as for alpha particles, beta particles, and gamma rays emitted during nuclear bombardment. They soon discovered that a number of light elements emitted positrons when bombarded by alpha particles from their radioactive source, polonium. Further studies

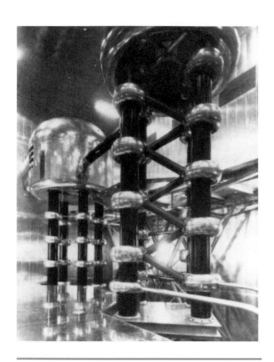

First high-voltage transformer-type accelerator used to produce a nuclear transformation (1932).

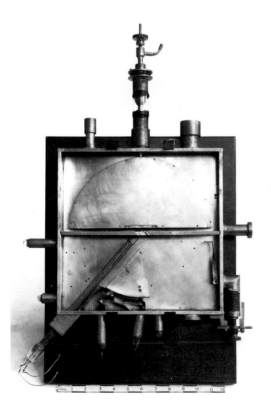

Ernest O. Lawrence (1901-1958) and his second cyclotron.[7]

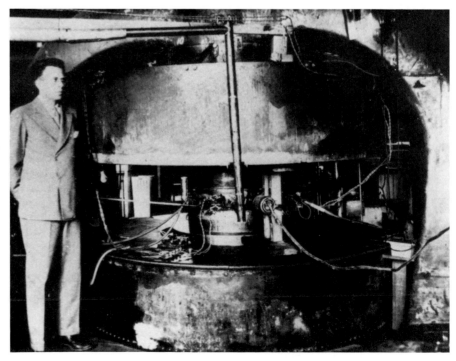

412

demonstrated that the bombardment of three elements—aluminum, boron, and magnesium—caused an emission of positrons that continued even after the polonium source had been taken away from the target. The only plausible explanation, as announced in a brief paper in *Nature* on February 10, 1934, was that "the transmutation of boron, magnesium, and aluminum by alpha particles has given birth to new radioelements (radioactive isotopes) . . ."[5]

Joliot and Curie deduced that the alpha bombardment of an aluminum nucleus (13 protons, 14 neutrons) resulted in the formation of a new nucleus of phosphorus-30 (15 protons, 15 neutrons), with one neutron emitted as radiation. However, this first artificially produced radioisotope was highly unstable (half-life of $3\frac{1}{4}$ minutes), and it soon transmuted into the stable nucleus of silicon-30.

The Joliot-Curie announcement revolutionized nuclear physics and prompted a mad scramble in the search for additional radioactive isotopes. Within a year, nearly 100 were discovered by European and American researchers.

The single most efficient source for the production of reasonably large amounts of artificial radioisotopes was Lawrence's cyclotron, which could produce a beam of high-energy protons, deuterons, and other particles vastly more intense than the radiation from the modest polonium source used by Joliot and Curie or the radium-beryllium sources used by Enrico Fermi in Italy and Niels Bohr in Denmark. The cyclotron could manufacture the new isotopes in far greater quantity and also could create new radioisotopes that could not be produced with the more primitive techniques. Indeed, using the cyclotron it was possible to manufacture new radioisotopes to meet specific needs.

The demand for radioactive materials soon exceeded the capacity of the few medical cyclotrons that were available. This problem was partially solved by the construction of the Oak Ridge reactor during World War II, although the secrecy of the Manhattan Project created some difficulties until the war was over. The reactor could not manufacture as wide a range of isotopes as the cyclotron, but it could produce many types in far larger quantities and at far lower cost.

Diagnostic procedures in nuclear medicine can be conveniently divided into four general groups. These techniques depend on localization, dilution, flow or diffusion, and biochemical and metabolic properties.[8] Many of these basic principles were first demonstrated by George Hevesy, a Hungarian-born physicist working in Denmark. The emergence of new artificially produced radioisotopes allowed Hevesy to make significant clinical contributions from research techniques that he had invented more than a decade earlier.

As related by the Brechers,[1] Hevesy's technique can best be illustrated by a story he told when receiving the Atoms for Peace Award of the Rockefeller Institute (1959):

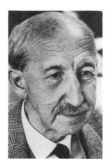

George Hevesy (1885-1966).

> While living in a boarding house in 1923, Hevesy had become suspicious of the cuisine. He therefore brought to the table with him a speck of one of the naturally occurring radioisotopes and deposited it on a scrap of meat which he left on his plate. Next day he brought a radiation detector—an electroscope—to the dinner table; sure enough, when the hash was served the electroscope revealed that it was radioactive. Hevesy had thus used a naturally occurring radioisotope as a *tracer* to follow the course of the meat scrap from his plate to the kitchen, through the meat chopper, through the hash pot, and back to the table again.

In more typical tracer experiments, Hevesy used a naturally occurring isotope of an element that participated in biochemical and physiological processes in precisely the same way as did the element itself. Thus by tracing the course of an isotope through a living cell or a complex organism, the course of the stable element was also revealed. For example, Hevesy grew bean plants in a solution containing a known amount of radioactive lead. At intervals he picked some of the plants, reduced their tissues (roots, stalks, leaves, beans) to ash, and measured the radioactivity in each tissue so as to trace the course of the lead through the plants.[9]

Hevesy's bean experiments also established the principles of *selective uptake* and *metabolic turnover*. When growing his beans in a solution containing only minimal amounts of lead, a large percentage of the lead was taken up by the roots. If Hevesy placed more substantial quantities of lead in the nutrient solution, a small percentage of it entered the bean plants. This implied that the maximum uptake of a substance was primarily determined by the organism and its state at the moment, rather than by the amount of the substance available. Hevesy also showed that when a lead atom entered a living tissue such as a bean leaf, it did not stay there indefinitely but was rather displaced by another atom of lead subsequently picked up by the roots and carried to the leaf. This showed that the living organism was the scene of an unceasing dynamic interchange with a characteristic turnover rate that could be measured. This rate could be expressed in terms of the *biological half-life*, the time it takes for one half of a dose of some substance administered to a living organism to depart from it.

The first tracer study in clinical medicine that used radioactivity was the work of Blumgart, Weiss, and Yens in Boston (1926).[10] After injecting minute amounts of radium C into a vein in a patient's right arm, they measured the time it took for the radioactive substance to affect a Wilson cloud chamber held close to the patient's left arm. This measured the blood circulation time, which ranged from 14 to 24 seconds in patients with normal circulation but rose to 71 seconds in a patient with cardiac decompensation. Circulation time measurements were reproducible and essentially unaffected by the amount of radioisotope injected for the test.[10]

The biological half-life and *isotope dilution* principles were illustrated clinically by experiments with "heavy water" (deuterium combined with oxygen). Hevesy and an associate (1934) drank small amounts of heavy water themselves, monitored its excretion in their urine, and thus established its biological half-life. By measuring the ratio of heavy water to ordinary water in the urine excreted, they were able to determine the total volume of body water with which the heavy water had been diluted.[11]

To fully exploit the tracer technique for physiological studies, Hevesy required radioactive isotopes of such biologically important elements as phosphorus, sodium, and carbon. Indeed, it is reported that Hevesy and his associate sometimes speculated on how much might be accomplished if these elements could by some unexpected miracle be rendered radioactive. The Joliot-Curie discovery of 1934 brought that miracle within reach.

However, the new phosphorus-30 had such a brief half-life that less than 1% (too little to measure) remained after 3 hours. The solution to this problem arrived soon afterward from Fermi's laboratory in Rome. In a mixture of radium and beryllium, the bombardment of beryllium nuclei by alpha particles from radium caused the emission of neutrons that in turn could be used to bombard other nuclei. Among the many new radioisotopes discovered with this technique was phosphorus-32, which had a half-life of 14.3 days that was far more useful than the 3¼-day half-life of phosphorus-30.[12]

The first biological experiments using a new artificial radioisotope were reported in 1935 by Hevesy and Chiewitz,[13] 12 years after Hevesy invented the tracer technique using a naturally radioactive isotope. By treating phosphorus-32 with nitric acid, Hevesy and Chiewitz produced phosphoric acid. They then treated a sodium compound with this radioactive phosphoric acid to secure *labelled* sodium phosphate—molecules of sodium phosphate that behaved chemically and physiologically like ordinary sodium phosphate but whose fate in living organisms could be traced by detecting the radiation emitted when a phosphorus atom in one of the molecules of the labelled compound decayed. After feeding their precious initial supply of labelled sodium phosphate to laboratory rats, they made careful daily determinations of the amount of radioactivity excreted in the urine and feces. They showed that the rat continued to excrete small additional amounts of radioactive phosphorus many days after it had last eaten the radioisotope.

> We have obviously to deal with the excretion of phosphorus which has already been deposited for a while in the skeleton, the muscles, or other organs, and which has been displaced again. From our experiment it follows that the average time which a phosphorus atom thus spends in the organism of a normally fed rat is about two months . . . The result strongly supports the view that the formation of the bones is a dynamic process, the bone continuously taking up phosphorus atoms which are partly or wholly lost again, and are displaced by other phosphorus atoms.[13]

When autopsying the rats, Hevesy and Chiewitz found that more than half of the phosphorus remaining in the rat after 20 days was lodged in its bones, a third was contained in the muscles and fat, and the small remainder was distributed in the liver and other organs. This *selective localization* of a particular radioisotope in specific tissues was to have far-reaching consequences in subsequent research.

The first application of artificially produced radioisotopes to a clinical problem was reported by two of Lawrence's colleagues, Joseph G. Hamilton and Robert S. Stone (1936). In reviewing the earlier literature on the intravenous injection of naturally radioactive substances, they came across the work of Proescher and Almquest, who in 1913 had injected radium chloride into the veins of patients suffering from various diseases, including chronic leukemia.[14] Although preliminary reports on these treatments were favorable, they discovered numerous incidents of radium poisoning, bone tumors following radium ingestion or injection, and other major hazards (see Chapter 30), which easily explained why the internal use of radium had quickly gone out of style. As they noted, "The amount which would be sufficient to be clinically effective probably would be fatal within a few years, due to the tendency of the radioactive elements to be deposited in the bones."[15]

Theoretically, a compound of sodium-24 should be much safer than radium salts, since the radioactive sodium was not fixed in body tissues and the duration of its effect was limited by its short half-life of only 14.8 hours. Accordingly, Hamilton and Stone decided to make a cautious clinical trial on patients with chronic leukemia. The selection of patients was easy, since the short half-life of sodium-24 required that it be administered to "the only patients with leukemia available at such times as the radiosodium could be obtained." Although there was no clinical improvement, there were no signs of toxic effects. In addition, the uptake, excretion, and course in the body of the radioactive sodium was successfully studied.[15]

More successful results were achieved by Lawrence, who administered the first dose of phosphorus-32 to a patient with chronic leukemia on Christmas Eve, 1936. Twenty years later, the patient was still alive and well. An even more impressive clinical cure was reported 3 years later (1939), when Lawrence and co-workers showed that the administration of phosphorus-32 to patients with polycythemia vera resulted in a dramatic decrease in their red cell counts and marked clinical improvement without objectionable side effects.

The first studies describing the use of radioactive iodine to treat thyrotoxicosis were presented independently at the 1942 meeting of the American Society for Clinical Investigation by Hertz and Roberts[16] and by Hamilton and Lawrence.[17] The use of radioactive iodine to treat hyperthyroidism soon became widespread, "except when contraindicated, as in young people, pregnant women, or patients with large goiters."[18] In the late 1940s, initial reports appeared demonstrating the use of radioactive iodine to treat functioning thyroid carcinomas and their metastases.

NUCLEAR MEDICINE INSTRUMENTATION

The first gamma-emitting radioisotope to be widely used in clinical diagnosis was iodine-131 (^{131}I). Unfortunately, this radionuclide emitted a principal gamma ray of such high energy (364 keV) that until about 1949 it could only be detected using the Geiger-Mueller (G-M) tube. Because of its high photon energy, most of the gamma rays passed through the detector without being absorbed, resulting in a detection rate of G-M tubes of only about 1%.

Detection of radiative iodine uptake in the thyroid using a Geiger-Mueller tube.[7]

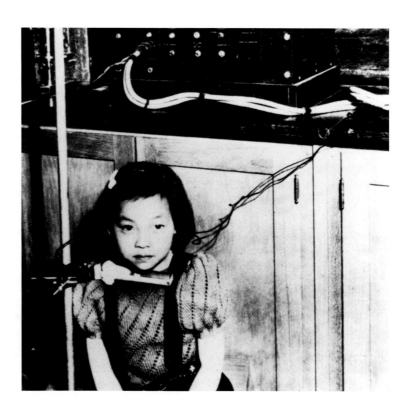

416

The earliest attempts at describing the spatial distribution of activity levels in a patient were a natural outgrowth of the "point measurements" for determining the radiation field around a radium needle. To evaluate patients with brain tumors, Moore pushed tiny Geiger tubes through needles inserted directly into the brain for detecting injected ^{32}P diiodofluorescein. When the label was changed to ^{131}I, the distribution of activity was mapped by taking Geiger counter measurements at multiple symmetrical, external counting positions. Using a collimated G-M tube, Veall (1950) succeeded in mapping the isoresponse curve image of the thyroid gland, though at a dose of ^{131}I of 1 to 2 mCi that was prohibitive for extensive clinical applications.[19] In 1952, Mayneord described a shielded Geiger counter for "point-by-point" counting for thyroid and distant metastases. Soon, many large hospitals had templates that would fit over the neck and were marked off in 1-cm squares. By drawing isodose lines between points of equal count levels, a "picture" of the distribution of the radioiodine in the thyroid gland was obtained.

The major breakthrough in radioisotope detection was the development of the *scintillation scanner* (scintiscan) by Benedict Cassen (1949) at the University of California, Los Angeles. The scintillation effects of ionizing radiation in solid substances had been described by Sir William Crookes as early as 1903 (see Chapter 1) and used by Rutherford and co-workers (1919) in their fundamental studies of the nature of radioactivity (see p. 409). However, broad application of this process required the development of photomultiplier tubes (1947) that could detect scintillations from a solid crystal at its cathode and generate a large electrical pulse as output. Cassen developed a moving solid-state detector utilizing a calcium tungstate crystal coupled to a photomultiplier tube.[20] Using a single-hole lead collimator, he was able to obtain a resolution of about

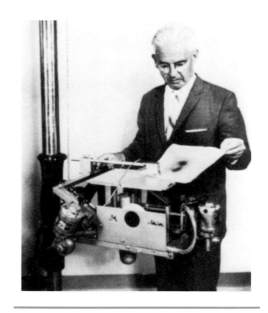

Benedict Cassen with his first rectilinear scanner.[7]

Arrangement for measuring ^{131}I uptake in the thyroid, showing the shadow projection method for positioning the patient (Veall, 1950).[19]

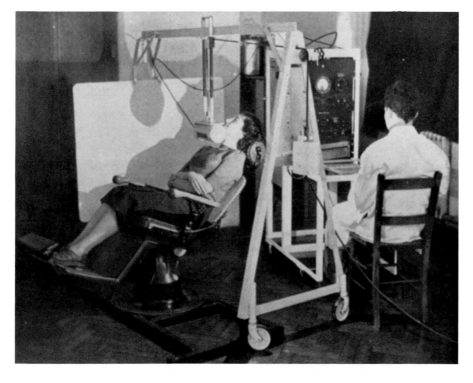

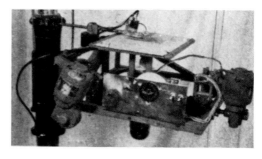

Automatic scintillation scanner and recorder (1951).[20]

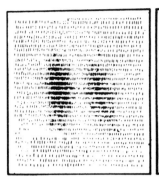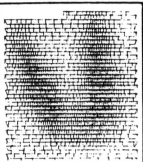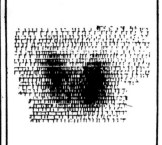

0.25 inches. In animal studies, Cassen showed that the thyroid gland could be easily and rapidly located after the administration of as little as 10 μCi of [131]I. His detection instrument was set on a stand, and point-by-point counts over the thyroid gland were made over a grid defining 400 positions. For human studies, Cassen first used a dose of 100 to 200 μCi of [131]I. Soon, the sensitivity of the UCLA scintillation scanner was so high that 6- to 24-hour thyroid uptake could be measured with an administered dose as low as 1 μCi. An examination of 1 to 1½ hours was required to make a complete mapping of the thyroid gland.

The detector was initially moved by hand. To facilitate this tedious process, Cassen produced an instrument that moved automatically—the first *rectilinear scanner*. This motorized scintillation scanner moved back and forth, dropping down a line at each sweep like a television scanning beam. Cassen coupled the output of the counter to an automatic pen, which moved synchronously with the counter, making a mark on a sheet of paper whenever a scintillation or a specified number of scintillations appeared on the calcium tungstate crystals. Thus as a radioactive area was scanned a map of the area appeared on the sheet of paper. Regions emitting large amounts of radiation appeared quite dark on the map because the pen made many marks close together; areas emitting little or no radiation appeared as only lightly shaded or white areas on the map. In studies of the thyroid gland, a cyst or tumor that did not take up ^{131}I appeared as a "cold spot," whereas a nodule concentrating the radioisotope excessively appeared on the scan as a "hot spot."

Refinements to the basic system were rapidly developed. Allen and co-workers introduced pulse height analysis to favorably alter the signal-to-noise ratio.[21] Newell and associates developed the multihole focusing collimator, the mechanical equivalent of a lens for gamma rays, which permitted higher sensitivity with smaller administered doses or a shorter scanning time.[22] The practical application of focused collimators required the production of large thallium-activated sodium iodide crystals that were specifically "grown" for this purpose.

A variation of the scintillation scanner was the *photoscan*, developed by David Kuhl in 1952, when he was a first-year medical student at the University of Pennsylvania. Instead of using an automatic pen and sheet of paper for recording, this device fed the output from the photomultiplier tube to a moving beam of light, the brightness of which at each moment was proportional to the number of scintillations on the face of the crystal at that time. A sheet of photographic paper or an x-ray film exposed to the moving light recorded point-for-point the amount of radioactivity emerging from the area scanned.[24] Photoscanning appealed to radiologists and was rapidly adopted because the scans were printed on standard-size

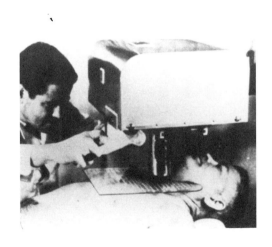

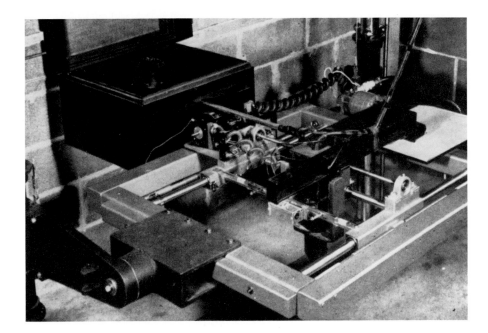

x-ray film, could be examined on conventional x-ray viewing boxes, and appeared to convey more information to the viewer than the "dot" scan printed on opaque paper.[25]

In conventional scintillation scanning using a moving detector, only one resolution element of the field of view was detected at a time. Gamma rays coming from the rest of the field of view were wasted. To address this problem, Hal Anger (1957) developed a stationary area detector or "scintillation camera" consisting of a sodium iodide crystal optically coupled to 19 photomultiplier tubes.[26] This device greatly improved the collection of gamma rays by viewing all the resolution elements in the field simultaneously, although each element was viewed with low efficiency. An absorbed gamma ray released light photons, some or all of which were detected by each photomultiplier tube.

Initially, the scintillation camera was not readily accepted. The process for localizing the x-y coordinates of an event required the use of a half-inch-thick NaI(Tl) crystal, which had poor detection efficiency for ^{131}I when compared with that achieved with the 2-inch detectors used with scanners. Because a pin hole was used for collimation and the detector size was small, only patients who had received therapeutic doses of ^{131}I could be imaged. In addition, there were no radionuclides available that could take advantage of the dynamic imaging capabilities offered by the camera.

The introduction of technetium-99m (^{99m}Tc) dramatically changed the requirements for imaging devices. The 140-keV gamma ray emitted by this radionuclide reduced the crystal thickness and collimator requirements for imaging. The development of a wide range of ^{99m}Tc-labelled radiopharmaceuticals in the late 1960s and 1970s, combined with improvement in collimator design, crystal characteristics, the number and type of photomultiplier tubes, and the use of solid-state circuitry, resulted in the scintillation camera becoming extremely popular, since it was an imaging device far superior to the rectilinear scanner.[28]

An alternative type of scintillation camera, termed the *autofluoroscope*, was devised by Bender and Blau in 1962.[29] The detector in this system was a mosaic of collimated sodium iodide crystals instead of a

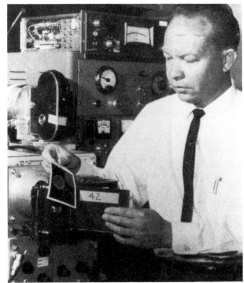

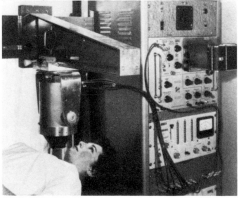

Hal Anger (*top*) and his first clinical scintillation camera in operation for thyroid imaging (*bottom*).[27]

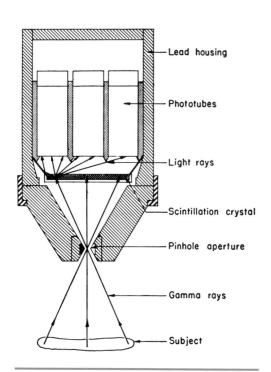

Sectional drawing of scintillation camera (1957).[26]

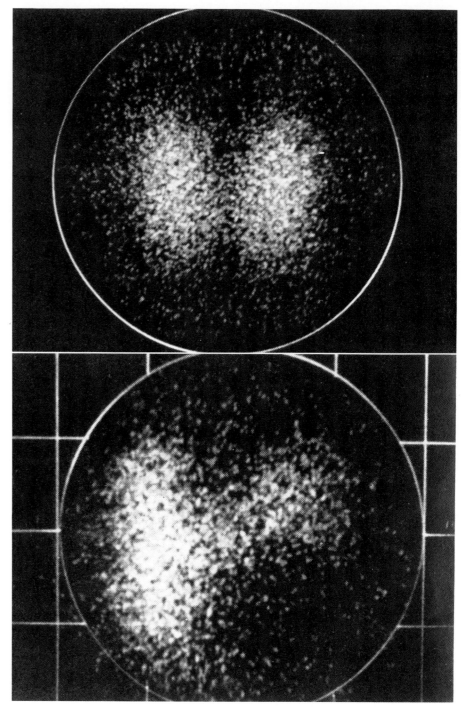

Early scintillation camera pictures. *Top*, Thyroid phantom. *Bottom*, Human thyroid in vivo.[26]

single large crystal. This device used 293 sodium iodide crystals, each of which was 2 inches thick. Thus the high-energy gamma rays could theoretically be much more efficiently detected than in the thin crystal of the scintillation camera.

Another method to enhance spatial resolution was the use of a positron scanner and "coincidence counting." The positron scanner was developed in 1953 by Brownell and Sweet at Massachusetts General Hospital[30]; extensive clinical tests were supervised there by Saul Aronow.[31] This technique was based on the fact that a number of chemical compounds are taken up more promptly by certain kinds of brain tumor than by normal brain tissue, although the difference in uptake is slight. If

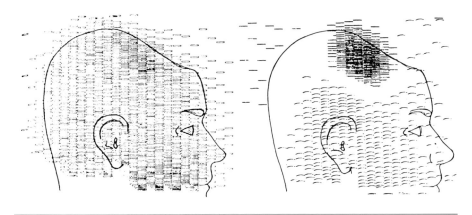

Coincidence scan (*left*) of patient showing recurrence of tumor under previous operation site and unbalance scan (*right*) showing asymmetry to the left (1953).[30]

a compound were labelled with ^{131}I in the usual way, the radiation emitted from the brain tumor would be masked by radiation from surrounding tissues. To solve this problem, the compound is labelled with a radio-isotope that emits positrons. A positron itself could not possibly be detected, since it travels only a few millionths of a centimeter through tissue before it captures an electron and the two annihilate one another. However, in this process of annihilation, two gamma rays are emitted at a specific voltage and leave the scene of annihilation in opposite directions. In coincidence counting, two scintillation scanning devices were stationed on opposite sides of the patient's head and the labelled compound was administered. The devices were arranged in a circuit that recorded radiation only when *both* devices were activated simultaneously by two gamma rays of the right energy emerging from the same positron annihilation. Thus the background radiation, or "noise," that would otherwise ruin the scan was totally ignored. This system could permit the detection of a deep-seated lesion with higher contrast, though less sensitivity, than the focused collimator.

Dynamic radionuclide studies were initially performed by observing a persistence oscilloscope, with hard copy provided by "pulling" Polaroid films in rapid succession. The introduction of electronic formatters increased the rate at which images could be acquired and improved image quality. The development of physiological gating and dedicated computer systems made possible the quantitative measurement of cardiac function.

The first instrument capable of giving multiple images at different depths from a single scan of a patient was the multiplane, longitudinal tomographic scanner built by Hal Anger (1965). A pair of scanning cameras provided a total of 12 longitudinal tomographic images equally spaced through the patient.[32] Longitudinal tomography also was performed using a rotating tomographic collimator (Muehllehner) and a seven-pinhole collimator (Vogel). However, all these devices provided blurring (limited-angle) tomography that did not offer a unique solution to the problem of the spatial distribution of activity.

The origin of *single photon emission tomography* (SPECT) can be traced to the work of Kuhl and Edwards (1963),[33] who utilized a computerized technique coupled with a transverse section imaging device to produce transaxial tomograms of the head using single gamma ray radionuclides. A pair of opposed collimated detectors were moved in angular

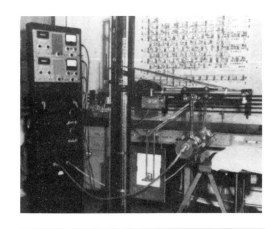

Scanning mechanism and electronic apparatus for positron scanner (1953). Components in relay rack (*top to bottom*): coincidence scaler, single-channel scaler, coincidence circuit, two linear amplifiers, scanning control panel, unbalanced circuit, and power supply.[30]

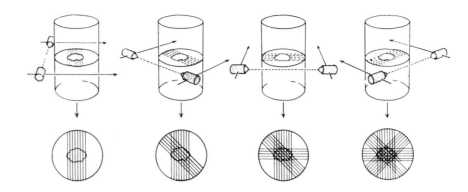

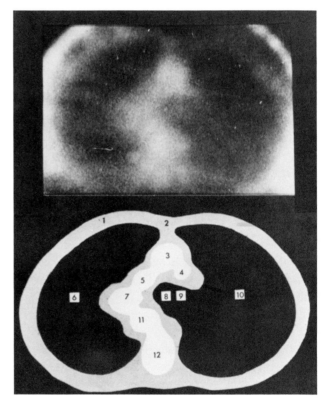

Right, First transmission section scan of living human thorax in May, 1965.[34]

Below, Mark II scanner for emission transverse tomography (1963).

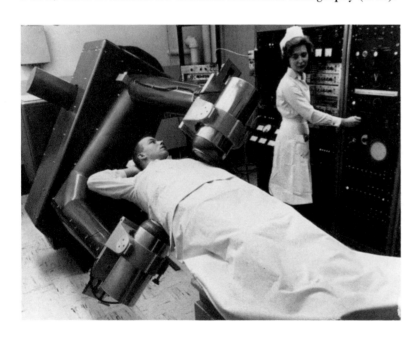

increments of 15 degrees around the subject, generating a sequence of tangential scans. Each back projection was displayed in real time on an oscilloscope, and multiple projections were integrated on photographic film. Within a few years, data acquired by rotating the patient in front of a stationary scintillation camera were fed into a computer and subsequently reconstructed into transaxial slices by complex algorithms analogous to those with x-ray computed tomography but capable of reconstructing multiple transaxial slices simultaneously. Subsequent design improvements resulted in scanners containing a single detector or multiple detectors surrounding the patient. Coronal and sagittal projections could be immediately obtained by simply reformatting so as to sample the data along these respective planes. By appropriately interpolating the initially acquired data, this technique also permitted imaging oblique views along arbitrarily selected axes, such as the long axis of the heart. The tomographic capabilities of SPECT scanning have proved invaluable in clinical imaging, especially of the heart, liver, and brain.

Early work by Brownell and co-workers introducing the idea of localizing positron emitters with dual detectors was revitalized in the mid-1970s with the development by Michel Ter-Pogossian of the first multicrystal positron emission transaxial tomographic system, now known as PET scanning.[35] Initially, a hexagonal array of crystals was placed around the patient to obtain tomographic images from the distribution of positron emitters within organs of interest. Later PET systems have employed circular rings of detectors, which typically contain large numbers of small detecting units that can produce spatial resolution of 5 mm. Most physiologically significant biochemical compounds are composed of carbon, nitrogen, and oxygen, all of which have positron-emitting isotopes. Consequently, it is possible with these isotopes to label small biologically active compounds that cannot be labelled by other externally detectable radionuclides and subsequently image their distribution in the living body over time.

Although PET was developed before SPECT, it is much less widely available because it requires access to a cyclotron for producing the ultrashort-lived positron-emitting radionuclides. During the mid-1980s, significant progress in miniaturization and simplification of cyclotron operation has increased the number of smaller hospital-based cyclotrons.

CLINICAL IMAGING

The first ^{131}I thyroid scintillation scans obtained on live human patients were reported by Cassen and Curtis in 1951.[36] One year later, Goodwin and associates in Cassen's laboratory noted that

> before the introduction of I^{131} into the diagnosis of thyroid disease, the only procedures available for the estimation of morphological characteristics of thyroid glands consisted of the very crude method of palpation or the much more drastic surgical exploration. After I^{131} became available on a large scale it was theoretically possible to map the I^{131} accumulating in the regions of the thyroid gland by means of gamma rays emitted

though for effective use of this procedure "it was necessary to develop suitable instrumentation." With the availability of scintillation scanning, they could report that

> the method described has become a routine clinical procedure in this hospital. It is being relied upon more and more by internists and surgeons who are interested in the size and shape of the patient's thyroid gland and in aberrant thyroid tissue. No other clinical method enables the surgeon to know whether a palpable nodule accumulates I^{131} or whether it does not. Clinically non-demonstrable nodular areas, I^{131} accumulating or non-accumulating, have been demonstrated by means of the scintigram. Substernal extension of thyroid tissue can also be brought to the attention of the surgeon before operation. Regeneration of thyroid tissue, both normal or carcinomatous, following ablative treatment can be accurately detected on follow-up examinations.[37]

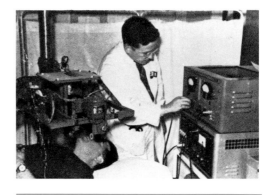

Equipment for thyroid scanning (1952). The patient is in supine position, the head of the directional scintillation tube is above the neck, and the rack, motors, table, and prints with the scintigram are shown.[37]

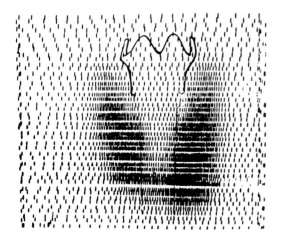

Scintigram of diffusely enlarged thyroid gland (1952).[37]

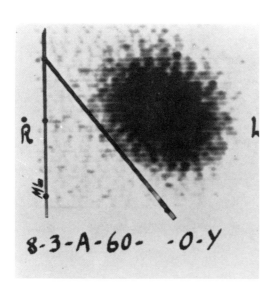

Early spleen scan (1960). Scan made 8 days after administration of 6 ml of sensitized red cells labeled with 200 μc of ^{51}Cr. The scan is viewed as if the patient were supine. The body midline (*ML*) and the lowest palpable left posterior rib (*oblique line joining ML*) are indicated. The symbols refer to factors used in the scan.[40]

For the past 25 years, the major radionuclide used in clinical work has been ^{99m}Tc. Technetium was discovered by Perrier and Segre (1937), who bombarded molybdenum with deuterons using the cyclotron at Berkeley.[38] However, its first biological use by Paul Harper did not occur until late 1961, 4 years before it came into widespread clinical practice. The circuitous path to the medical applications of technetium began with the development of a series of isotope generator systems (cows) at the Brookhaven National Laboratories. In 1957, they developed a molybdenum-technetium system that initially was used to help an oil company solve mixing problems in large vats. In 1960, Powell (Jim) Richards first suggested the use of the molybdenum-technetium cow for medical purposes. Soon afterward, Richards tried to sell Harper on this new system. One year later, the first generator was shipped to the Argonne Cancer Research Hospital, where Harper and Katherine Lathrop "milked" the cow, injected the material into a mouse, and scanned it. To their surprise, there was pertechnetate uptake in the stomach, salivary glands, and thyroid.

The physical characteristics of ^{99m}Tc are almost ideal for external detection. The radionuclide has a physical half-life of only 6 hours, no beta emission, and a gamma emission of 140 keV. Larger quantities of radioactivity could be injected to improve image quality, yet patient dose would be reduced. Within 3 years, technetium compounds became the standard radionuclide agents for a broad spectrum of nuclear medicine procedures.

Radionuclide scanning of the liver probably began with the work of Dobson and Jones (1952), who determined that a colloidal size of 30 to 100 μm was ideal for Kupffer cell clearance to quantitate hepatic blood flow. They used particles labelled with ^{32}P, whose beta emission could not be detected externally. In the next year, Vetter tagged particles with gold-198 (^{198}Au) and easily detected their distribution using external counters. In 1954, Stirrett and co-workers reported the first liver scan using radioactive gold. Two years later, Helpern and associates recorded the successful use of albumin aggregates as colloidal particles for liver scanning.

While seeking an appropriate agent to study hepatic reticuloendothelial function, George Taplin found a 30-year-old article describing the excretion of rose bengal into the biliary system, presumably by way of the Kupffer cells. After initial tests with ^{131}I-labelled rose bengal, Taplin[39] discovered that this agent was not excreted by the Kupffer cells but rather by the polygonal cells. In addition, it was not absorbed by the bowel. Although rose bengal could not be used as an effective reticuloendothelial agent, Taplin realized that it could be readily applied to the problem of neonatal jaundice in biliary atresia, as well as for the dynamic assessment of extrahepatic biliary patency in adults.[36] This radionuclide was later replaced by the iminodiacetic acid derivatives as the standard test for acute cholecystitis (see Chapter 16).

In 1962, Harper gave a paper on an improved liver scanning agent, a ^{99m}Tc-thiocyanate-fat emulsion. Soon afterward, Richards perfected the technetium sulfur colloid preparation that supplanted the fat emulsion sulfide technique for liver imaging.

Imaging of the spleen was initially based on the function of this organ to remove damaged red cells from the bloodstream. Preliminary studies described the labelling of chromium-51 (^{51}Cr) to red blood cells and the splenic sequestration of immunologically injured red cells carrying the chromium label. In 1960, Philip Johnson and associates made the first

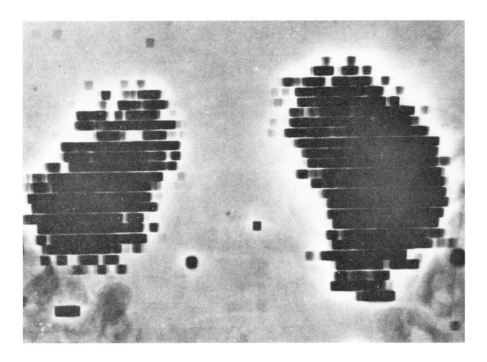

radionuclide scans of the spleen using immunologically damaged red cells.[40] This technique was later simplified by using heat-treated red cells. Currently, radionuclide scans of the spleen are generally performed with technetium sulfur colloid.

The first kidney scan was performed by McAfee and Wagner in 1960 using mercury-263 (^{263}Hg)-labeled Neohydrin.[41] This technique could detect focal lesions of the kidney, such as infarcts and ischemic segments, and was valuable in assessing renal size in patients with severe chronic renal failure. In the same year, Tubis and co-workers used ^{131}I-labelled Hippuran for renal function tests.[42] This agent later became widely used for kidney imaging, especially with the increased availability of scintillation cameras.

Radionuclide imaging of the pancreas was championed by Monte Blau. After noting that many amino acids concentrated in the pancreas to a far higher degree than any other organ, Blau attempted to use several different radioactive amino acids as scanning agents. When these proved unsuccessful, he decided to develop a true amino acid analog. Using selenium as a substitute for the sulfur in methionine, Blau succeeded in biologically synthesizing selenium-75 (^{75}Se)-labelled selenomethionine using yeast grown in a sulfur-poor medium. Although Blau's initial results were encouraging,[44] radionuclide imaging of the pancreas never achieved substantial success.

In 1963, Taplin introduced the use of human serum albumin macro-aggregates tagged with ^{131}I for demonstration of the pulmonary circulation and the diagnosis of pulmonary embolism.[45] The image quality of lung

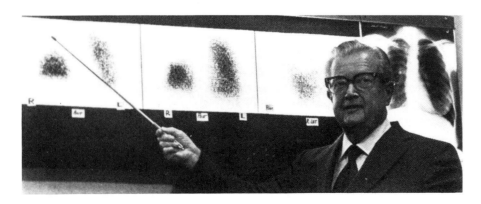

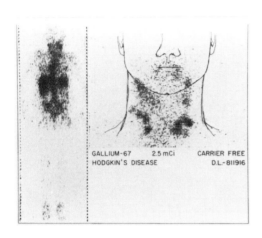

Tumor scanning with [67]Ga (1969). *Left*, Posterior whole-body photoscan obtained 6 days after injection of 2.5 mCi of ^{67}Ga in a patient with Hodgkin's disease revealed no bone lesions but an unexpected concentration of the isotope in the neck. A more detailed scan (*right*) showed that the distribution of the isotope corresponded to the localization of the palpable cervical lymph nodes.[50]

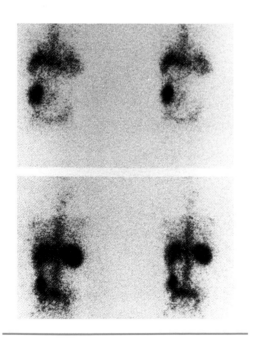

Abscess scanning with [111]In (1979). Tomographic scan about 20 hours after intravenous injection of 600 Ci of ^{111}In leukocytes demonstrates intense accumulation in a right-sided abdominal abscess.[54]

scanning was subsequently improved by the use of ^{99m}Tc as the label. Using [15]CO$_2$, West and Dallery (1960) demonstrated a normal gradient of pulmonary ventilation distributed from the diaphragm to the first rib in erect humans.[46] Two years later (1962), Ball and associates demonstrated the value of radioactive xenon in assessing regional pulmonary ventilation.[47] For the use of radionuclide imaging in cardiac disease, see Chapter 13.

The diagnosis of pernicious anemia was greatly facilitated in 1953, when Schillings described the vitamin B$_{12}$ absorption test. In patients with this condition, an orally administered radioactive dose of the vitamin was excreted in the feces, rather than being absorbed via the alimentary tract and excreted in the urine as in normal individuals.

Interest in the radioisotopes of gallium began with the work of Dudley and Maddox (1949), who demonstrated localization of gallium citrate in bone.[49] Twenty years later, while using gallium-67 (^{67}Ga) citrate as a bone-scanning agent in a patient with malignant disease, Edwards and Hayes (1969) noted a localization of the radionuclide in malignant nodes in the neck.[50] Subsequent studies showed that gallium also localized in inflammatory disorders, including abscesses.[51] This nonspecificity has proven to be a major disadvantage, as is the prolonged time course for a complete examination (72 to 96 hours). In addition, a considerable amount of the injectable material is excreted through the gut, so that considerable caution must be exercised in evaluating an abdominal collection of the radionuclide. The slow blood clearance and four energy peaks of its gamma emissions are added problems.

For many years, investigators have discussed the possibility of using labelled white blood cells to localize abscesses. However, the clinical usefulness of this approach was thwarted by the lack of a suitable gamma-emitting label. In the late 1970s, McAfee, Thakur, and others demonstrated conclusively that leukocytes could be labelled efficiently with indium-111(^{111}In) and still retain their functional capabilities of host defense against pyogenic infections.[52,53] Thus indium-labelled leukocytes could provide a specific homing marker to label abscesses or other inflammatory conditions associated with the accumulation of white blood cells. Further clinical studies showed the value of whole body scanning with this radionuclide for the detection of abscesses anywhere in the body.[54]

Early work on bone metabolism using calcium-45 ([45]Ca) and strontium-89 (^{89}Sr) was accomplished during the 1940s and early 1950s. However, these radionuclides were pure beta emitters and not detectable externally. Clinical bone imaging began with the use of strontium-85 ([85]Sr), a pure gamma emitter, which was soon replaced by strontium-87m ([87m]Sr), which has a much shorter half-life.[55] In areas that had access to cyclotron-produced isotopes, fluorine-18 (^{18}F) became an important bone-scanning agent because of its shorter half-life and positron emission.[56] The value of bone scanning for the early diagnosis of metastatic disease was stressed in a study by Arnot and co-workers (1969), in which radionuclide scanning demonstrated skeletal metastases in a significant number of patients who were thought to have only primary breast neoplasms.[57] This stimulated the search for a bone-specific radiopharmaceutical of sufficiently short half-life, high photon yield, and wide availability to be used to screen for metastatic disease. With the development of ^{99m}Tc stannous polyphosphate (STPP) by Subramanian and McAfee in 1971[58] and subsequent technetium compounds containing pyrophosphate and diphosphonate, radionuclide bone scanning became the major modality for the early detection of skeletal metastases.

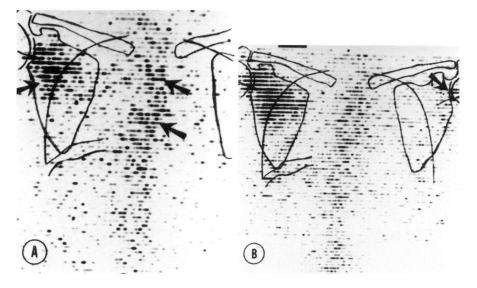

Strontium bone scanning (1964). *Left*, Posterior chest scan of an elderly woman using [87m]Sr shows extensive uptake in the right scapula (*arrow*) representing metastatic breast carcinoma. *Right*, Repeat scan using [85]Sr 8 days later again shows the metastasis to the right scapula that had been overlooked on initial chest radiographs. Note the slight but normal increase in strontium deposition in the left glenoid fossa and humeral head (*arrow*) and abnormal uptake in the mid-dorsal spine (*arrows*).[55]

The flow of cerebrospinal fluid after the injection of ^{131}I-labelled human serum albumin in the subarachnoid space was first described by DiChiro in 1964. Subsequently, this technique has been used to assess cerebrospinal fluid leaks, communicating and normal pressure hydrocephalus, and porencephalic cysts.

The rapid growth of nuclear medicine during the decade of the 1960s was due in part to the widespread use of technetium scanning for the evaluation of brain tumors. This method was almost completely replaced by computed tomography in the mid-1970s and by magnetic resonance imaging in the 1980s.

Since that time, the role of nuclear medicine in neurological disease has shifted from the imaging of brain tumors to an evaluation of brain function and cerebral blood flow using PET and SPECT. Using principles developed by Kety and Schmidt in the late 1940s,[60] numerous investigators in the 1960s showed that it was possible to measure regional cerebral blood flow using krypton-85 ([85]Kr) and xenon-133 (^{133}Xe). At Washington University in St. Louis, Michel Ter-Pogossian established the first medical cyclotron installation and developed methods for the production of carbon-11 (^{11}C)-labelled glucose to measure regional brain glucose utilization. Subsequently, it was shown that fluorodioxyglucose had biological properties similar to ^{11}C-glucose, providing an opportunity to use the longer-lived fluorine-18 label as a positron emitter to assess regional brain function.

More recent experiments, particularly with visual and audio stimulation, have produced great insight into the localization of brain metabolism under a variety of conditions, and PET scanning has begun to demon-

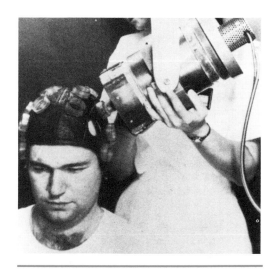

Brain tumor localization with a shielded and collimated scintillation detector (1958).[59]

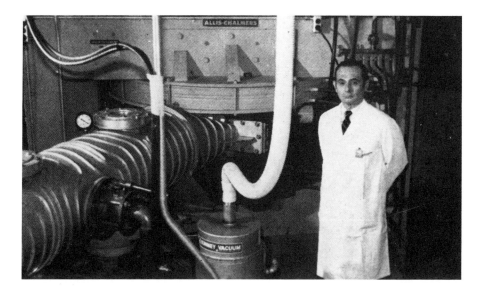

Michel Ter-Pogossian with the first American medical cyclotron.[63]

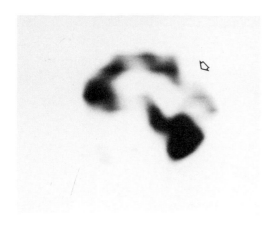

SPECT scan of Alzheimer's disease. Decreased blood flow to the posterior parietal cortex (*arrow*).

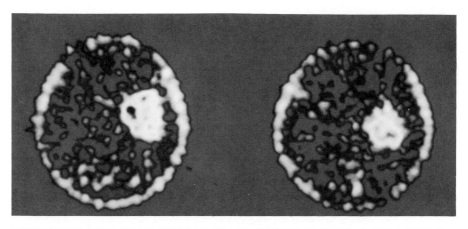

PET scan of high-grade brain tumor using F-18 fluorodeoxyuridine.[64]

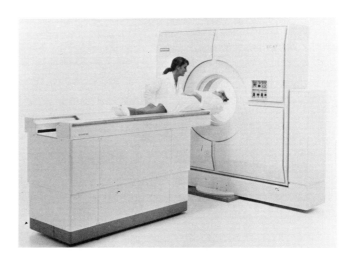

Modern PET scanner. Patient table and gantry resembling a standard CT scanner.[64]

strate diagnostic potential in dementia, epilepsy, and psychosis.[61] The high cost of a dedicated cyclotron and radiopharmaceutical laboratory for PET scanning is not required with SPECT, which can offer similar capability for regional brain function assessment in diagnostic nuclear medicine. Holman and Hill[62] have shown that SPECT not only performed functions similar to PET but also could study cerebral blood flow and neuroreceptor binding using ^{123}I-iodoamphetamine.

Among recent developments in nuclear medicine are radiolabelling techniques for cells (e.g., labelled lymphocytes), which have resulted in cell-specific imaging methods, and improved protein labels (e.g., monoclonal antibody labelling), which have led to the development of specific antibody techniques.[64]

Bibliography

Graham LS, Kereiakes JG, Harris C, and Cohen MB: Nuclear medicine from Becquerel to the present. RadioGraphics 9:1189-1202, 1989.

Lindeman JF: The recent history of nuclear medicine instrumentation. In Gottschalk A, Hoffer PD, and Potchen EJ (eds): Diagnostic nuclear medicine. Baltimore, Williams & Wilkins, 1988.

Lindeman JF and Quinn JL: The recent history of clinical procedures in nuclear medicine. In Gottschalk A, Hoffer PB, and Potchen EJ (eds): Diagnostic nuclear medicine. Baltimore, Williams & Wilkins, 1988.

References

1. Brecher R and Brecher E: The rays. A history of radiology in the United States and Canada. Baltimore, Williams & Wilkins, 1969.

2. Abbe R: Illustrating the penetrating power of radium. Arch Roentgen Ray 11:247, 1907.

3. Cleaves MA: Light energy. New York, Rebman, 1904.
4. Beck C: Rontgen ray diagnosis and therapy. New York, Appleton, 1904.
5. Curie I and Joliot F: Artificial production of a new kind of radio-element. Nature (London) 133:201-202, 1934.
6. Aebersold PC: The development of nuclear medicine. AJR 75:1027-1039, 1956.
7. Wagner H: Nuclear medicine. New York, HP Publishers, 1975.
8. Leucutia T: Nuclear medicine. AJR 75:1195-1198, 1956.
9. Hevesy G: The absorption and translocation of lead by plants. Biochem J 17:439, 1923.
10. Blumgart HL, Weiss S, and Yens OC: Studies on the velocity of blood flow. J Clin Invest 4:1-31, 1927.
11. Hevesy G: Nature 134:879, 1934.
12. Fermi E: Radioactivity induced by neutron bombing. Nature (London) 133:757, 1934.
13. Hevesy G and Chiewitz D: Letter to the editor. Nature 136:754-755, Nov. 9, 1935.
14. Proescher F and Almquest BR: Contribution on the therapeutic value of the intravenous injection of soluble radium salts in the treatment of pernicious anemia and leukaemia. Radium 6:85-96, 1916.
15. Hamilton JG and Stone RS: The intravenous and intraduodenal administration of radiosodium. Radiology 28:178-188, 1937.
16. Hertz S and Roberts A: Application of radioactive iodine in therapy of Graves' disease. J Clin Invest 21:624, 1942.
17. Hamilton JG and Lawrence JH: Recent clinical developments in the therapeutic application of radio-phosphorus and radioiodine. J Clin Invest 21:624, 1942.
18. Means JH, DeGroot LJ, and Stenburg JB: The thyroid and its diseases. New York, McGraw-Hill, 1963.
19. Veall NL: Diagnostic and therapeutic use of radioactive isotopes. Brit J Radiol 23:527-534, 1950.
20. Cassen B and Curtis L: The in vivo delineation of thyroid glands with an automatically scanning record. University of California, Los Angeles, Report 130, 1951.
21. Allen HC, Reiser JR, and Green JA: Improvements in outlining of thyroid and localization of brain tumors by the application of sodium iodide gamma-rays spectrometry techniques. In Proceedings of the Second Oxford Radioisotope Conference, New York, Academic Press, 1954.
22. Newell R, Saunders W, and Miller E: Multichannel collimators for gamma scanning with scintillation counters. Nucleonics 10:36, 1952.
23. Blahd WH: History of external counting procedures. Semin Nucl Med 9:159-163, 1979.
24. Kuhl DE, Chamberlain RH, Hale J, et al: A high contrast photographic recorder for scintillation counter scanning. Radiology 66:730-739, 1956.
25. Cassen B: The evolution of scintillation imaging. In Freeman LM and Johnson PM (eds): Clinical scintillation scanning, New York, Hoeber, 1969.

26. Anger HO: Scintillation camera. Rev Sci Instrum 29:27-33, 1958.
27. Powell MR: H.O. Anger and his work at the Donner laboratory. Semin Nucl Med 9:164-168, 1979.
28. Rollo FD, Patton JA, and Cassen B: The evolution of radionuclide imaging. In Freeman LM (ed): Freeman and Johnson's clinical radionuclide imaging. Orlando, Fla., Grune & Stratton, 1984.
29. Bender M and Blau M: Autofluoroscopy: The use of a nonscanning device for tumor localization with radioisotopes (abstract). J Nucl Med 1:105, 1960.
30. Brownell GL and Sweet WH: Localization of brain tumors. Nucleonics 11:40-45, 1953. See also JAMA 157:1183-1186, 1955.
31. Aronow S, Brownell GL, Lovo SL, and Sweet WH: Statistical analysis of eight years' experience in positron scanning for brain tumor localization (abstract). J Nucl Med 3:198, 1962.
32. Anger HO: Tomographic gamma-ray scanner with simultaneous readout of several planes. U.C.R.L. Report 16899, Lawrence Radiation Laboratory. Berkeley, University of California Press, 1966.
33. Kuhl DE and Edwards RQ: Image separation radioisotope scanning. Radiology 80:653-662, 1963.
34. Kuhl DE, Hale J, and Eaton WL: Transmission scanning. Radiology 87:278-284, 1966.
35. Ter-Pogossian MM, Phelps ME, and Hoffman EJ: A positron-emission transaxial tomography for nuclear imaging (PETT). Radiology 114:89-98, 1975.
36. Cassen B, Curtis L, Reed C, and Libby R: Instrumentation for ^{131}I use in medical studies. Nucleonics 9:46-50, 1951.
37. Goodwin WE, Bauer FK, Barrett TF, and Cassen B: A method using I^{131} for the determination of abnormal thyroid morphology. AJR 68:963-970, 1952.
38. Perrier C and Segre E: Radioactive isotopes of element 43. Nature 140:193, 1937.
39. Taplin GV: The radioactive (I-131 tagged) rose bengal uptake excretion test for liver function using external gamma-ray scintillation counting technique. J Lab Clin Med 45:665-673, 1955.
40. Johnson PM, Wood EH, and Mooring SL: Scintillation scanning of the normal human spleen utilizing sensitized radioactive erythrocytes. Radiology 74:99-101, 1960.
41. McAfee JG and Wagner HN: Visualization of renal parenchyma: Scintiscanning with Hg-203 Neohydrin. Radiology 75:820-821, 1960.
42. Tubis M, Posuick E, and Nordyke RA: Preparation and use of ^{131}I labeled sodium iodohippurate in kidney function tests. Proc Soc Exp Biol Med 103:497, 1960.
43. Winter CC: A clinical study of a new renal function test: The radioactive diodrast renogram. J Urol 76:182, 1956.
44. Blau M and Manske RF: The pancreas specificity of ^{75}Se-selenomethione. J Nucl Med 2:102-105, 1961.

45. Taplin GV, Dore EK, and Johnson DE: Suspensions of radioalbumin aggregates for photoscanning the liver, spleen, lung and other organs. UCLA report 519, 1963.
46. West JB and Dallery CT: Distribution of blood flow and ventilation/perfusion ratio in the lung measured with radioactive CO_2. J Appl Physiol 15:405-410, 1960.
47. Ball WC, Stewart PB, Newsham LGS, and Bates DV: Regional pulmonary function studies with Xe-133. J Clin Invest 41:519-531, 1962.
48. Taplin GV: The history of lung imaging with radionuclides. Semin Nucl Med 9:178-185, 1979.
49. Dudley HC and Maddox GE: Deposition of radiogallium (Ga^{72}) in skeletal tissues. J Pharm Exper Therap 96:224-227, 1949.
50. Edwards CL and Hayes RL: Tumor scanning with ^{67}Ga citrate. J Nucl Med 10:103-105, 1969.
51. Lavender JP, Barker JR, and Chaudhri MA: Gallium 67 citrate scanning in neoplastic and inflammatory lesions. Br J Radiol 44:361-366, 1971.
52. McAfee JG and Thakur ML: Survey of radioactive agents for in vitro labeling of phagocytic leucocytes. I. Soluble agents. J Nucl Med 17:480-487, 1976.
53. Thakur ML, Coleman E, Mayhall CG, and Welch MJ: Preparation and evaluation of ^{111}In-labeled leukocytes as an abscess imaging agent in dogs. Radiology 119:731-732, 1976.
54. McDougall IR, Baumert JE, and Lantieri RL: Evaluation of ^{111}In leukocyte whole body scanning. AJR 133:849-894, 1979.
55. Charkes ND, Sklaroff DM, and Young I: Detection of metastatic cancer bone by scintiscanning with 87m-Sr. AJR 91:1121-1127, 1964.
56. Blau M, Nagler W, and Bender M: Fluorine-18: A new isotope for bone scanning. J Nucl Med 3:332-334, 1962.
57. Arnot RN, Glass HI, and Williams ED: Clinical applications for short-lived cyclotron-produced isotopes. J Physiol 202:17, 1969.
58. Subramanian G and McAfee JG: A new complex of ^{99m}Tc for skeletal imaging. Radiology 99:192-196, 1971.
59. Blahd WH, Cassen B, and Bauer FK: The practice of nuclear medicine. Springfield, Ill, Charles C Thomas, 1958.
60. Kety SS and Schmidt CF: The nitrous oxide method for determination of cerebral blood flow in man: Theory, procedure, and normal values. J Clin Invest 27:476-483, 1948.
61. Walker MD: Research issues in positron emission tomography. Ann Neurol 15 (Suppl), 1984.
62. Holman BL and Hill TC: Functional imaging of the brain with SPECT. Appl Radiol 13:21-27, 1984.
63. Grigg ERN, et al: The RSNA historic symposium on American radiology: Then and now. Radiology 100:1-26, 1971.
64. Akin JR: Positron emission tomography (PET): The future is now. Berkeley, University of California Press, 1990.

CHAPTER 24

Tomography

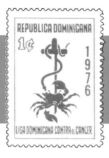
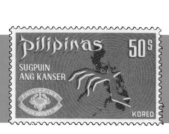
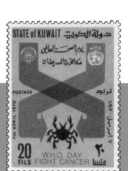

The early x-ray pioneers soon realized that the images produced on radiographic plates and film represented a combination of the shadows of all the various tissues of the body through which the rays passed. The shadow of one dense object, such as a bone, could blot out the fainter shadows of tissues above and below it. In regions such as the skull, where there are multiple small structures of variable densities situated within a relatively small space, areas of primary interest were often obscured by overlying shadows. Various techniques were recommended to solve this problem. Multiple projections and optical separation of superimposed images by stereoscopy were suggested, as was the continuous motion of fluoroscopy and changes in density produced by introducing more or less opaque contrast material.[1]

The most effective solution was the tomographic principle, borrowed from optics, in which the x-ray tube and the film move synchronously in opposite directions during the exposure. Thus when the tube is moving from left to right with respect to the region of interest in the patient being radiographed, the film is moving in a parallel plane from right to left; when the tube moves back or forward, the film moves forward or back. The images of all points in a plane through the fulcrum and parallel to the film are clearly recorded as they occupy unchanging positions on the moving film. The images of all other points are blurred by the movement, with the degree of blurring increasing with the distance from the selected plane. A thinner section can be obtained with a longer tube movement or a shorter focus-film distance. The central ray may move perpendicular to the plane of the section throughout or be continuously directed to the center of this plane.[1-3]

The name *tomography,* derived from the Greek word *tomos,* meaning a section or cut, was coined by Grossmann[4] in 1935 for his specific apparatus. This must have come as a shock to Speed and Brackin,[5] who in 1955 asserted that the "tomogram was first used by Sir John Tomes, an English dentist, in 1889 and named after him"—a remarkable achievement since Roentgen made his discovery 6 years later![3] The more inclusive term, *body section roentgenography*, was introduced in 1936 by Andrews.[6]

The history of the development of tomography is fascinating in that it was independently "discovered" in five countries by at least nine investigators and had been patented at least six times in five countries! The earliest recorded application of the tomographic principle was made by a Polish radiologist, Karol Mayer, in 1914. In an attempt to visualize the heart without the distracting shadows cast by the superimposed ribs, Mayer moved the x-ray tube back and forth during the exposure. This technique blurred all of the images on the plate, but since the heart was farther from the tube, its shadow was less blurred than the rib shadows. Since the plate remained stationary throughout the image, this was not true tomography.[1]

One year later (1915), an Italian engineer, C. Baese, patented a device for linking an x-ray tube and a fluorescent screen in such a way as to impart to them a proportional, reciprocal motion. Baese's purpose, however, was to locate bullets and other foreign objects; he apparently did not realize that this technique could "erase" unwanted shadows.[1]

The originator of the true tomographic process was a Parisian physician, André Edmund Marie Bocage. In 1921, Bocage applied for a patent on a device for moving both an x-ray tube and a plate reciprocally and proportionately. His invention contained almost all the essential features of modern tomographic devices, but for 17 years he was unable to get a workable unit constructed. Four months later, two fellow countrymen, Portes and Chausse, applied for a similar patent; in 1927, Pohl obtained a German patent along the same lines. However, none of these early proposals led to the manufacture of a true tomographic device.[3]

In 1930, Alessandro Vallebona of Genoa introduced *stratigraphy* (from *stratum*, meaning a layer). In his original technique, both the tube and film were stationary, and the object was placed on a simple platform that rotated in the x-ray beam.[7] This was the basic principle of *autotomography*, a technique that was used in pneumoencephalography to show the air-filled third and fourth ventricles free of overlying skull shadows. However, this method could not easily be used for other diagnostic studies because of the practical difficulty encountered in placing and fixing the patient on the rocker. In Vallebona's later apparatus, the patient remained immobile, while the tube and film (fixed to the ends of a pendulum) described arcs.[1]

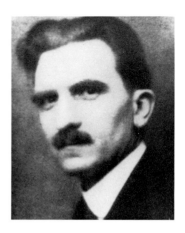

André Edmund Marie Bocage (1892-1953).[3]

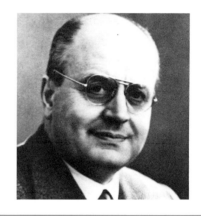

Alessandro Vallebona.

Left, Photographs[7] and *right* schematic drawing of Vallebona's original stratigraphic apparatus (1930).[6]

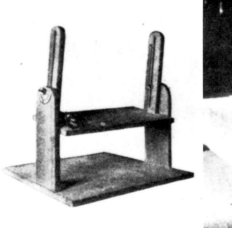 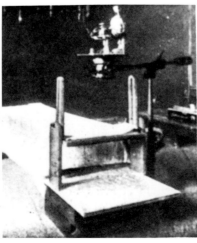 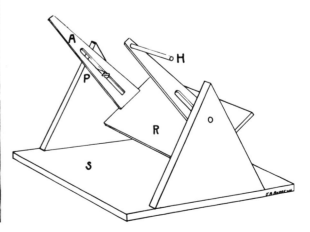

431

Planigraphic apparatus of Ziedses des Plantes. "A, Supporting frame; R, x-ray tube; K, carrier that can slide the length of the table while the frame (A) moves perpendicularly to it; H, level that pivots at point F. The lower moving bar of the frame was attached by a cord (D) to a peg (T) on the floor. Manual turning of this lower bar of A during the exposure provided the motive power for the moving system. The turning movement caused the cord to wind around the peg so that the moving bar and the whole frame came gradually to the center with a spiral motion. When a heavier peg was used, the spiral turns were farther apart and thus pegs of different sizes were provided."[6]

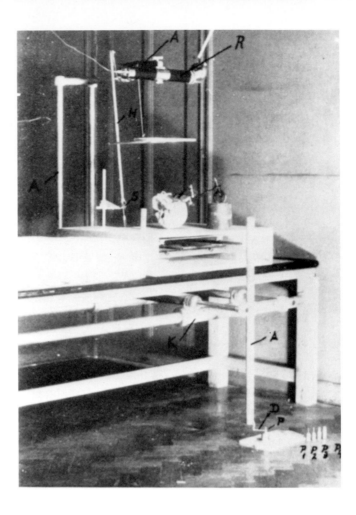

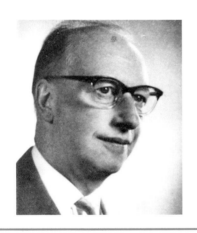

Bernard Ziedses des Plantes.

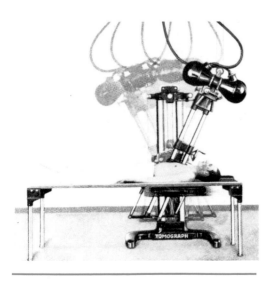

Tomograph of Grossmann (1935).[4]

Bernard Ziedses des Plantes presented his Dutch doctoral thesis on "plani-graphy" (from *planus*, meaning flat) in 1931. In his planigraph, the tube and the film moved in horizontal planes and described spiral, circular, or linear paths. The central ray was directed by simultaneous rotation of the tube toward the same point on the film at all times during the exposure. The focal plane was changed by raising or lowering the mechanical point of rotation. To accurately note the focal plane being projected, Ziedses des Plantes attached a simple wood cylinder phantom in which metal numerals had been placed, each indicating its own height. He suggested that a pleuridirectional movement, such as the spiral, was a basic requirement for satisfactory tomography, which could not be fulfilled with a simple linear movement. In addition, Ziedses des Plantes was the first to define *zonography* as a special radiographic method, referring to tomography with exposure angles of 10 degrees or less. This method was proposed to provide a "thicker section" and was particularly applicable where the object of interest was situated some distance from the disturbing shadows to be blurred.[8]

Gustav Grossmann, in Berlin, made an extensive study of the mathematical and geometric principles of tomography and concluded that the available equipment was too complicated. He noted that circular movements required 3 to 5 times the normal exposure required for a plain radiograph, and that 10 to 15 times as much radiation was necessary for the spiral movement. In Grossmann's "tomograph" (1935), the tube and film rotated through arcs and the central ray was at all times directed to the center of the film.[4] He suggested that overlying shadows would be most effectively blurred by applying a pendular motion of the tube. As long as the total excursion was sufficiently great, Grossmann considered the degree of blurring to be equal to that obtained with circular or spiral movements. Grossmann's work led to the first commercial production of a body-section machine.

The scene now shifted to the United States, where Jean Kieffer, a self-taught technician, secured employment in the x-ray department of a Connecticut tuberculosis sanitarium after he had recovered from a bout of the disease. During a relapse he suffered in 1928, Kieffer spent many months in bed suffering from tuberculous involvement of the mediastinum, an area that was difficult to visualize with conventional radiographic techniques because of surrounding bony structures. Kieffer spent his convalescence conceiving of a method of body-section radiography that would permit x-ray visualization of his own mediastinum.

As the Brechers[2] described Kieffer's device:

Tube and film were linked together by a pivoted system somewhat resembling a teeter-totter. By moving the pivot-point or fulcrum in one direction or the other, he could "bring into focus" any desired plane of the object under study. The linked tube and film, moreover, could be moved back and forth, or in a circle, or along a sine curve or spiral, or in any combination of these paths; the motions remained always reciprocal and proportional. This wide variety of motions made possible a more complete erasure of the unwanted shadows under varying circumstances. The thickness of the unblurred section could be changed by varying the amplitude of the movement; the more ample the movement of tube and film, the thinner the section reported on the film without blurring and the more complete the erasing of shadows cast by objects above and below that plane. Kieffer even worked out a way to combine his device with a Potter-Bucky grid.

After applying for a patent for his "x-ray focusing machine" in 1929, Kieffer tried unsuccessfully for several years to interest an x-ray manufacturer to build his machine. Thus his theoretical design of a tomographic device lay dormant for 8 years, until September 29, 1936, when he was shocked to read the following account in the New York Times[2]:

NEW X-RAY DEVICE "DISSECTS" BY FILMS
Machine Makes Possible Photographs of Parts of Organs
Unobscured by Tissue

TAKES "SLICES" OF BODY

Shown at Roentgen Ray Meeting, It Enables Demonstration of
Diseased Portion

Under the headline was an Associated Press dispatch from Cleveland, which began:

A new X-ray machine which makes picture slices of the head or organs of the body was demonstrated today to early arriving members of the American Roentgen Ray Society.

Known technically as a "tomograph," the device makes possible for the first time effective photography of separate parts of particular organs without such parts being obscured by shadows of intervening tissue.

Dr. J. Robert Andrews and Robert J. Stava, of the Cleveland University Hospitals who perfected the machine, demonstrated with their x-ray pictures how sections of the human skull, for example, could be pictured clearly to show the presence or absence of diseased conditions. By a simple adjustment, sections could be made one inch back of the forehead, two inches back, or at any similar point . . .

More than 3,000 members of the X-ray society were expected to attend the scientific sessions opening tomorrow . . .

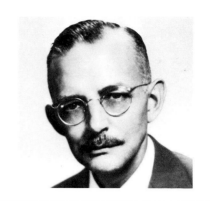

Jean Kieffer.

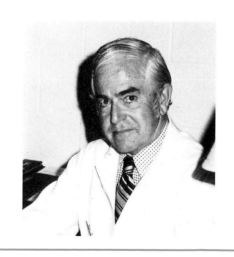

J. Robert Andrews.

433

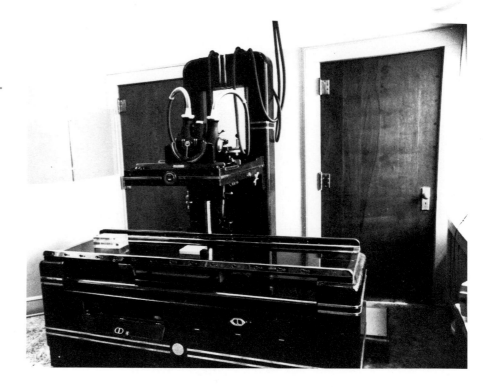

Laminagraph manufactured by the Keleket Company.

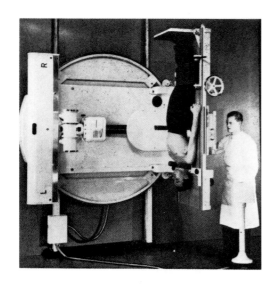

SRW Universal Planigraph (1949). The ring stand permitted body section radiography in any desired position.

A shocked Kieffer set off at once for Cleveland to meet Andrews, who as a resident in radiology at the University of Pennsylvania had noted an abstract of a paper in a European journal describing a tomographic device. Needing a subject for his postdoctoral thesis, Andrews decided to review the topic of body-section imaging.[6] After moving to Cleveland University Hospitals, Andrews and Stava (of the Picker X-ray Corporation), both still ignorant of Kieffer's patent, constructed the first workable American tomographic unit.

Although Kieffer was chagrined when Andrews told him of the many other inventors who had predated him, all eventually turned out well. Andrews' exhibit attracted the attention of Sherwood Moore, Director of the Mallinckrodt Institute of Radiology in St. Louis. Andrews introduced Kieffer to Moore, who was "deeply impressed with both Kieffer's personality and his detailed plans for a tomographic device." Moore arranged for its construction at Mallinckrodt, and by 1939 a commercial "laminagraph" unit was manufactured by the Keleket Company.[1]

In a later publication describing in greater detail the analysis of tomographic movements and their values, Kieffer (1938) offered some interesting insights[9]:

A satisfactory roentgenographic "tomographic" study, therefore, should give maximum positive information consistent with the absence of false information.

. . . a satisfactory roentgenograph depends on who is looking at it and what he is looking for. A well trained roentgenologist will be better able to notice positive findings and discount possible false shadows than one not so trained, so that a roentgenograph barely satisfactory for the trained man is entirely unsatisfactory for the untrained. Yet it is the less trained man who most often interprets unsatisfactory roentgenographs.

It can then hardly be gainsaid that it is better if the roentgenograph is not clear than if it is not truthful. It is better that no deduction be possible, due to lack of clarity, than that an erroneous statement be made because the roentgenograph is not a true representation of the anatomical part under observation.

Other variations on the theme of tomography were introduced. Kieffer described "stereolaminagrams" for situations in which the layer in focus was relatively thick (thin sections would be virtually two dimensional).

434

Baese used "tomoscopy," in which he fluoroscopically determined the depth of an object in the body (and thus the desired body-plane) before tomography. This film-sparing, but time-consuming, variation received an unenthusiastic response.

A complex innovation was transverse axial, or cross-sectional, tomography, which was initially described by a technologist, William Watson (1937)[10] and by Jean Kieffer (1938)[9]. In the first practical use of this technique reported by Vallebona (1950),[11] the vertical patient and the horizontal film were turned synchronously a full circle in the same direction. The angle of the x-rays to the film was extremely oblique, and high exposures were required. Another variation was *pantomography*, originated by Paatero in 1949, in which a curved layer of the subject was sharply imaged on a curved film, with both being vertical and rotating in opposite directions.[12] This device, marketed commercially as Panorex, is employed primarily in studies of teeth and temporomandibular joints.

In *multisection tomography*, multiple planes through the body were recorded during a single x-ray exposure by loading several films fixed specific distances apart. Progressively faster intensifying screens were required as the table-screen distance increased, to compensate for the absorption of intervening screens and, to a lesser extent, for the greater distance. Although described in theory and used on a postmortem specimen in 1931 by Ziedses des Plantes, the first studies in living patients were made of lung cavities by Manoel de Abreu in 1947.[14] Major advantages of this technique were less radiation, shorter procedure time, and the ability to ensure the same phase of respiration for chest work. A minor disadvantage was that a "single cut" provided slightly better detail and often was still required as a supplementary view at the depth of interest indicated by the multisection.

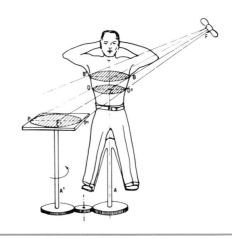

Geometrical factors involved in axial transverse laminagraphy (1950). "The x-ray beam is directed with considerable obliquity to the center of the desired cross-section and reaches a film, which is carried on a horizontal platform that rotates simultaneously in the same direction as the patient during the exposure. All shadows in plane D-D' will fall on the same points of the film during this rotation, while all shadows in other planes, such as B'-B, will either move on the film or be projected completely outside of the film."[11]

Top, Pantomography (1954). Jaw film cassette bent on its support.[12] *Bottom*, Pantomogram (1954).[12]

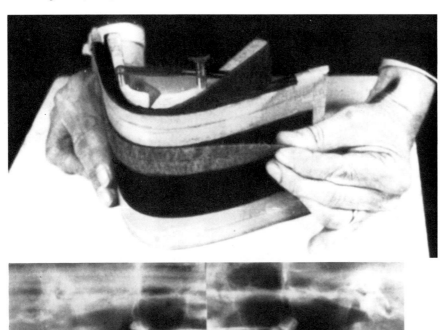

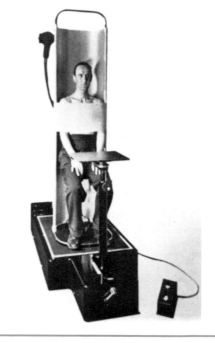

Watson's first commercially available apparatus for transverse tomography (1938).[10]

435

Polytome. First of the modern pluridirectional units to be installed in the United States. Shown with the instrument are C. L. Rumbaugh, J. T. Littleton, and Virginia Wilcox.[1]

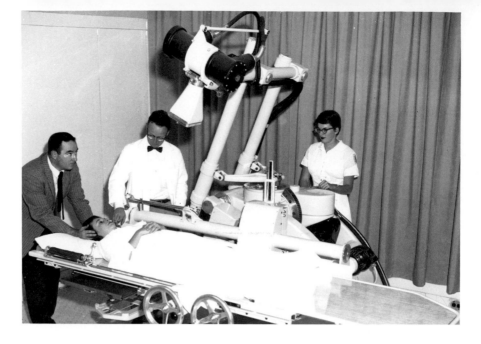

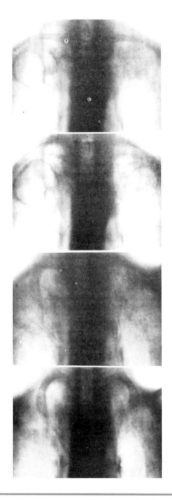

Multisection tomography (1948). Simultaneous tomograms with one front screen per film and balsa wood separations of 1.5 cm. The sections are posterior at 7.0, 8.5, 10.0, and 11.5 cm.[14]

An ongoing debate regarding tomography concerned the best path to be followed by the x-ray focal spot. Linear, circular, and spiral motions were strongly defended by their proponents. Kieffer suggested that no single type of focus movement was best for all tomographic problems and that any might be superior for a given case. Perhaps his view was influenced by the fact that only *his* apparatus happened to be capable of all these possible focal paths. The most complex tomographic device was the Polytome (introduced in 1952), which also offered hypocycloidal motion with a rotating grid and a fine focus tube.[7]

In the early days, tomography was mainly used for diseases of the chest, especially for detecting cavities in areas of tuberculous infiltration and bronchial narrowing secondary to bronchogenic carcinoma. Other pulmonary indications included verifying the presence of calcium in a solitary pulmonary nodule and visualization of abnormal feeding and draining vessels communicating with an arteriovenous fistula of the lung. Since the 1940s, tomography has been applied in many areas, including skeletal disorders (detection of fractures and their complete healing, identifying the elusive sequestrum or a nidus in osteoid osteoma), assessing the extent of cancer of the larynx, and improving visualization of abnormalities of temporomandibular joints and middle ear structures. Tomography of the kidneys during the nephrogram phase (nephrotomography) became an indispensable part of excretory urography; tomography of the bile ducts was an integral part of intravenous cholangiography.[3]

With the development of computed tomography, the use of conventional tomography has dramatically decreased.

References

1. Littleton JT (ed): Tomography: Physical principles and clinical applications. Baltimore, Williams & Wilkins, 1976.
2. Brecher R and Brecher E: The rays. A history of radiology in the United States and Canada. Baltimore, Williams & Wilkins, 1969.
3. Bricker JD: Tomography. In Bruwer AJ: Classic descriptions in diagnostic roentgenology. Springfield, Ill, Charles C Thomas, 1964.
4. Grossmann G: Lung tomography. Brit J Radiol 8:733-751, 1935.
5. Speed K and Brackin RE: Use of the tomogram after attempted joint fusion. Am J Surg 89:872-874, 1955.

6. Andrews JR: Planigraphy I. Introduction and history. AJR 36:575-587, 1936.
7. Vallebona A: A modified technique of roentgenographic dissociation of shadows applied to the study of the skull. Radiol Med 17:1090-1097, 1930.
8. Ziedses des Plantes BG: A new method of obtaining roentgenograms of the skull and vertebral column. Nederl Tijdschr Geneesk 75:5218-5222, 1931.
9. Kieffer J: The laminagraph and its variations. Applications and implications of the planigraphic principles. AJR 39:497-513, 1938.
10. Watson W: Axial transverse tomography. Radiography 28:179-189, 1962.

11. Vallebona A: Axial transverse laminagraphy. Radiology 55:271-273, 1950.
12. Paatero YV: Pantomography in theory and use. Acta Radiol 41:321-335, 1954.
13. Glenner RA: The dental office: A pictorial history. Missoula, Mont, Pictorial Histories, 1984.
14. de Abreu M: Theory and technique of simultaneous tomography. AJR 60:668-674, 1948.
15. Krohmer JS: Radiography and fluoroscopy, 1920 to the present. RadioGraphics 9:1129-1153, 1989.

CHAPTER 25

Angiography

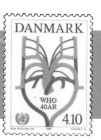
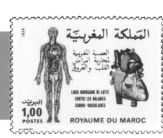
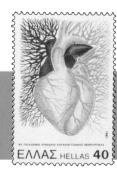
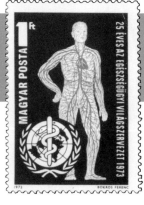

The history of the radiographic study of arteries and veins goes back to January, 1896, the month after the announcement of Roentgen's discovery, when Hascheck and Lindenthal[1] injected a contrast material into the blood vessels of an amputated hand. Since that time, improved contrast material, technical advances, and new puncture and catheter techniques have dramatically widened the role of angiography in both diagnosis and therapy.

Many developments in angiography had their initial impact on the study of the heart and great vessels and therefore are included in Chapter 13 on cardiac radiology.

CONTRAST MATERIAL

Of all the elements in the periodic table, only iodine has been found suitable for injection into the circulation as a radiographic contrast agent. Although many elements are much more radiopaque than iodine, none has yet been found that can be injected as safely as iodine into the circulation in sufficient concentrations and in sufficient dose to produce radiopacity of diagnostic quality.[2] Before achieving the first carotid arteriogram in a human using sodium iodide, Egas Moniz conducted many experiments, mainly on rabbits, monkeys, and dogs, using bromine and iodine salts of sodium, potassium, lithium, strontium, and even rubidium. After much disappointment with the halogen compounds, Moniz introduced a suspension of thorium dioxide that had little acute intravascular toxicity, was almost painless on arterial injection, and was intensely radiopaque. Unfortunately, thorium was later abandoned as a diagnostic contrast agent because it produced dangerous alpha radiation that could lead to the development of malignant tumors 20 to 30 years later in the reticuloendothelial organs (liver, spleen, and lymph nodes) in which it was stored.

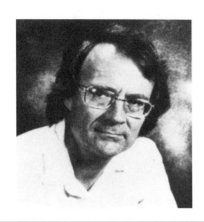

Torsten Almen.

The first major achievement in the development of contrast media was the introduction by Moses Swick (1929) of iodides of the pyridine nucleus for use in excretory urography (see Chapter 17). This led to the production of Hypaque, Renografin, and Conray, the three major currently employed contrast media that are ionic monomeric salts of tri-iodinated substituted benzoic acids.

The next major advance in the synthesis of contrast media was the work of Torsten Almen, a Swedish radiologist who was determined to find a contrast material that would produce less pain during arteriography than the available substances.[3] In 1968, Almen theorized that a contrast agent with lower osmotic effects would produce less peripheral vasodilatation and decrease the damage to endothelial cells. Decreasing the osmotic effects could be accomplished by (1) increasing the number of iodine atoms per particle in solution; (2) producing dimers, trimers, or polymers of the existing anions; or (3) avoiding the use of cations by including a sufficient number of hydrophilic hydroxyl groups to increase the water solubility. Almen decided on the latter approach but was unable to achieve support from any major pharmaceutical company. Turning to a relatively small Norwegian company (Nyegaard) with a good reputation for contrast medium research, Almen developed metrizamide (Amipaque), the first nonionic contrast agent. Metrizamide permitted virtually painless arteriography, as well as apparently decreased toxicity. Modifications of the metrizamide formula made by substituting different side chains have resulted in a second generation of low-osmolality products such as Iopamidol and Iohexol, as well as Hexabrix (ioxaglate), which is essentially a salt of a monoacid dimer.

The major limiting factor of the new ionic contrast media is their substantial expense, and major efforts are underway to produce similar but less costly agents. Meanwhile, controversies continue over the precise indications for the clinical use of these costly pharmaceuticals.[3]

TECHNICAL ADVANCES

The development of arteriography required an ability to obtain multiple images of the vascular tree following a single injection of contrast material. The development of rapid film changers permitted a filming rate of two or more radiographs per second. Other important technical developments leading to the growth of arteriography included the application of cine techniques, the development of biplane film changers, and the introduction of practical imaging amplification.

In the early days of arteriography, rubber ureteral catheters were the only ones available. Advances in plastic chemistry led to the development of materials that lose both shape and form when heated and regain them when cooled. Because polyethylene does not soften significantly at body temperature, it has remained a favorite material for selective catheterization. Arteriographers have the option of using preshaped molded catheters or less expensive catheters that are supplied in long rolls, custom-made by the radiologist for a particular case, and discarded after one use. Thermoplastic preshaped catheters with excellent torque are now available. An interlacing braided steel-wire mesh sandwiched between the walls of the catheter provides this control, while the outer and inner surfaces retain all of the inherent softness, elasticity, and smoothness of thermoplastic material.[4]

Examples of the shapes of some preformed ready-made catheters. *Left to right,* Simmons catheter for common carotid arteries; Cobra catheter for abdominal visceral vessels (renal and superior mesenteric arteries); Newton 4 catheter for the left carotid artery; pig-tail catheter for aortic injection; and Harwood-Nash catheter for cerebral arteries in children.

To minimize the dilution of contrast material that occurs when it is injected into the vascular system, various types of pressure injectors have been devised to increase the rate and amount of contrast material being injected. Early hand injectors incorporated movable levers that transmitted force to a steel or reinforced-glass syringe. These simple instruments delivered an inconstant force that was difficult to reproduce on multiple injections. In addition, the maximum pressure was generally inadequate for injections through small catheters.

Hand injectors were replaced by pneumatic power injectors, which utilized compressed gases to transmit pressure directly to a cylinder connected to the injector syringe. The high pressures generated by this system made it necessary to use specially designed stainless steel syringes that tolerated high pressures. Because the syringes were not transparent, special features had to be built in to avoid the inadvertent injection of any air that might enter the syringe while it was being filled with contrast material.[4]

In 1956, Gidlund[6] described a compressed-air injector with a stainless steel syringe that could be placed in a vertical position, which facilitated the addition of a valve for air removal at the top of the syringe. The contrast material was kept at body temperature by a thermostatically controlled water bath that surrounded the injector syringe. Four years later (1960), Kurt Amplatz[7] described a cardiovascular injector powered by carbon dioxide cartridges such as those commonly used for the preparation of carbonated beverages. The major advantage of this system was that the injector weighed only 5 kg.

A mechanical injector powered by a series of springs (Tavaras injector) permitted the speed of injection to be controlled by an adjustable valve. In this device, the syringe was pointed downward so that air bubbles in the system rose to the surface and were not injected. As additional insurance against inadvertent injection of air, the unit retained approximately 3 to 6 ml of contrast material within the syringe.[4]

Current pressure injectors are electronically powered and mechanically driven and can be programmed with the electrocardiogram so that multiple small injections can be made during specific phases of the

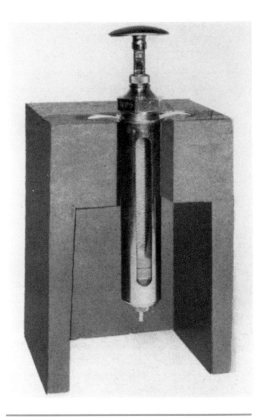

Simple wooden injection block to allow rapid injection of contrast material (1957).[5]

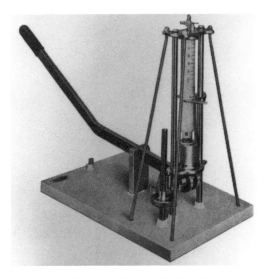

Lehman manual injector (Hogan X-Ray Company).[4]

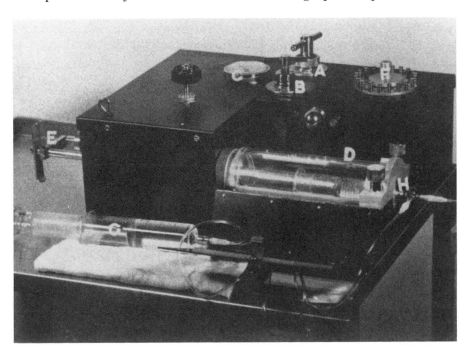

Pneumatic cardiovascular injector powered by carbon dioxide cartridges (1960).[7]

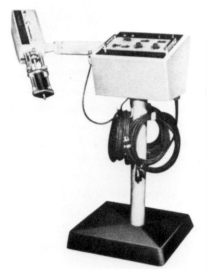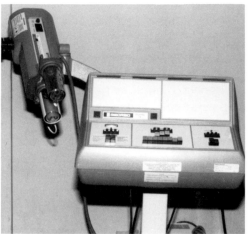

Pressure injectors. *Left*, Viamonte-Hobbs injector (Barber-Colman Electro-Mechanical Products). *Right*, Medrad injector (Medrad Inc).[4]

cardiac cycle. They contain built-in safeguards to prevent ventricular fibrillation resulting from inadequate grounding of an electric injector at the time the patient's catheter is connected to a syringe. Specific dials on the control panel permit selection of the duration of the injection and the delivery rate.[4]

PUNCTURE AND CATHETER TECHNIQUES

Arteriographic procedures were initially performed by injecting contrast material through a needle that was placed by a surgical cutdown into the artery leading to the clinical area of interest. Following the procedure, the artery was either ligated or repaired.

Translumbar aortography was first described by the Portuguese surgeon, Reynaldo dos Santos, in 1929.[8] While experimenting with lumbar ganglionic blockade, dos Santos on several occasions accidentally punctured a human aorta. Noting that this unplanned procedure seemed to cause no substantial complications, dos Santos began deliberately puncturing the aorta with the apparent intention of using this daring route for parenteral drug therapy. By 1937, dos Santos had performed more than

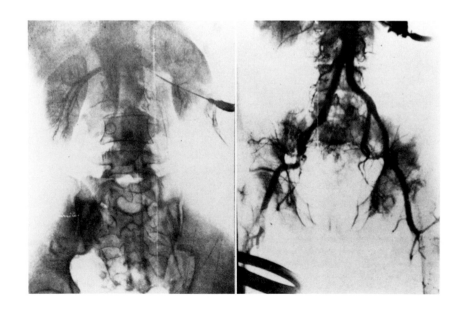

Translumbar aortography (1929). *Left*, Direct injection of sodium iodide at the level of the first lumbar vertebra in the supine position. The right renal circulation is normal in contrast to the diffuse opacity of the left kidney (left renal tuberculosis). *Right*, In this patient, note the wealth of detail of the lumbar and pelvic circulation, especially the branches of the hypogastric arteries.[8]

1,000 translumbar aortograms. However, the popular appeal of this diagnostic procedure was limited because of reluctance to blindly puncture the aorta and the lack of a suitably benign, easily injectable, and densely opaque contrast material.[9] Direct puncture of the thoracic aorta was first performed in humans by Nuvoli (1936),[10] who succeeded in demonstrating aneurysms, tortuosity, and other abnormalities.

Retrograde arteriography was first reported by Saito and Kamikawa (1932),[11] who described the successful visualization of the major vessels by retrograde injection of an emulsion of iodized oil into peripheral arteries or collateral branches. The major early developers of retrograde arteriography were Castellanos and Pereiras,[12] who in 1939 described visualization of the thoracic aorta via a "countercurrent" (retrograde) brachial approach.

The radiographic examination of the abdominal aorta exclusively utilized the translumbar approach until 1941, when Pedro Fariñas[13] of Cuba wrote that

> to avoid the blind puncturing of the aorta, we recommend the arteriographic study of the abdominal aorta and its branches by the puncture and catheterization of the femoral artery at Scarpa's triangle. After local anesthesia the femoral artery is exposed by blunt dissection, mounted in two catguts, and punctured with a trocar through which a catheter is passed, it being introduced to the desired level in the aorta. The patient is placed in position according to the organ to be roentgenographed so that its selective arteriogram may be obtained. A compression at the root of the opposite member is made with a tourniquet, in order to compress the femoral artery and to obtain an ectasis in the abdominal circulation.

Although this method of arteriography of the aorta and visceral vessels proved highly satisfactory, the arteriotomy required was extremely time-consuming and difficult, requiring a certain amount of surgical experience and skill on the part of the physician performing the examination.

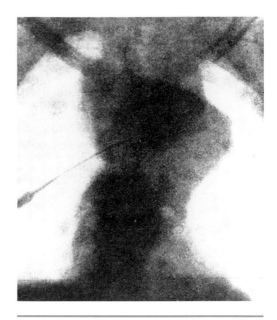

Aortic aneurysm demonstrated by direct puncture of the thoracic aorta (1936).[10]

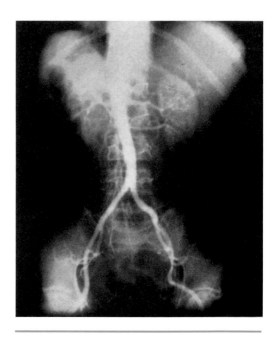

Early retrograde aortogram via catheterization of the femoral artery (1941). In a patient with abdominal Hodgkin's disease, multiple compressions of the aorta and its branches are caused by enlarged nodes.[13]

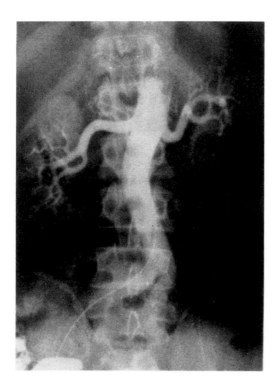

Early percutaneous aortogram via a femoral artery approach (1951). Mild aortic tortuosity in this patient with severe hypertension.[14]

In 1951, E. Converse Peirce[14] developed "a method of introducing a disposable polyethylene catheter of fairly large caliber into the femoral percutaneously and passing it to any desired aortic level." Using this technique, Peirce noted that "contrast aortography may be effected simply with a minimum of equipment and personnel. The examiner can be outside the x-ray field, the patient readily positioned, and repeated exposures made with no necessity for haste. At the completion of the procedure the catheter is withdrawn without the necessity for surgical repair of an artery." In the same year, Donald and co-workers[15] used a similar percutaneous technique in cerebral arteriography by catheterizing the common carotid artery with a large-bore needle through which they passed a thin-walled polyethylene catheter.

The revolutionary development that paved the way for modern arteriography was the significant modification of the percutaneous catheter technique introduced by Sven Ivar Seldinger in 1953. In his classic article, Seldinger[16] noted that

> the catheter method of angiography has become more popular in the past few years, as it provides the following advantages over the method of injecting the contrast medium by means of a simple needle:
> 1. The contrast medium may be injected into a vessel at any level desired.
> 2. Risk of extravascular injection of the contrast medium is minimized.
> 3. The patient may be placed in any position required.
> 4. The catheter may be left in situ without risk while the films are being developed, thus facilitating re-examination if necessary.

However, the techniques of Peirce and Donald and his colleagues both required

> the use of a large bore needle which may make puncture difficult and limits its use to comparatively large arteries . . . There is also damage to the artery and, as the hole in the artery is larger than the catheter, hemorrhage after removal of the needle may be troublesome. To prevent bleeding, the needle may be kept in situ during the investigation; this, however, increases the risk of injury to the patient during movement.

Seldinger's solution was

> a simple method . . . of using a catheter the same size as the needle . . . The main principle consists in the catheter being introduced on a flexible leader [guidewire, author's note] through the puncture hole after withdrawal of the puncture needle . . . The leader should have a diameter slightly less than the bore of the needle and the catheter, so that it is capable of passing through both, and should be at least 8-9 cm longer than the latter; on the other hand it should just fit the lumen of the catheter.

Once the artery was punctured percutaneously,

> the supple tip of the leader is inserted a very short distance into the lumen of the artery through the needle. The leader is held in place and the needle removed. At this moment bleeding should be controlled by pressure on the artery proximal to the puncture site, because the diameter of the leader is smaller than the hole in the artery. The catheter is threaded on to the leader; when the tip reaches the skin the free end of the leader must protrude from the catheter. The catheter and leader are gripped near the skin through which they are inserted. The catheter enters the artery easily as an

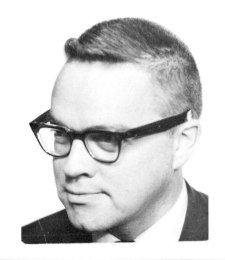

Sven Ivar Seldinger.

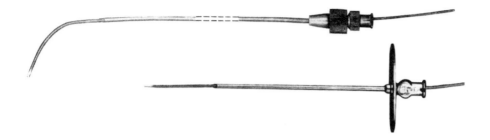

opening has already been made by the needle. The catheter and leader are pushed just far enough to ensure that the tip of the former is in the lumen of the vessel. The leader is removed and the catheter directed to the level required, after good arterial bleeding through the catheter has been obtained. The unsupported catheter is usually pushed up the vessel without difficulty, but occasionally the leader must be reintroduced into the catheter in order to support it. The leader should not be passed beyond the tip of the catheter.

Seldinger noted that the

polyethylene tubing is unfortunately not radio-opaque. For this reason, in aortography via the femoral artery, a small amount of contrast medium may be injected and followed by a test exposure. This will show the position of the catheter and also the exact situation of the renal arteries and the iliac bifurcation. When the brachial artery is catheterized, the procedure is carried out in the fluoroscopy room

Clinical example of Seldinger technique (1953). Occlusion of the right external iliac artery with collaterals from the superior gluteal to the deep femoral artery. The catheter was inserted through the left femoral artery with its tip at the bifurcation.[16]

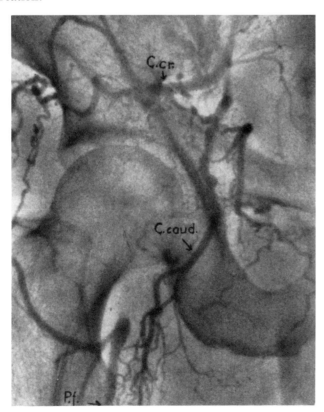

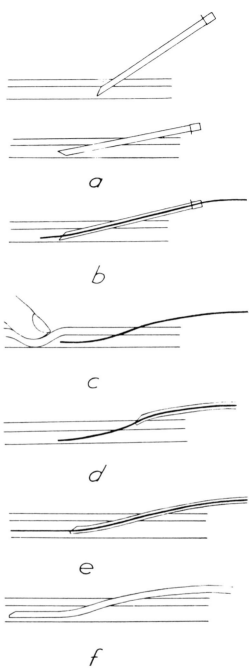

Seldinger technique (1953). *Top left,* "The equipment. The stilette is removed and the leader inserted through the needle (*left*) and the catheter (*right*)." *Top right,* "Diagram of the technique used. *a,* The artery punctured. The needle pushed upwards. *b,* The leader inserted. *c,* The needle withdrawn and the artery compressed. *d,* The catheter threaded onto the leader. *e,* The catheter inserted into the artery. *f,* The leader withdrawn."[16]

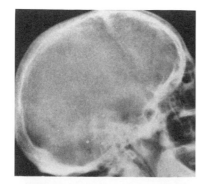

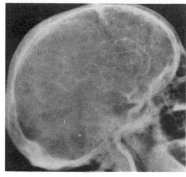

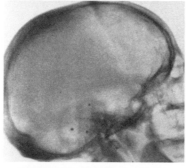

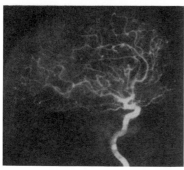

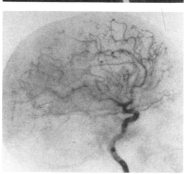

Principle of the subtraction method (1963). *Top to bottom*, Conventional roentgenogram of the skull; angiogram; diapositive print; result of covering the angiogram with the diapositive; and print of the superimposed films.[19]

and the leader used as an indicator of position; the catheter is then kept free from blood by the injection of saline solution.

Not everyone was convinced of the value of the Seldinger technique or even aortography itself. In 1963, McGraw[17] wrote,

> Except for visualization of the renal arteries, or due to inability to needle the small aorta in children, retrograde abdominal aortography offers no advantages over the translumbar method, and there are definite practical disadvantages . . . Retrograde arteriography should be restricted to those patients in whom it is difficult or impossible to introduce the radiopaque material into the artery proximal to the lesion.

As late as 1957, prominent surgeons in the United States stated that[18]

> In the great majority of cases of aneurysms of the abdominal aorta, for example, there is little or no need to perform aortography for these purposes. Similarly, in complete occlusive disease of the aorta, aortography has been found unnecessary for these purposes. Its usefulness lies primarily in patients with incomplete aortic occlusion and in the few patients in whom the diagnosis remains doubtful . . . the necessity for aortography may be eliminated in the majority of patients with aneurysms and occlusive disease of the abdominal aorta, approximately two-thirds of the cases, with commensurate reduction in the occurrence of complications.

A significant technical development permitting visualization of small vessels and subtle capillary blushes was radiographic subtraction, first described by Bernard Ziedses des Plantes[19] in 1963. As he wrote,

> The object of the subtraction method is to produce a separate image of the difference between two roentgenograms obtained under similar conditions and is effected by covering one roentgenogram with a diapositive print of the other. In carotid angiography, for instance, a conventional roentgenogram of the skull and one or more angiograms are obtained in exactly the same position. A diapositive print of the conventional roentgenogram and in the same size is then made on a normal photographic film; this film is exposed and developed in such a way that its contrast is as it were, inversely, that of the roentgeno-

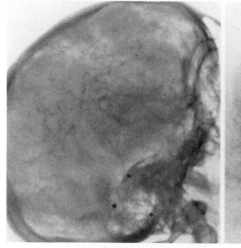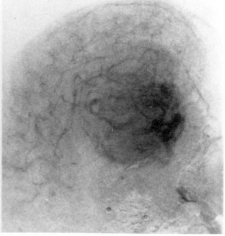

Value of subtraction method in arteriography (1963). Meningioma. *Left*, Common carotid arteriogram. *Right*, Result of subtraction.[19]

gram. If the roentgenogram is covered with this diapositive print the result will be that the image of the skull is completely blotted out but if the angiogram is covered with the diapositive only the contrast medium in the vessels will be evident. A final print of the superimposed films will be useful and will depict the filled vessels as dark structures against a light background. The contrast outside the image of the contrast medium being very low, the final print may be made on a material of high contrast.

PHARMACOANGIOGRAPHY

The earliest experience with pharmacoangiography was reported in 1937 by Sgalitzer,[20] who performed peripheral arteriography after papaverine infusion. That same year, Ratschow[21] attempted to enhance the visualization of the small arteries and collaterals in the lower extremities by performing peripheral arteriography after reactive hyperemia was produced by means of transient arterial compression. Ratschow noted that the increase in blood flow after release of compression caused sufficient vasodilatation to improve the quality of the arteriograms.

Bierman, Kelly, and Byron (1961)[22] were among the first to perform arteriography in conjunction with a vasoconstrictor when they used epinephrine during hepatic arteriography in a patient with metastatic breast carcinoma. One year later (1962), Abrams, Boijsen, and Borgstrom[23] published their classic paper describing the effects of epinephrine on the renal circulation. The first clinical article that laid the foundation for modern pharmacoangiography was published 2 years later by Herbert Abrams.[24] He hypothesized that neoplastic vessels, which were deficient in wall musculature, would constrict only weakly following selective infusion of epinephrine into the renal artery. In patients with kidney malignancies, Abrams found that

> following the injection of 25 micrograms of epinephrine into the renal artery, there was cessation of normal flow through the vessels supplying normal parenchyma, while the tumor vessels were densely opacified, although at a slower rate than during the control study.

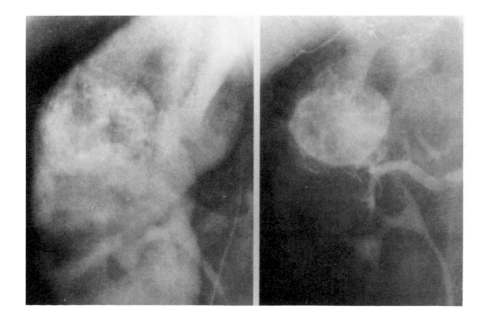

Epinephrine renal arteriogram. *Left*, Capillary phase suggests tumor vasculature in the superolateral aspect of the renal parenchyma. *Right*, An epinephrine arteriogram enhances the appearance of the tumor vasculature and clearly outlines a small renal cell carcinoma.[25]

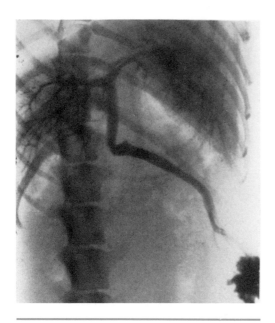

Direct splenoportography (1951). Radiograph obtained 4 seconds after the end of an injection of 8 cc of contrast material directly into the spleen (*lower right*).[28]

This constitutes the first evidence in man that the response of neoplastic renal vessels to humeral stimuli differs from that of normal vessels.

Since that time, numerous reports have been published on pharmacoangiography with a variety of vasodilators and vasoconstrictors, although it has been stressed that this effect may vary depending on dosage, timing, and individual patient responsiveness; thus the test is not completely reliable for differentiating malignant from benign conditions.

SPLENOPORTOGRAPHY AND ARTERIAL PORTOGRAPHY

Before the advent of ultrasound and computed tomography, the relative inaccessibility of the portal venous system prompted the search for a variety of techniques, both intraoperative and nonsurgical, to explore this circulation in patients with portal hypertension and its complications to determine the anatomical patency of the splenoportal axis and the hemodynamic alterations from the development of extrahepatic portosystemic collateral channels.[26] The earliest technique for portal vein visualization in humans was devised by Blakemore and Lord (1945),[27] who directly injected contrast material into the portal vein or one of its mesenteric tributaries at laparotomy. Further reports in the early 1950s confirmed the value of operative portal venography at laparotomy, but it quickly became apparent that this method was cumbersome, time-consuming, and less than satisfactory. Of more importance, it did not aid in the preoperative diagnosis of the patient and therefore was of no use in planning the surgical approach.[26]

In 1951, Abeatici and Campi[28] showed in dogs that contrast material injected directly into the spleen flowed into the splenic and portal veins. In that same year, Leger[29] performed the first successful percutaneous splenoportogram in humans. Soon, this method became firmly entrenched as the major preoperative diagnostic technique for investigating patients with portal hypertension. However, direct puncture of the splenic pulp for portal venography was limited by serious postpuncture complications (splenic bleeding or rupture), was contraindicated in cases of infec-

Modern biplane angiography suite.

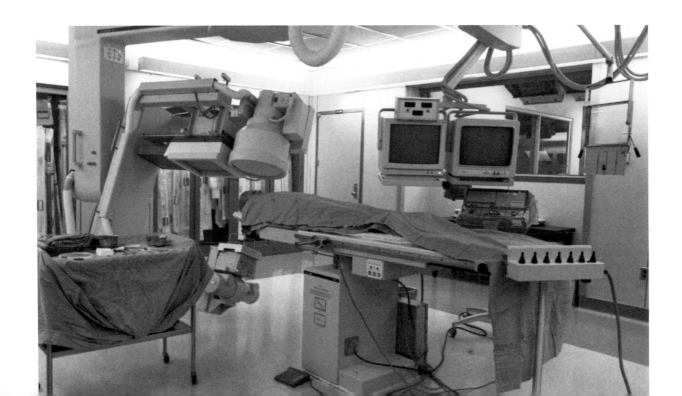

tive splenomegaly, and obviously could not be performed when the spleen had been resected.[30]

Arterial portography, as an alternative nonoperative technique, developed gradually after the observation by Rigler and co-workers (1953)[31] that the portal venous system was occasionally visualized after the injection of contrast material into the upper abdominal aorta. This technique was largely neglected because the low concentration of contrast made visualization of the portal circulation by aortic injection poor.[26] In 1958, Odman[32] refined the technique by selective catheterization of the celiac axis and was able to obtain excellent splenic and portal visualization. Improved portal vein visualization by arterial portography was later demonstrated following simultaneous selective contrast injection of the celiac and superior mesenteric arteries[33] and selective splenic artery injection.[30]

DIGITAL SUBTRACTION ANGIOGRAPHY

Although radiographic visualization of the arterial circulation using intravenously administered contrast material achieved some success in the 1960s,[34] this technique never achieved general popularity because of the necessity of using large-bore needles for the injection of large amounts of contrast material, the lack of a convenient method to accommodate substantial variations in tissue thickness, and an inability to rapidly or conveniently perform subtraction on large numbers of films.[35] In the early 1970s, analog subtraction systems were developed that permitted the demonstration of arterial structures after the intravenous injection of contrast material, but they had such poor reliability that they were unsuitable for clinical use. By the end of the decade, several digital video imaging programs for intravenous digital subtraction angiography (DSA) were developed, especially by Mistretta and associates at the University of Wisconsin[36,37] and by Ovitt and co-workers at the University of Arizona.[38]

Intravenous DSA could be performed on an outpatient basis because it required only a venipuncture. However, because intravenous DSA was sensitive to motion, it was impossible to perform this procedure in uncooperative patients. Dilution of the contrast bolus often precluded a successful examination in patients with poor cardiac output or cardiac dysrhythmia. These limitations were overcome by the use of intraarterial

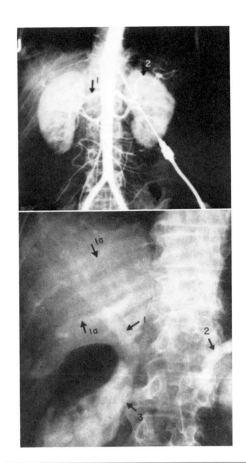

Arterial portography (1953). *Top*, "Aortogram obtained just at the end of contrast injection clearly shows the hepatic artery (*arrow 1*), the splenic artery (*arrow 2*), the superior mesenteric, renal, and iliac arteries." *Bottom*, "Radiograph made 5 seconds after the end of injection shows the normal liver with portal vein circulation. Arrow 1 indicates the portal vein and branches within the liver (la); arrow 2 the splenic vein; arrow 3 the opacity of the right kidney."[31]

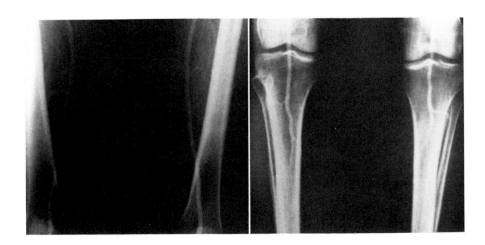

Intravenous angiography (1964). Single arm pressure injection of contrast material studied with an automatic table. *Left*, The superficial femoral arteries are intact. *Right*, The last of the serial roentgenograms shows excellent run-off below both knees.[34]

447

DSA, which in comparison with conventional film angiography provided increased speed and flexibility in performing procedures, less patient discomfort, and, in certain instances, greater diagnostic accuracy.[39]

LYMPHOGRAPHY

The first radiographic visualization of the lymphatics was reported in 1930 by Funaoka of Japan[40] and in 1931 by de Carvalho of Portugal.[41] They performed lymphography by injecting thorotrast into the lymph nodes and subcutaneous tissues of animals and cadavers. In 1932, Pfahler[42] introduced the *indirect* method of lymphography in humans. One week after the injection of Lipiodol into the maxillary sinuses, the lymphatics leading from that region were observed. Other investigators injected contrast material into subcutaneous tissues and subsequently examined adjacent nodes for uptake of the opaque material. Unfortunately, this indirect method was impractical because the lymphatics did not absorb contrast material rapidly enough to adequately visualize the vessels and nodes.[43]

The *direct* method of lymphography involved the injection of contrast material into large palpable nodes and lymph vessels. Teneff and Stoppani (1936)[44] and Servelle (1945)[45] visualized the lymphatic channels and nodes in the pelvis by injecting thorotrast into the inguinal nodes.

However, lymphography did not become a clinically useful procedure until Kinmonth (1952)[46] developed a method of cannulating lymphatic

Earliest radiographic visualization of the lymphatics (1931). "*Left*, Opacification of the draining lymph channels following injection of contrast into the submaxillary nodes. *Right*, Opacification of a left-sided lymphatic following contrast injection into the left inguinal node."[41]

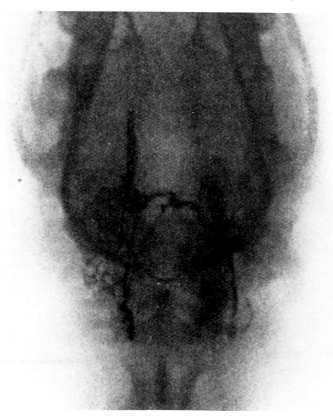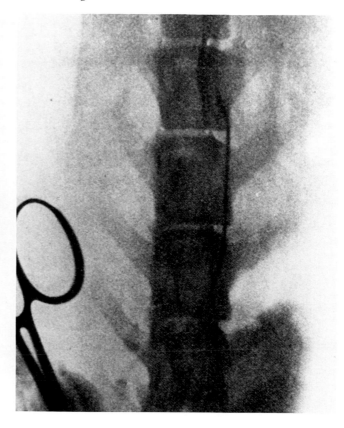

vessels and injecting contrast material directly into them. As he wrote, "lymph vessels, or at least normal ones, are much smaller than the arteries or veins used in angiography. They contain colourless lymph, which makes them difficult to see, and under normal circumstances they may be empty or nearly so, existing as potential spaces like the pleura or peritoneum." In studying patients with lymphedema, Kinmonth noted that when he injected an 11% solution of blue dye into the subcutaneous tissue between the toes, lymphatic vessels on the dorsum of the foot took up the dye and became clearly visible. A simple surgical cutdown permitted relatively easy cannulation of the lymphatic vessels and injection of contrast material.[47]

It is interesting to note that Hudack and McMaster (1933) at the Rockefeller Institute had outlined the subcutaneous lymphatics in humans using a similar blue violet dye. However, they apparently did not conceive of the possibility of directly injecting contrast material into the lymphatic vessels, and thus clinical lymphography did not appear until almost 20 years later.[43]

Contrast material injected into the dorsum of the foot flowed proximally to successively outline lymphatic vessels and lymph nodes in the inguinal, iliac, and paraaortic regions to about the level of the second lumbar vertebra. At this point, the contrast entered the cisterna chyli and then the thoracic duct. Lymphatic drainage of the upper extremity, head and neck, tongue, and breast also could be studied with this technique by injecting contrast material into the adjacent regional peripheral lymphatic vessels.[48] Although water-soluble contrast material was initially used, it proved unsatisfactory for studying the nodes and, in addition, was diluted by lymph in the lumbar area. Oil-soluble material became the contrast agent of choice, since it provided excellent opacification of lymph nodes, as well as good visualization of the paraaortic lymph channels and nodes and the thoracic duct.[43]

The first major publications describing the use of oil-based contrast material for lymphography appeared almost simultaneously in 1961.[49,50] Sidney Wallace and co-workers[49] stressed the value of lymphography as both a diagnostic tool and a therapeutic aid. They stated that "the procedure requires a minimum of surgical proficiency, so that under the

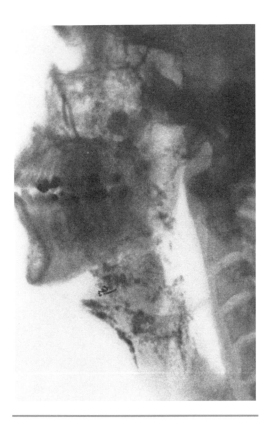

Indirect lymphography (1931). Lateral view of the sinuses and neck obtained 10 weeks after injection of Lipiodol into the maxillary sinuses.[42]

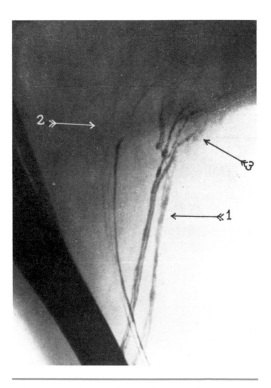

Direct lymphography (1936). Radiograph obtained 15 minutes after contrast injection demonstrates the popliteal lymph node (2) and its "efferent" (1) and "afferent" (3) lymphatic channels.[44]

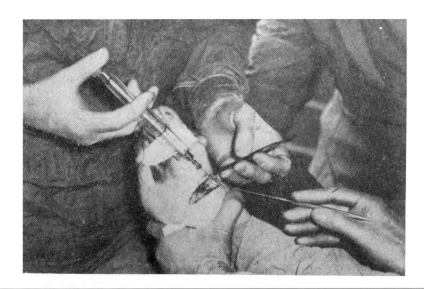

Method of contrast material injection into a lymphatic (1955).[47]

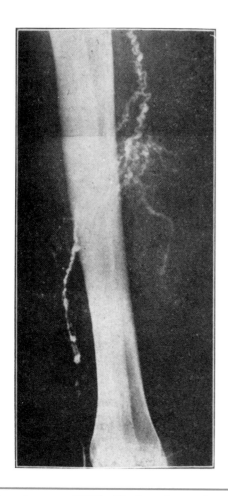

Lymphogram (1955). The lymph vessels are tortuous and wide in this patient with idiopathic lymphedema.[47]

usual circumstances the technical aspects are accomplished in approximately half an hour." In subsequent years, many radiologists have considered this appraisal far too optimistic as they struggled with this often time-consuming and frustrating procedure.

Wallace and co-workers showed examples in which they clearly demonstrated the pelvic, paraaortic, axillary, and supraclavicular nodes, as well as the thoracic duct. They noted that

> in lymphedema the findings vary from an increase to an almost complete absence of channels. Extensive collateral pathways in the face of obstruction to lymph flow have been shown. Normal nodes exhibit a homogeneous reticular pattern. In lymphadenitis, the nodes are larger but normal in architecture; in lymphomas there are enlarged, lacy, ghost-like nodes; in carcinoma the nodes have a moth-eaten appearance.

In patients with malignancy, Wallace and associates showed that lymphography was valuable in determining the extent of disease. They noted the detection of unsuspected metastatic disease, often situated out of the reach of the palpating finger, which could alter the therapeutic approach. In patients with lymphoma, lymphograms frequently revealed diffuse malignant involvement where only local disease was manifest clinically. As a preoperative study, lymphography could provide the surgeon with a more exact visual picture of the location and status of the nodes. Postoperative radiographs could reveal abnormal lymph nodes that were inadvertently left behind. Radiotherapy treatment portals could be more accurately placed after lymphography, and the prolonged presence of contrast material within lymph nodes could aid in determining the efficacy of radiotherapy or chemotherapy.

In most centers, computed tomography has now supplanted lymphography as the modality of choice for assessing lymphadenopathy.[51]

VENOGRAPHY

Radiographs of veins after injection of radiopaque substances were first made by Berberich and Hirsch (1923),[52] using strontium bromide, and by

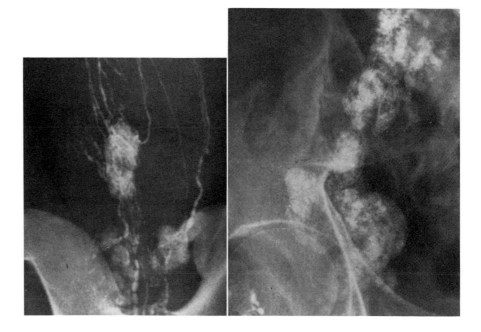

Lymphangiography (1961). *Left*, Normal femoral nodes and lymphatics. *Right*, Lymphomatous involvement.[49]

McPheeters and Rice (1929)[53] with Lipiodol. However, this procedure was infrequently performed until iodinated contrast media used for intravenous pyelography was available. *Indirect* venography after intraarterial injection of contrast material was described by Allen and Barker (1934), although this technique was rarely applied to the lower limbs because of their large bulk and the consequent dilution of contrast leading to nondiagnostic radiographs.[54] *Direct*, or *ascending*, venography was first reported by dos Santos (1938), who succeeded in outlining both the deep and superficial venous systems by injecting contrast material into the superficial vein behind the external malleolus.[55] Several other authors described technical improvements such as using a tourniquet above the ankle to force the contrast into the deep veins and conducting the examination in the vertical or semivertical position so that gravity aided in filling the deep venous system. The major limiting factor of venography was its reliance on "blind" overhead radiographs that had to be obtained with no knowledge of the speed of venous blood flow. Venography became a widely accepted technique with the development of image intensification and improved fluoroscopy, which permitted films to be taken when the veins were optimally filled. Coupled with small focal-spot tubes, venography became the major technique for detecting and assessing the effects of treatment of deep vein thrombosis that could be a source of pulmonary emboli.[54]

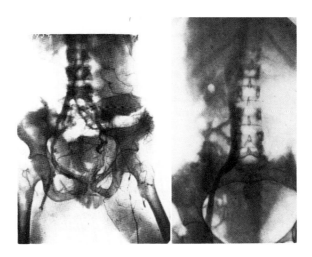

Left, Direct venography showing thrombosis of the left external iliac vein (1938). *Right,* Direct venography of a normal right iliac vein and inferior vena cava.[55]

References

1. Hascheck E and Lindenthal OT: A contribution to the practical use of the photography according to Röntgen. Wien Klin Wochenschr 9:63-64, 1896.
2. Grainger RG: Intravascular contrast media: the past, the present and the future. Brit J Radiol 55:1-18, 1982.
3. Lasser EC: Contrast media for urography. In Pollack HM (ed): Clinical urography. Philadelphia, WB Saunders, 1990.
4. Baum S: Catheters and injectors. In Abrams HL (ed): Vascular and interventional radiology. Boston, Little, Brown, 1983.
5. Thal AP, Lester RG, Richards LS, et al: Coronary arteriography in arteriosclerotic disease of the heart. Surg Gynec Obstet 105:457-464, 1957.
6. Gidlund A: Development of apparatus and methods for roentgen studies in haemodynamics. Acta Radiol (suppl) 130:1, 1956.
7. Amplatz K: A vascular injector with program selector. Radiology 75:955-956, 1960.
8. dos Santos R, Lamas A, and Pereira-Caldas J: Arteriografia da aorta e dos vasos abdominais. Med Contemp 47:93-97, 1929.
9. Lipchik EO and Rogoff SM: Abdominal aortography: Translumbar, femoral, and axillary artery catheterization techniques. In Abrams HL (ed): Vascular and interventional radiology. Boston, Little, Brown, 1983.
10. Nuvoli I: Arteriografia del'aorta toracica mediante punctura dell'aorta ascendente o del ventricolos. Policlinico (Prat) 43:227-237, 1936.
11. Saito M and Kamikawa K: A new modification for the injection method for arteriography (injection in refluence). Am J Surg 17:16-19, 1932.

12. Castellanos A and Pereiras R: Countercurrent aortography. Rev Cuba Cardiol 2:187-201, 1939.

13. Fariñas PL: A new technique for the arteriographic examination of the abdominal aorta and its branches. AJR 46:641-645, 1941.

14. Peirce EC: Percutaneous femoral artery catheterization in man with special reference to aortography. Surg Gynec Obstet 93:56-74, 1951.

15. Donald DC, Kesmodel KF, Rollins SL, and Paddison RM: An improved technic for percutaneous cerebral angiography. Arch Neurol Psych 14:508-510, 1951.

16. Seldinger SI: Catheter replacement of the needle in percutaneous arteriography: A new technique. Acta Radiol 39:368-376, 1953.

17. McGraw JY: Arteriography of peripheral vessels: A review with report of complications. Angiology 14:306-318, 1963.

18. Crawford ES, Beall AC, Moyer JH, and DeBakey ME: Complications of aortography. Surg Gynec Obstet 104:129-141, 1957.

19. Ziedses des Plantes BG: Application of the roentgenographic subtraction method in neuroradiology. Acta Radiol 1:961-966, 1963.

20. Sgalitzer M: Unterscheidung funktioneller und organischer Erkrankungen der Extremitatenarterien durch die Rontenuntersuchung. "Das Doppelinjektionsverfahren." Fortschr Rontgenstr 56:387-404, 1937.

21. Ratschow M: Leistung und Bedeutung der Vasographie als Funktionsprufung der peripheren Blutgenfasse. Fortschr Rontgenstr 55:253-266, 1937.

22. Bierman HR, Byron RL, Kelly KH, et al: Studies on the blood supply of tumors in man: Vascular patterns of the liver by hepatic arteriography. J Nat Cancer Inst 12:107-131, 1951.

23. Abrams HL, Boijsen E, and Borgstrom KE: Effect of epinephrine on renal circulation: Angiographic observations. Radiology 79:911-922, 1962.

24. Abrams HL: The response of neoplastic renal vessels to epinephrine in man. Radiology 82:217-224, 1964.

25. Novelline RA: Pharmacoangiography. In Athanasoulis CA, Pfister RC, Greene RE, and Roberson GH (eds): Interventional radiology. Philadelphia, WB Saunders, 1982.

26. Bron KM: Arterial portography. In Abrams HL (ed): Vascular and interventional radiology. Boston, Little, Brown, 1983.

27. Blakemore AH and Lord JW: Technique of using vitallium tubes in establishing portacaval shunts for portal hypertension. Ann Surg 122:476-480, 1945.

28. Abeatici S and Campi L: On the possibilities of hepatic angiography—visualization of the portal system (experimental studies). Acta Radiol 36:383-392, 1951.

29. Leger L: Portal phlebography by intraparenchymal splenic injection. Mem Acad Chir (Paris) 77:712, 1951.

30. Pollard JJ and Nebesar RA: Catheterization of the splenic artery for portal venography. N Engl J Med 271:234-237, 1964.

31. Rigler LG, Olfelt PC, and Krumbach RW: Roentgen hepatography by injection of a contrast medium into the aorta. Radiology 60:363-367, 1953.

32. Odman P: Percutaneous selective angiography of the coeliac artery. Acta Radiol (Suppl) 159, 1958.

33. Boijsen E, Eckman CA, and Olin T: Coeliac and superior mesenteric angiography in portal hypertension. Acta Chir Scand 126:315-325, 1963.

34. Steinberg I and Stein HL: Intravenous angiocardiography, abdominal aortography, and peripheral arteriography with single arm pressure injection. AJR 92:893-906, 1964.

35. Mistretta CA, Crummy AB, and Strother CM: Digital angiography: A perspective. Radiology 139:273-276, 1981.

36. Mistretta CA, Ort MG, Kelcz F, et al: Absorption edge fluoroscopy using quasimonoenergetic x-ray beams. Invest Radiol 8:402-412, 1973.

37. Strother CM, Sackett JF, Crummy AB, et al: Clinical applications of computerized fluoroscopy: The extracranial carotid arteries. Radiology 136:781-783, 1980.

38. Ovitt TW, Christenson PC, Fisher HD, et al: Intravenous angiography using digital video subtraction: X-ray imaging system. AJNR 1:387-390, 1980.

39. Foley WD and Milde MW: Intra-arterial digital subtraction angiography. Radiol Clin North Am 23:293-319, 1985.

40. Funaoka S, Tachikawa R, Yamaguchi O, and Fijita S: Kurze Mitteilung über die Roentgenographie des Lymphagefasssystems sowie über den Mechanismus der Symphströmung. Ab Dritten Abst Inst Kaiserlich und Univ Kyoto 1:11, 1930.

41. de Carvalho R, Rodrigues A, and Pereira S: La mise en évidence par la radiographie du système lymphatique chez le vivant. Annales d'Anatomie Pathologique 8:193-197, 1931.

42. Pfahler GG: A demonstration of a lymphatic drainage of the maxillary sinuses. AJR 27:352-356, 1931.

43. Clouse ME: History. In Clouse ME (ed): Clinical lymphography. Baltimore, Williams & Wilkins, 1977.

44. Teneff S and Stoppani F: A propos de la lymphographie. J Radiologie 20:74-77, 1936.

45. Servelle M: A propos de lymphographie expérimentale et clinique. J Radiologie 26:165-169, 1944.

46. Kinmonth JB: Lymphangiography in man: Method of outlining lymphatic trunks at operation. Clin Sci 11:13-20, 1952.

47. Kinmonth JB, Taylor GW, and Harper RK: Lymphangiography: A technique for its clinical use in the lower limb. Brit Med J 1:940-942, 1955.

48. Miller WE: Lymphography. In Witten DM, Myers GH, and Utz DC (eds): Clinical urography. Philadelphia, WB Saunders, 1977.

49. Wallace S, Jackson L, Schaffer B, et al: Lymphangiograms: Their diagnostic and therapeutic potential. Radiology 76:179-199, 1961.

50. Hreshchyshyn MM, Sheehan FR, and Holland JF: Visualization of retroperitoneal lymph nodes: Lymphangiography as an aid in the measurement of tumor growth. Cancer 14:205-209, 1961.

51. Lee JKT: Retroperitoneum. In Lee JKT, Sagel SS, and Stanley RJ (eds): Computed body tomography with MRI correlation. New York, Raven Press, 1989.

52. Berberich J and Hirsch S: Klin Wschr 2:2226, 1923.

53. McPheeters HO and Rice CO: Varicose veins. Surg Gynec Obstet 49:29-33, 1929.

54. Dodd H and Cockett FB: Pathology in surgery of the veins of the lower limb. New York, Churchill-Livingstone, 1976.

55. dos Santos JC: La phlébographe directe. J Int Surg 3:625-669, 1938.

CHAPTER 26

Ultrasound

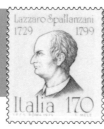

In contrast to the early acceptance and rapid application of x-rays to medical diagnosis, the development of diagnostic ultrasound has been comparatively slow and beset with technological difficulties. Progress has depended on the development of efficient ultrasound transducers, powerful amplifiers, and complex electronic display devices.[1]

In 1794, Spallanzani observed bats flying in the dark and successfully avoiding obstacles. He correctly assumed that they were guided by sound, rather than by light, and theorized that the sound produced by bats could not be perceived by the human ear.[2] Almost a century later (1880), Pierre and Jacques Curie discovered the piezoelectric effect, in which an electric charge is produced in response to the application of mechanical pressure on materials such as quartz and some ceramics. A year later, the Curie brothers showed that an oscillating electrical potential applied across a quartz crystal caused it to alternately contract and expand. This produced vibrations that were transmitted to the surrounding medium as sound waves, which could be recorded with appropriate devices. Thus was born the principle of ultrasonic transducers for both the generation and detection of ultrasound energy.[2]

Clinical ultrasound imaging had its origin in the wake of the Titanic disaster of 1912, when efforts began to develop a method for detecting undersea obstacles.[3] The first practical application was the effort by French physicist, Paul Langevin, and associates, who were commissioned by the French government in World War I to use high-frequency ultrasound in the detection of submerged enemy submarines. Extensive technical improvements on Langevin's original apparatus led to the development of the *SONAR* (*SO*und *N*avigation *A*nd *R*anging) system of underwater detection of objects developed by the United States Navy during World War II.

Between the wars, ultrasound waves were applied to medicine, as well as industry. Langevin's observation[4] that an ultrasound beam could destroy small fish that came in contact with it led to the use of high-intensity ultrasound for cancer treatment, especially in Germany. Elsewhere in Europe and in the United States, ultrasound was used in physical therapy because of a variety of suspected tonic, restorative, and balancing effects.

Medical practitioners focused on the therapeutic applications of ultrasound, whereas in industry the use of sound waves was "diagnostic" in nature—to detect flaws in materials and construction. In medical therapeutics, the generation of ultrasound waves was essential, but subsequent detection of these waves and retrieval of information played no role. In contrast, the detection of otherwise hidden flaws in industry (first suggested in 1928 by Soviet physicist, S.Y. Sokolov) required retrieval of information from the interaction of the ultrasound waves with the materials being examined. Flaw detection in industry was based on a "through transmission" technique. A transmitter on the opposite side of the material being tested recorded "shadows" produced as waves generated by another transducer passed through the material. During World War II, researchers in several countries investigated the application of pulsed reflective ultrasound for industrial purposes. In England, Donald Sproule (1941) developed a system in which a second nongenerating transducer detected returning echoes in the interval between generated pulses. In the United States, Floyd Firestone (1944)[5] patented the *Reflectoscope*, in which the same transducer picked up the echoes returning in the interval between generated pulses.

PIONEERS IN DIAGNOSTIC ULTRASOUND

As Barry Goldberg and Barbara Kimmelman noted in their extensive 1988 retrospective,

> In virtually all the early investigations involving diagnostic applications of ultrasound (1948–1958) direct contact and/or collaboration with military or industrial personnel and equipment facilitated the research. And, in each case, close collaboration between physicians and engineers produced technical applications of ultrasonic equipment with diagnostic applications in mind; in several cases, this collaboration led to fruitful commercial innovation.

Probably the first successful application of ultrasound to medical diagnosis was reported by the Austrian physician, Karl Dussik, and his physicist brother, Friederick.[6] During 1947-1948, the Dussiks introduced *hyperphonography*, a through-transmission technique that produced what they believed were *ventriculograms*, or echo pictures of the ventricles of the brain. Deformity of the normal shape and position of the ventricular system of the brain suggested the presence and location of an intracerebral mass lesion. However, 4 years later (1952), Guttner[7] in Germany showed that this technique actually did not image the ventricles at all but was merely showing variations in attenuation caused by the overlying skull.

In the United States, George Ludwig (1949),[8] at the Naval Military Research Institute, experimented with the detection of gallstones and foreign bodies embedded in tissues, using a method similar to the flaw detection approach. Ludwig[9] investigated fundamental problems in the

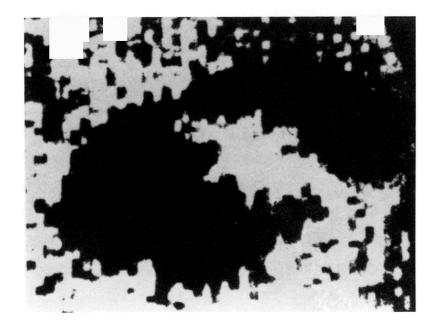

physical interaction of ultrasound waves and tissues with the intent of determining their characteristic acoustic properties. His findings concerning the velocity of ultrasound in various animal tissues served as standards for later investigators.

At the University of Minnesota, a transplanted Englishman, John J. Wild,[10] attempted to use ultrasound to measure the thickness of the intestinal wall in the diagnosis of acute crises of the bowel, his area of specialty. Wild showed that different echo patterns could be obtained from each of the different layers of his intestinal specimen. Of greater importance was the discovery that echoes from tumor-invaded tissue were distinguishable from those produced by normal tissue in the same piece of excised bowel. Wild also noted significant echo changes as the sound beam traversed areas approaching the tumor but in which neither the eye nor palpation had detected invasion by cancer. This suggested that ultrasound might not only detect differences between normal tissues and malignant lesions but that this modality might identify tumor-invaded tissue earlier than any detection technique then available.

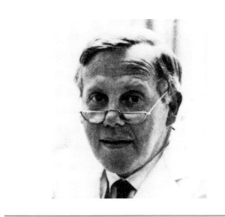

John J. Wild.[1]

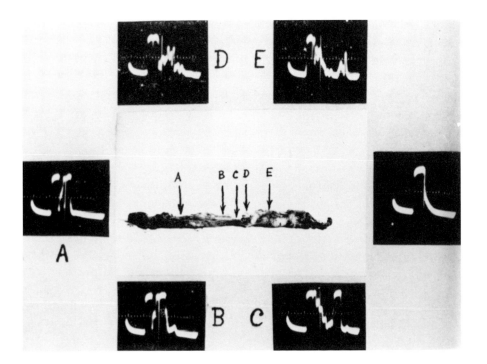

Results of experiments with a fresh strip of human stomach containing a carcinomatous ulcer (1950).[10] "*Top left*, Two strong signal returns from the normal stomach wall; *top middle*, tracing through the infiltrative area near the ulcer shows widening of the base-line interval, which indicates a denser tissue, since the thickness of the stomach wall at this point was approximately the same as top left; *top right*, further widening of the base-line interval. *Bottom left and right*, Sections through the everted edge of the tumor and through the tumor mass, respectively, show not only a still wider base-line interval but also many interface returns from within the tumor substance. (Tracing bottom right is the rubber membrane only.)"

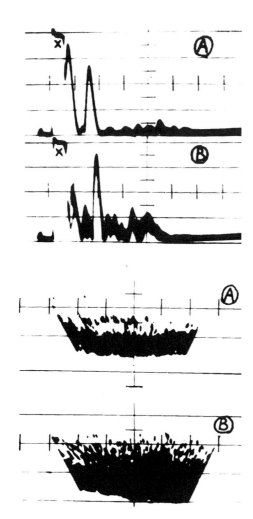

Early one-dimensional (*top*) scan of the breast (1952). *A*, Normal scan, and *B*, sarcoma of the breast. Two-dimensional scan (*bottom*) of normal breast (*A*) and sarcoma of the breast (*B*) (1952).[13]

In collaboration with engineer John M. Reid, Wild[11] developed a two-dimensional B-mode scanning system. For breast scanning, Wild introduced the first hand-held "contact" scanner, a sloping plastic chamber with its smaller end covered with a rubber diaphragm that was applied directly over the breast. Sonic contact was achieved by the use of an aqueous jelly, in contrast to the immersion bath or enclosed water tanks employed by other pioneers of contact scanning. The transducer was moved back and forth to produce ultrasound echoes in real time, which permitted rapid generation and interpretation of clinical information. Using this device, Wild and Reid[12] reported a 90% accuracy in the diagnosis of benign versus malignant lesions. Wild also developed both rigid and flexible probes for transrectal and transvaginal scanning.

Wild's most significant insight was the recognition that malignant tissue might be distinguished from nonmalignant tissue by means of their echo patterns, a problem that has intrigued subsequent investigators. By calculating the area under their A-mode displays, Wild and Reid found that malignant tissue seemed consistently more echoic than normal tissue and nonmalignant tumors.

In Colorado, Douglass Howry (in collaboration with engineer Roderic Bliss) began investigating the idea that ultrasound beams directed into the body would be reflected from tissue interfaces. Their system was constructed from surplus Navy sonar equipment, a radar amplifier, a Heathkit oscilloscope, and a high-fidelity recorder power supply. Scans were made with the transducer immersed in water, which permitted transmission of the sound waves to the object being examined. Initially, a laundry tub was used for this purpose. Later they used a metal cattle watering trough with the transducer running along hardwood rails attached to the side of the tank.

Demonstration of foreign bodies by ultrasound (1952). *Top*, A nail, plastic rod, and matchstick have been embedded deeply into a block of liver to demonstrate the ability of the ultrasonic unit to reveal foreign bodies in tissue. *Bottom*, The strong signals from the foreign bodies are well seen within the liver tissue. The rear surface of the liver was shown by placing a flat cork sheet against it to increase the amplitude of the signal for identification purposes.[16]

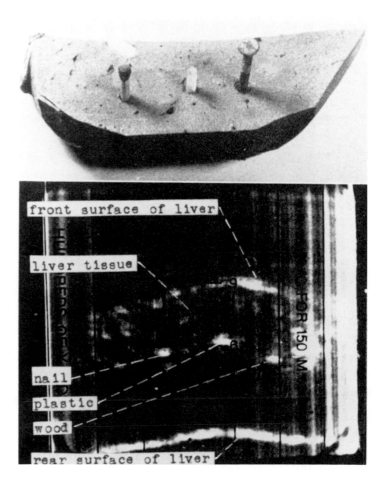

In a later version (1954), the scanning tank was the rotating ring gear from a B-29 gun turret.[15] The transducer carriage was mounted on a metal ring, immersed in water, and rotated 360 degrees around the tank. During rotation of the carriage around the tank, the 2½-inch focused transducer moved back and forth across the carriage in a 4-inch linear scan. The combined linear and circular motions of this "Somascope" produced a compound scan in a plane of cross-section parallel to the surface of the water. The patient under examination sat in the tank holding lead weights to maintain his position. The echoes received were displayed as intensity-modulated dots in their appropriate orientation on the large screen and photographed by the camera mounted above it. A long persistent phosphor screen was used and provided a form of gray scale to record variations in echo intensity.[1]

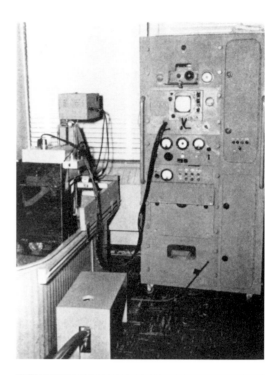

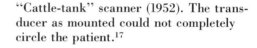

"Cattle-tank" scanner (1952). The transducer as mounted could not completely circle the patient.[17]

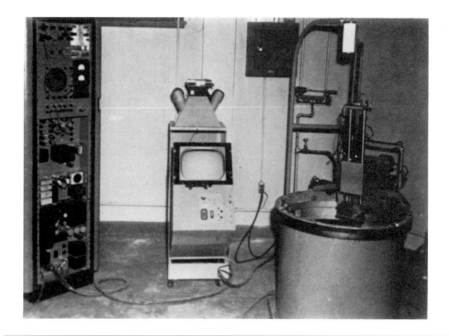

B-29 gun turret water-bath scanner (1954).[17]

Scanning positions for patients in the fluid-filled B-29 gun turret scanner (1954). *Left*, For a transverse cross-section of the neck, the 2½-inch focus transducer is seen just below the water level. The transducer carriage travelled around the tank on the outside track.[1] *Right*, Examination of the leg obtained with the subject standing in the scanner.[14]

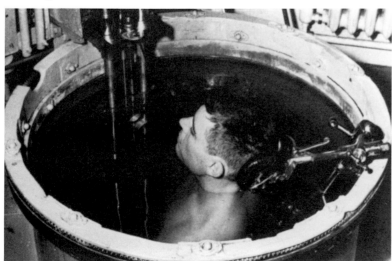

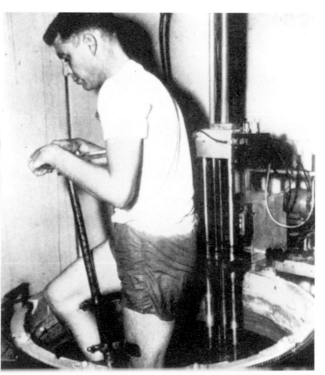

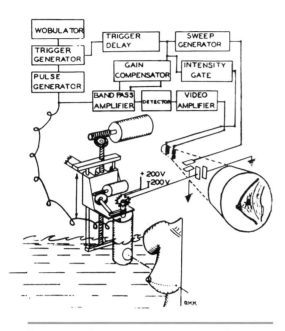

Diagram of cross-section somagraphy (1955).[18]

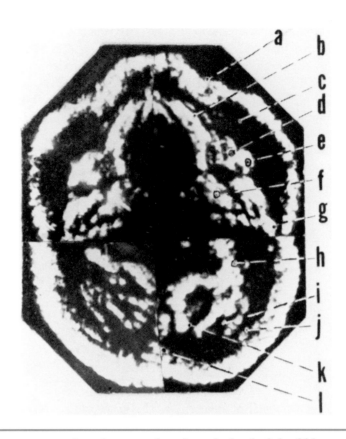

Somagram cross-section of a normal neck at the level of the fifth cervical vertebra (1955). *a*, Skin surface; *b*, trachea; *c*, sternocleidomastoid muscle; *d*, carotid artery; *e*, internal jugular vein; *f*, vertebral vessels; *g*, fascia colli lateralis; *h*, transverse process of fifth cervical vertebra; *i*, splenius capitis muscle; *j*, trapezius muscle; *k*, spinous process; *l*, ligamentum nuchae.[18]

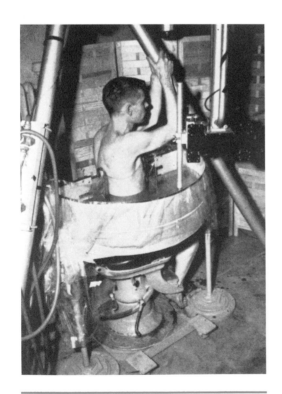

"Pan scanner" (1957-58). The patient is seated on a modified dental chair strapped against the plastic window of a semicircular pan filled with a saline solution. The transducer rotated through the solution in a semicircular arc around the patient.[19]

Although excellent results were obtained with this circular water-path scanner, seriously ill patients could not be examined and the need to keep the anatomical area of interest under water made this technique too cumbersome for routine clinical use. These difficulties were partly circumvented by construction of a modified water-path scanner ("pan scanner"), using a semicircular tank with a rectangular window cut into its flat surface. The tank was lined with heavy plastic and the patient positioned against the plastic in a sitting position. A modified dental chair was used that could be easily raised or lowered to obtain serial cross-sections at multiple levels. The transducer carriage was suspended from an overhead tripod and rotated through a 140-degree path.[1] Using mineral oil as a coupling agent, reasonably good images were obtained for the breast and such abdominal and pelvic organs as the liver, spleen, kidneys, and bladder. Nevertheless, this system still was cumbersome for use on very sick patients and pregnant women. Therefore Howry and co-workers began construction of a compound contact scanner. The instrument, completed in 1962, employed a scanning carriage suspended from an overhead framework. The transducer, mounted within the scanning head, was capable of continuous contact with the patient's body surface and could pivot at any point within the cross-sectional plane of the scan. The scanning arm used a system of pulleys and potentiometers to translate the vertical and horizontal positions of the transducer, as well as the angle of the ultrasound beam at any point in space. This permitted free movement of the transducer in one continuous sweep over the abdomen, recording echoes from any point within the body.[20]

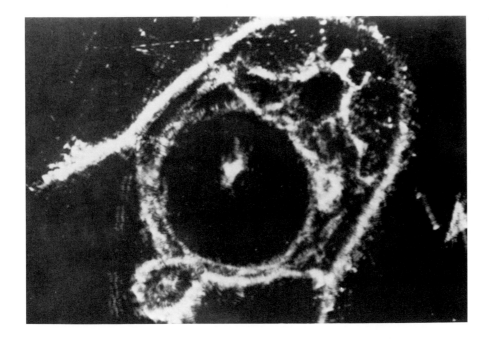

Transverse cross-section of a dog urinary bladder (c. 1960). The circular structure is the distended urinary bladder, while the flank folds and penis are at the bottom. The group of echoes within the bladder arises from an intravesical catheter.[1]

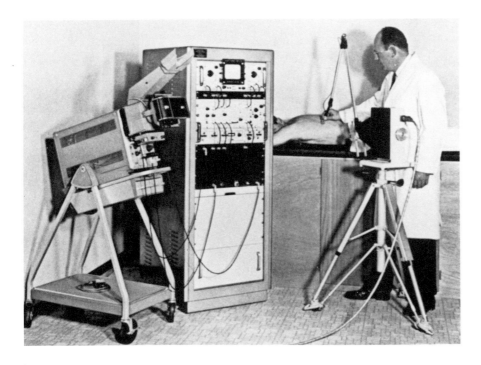

First commercial ultrasonic scanner manufactured in the United States of America. The pivot-arm scanner is mounted on a tripod at the right. The electronics and display oscilloscope are in the rack and cart at the left.[1]

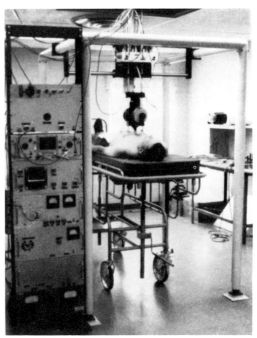

First compound contact scanner developed at the University of Colorado (1960-1962). The electronics and display oscilloscopes are in the rack at the left.[1]

Howry initially worked (as did John Wild) in his own basement. Later, he joined forces with Joseph Holmes, who was Acting Director of the Medical Research Laboratory of the Veterans Administration Hospital where Howry was a resident. Holmes served as a liaison between Howry and the institutional support needed so badly if the project was to gain financial support and proceed further.

Using different approaches, the Howry-Holmes and Wild-Reid groups provided invaluable contributions to the development of diagnostic ultrasound. The commitment of Howry and co-workers to cross-sectional imaging has remained the center of diagnostic ultrasound. Wild's emphasis on differentiation between benign and malignant tissue ("tissue characterization") remains the ultimate goal of this imaging modality. In addition, their real-time concept has replaced compound scanning as the basis of current ultrasound diagnosis.

ECHOENCEPHALOGRAPHY

After the Dussik brothers' hyperphonography using transmitted ultrasound was shown to be ineffective, French, Wild, and Neal (1950)[21] extended their investigation of echo patterns using pulsed-echo technique from the breast and abdomen to the brain. As in their previous studies, they showed that the echo pattern of a tumor in a freshly excised brain was indeed different from adjacent normal brain. In addition, a second unexpected tumor within the brain was identified and later verified. After trials with experimental animals indicated the safety of the method, a hand-held transducer was applied directly to a human brain after removal of part of the skull during surgery. Again, echoes from the area over the already diagnosed malignancy were more numerous and stronger than echoes from adjacent normal brain tissue.

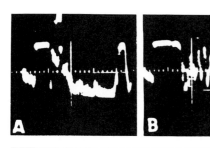

Echoencephalography (1951). *Left*, Normal cerebral tissue. *Right*, Neoplastic tissue (glioblastoma multiforme).[21]

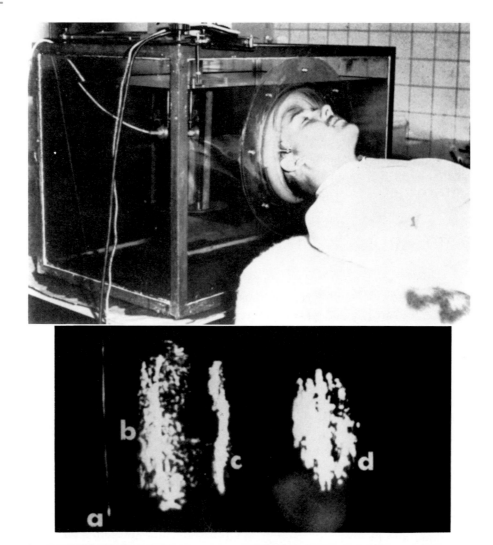

Two-dimensional echoencephalography (1963). *Top*, Arrangement for immergent scanning in a tank with water. *Bottom*, Echoencephalogram of a patient with hydrocephalus. *a*, Skull; *b*, lateral wall of ventricle; *c*, medial wall of ventricle and midline structures; *d*, skull.[23]

Nevertheless, it was still impossible to obtain clinically useful ultrasound images through the *intact* skull. In 1953, Lars Leksell[22] of Sweden was asked to help solve the clinical dilemma of a 16-month-old infant in a coma. Using borrowed flaw-detection equipment, Leksell demonstrated the midline echo and showed that a shift of position in the echo was diagnostic evidence of an intracranial mass, in this case a life-threatening hematoma. Later he was able to diagnose intracranial pathology following head trauma in four children by demonstrating a shift of the midline echoes. Leksell was more successful than other early investigators because many of his initial subjects were children, who had thinner skulls less likely to scatter the ultrasound waves. In addition, he used a lower-frequency transducer that permitted deeper penetration with less scattering.

Also in Sweden, Marinus de Vlieger (1963)[23] introduced two-dimensional echoencephalography. He recognized that reflection and absorption of ultrasound by the adult skull seriously interfered with the acquisition of informative echoes from within the brain. Accordingly, like Leksell, he did much of his research and clinical work on infants and young children.

Despite the clinical success of midline echoencephalography, ultrasonic imaging of the brain itself remained a challenge. In Canada, David Makow and D.N. White attempted to solve the problem by constructing a compound B-mode machine that included water bath coupling and two transducers scanning simultaneously from either side of the head.

Although the advent of new techniques such as computed tomography (CT) and magnetic resonance (MR) imaging has diminished the importance of echoencephalography, it is still used today in evaluating the surgically exposed brain and spinal cord. However, the major value of this technique is in neonates and young children with open fontanels, which permit good demonstration of intracranial pathology without the detrimental effect of overlying skull.

ECHOCARDIOGRAPHY

The collaboration of physician Inge Edler and physicist C. Hellmuth Hertz[25] launched clinical echocardiography using the pulse-echo technique. As a cardiologist, Edler was interested in noninvasive diagnostic techniques, especially for the evaluation of mitral valve disease. Following a chance meeting at lunch in 1953, Hertz suggested to Edler (after Edler's speculations concerning radar) that ultrasonic pulses might provide a means for obtaining the desired information. They borrowed an ultrasound flaw detector from a local shipyard and used it to demonstrate echoes from the moving heart. Using a B-mode scanner, Edler and Hertz developed the M-mode technique, in which the echo information was projected as a bright dot on the oscilloscope screen. The dot would move as the echo from the moving structure shifted position. Employing a continuous moving film and special camera, they displayed in wave form the motion of the echo dot reflected from the intracardiac structures. By 1955, Edler[26] reported the ability to diagnose mitral stenosis, left atrial thrombus, and pericardiac effusion. The development of barium titanate transducers permitted recording of not only stenotic mitral valve motion but also the more rapid motion of the normal mitral leaflet. By using needles at the autopsy table, Edler and co-workers[27] demonstrated the anatomical source of the cardiac echo patterns.

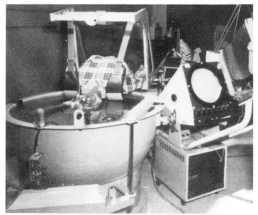

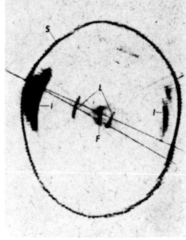

Symmetric immergent ultrasound scanning of the head (1968). *Top*, The patient's head is immersed in the water to the level of the eyebrows and ears. Two transducers scan the head symmetrically in two semicircles. A true-scale sonechogram of a head section is being formed on the cathode-ray screen and is photographed on medical x-ray film by the camera above. *Bottom*, Horizontal scan shows distorted lateral ventricles from two tumors, one in the left and one in the right half of the brain, but in different locations. *F*, Falx; *L*, lateral ventricles; *I*, brain-bone interface; *S*, compressed hair- or scalp-water interface.[24]

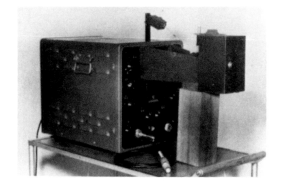

Ultrasonic flaw detector adapted for use as an M-mode echocardiograph with home-built camera attached (1954).[25]

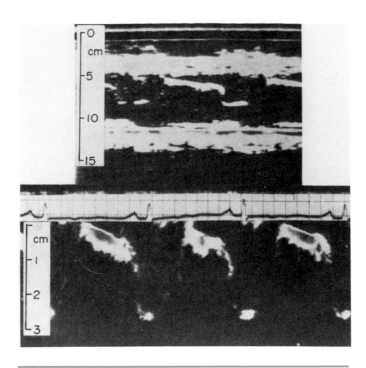

First successful recording of mitral valve motion in a case of mitral stenosis (1955).[26]

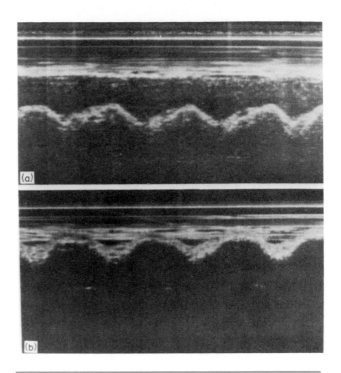

Early recording of pericardial effusion (1954). *Left*, Before and (*right*) after pericardial puncture.[28]

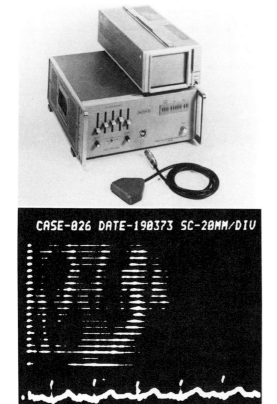

Two-dimensional echocardiography (1973). *Top*, Prototype equipment including multiscan cabinet, display monitor, and transducer. *Bottom*, Multiscan echocardiogram frame of a sagittal cross-section of the heart. Patient identification data are printed at the top, and the electrocardiogram is recorded at the bottom of the frame. Anterior chest wall echoes are to the left, and the bright dots to the left indicate the transducer position.[32]

In the United States, cardiologist Claude Joyner and engineer John Reid[29] succeeded in displaying both the electrocardiogram and echocardiogram simultaneously. Joyner confirmed the diagnosis of mitral valvular disease based on ultrasound echoes, identified the tricuspid valve, and began clinical treatments based on the echocardiogram. Harvey Feigenbaum (1965)[30] emphasized the role of ultrasound as a valuable and relatively simple technique for demonstrating pericardial effusion. He greatly stimulated interest in ultrasound among cardiologists and developed courses and provided training fellowships in echocardiography at Indiana University.

The use of contrast media in echocardiographic diagnosis was pioneered by Ray Gramiak.[31] In the mid-1960s, a central problem in echocardiography was the accurate identification of echoes from the various cardiac structures. In 1968, Gramiak and associates introduced the intracardiac injection of indocyanine green dye to aid in the echographic recognition of the aortic root and aortic valve. The microbubbles formed by cavitation at the needle's tip provided a strongly echoic contrast medium, and the location of the imaged cardiac structures could be directly correlated with the site of injection.

The development of two-dimensional imaging in the late 1960s and early 1970s led to more widespread clinical acceptance and application of echocardiography. Major researchers in the development of this approach included Donald King and F.L. Thurstone in the United States and Nicolaas Bom in the Netherlands.

DOPPLER ULTRASOUND

In 1842, Johann Christian Doppler, an Austrian physicist and mathematician, noticed that when a source of wave motion itself moved, the apparent frequency of the emitted waves changed. Other scientists later demonstrated the Doppler effect for both sound waves and electromagnetic waves.

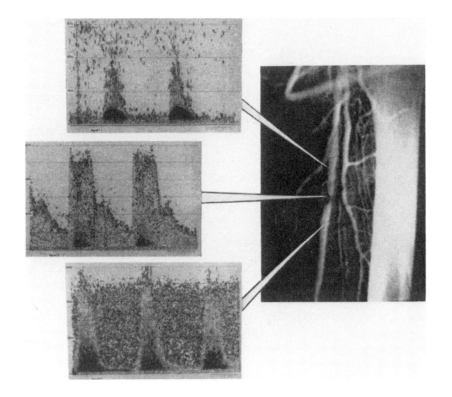

The earliest work in Doppler ultrasound dates back to the 1950s, when Shigeo Satomura and Yasuharu Nimura in Japan pioneered its application to cardiovascular investigation. In 1955, they and other colleagues in Osaka began their studies of the motions of the human heart with Doppler ultrasound.[33] Within 5 years, the group had detected motion of the mitral, aortic, and pulmonary valves.

In the United States, the major work in Doppler ultrasound took place at the University of Washington, where D. Eugene Strandness[34] began clinical trials using continuous-wave Doppler around 1964. Within 3 years, Strandness published spectrographic analysis of normal and abnormal wave profiles of the peripheral vascular system, an initial step toward assigning particular wave forms to specific diseases.

However, continuous-wave Doppler could not separate arteries or distinguish moving structures from one another. With the arrival of Reid, work on pulsed Doppler equipment began. The Seattle group was primarily interested in Doppler identification and measurement of blood flow. Later, actual Doppler imaging was introduced, and color Doppler was developed to graphically distinguish between flow toward and away from the detector.

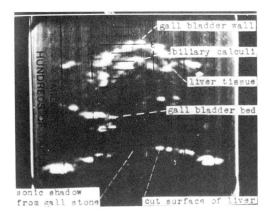

Early ultrasound studies on a pathologic gallbladder (1952). Cross-section of a thick, fibrotic, contracted gallbladder containing numerous large faceted and small gravellike calculi. The thick fibrous wall of the gallbladder is well seen. Inside the gallbladder, strong echoes from the large faceted stones and gravel appear. The broken line of the gallbladder bed and the cut surface of the liver is the result of the areas of sonic shadow produced by the highly reflecting calculi.[16]

OBSTETRICAL ULTRASOUND

A thorough discussion of the use of ultrasound in obstetrics and gynecology can be found in Chapter 19.

EARLY ABDOMINAL APPLICATIONS

The first attempts to use ultrasound in the diagnosis of intraabdominal conditions were made by George Ludwig, who in the late 1940s and late 1950s used a unidimensional technique to detect gallstones and other foreign bodies that had been embedded in the muscles of dogs.[8] Using

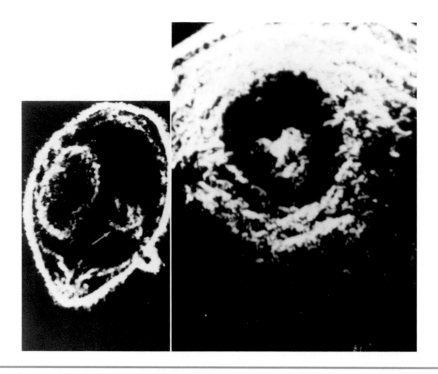

Early clinical applications of ultrasound to imaging abdominal structures. *Left*, Transverse cross-section of a cat liver following creation of an hepatic abscess (*arrow*).[19] *Right*, Transverse cross-section of a kidney. The skin surface is at the top. The renal cortex appears echo-free. Central echoes arise from the vessels and collecting system.[1]

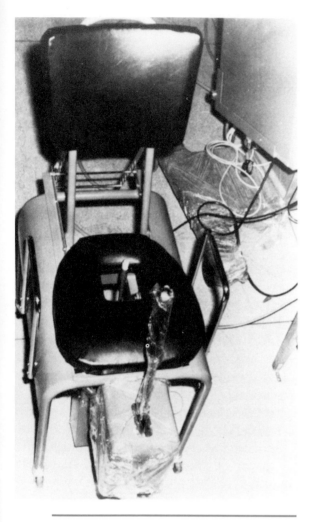

Transrectal ultrasonography (1974). A transducer with the attached scanner is pushed up through a hole in the chair.[35]

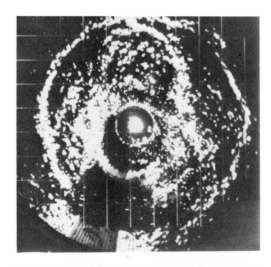

Early prostatic sonogram (1974). Advanced prostatic cancer. The cancer infiltration can be localized.[35]

their "Somascope," Howry and Bliss succeeded in demonstrating gallstones within a freshly excised gallbladder.[16] This demonstration suggested that it might some day be possible to visualized even the deep-lying organs such as the kidney, liver, and spleen in the living subject. Using their pan scanner and cross-sectional techniques, by the late 1950s the Denver group was producing scans of abdominal organs through the abdominal wall.

In China, Chou Yung Chang attempted to break up ureteral calculi with ultrasound beams. Although the therapy proved ineffective, during clinical trials Chou noted that the beams seemed able to detect space-occupying lesions in the liver and kidney.

In the 1960s, the clinical application of ultrasound to imaging abdominal structures and assessing abdominal diseases expanded rapidly. In addition to the University of Colorado team, major research efforts were undertaken by Hans Holm in Copenhagen, R. Uchida and Hiroki Watanabe in Japan, J. Stauffer Lehman and Barry Goldberg in Philadelphia, George Leopold in Pittsburgh (later San Diego), and Atis Freimanis in Columbus.

Transrectal and transvaginal scanning offered an opportunity to insert an ultrasound probe close to deep-lying abdominal structures. The first transducer probes for entry into the body rectally and vaginally were designed by Wild in the early 1950s. In the mid 1970s, Watanabe and associates[35] developed the "ultrasonic chair." The patient sat on the chair, through the seat of which protruded a thin rigid probe equipped with an ultrasonic transducer that passed through the anus and entered the rectum. Scans of the prostate and bladder were made that were of particular value in the diagnosis of prostatic cancer. Martin Resnick soon developed another transrectal probe for prostatic cancer that could be inserted with the patient in the lithotomy position. Initially providing only B-mode imaging, later versions added gray scale.

OPHTHALMOLOGICAL APPLICATIONS

The major development of two-dimensional imaging of the eye and orbit was by Gilbert Baum of New York. Although Mundt and Hughes (1956)[36] had published the initial account of the use of an industrial unidimensional A-mode technique for recording echoes from an intraocular neoplasm, Baum was the first to produce a graphic cross-sectional image. Working with engineer Ivan Greenwood, Baum constructed a sophisticated scanning apparatus using a water-path coupling system. The patient placed his face in a swimmer's mask built into the side of a saline-filled plastic tank. The 15-MHz transducer, positioned in front of the eye, oscillated through approximately a 30-degree sector scan in a horizontal or transverse plane. The higher frequencies permitted greater resolution in an area in which low frequencies were of no advantage, since absorption and scattering by bone and intervening structures were not a problem. With this apparatus, Baum[37] was able to produce the first cross-sectional ultrasound images of the eye showing retinal detachment, intraocular tumors, and foreign bodies. Later, he reported the first ultrasound demonstration of orbital tumors and foreign bodies.[38]

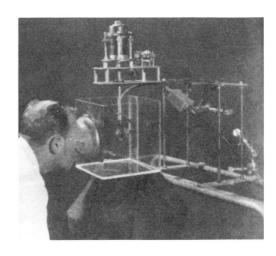

Early apparatus for ophthalmic imaging with ultrasound (1958).[37]

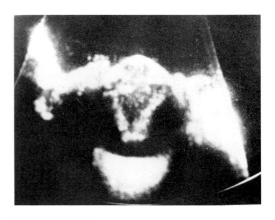

Echogram of the right eye in a patient with haziness of the cornea and hyphema (1960).

LATER DEVELOPMENTS

As contact compound B-mode scanning was refined during the 1960s, sonography became recognized as the primary imaging modality in obstetrics, and echocardiography was acknowledged to be important for detecting abnormal cardiac conditions. In addition, sonography was considered an adjunctive diagnostic technique in the abdomen. However, long scanning times of several seconds led to a loss of spatial resolution because of motion. In addition, sonography was more an art than a science, since the quality of the image depended as much on the skill of the operator as on the sophistication of the equipment. Technologists who could consistently obtain decent images were difficult to find. Consequently, image quality often varied widely from examination to examination and among institutions. Furthermore, the persistence oscilloscopes available provided little gray-scale information, and the resulting ultrasonic images were termed *bistable*, since each part of the image was either black or white. In the early 1970s, analog and then digital scan converters were introduced. These devices could record and display gray-scale information, thus leading to significant improvements in the ability of ultrasonic images to reveal subtle differences among tissues. The scan converter greatly improved the clinical usefulness of ultrasonic imaging, especially for obstetrical and abdominal applications.[3]

The time required to compile the data for an ultrasonic image was determined primarily by the need to move the transducer across the patient's body in a series of complex motions. Two ways were developed for reducing the imaging time. One involved replacement of manual motion by mechanically controlled, automated motion of the transducer. The resulting mechanical sector scanners produced "real-time" ultrasonic images. The other approach was the use of multiple transducers operated as a linear or phased array. These systems also became avail-

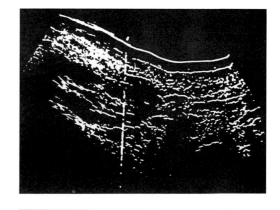

Early bistable scan of the kidney.

able in the late 1970s and have proved especially popular for obstetrical and cardiac imaging. With these developments, real-time ultrasound scanning has become a reality, and static B-mode scanners have gradually been replaced by real-time units over the past decade. This replacement partially automated the scanning process and reduced the dependence of image quality on the skill of the operator.

Bibliography

Goldberg BB and Kimmelman BA: Medical diagnostic ultrasound: A retrospective on its 40th anniversary. Eastman Kodak Company, 1988.

References

1. Holmes JH: Diagnostic ultrasound: Historical perspective. In King DL (ed): Diagnostic ultrasound. St. Louis, CV Mosby, 1974.

2. Azimi F, Bryan PJ, and Marangola JP: Ultrasonography in obstetrics and gynecology: Historical notes, basic principles, safety considerations, and clinical applications. CRC Crit Rev Clin Radiol Nucl Med 8:153-253, 1976.

3. Rosenfield AT, Rigsby CM, Burns PN, and Romero R: Ultrasonography of the urinary tract. In Pollack HM (ed): Clinical urography, Philadelphia, WB Saunders, 1990.

4. Wood W and Loomis AL: The physical and biological effects of high-frequency sound waves of great intensity. Phys Rev 29:373, 1927.

5. Firestone FA: The supersonic reflectoscope for interior inspection. Metal Progress 48:505, 1945.

6. Dussik KT, Dussik F, and Wyt L: Auf dem Wege zur Hyperphonographie des Gehirns. Wien Med Wochenschr 97:425, 1947.

7. Guettner W, Von Fiedleg G, and Patzold J: Über Ultraschallabbildungen am menschlichen Schädel. Acustica 2:148, 1952.

8. Ludwig GD and Struthers FW: Considerations underlying the use of ultrasound to detect gallstones and foreign bodies in tissues. Naval Med Res Inst Reports, Project #004 001, Reports No. 4 (June 1949).

9. Ludwig GD: The velocity of sound through tissues and the acoustic impedance of tissues. J Acoust Soc Am 22:862, 1950.

10. Wild JJ: The use of ultrasonic pulses for the measurement of biologic tissues and the detection of tissue density changes. Surgery 27:183-188, 1950.

11. Wild JJ and Reid JM: Application of echoranging techniques to the determination of structure of biological tissues. Science 115:226-230, 1952.

12. Wild JJ and Reid JM: Diagnostic use of ultrasound. Br J Phys Med 19:248-257, 1956.

13. Wild JJ and Reid JM: Echographic studies on tumors of the breast. Am J Path 28:839-861, 1952.

14. Holmes JH: Early applications of ultrasound in study of kidney and bladder. In Watanabe H, Holmes JH, Holm HH, and Goldberg BB (eds): Diagnostic ultrasound in urology and nephrology. Tokyo, Igako-Shoin, 1981.

15. Howry DH, Stott DA, and Bliss WR: The ultrasonic visualization of carcinoma of the breast and other soft tissue structures. Cancer 7:354-358, 1954.

16. Howry D and Bliss WR: Ultrasonic visualization of soft tissue structures of the body. J Lab Clin Med 40:579-592, 1952.

17. Howry DH: A brief atlas of diagnostic ultrasonic radiologic results. Radiol Clin North Am 3:433-452, 1965.

18. Howry DH, Holmes JH, Cushman CR, et al: Ultrasonic visualization of living organs and tissues. Geriatrics 10:123-128, 1955.

19. Holmes JH and Howry DH: Ultrasonic diagnosis of abdominal disease. Am J Dig Dis 8:12-32, 1963.

20. Holmes JH, et al: Ultrasonic contact scanner for diagnostic application. Am J Med Electron 4:147-152, 1965.

21. French LA, Wild JJ, and Neal D: The experimental application of ultrasonics to the localization of brain tumors. Preliminary report. J Neurosurg 8:198-203, 1951.

22. Leksell L: Echoencephalography: Detection of intracranial complications following head injury. Acta Chir Scand 110:301-315, 1955-1956.

23. de Vlieger M: Ultrasound for two-dimensional echoencephalography. Ultrasonics 1:148-151, 1963.

24. Makow DM and McRae DL: Symmetrical scanning of the head with ultrasound using water coupling. J Acoust Soc Am 44:1346-1352, 1968.

25. Edler I and Hertz CH: The use of ultrasonic reflectoscope for the continuous recording of movements of heart walls. Kungl Fysiogr Sallsk i Lund Forhandl 24:1-19, 1954.

26. Edler I: The diagnostic use of ultrasound in heart disease. Acta Med Scand, Suppl 308, 32-36, 1955.

27. Edler I: Ultrasound cardiography. Acta Med Scand, Suppl 370, 1961.

28. Hertz CH: The interaction of physicians, physicists and industry in the development of echocardiography. Ultrasound Med Biol 1:3-11, 1973.

29. Joyner CR, Hey ED, Johnson J, and Reid JM: Reflected ultrasound in the diagnosis of tricuspid stenosis. Am J Cardiol 19:66-73, 1967.

30. Feigenbaum H, Waldhausen JA, and Hyde JP: Use of ultrasound in the diagnosis of pericardial effusion. JAMA 191:711-714, 1965.

31. Gramiak R and Shah PM: Echocardiography of the aortic root. Invest Radiol 3:356, 1968.

32. Bom N, Lancee CT, Van Zwieten G, et al: Multiscan echocardiography. Circulation 48:1066-1074, 1973.

33. Satomura S: Ultrasonic Doppler method for the inspection of cardiac functions. J Acoust Soc Am 29:1181, 1957.

34. Strandness DE, Schultz RD, Sumner DS, and Rushmer RF: Ultrasonic flow detection: A useful technique in the evaluation of peripheral vascular disease. Am J Surg 113:311-320, 1967.

35. Watanabe H, Ingari D, Tanahashi Y, et al: Development and application of new equipment for transrectal ultrasonography. J Clin Ultrasound 2:91-98, 1974.

36. Mundt GH and Hughes WF: Ultrasonics in ocular disease. Am J Ophthal 41:488-498, 1956.

37. Baum G and Greenwood I: The application of ultrasonic locating techniques to ophthalmology. Arch Ophthal 60:263-279, 1958.

38. Baum G and Greenwood I: Ultrasonography: An aid in orbital tumor diagnosis. Arch Ophthal 64:180-194, 1960.

CHAPTER 27

Computed Tomography

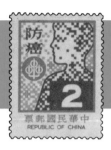
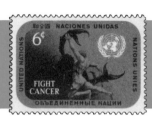
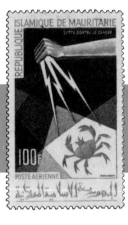

Computed tomography (CT) was first introduced in 1972 by Godfrey Hounsfield of EMI Limited in London. As Hounsfield[1] noted in his 1979 Nobel Prize lecture:

When we consider the capabilities of conventional x-ray methods, three main limitations become obvious. First, it is impossible to display within the framework of a two dimensional x-ray picture all the information contained in the three-dimensional scene under view. Objects situated in depth, i.e., in the third dimension, super-impose, causing confusion to the viewer.

Second, conventional x-rays cannot distinguish between soft tissues. In general, the radiograph differentiates only between bone and air, as in the lungs. Variations in soft tissues such as the liver and pancreas are not discernible at all, and certain other organs may be rendered visible only through the use of radio-opaque dyes.

Third, when conventional x-ray methods are used, it is not possible to measure in a quantitative way the separate densities of the individual substances through which the x-rays pass. The radiograph records the *mean* absorption by all the various tissues which the x-ray has penetrated. This is of little use for quantitative measurement.

Computed tomography, on the other hand, measures the attenuation of x-ray beams passing through sections of the body from hundreds of different angles, and then, from the evidence of these measurements, a computer is able to reconstruct pictures of the body's interior.

Pictures are based on the separate examination of a series of contiguous cross sections, as though we looked at the body separated into a series of thin "slices." By doing so, we virtually obtained total three-dimensional information about the body.

However, the technique's most important feature is its enormously greater sensitivity. It allows soft tissue such as the liver and kidneys to be clearly differentiated, which radiographs cannot do . . . It can also very accurately measure the values of x-ray absorption of tissues, thus enabling the nature of tissue to be studied.

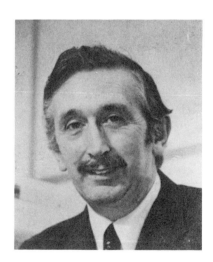

Godfrey Hounsfield (1919-   ).

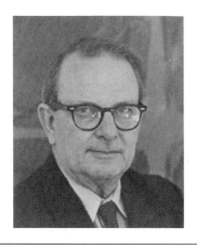

Allen M. Cormack.

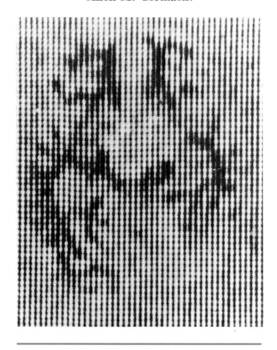

Picture of the first brain scanned on the laboratory CT machine.[1]

The principle of CT evolved from the work of an Austrian mathematician, Radon, who demonstrated in 1917 that the image of a three-dimensional object could be reconstructed from an infinite number of two-dimensional projections of the object.[2] Rather than applying this concept to medical images, Radon was working with equations that described gravitational fields. In the 1950s and 1960s, Radon's mathematics, modified for a finite number of projections, were applied to several imaging problems such as solar astronomy, electron microscopy, and holographic interferometry. In 1961, Oldendorf explored the potential of producing images from transmission projections produced with gamma rays from an iodine-131 source. He constructed a scintillation detector to measure the intensity of radiation transmitted through an object rotating between the source and the detector.

In the 1950s, Allen M. Cormack of Capetown, South Africa, became interested in the changes in radiation therapy dose distributions caused by inhomogeneous regions of the body. He realized that these changes could be predicted if the distribution of attenuation coefficients, which could be displayed as a gray-scale image, were known across the body region of interest. In 1964, Cormack[3] (who shared the Nobel Prize with Hounsfield) published his first experimental results in which the attenuation coefficients of a slice of an object were reconstructed from a series of angular projections obtained at 7½-degree increments. However, his publication received little attention at that time.[4]

As Hounsfield[1] recalled some time later:

I investigated the possibility that a computer might be able to reconstruct a picture from sets of very accurate x-ray measurements taken through the body at a multitude of different angles. Many hundreds of thousands of measurements would have to be taken, and reconstructing a picture from them seemed to be a mammoth task as it appeared at the time that it would require an equal number of many hundreds of thousands of simultaneous equations to be solved. When I investigated the advantages over the conventional x-ray techniques, however, it became apparent that conventional methods were not making full use of all the information the x-rays could give. On the other hand, calculations showed that the new system used the data very efficiently and would be two orders of magnitude more sensitive than conventional x-rays.

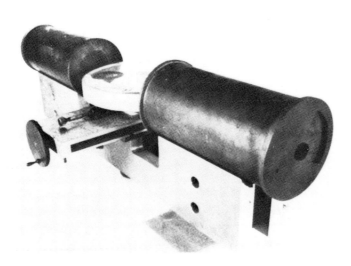

CT scanner of 1963 vintage, cost approximately $100.[4]

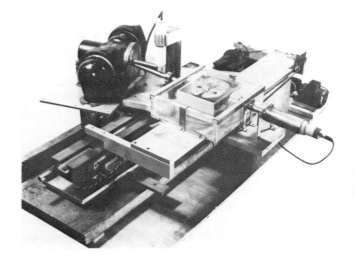

Original laboratory CT scanner (1968) showing the x-ray tube and detector on a lathe bed with a preserved section of the human brain in between.[1]

In Hounsfield's initial experiments using a gamma-ray source, it took 9 days to acquire the data (about 28,000 measurements) and 2.5 hours to reconstruct the image on a large main-frame computer. Replacing the gamma-ray source with an x-ray tube reduced the scanning time to 9 hours. The x-ray tube and detector were mounted on a lathe bed with a preserved section of human brain in between. At the end of a translational stroke, the brain specimen was rotated 1 degree, and the translational stroke of the x-ray tube and detector repeated. With this apparatus, Hounsfield was able to differentiate gray and white matter on the preserved specimen.[5]

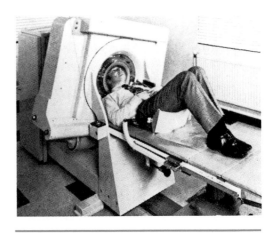

First clinical prototype EMI brain scanner installed at Atkinson Morley's Hospital, London. Note the water bag surrounding the patient's head.[1]

The first clinical prototype EMI head scanner (Mark I) was installed in early 1972 at Atkinson Morley's Hospital, London.[6] It proved to be an immediate success, and an improved version was introduced at that year's meeting of the Radiological Society of North America. The scanner consisted of a stationary-anode x-ray tube cooled by circulating oil. The x-ray output was collimated to a pencil beam and, after passing through the patient's head and a water bath (to provide a constant tissue-equivalent path length), it was detected by a sodium iodide crystal coupled to a photomultiplier tube attached to a rigid metal frame called the *gantry.* Two side-by-side detectors, each with an aperture of 5 × 13 mm, were used so that two slices could be obtained simultaneously.

The x-ray tube and detectors were rigidly coupled by means of a yoke. This complex moved along in a linear traverse, sweeping across the patient to obtain a set of parallel measurements determining the amount of radiation that could penetrate through the patient along each set of parallel lines. After this linear traverse, the gantry rotated by 1 degree. This translate-rotate movement was repeated until 180 attenuation profiles, each 1 degree apart, were obtained. The acquisition of data took 4½ minutes. Another 1½ minutes were required to reconstruct the 80 × 80 matrix (3-mm pixel) images of the two slices.[5]

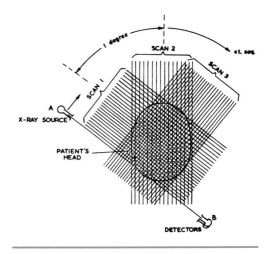

Simplified illustration of the scanning sequence (1973).[6]

The EMI scanner was designed for brain scanning, and its applications were limited to the head. In the United States, a dentist named Ledley became intrigued with the possibility of applying the technique to other regions of the body. He parlayed this interest into funding for construction of the first whole-body scanner. The first clinical unit was named the ACTA scanner and installed at the University of Minnesota in 1973. However, anatomical motion remained a significant problem in applications of this scanner to regions other than the head and extremities.[7]

Since the development of first-generation CT scanners, the major technical advances have been designed to dramatically increase the speed of scanning and image reconstruction. This has been accomplished by simultaneously acquiring data through more extensive detector arrays.[6] The pencil beam employed in the Mark I scanner resulted in poor geometrical utilization of the x-ray beam and consequently long scanning times. In the second-generation EMI 5000 scanner, the x-ray beam was collimated to a 10-degree fan, which encompassed an array of 8 to 30 radiation detectors rather than the previous pencil beam with only a single detector. Although the second-generation scanner also used the complicated translate-rotate mechanical motion, the fan beam permitted multiple angles to be obtained with a single translation across the patient. Using a fan 10 degrees wide, only 18 passes were needed at 10-degree angular increments to obtain the full 180 degrees of data.[5]

The fastest second-generation CT units could achieve a scanning time of 18 seconds per slice. The image quality was substantially improved over the Mark I scanner because of the additional views, finer ray sam-

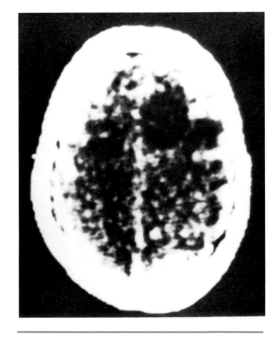

First clinical image obtained from EMI prototype unit. In a woman with a suspected brain lesion, the scan clearly shows a dark circular cyst.[1]

469

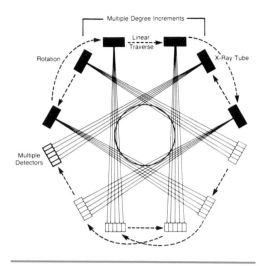

Second-generation CT scanner. There are a small number of beams (approximately 8 to 30) in a narrow fan configuration with the same translate-rotate motion used in first generation machines. Each linear traverse produces several projections at differing angles, one view for each x-ray beam.[8]

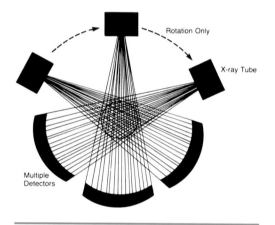

Third-generation CT scanner. There are a large number of x-ray beams (approximately 500 to 700) in a wide fan configuration. Both the x-ray tube and the detectors rotate.[8]

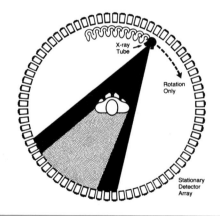

Fourth-generation CT scanner. There are an intermediate number of x-ray beams (approximately 50 to 200) in a wide fan configuration with a rotating x-ray tube and a stationary circular array of approximately 600 to 2,400 detectors surrounding the patient.[8]

pling, larger image matrix (i.e., 320 versus 80), smaller detector aperture, and reduced scan time. In addition, the cumbersome water bag was omitted on this and subsequent CT scanners. However, the second-generation units had definite speed limitations resulting from the inertia of the heavy x-ray tube and gantry, as well as the use of the complicated translate-rotate motion.

To increase speed, third- and fourth-generation systems were developed that used rotation only. These devices eliminated the necessity for a back-and-forth translation and permitted the rotation to be accomplished in a continuous smooth motion. Because the back-and-forth motion was eliminated, it was necessary for the fan of the x-ray beam to be wide enough to completely envelop the patient from side-to-side.[8]

The major difference between the third- and fourth-generation rotational scanners is the motion of the detectors. In the third-generation system, the x-ray tube and detector array are mounted opposite one another and pivot around the patient in a single rotational movement during which the views are acquired. The rays of a view are all acquired simultaneously with each active detector (the number of which is determined by the scan field of view) associated with a ray.[5] In fourth-generation systems, the detector array is a stationary circle, and only the x-ray tube rotates through a circle within the array. As many as 1,200 to 2,400 detectors may be used, compared with 500 to 700 in third-generation units.[8] Both third- and fourth-generation scanners can obtain individual slices in 2 to 4 seconds.

A variation on the fourth-generation design is the "ultrafast" CT scanner. Designed by Douglas Boyd and collaborators at Imatron for the purpose of imaging the heart, this unit has no moving parts and can acquire an image in as little as 17 msec. By successively steering a small focal-spot size electron beam at four fixed tungsten target rings, the heart can be imaged without moving the patient and virtually free of motion artifacts.[5]

IMAGING OPTIONS

Several techniques have been developed to provide information in addition to that offered by the basic CT cross-sectional image. Virtually all CT units can generate an image-projection radiograph analogous to a plain film. This is accomplished by moving the scan couch through the gantry aperture while the CT x-ray tube is rapidly pulsed, thus producing a series of thin slit sections that can be reconstructed in a plain-film format. Any of four views (posteroanterior, anteroposterior, lateral, and oblique) can be obtained by appropriate positioning of the x-ray tube. The resulting digital radiographic images are often of sufficient detail and quality to be used as a preliminary plain radiographic film. They can be employed to detect retained barium or other extraneous high-density objects that could produce image-degrading artifacts, to quickly localize lesions for CT-guided biopsy procedures, and to serve as a guide for radiation therapy.[9]

Dynamic imaging refers to rapid, repetitive image acquisitions, usually without image processing between scans. Rapid sequential imaging can be performed at a single level or at several levels (with incremental movement of the table between each scan). Dynamic scanning at a single level after a bolus injection of contrast material provides phasic information regarding blood flow and the "vascularity" of a lesion or structure at that level. It ensures that dense opacification of any potential vascular

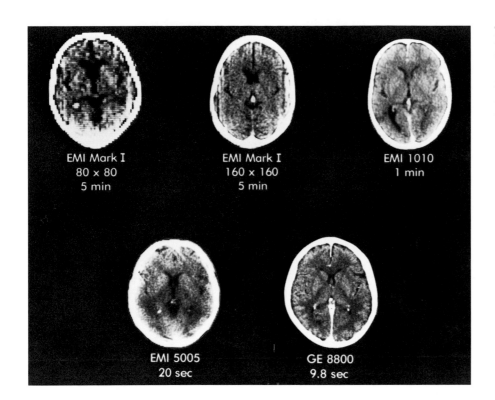

Five CT brain scans through the same level of the mid brain in five different patients. *Top left,* 1974; *top middle,* 1976; *top right,* 1977; *bottom left,* 1978; and *bottom right,* 1980. The difference in quality is apparent.[10]

EMI Mark I
80 x 80
5 min

EMI Mark I
160 x 160
5 min

EMI 1010
1 min

EMI 5005
20 sec

GE 8800
9.8 sec

structure will occur on at least one of the images. Rapid serial scanning at contiguous levels during a bolus injection provides anatomical information about a larger area and can aid in confidently distinguishing blood vessels from nonvascular structures or masses.[9]

Multiplanar reconstruction permits reorientation of CT data in other planes, typically coronal or sagittal. These alternate images are primarily of value in complex anatomical regions such as the spine, appendicular skeleton, and pelvis. However, the ability of magnetic resonance (MR) imaging to provide sagittal and coronal images without the need for reconstruction has greatly limited this CT imaging option.

Three-dimensional (3-D) imaging is a relatively new CT (and MRI) technique that is most applicable in complex anatomical regions. Major uses of 3-D CT imaging are in evaluating complex fractures of the spine, pelvis, shoulder, and face and in assessing articular disorders of the hip and spinal stenosis. Because of the need for multiple thinly collimated contiguous or overlapping sections, 3-D imaging requires additional acquisition time and radiation exposure (although in selected bone reconstructions a dramatic decrease in exposure factors may result in a radiation dose identical to that incurred during routine CT imaging).[8]

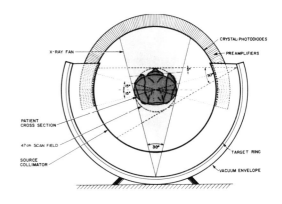

Cross-sectional view of "ultrafast" CT scanner. The unit employs a stationary detector array and is based on the fourth-generation principle. Each view is acquired by sampling a detector as the x-ray focus goes through its arch.[4]

References

1. Hounsfield GN: Computed medical imaging: Nobel lecture, December 8, 1979. J Comput Assist Tomogr 4:665-674, 1980.
2. Radon JH: Über die Bestimmung von Funktionen durch ihre Integralwerte länges gewisser Mannigfaltigkeiten. Ber Vehr Sachs Adad Wiss 69:262-277, 1917.
3. Cormack AM: Representation of a function by its line integrals with some radiological applications. J App Phys 35:2908-2913, 1964.
4. Cormack AM: Early two-dimensional reconstruction (CT scanning) and recent topics stemming from it: Nobel lecture, December 8, 1979. J Comput Assist Tomogr 4:658-664, 1980.
5. Barnes GT and Lakshminarayanan AV: Computed tomography: Physical principles and image quality considerations. In Lee JKT, Sagel SS, and Stanley RJ (eds): Computed body tomography with MRI correlation. New York, Raven Press, 1989.
6. Hounsfield GN: Computerized transverse axial scanning (tomography): Part I. Description of system. Br J Radiol 46:1016-1022, 1973.
7. Hendee WR: Cross sectional medical imaging: A history. RadioGraphics 9:1155-1180, 1989.
8. Winter J and King W: Basic principles of computed tomography. In Greenberg M (ed): Essentials of body computed tomography. Philadelphia, WB Saunders, 1983.
9. Anderson DJ and Berland L: CT techniques. In Lee JKT, Sagel SS, and Stanley RJ (eds): Computed body tomography with MRI correlation. New York, Raven Press, 1989.
10. Margulis AR: Radiologic imaging: Changing costs, greater benefits. AJR 136:657-665, 1987.

CHAPTER 28

Magnetic Resonance Imaging

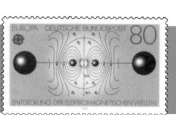
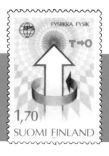
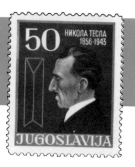

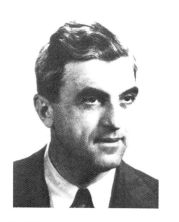

Felix Bloch (1905-1983).[27]

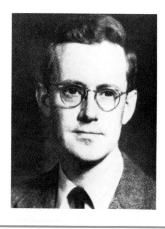

Edward Purcell (1912-   ).[27]

The first successful demonstrations of nuclear magnetic resonance (NMR) in bulk matter were published in consecutive issues of *Physical Review* in 1946 by two independent groups working in physics laboratories on opposite coasts of the United States. Felix Bloch and co-workers[1] at Stanford and Edward Purcell and associates[2] at Harvard noted that nuclei precessing in the radiofrequency range could emit a radiofrequency signal that could be detected by a radio receiver. They also showed that certain nuclei with odd numbers of protons, odd numbers of neutrons, or both tended to align themselves with a powerful magnetic field. If, for any reason, these atoms were displaced from the direction of the primary magnetic field, they tended to precess about the direction of the magnetic field at a specific (resonant) frequency termed the *Larmor frequency*. A radiofrequency stimulus applied to the atoms at right angles to the magnetic field caused the nuclei to precess at a wider and wider angle from the magnetic field. When the radiofrequency stimulus was discontinued, the precessing nuclei emitted a radiofrequency signal for a short time that was at the same frequency as the precession frequency and could be detected by using an appropriate antenna and radio receiver.[3] The importance of the discovery of nuclear magnetic resonance was recognized by the joint award of the 1952 Nobel Prize for Physics to Bloch and Purcell.

Initial interest in the NMR phenomenon centered on the discovery of *chemical shift*, a small but specific change in the resonant frequency of a particular nucleus in different chemical compounds. The demonstration that a molecule with nuclei in several chemical environments generated a spectrum with several distinct NMR responses led to the development of NMR spectroscopy. Because the NMR spectrum was in essence a fingerprint of the chemical compound, NMR spectroscopy became one of the chemist's most valuable structural and analytical tools.

The earliest biological NMR experiments took place at Stanford soon after the discovery of the phenomenon, when Bloch[1] obtained a strong proton NMR signal by inserting his finger into the radiofrequency coil of his spectrometer. At Harvard, Purcell and Ramsey (1948) inserted their heads into a 2 Tesla (T) field; around their heads was a coil connected to a powerful radiofrequency generator tuned to the proton NMR frequency. The only sensation recorded was that of induced electromotive force in the surrounding radiofrequency coil generated within the metal fillings of their teeth and detected by their tongues as the heads of the experimenters were moved into and out of the magnet.

The first application of high-resolution NMR spectroscopy to living systems was reported by Moon and Richards,[5] who published phosphorus-31 (^{31}P) NMR studies of intact red blood cells in which they could assign lines to individual metabolites. This was followed by the work of Hoult and associates,[6] who recorded a ^{31}P NMR spectrum from an intact freshly excised muscle from a rat's leg. At this stage in its development, the major limitation to NMR spectroscopy was the small bore (5 cm in diameter) of conventional NMR superconducting magnets. As the access width increased, studies could be performed on intact living animals. By 1980, the Oxford Instrument Company in England, a pioneer of many NMR magnet developments, provided superconducting magnets with a field of 2 T, a 30-cm diameter horizontal bore, and a high-resolution capability over a region 2 to 4 cm in extent. It was possible to insert the human hand and arm or foot and leg into such a magnet, and many high-resolution NMR spectra were recorded of ^{31}P as well as of carbon-13 (^{13}C) and hydrogen-1 (^{1}H) nuclei. The metabolism of both normal and diseased human limbs could be monitored. The effects of exercise and a tourniquet could be followed; diseased muscles could be diagnosed and their treatment and course followed in biochemical detail. Eventually, magnets with 100-cm diameter bores and high-resolution capability became available so that the whole human body could be inserted and a high-resolution NMR spectrum obtained from any desired part of the anatomy.[5]

MEDICAL IMAGING

In 1973, Paul Lauterbur[8] published the first NMR image of a heterogeneous object. He placed two thin-walled glass capillary tubes (1 mm inner diameter) containing water inside another larger glass tube (4.2 mm inner diameter) filled with D_2O. By applying a second magnetic field to the powerful primary magnetic field in such a way that the NMR response was only produced in a limited region, Lauterbur obtained a one-dimensional projection of nuclear density along the gradient direction. To generate a two-dimensional image of the object, Lauterbur devised an algorithm for combining the data from several projections, obtained by rotating the object about an axis perpendicular to the gradient direction.

Lauterbur recognized that, unlike traditional microscopy, the resolution of detail in NMR images was not related to the wave length of the illuminating radiation. The resolution and spatial discrimination were determined by the magnetic field and its gradient, whereas the radiofrequency electromagnetic field served to detect the NMR phenomenon. Because both fields must be conjoined in the object, Lauterbur coined the term *zeugmatography* from the Greek word *zeugma*, meaning "that which joins together." However, the term *zeugmatography* never became

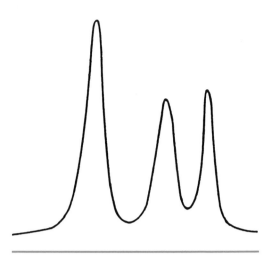

Proton NMR spectrum from ethyl alcohol (1951).[4] Reading from left to right, the three peaks correspond to CH_3, CH_2, and OH groups.[4]

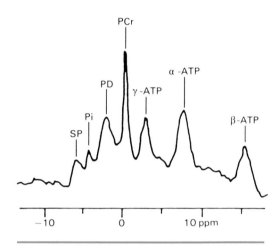

^{31}P NMR spectra from a live human head in a field of 1.5 T using a surface coil placed over the temple (1983).[7]

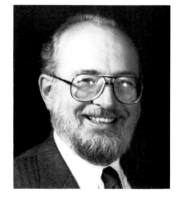

Paul Lauterbur.

473

First proton nuclear magnetic resonance zeugmatogram of tubes of water (1973).[8]

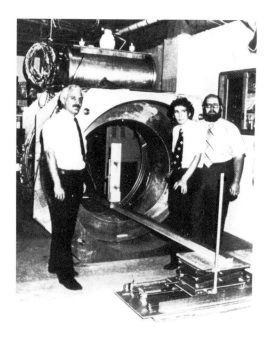

First NMR scanner for humans. *Left to right*, R. Damadian, L. Minkhoff, M. Goldsmith (1988).[28]

First human scan (1977). "Cross-section through the chest at the level of the eighth thoracic vertebra. The image shows the body wall; the right and left lung field; the heart encroaching on the left lung field; the cardiac chambers, right atrium, and a ventricle; and a section across the descending aorta."[11]

popular and the technique was generally called nuclear magnetic resonance (NMR) imaging. However, in the mid-1980s, to eliminate the word "nuclear" with its unpopular public connotation, the name was changed to the now universally accepted magnetic resonance imaging (MR imaging or MRI).

The concept of using the NMR technique for detecting neoplasms was first introduced by Raymond Damadian,[9] who in 1971 demonstrated that relaxation constants (T1 and T2) of water (i.e., hydrogen) were significantly longer in malignant rat tumors than in corresponding normal tissue. He even suggested that NMR should be present in the operating room as an aid in identifying malignant disease in excised tissues.

The initial work of Lauterbur and Damadian stimulated more skepticism than interest among seasoned researchers in diagnostic imaging. NMR signals were extremely weak and susceptible to noise interference from a variety of sources. In the chemistry laboratory, this problem could be solved by acquiring NMR data over several hours and adding thousands of measurements to obtain the result. However, in the clinical setting such long periods of data acquisition were impractical. In addition, chemical samples analyzed by NMR were small and homogeneous, whereas the living body was much larger and much less homogeneous. To develop NMR into a clinically useful imaging technology, it would be essential to make major investments in new instrumentation, including extremely uniform and intense magnetic fields.

In 1974, the first image of a biological specimen (a mouse) was obtained at the University of Aberdeen. Not only were the mouse's organs visible, but the darkest areas in the image corresponded to edema around a neck fracture. Two years later (1976), Damadian and colleagues[10] published the first NMR image of a live animal, a mouse with a tumor surgically implanted in the anterior chest wall. In the next year (1977), Damadian and co-workers[11] published the first human image, a cross-sectional visualization through the torso at the level of the eighth thoracic vertebra. Although these images were crude, they indicated that NMR imaging of the body was possible and a subject worthy of intensive research effort.

Damadian's FONAR (field focusing NMR) technique was time-consuming, since the tissue region of interest was sampled one point at a time. If NMR imaging were to be clinically important, a way had to be found to speed up the data-acquisition process. Mansfield and associates at the University of Nottingham in England developed a procedure to sample a region one line (rather than a point) at a time. Using this procedure, a planar region of tissue could be sampled by incrementally moving the data-acquisition line. Mansfield succeeded in producing crude images of a finger (1976)[13] and the abdomen (1978)[14] in greatly shortened time, but these images were barely recognizable.

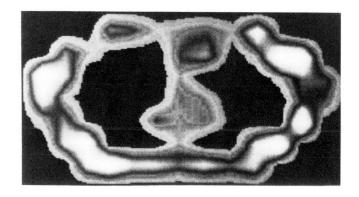

At Aberdeen, advances in the line-scale technique produced human images that were substantially better than those from Nottingham. Nevertheless, motion artifacts were a problem because in the Aberdeen approach two signals obtained at slightly different times were subtracted to produce the image. This problem was eventually resolved, primarily by stimulating the sample with radiofrequency pulses of constant duration but different amplitudes, rather than of constant amplitudes but different durations ("spin-warp" method).

Meanwhile, a second group of Nottingham researchers led by Moore and Hinshaw[16] employed a new technique in which alternating magnetic gradients were used to select and move a data-acquisition line in the specimen. In early images of the wrist and forearm, bones, muscles, tendons, and arteries were clearly visible. In 1980, this group produced the first recognizable pictures of the human brain.

Reports of the first patients studied using the new NMR technique were published in 1981. At Aberdeen, Smith and co-workers[17,18] published several reports indicating the ability of NMR to differentiate malignant from benign tissue and its superiority over ultrasound and the radionuclide liver scan for the diagnosis of a wide spectrum of hepatic diseases. At Hammersmith, Young and associates[19] used a variety of pulse sequences to produce images that provided different information. They showed that NMR was superior to computed tomography (CT) scanning for demonstration of small areas of demyelination in patients with multiple sclerosis[19] and for depicting the posterior fossa and its contents.[20]

In North America, NMR imaging research proceeded relatively slowly. By the early 1980s, spurred on by the emigration of British physicists to the United States, significant advances were made. Kaufman and Crooks, at the University of California at San Francisco, developed a sophisticated imaging system using a "multi-slice" approach, in which data were collected from nearby slices of tissue while the tissue in a previously sampled slice was given time to recover.

Three different types of magnet units were developed. Permanent magnets (e.g., FONAR) were made of ferromagnetic materials in which a large intrinsic magnetic field was induced at the time of manufacturing. Initially, these magnets were exceedingly heavy; one commercially available 0.3 T magnet weighed 100 tons. More recent permanent magnets have been constructed using rare earth alloys to produce higher fields

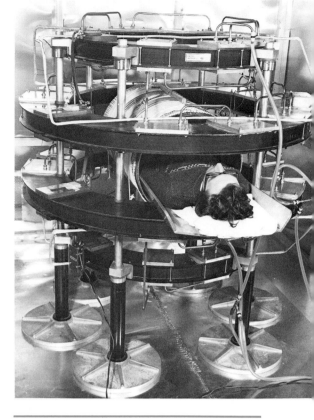

Aberdeen NMR imaging machine (1979).[15]

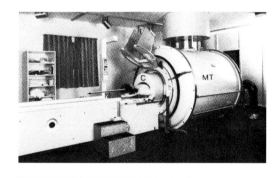

NMR imaging machine at Hammersmith (Steiner and Bydder, 1984). The machine is constructed around a large magnet (*MT*). The patient lies within the combined transmitter and receiver coil (*C*). The magnet induces a net magnetization (*M*) in the long axis of the patient.[22]

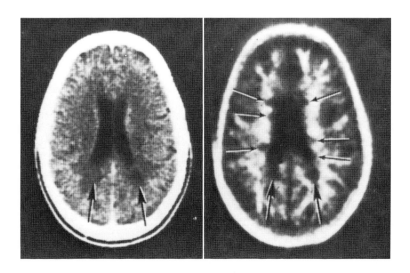

NMR imaging of the brain in multiple sclerosis (1981). "Comparable CT (*left*) and NMR (*right*) scans at the midventricular level. The two posterior periventricular lesions seen on the CT scan are also seen on the MR scan (*large arrows*). In addition, six smaller lesions are seen on the NMR scan at the lateral margin of the lateral ventricles (*small arrows*). The sharply defined area on the medial margin of the left posterior horn is a circular artifact."[19]

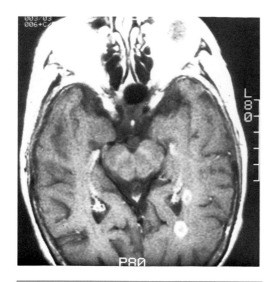

Gadolinium-enhanced MR. T1-weighted axial scan shows several rings of increased signal representing metastases that were not detectable on unenhanced T1- or T2-weighted images.

MR images and spectra from an untreated, low-grade astrocytoma. "*Left*, Axial T2-weighted image shows a tumor in the right frontal lobe, extending across the midline. *Middle*, Short flip angle image shows MR spectroscopic volumes of interest (squares) of the tumor and the mainly normal contralateral brain. *Right*, Hydrogen MR spectra from the lesion (*bottom*) and the normal control tissue (*top*). There is elevation of the choline (3.25 ppm) and creatine (3.05 ppm) levels and a marked decrease in the NAA peak (2.02 ppm) in the lesion spectrum compared with the control."[26]

with less weight. Resistive magnets generate their magnetic field by the flow of current within multiple turns of wire or ribbon of conductors such as aluminum or copper, both of which have significant resistance. As a result of the presence of this resistance, there is significant power dissipation and heating of the magnet. This limits the magnet's strength, since at high-field power the cooling requirements become excessive.[23]

The most popular design for an MR imaging unit is the superconducting magnet, which operates at relatively high field strength (0.35 to 2 T). Although the magnetic field of superconducting magnets is also produced by current flowing in wires, unlike resistive magnets the wire is made from one of a number of "superconducting" materials that have no measurable resistance. Thus there is no loss of power, and the current theoretically flows "forever," although there is a small loss of current with time in real magnets. To remain superconducting, the wire must be immersed in a bath of liquid helium, which must be surrounded by liquid nitrogen to slow the evaporation ("boil-off") of the considerably more expensive liquid helium. Superconducting magnets can attain considerably higher field strengths than resistive magnets but are substantially more expensive and must have their supply of liquid helium and nitrogen replenished periodically.[23]

By the end of 1982, MR imaging was gaining increasing practical acceptance, and within a few years it became the imaging examination of choice for the central nervous system and other body regions. Noninvasive and free of ionizing radiation, MR imaging yielded additional diagnostic insights through relaxation parameters that were not available from other imaging modalities. Unlike ultrasound, overlying bony structures caused no degradation of the image. In contrast to x-ray CT scanning, MR imaging could directly provide images of transverse, coronal, or sagittal slices or slices of any arbitrary orientation. By showing flow voids or localized rounded areas of high signal intensity, MR imaging could indicate vascular patency or obstruction without the need for iodinated contrast material.

More recent major advances in MR imaging include the development of intravenous contrast media and fast scanning techniques. The use of paramagnetic metal ion chelates in MR imaging was first advocated by Runge and co-workers,[24] who showed that trace amounts of these substances could reduce the T_1 relaxation time of nuclei in the surrounding environment because of the strong electron-nuclear magnetic moment interaction. This led to the rapid development of gadolinium (Gd) DTPA as an effective contrast agent, which showed breakdown of the blood-brain barrier similar to the iodinated contrast used in CT. Although initially used in MR imaging of the head, gadolinium is now being applied to numerous studies elsewhere in the body.[24]

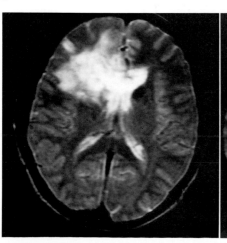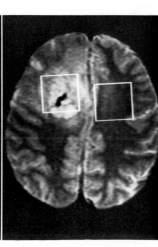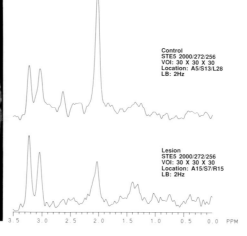

Because MR examinations were often prolonged, requiring patients to lie motionless for up to an hour, intensive investigations were undertaken to develop fast imaging techniques that could permit successful examinations even in patients with tremors or nervousness who could cooperate for only short periods, as well as allowing studies of the chest and abdomen where even a cooperative patient could not consciously halt cardiovascular functions, peristalsis, and respiration. In essence, the fast techniques combine small flip angles and gradient focusing to produce images in less than 1 second. MR angiograms can also be generated in which flowing blood appears much brighter than stationary tissues.[25]

Initially, hospital installations were difficult, if not nearly impossible, because of environmental radiofrequency interference. In addition, stray magnetic fields produced by the magnet affected the performance of nearby equipment. To meet this challenge, commercial manufacturers developed and implemented shielding approaches for hospital suites that, for the most part, were extensions of the radiofrequency and magnetic shielding developed for top-secret military electronics installations.[4]

Investigations are now underway to couple MR imaging with spectroscopy to precisely localize the source of in vivo metabolic activity. In the not-too-distant future, MR imaging and spectroscopy will probably become so closely linked that it may be possible to accumulate simultaneously imaging and spectroscopic data from several elements.

Bibliography

Andrew ER: A historical review of NMR and its clinical applications. Brit Med Bull 40:115-119, 1984.

Hendee WR: Cross sectional medical imaging: A history. RadioGraphics 9:1155-1180, 1989.

Partain CL, Price RR, Patton JA, et al (eds): Magnetic resonance imaging. Philadelphia, WB Saunders, 1988.

References

1. Bloch F, Hansen WW, and Packard ME: Nuclear induction. Phys Rev 69:127-129, 1946.
2. Purcell EM, Torrey HC, and Pound RV: Resonance absorption by nuclear magnetic moments in a solid. Phys Rev 69:37-38, 1946.
3. Smith FW: NMR—Historical aspects. In Newton TH and Potts DG (eds): Modern neuroradiology. San Anselmo, Calif, Clavadel, 1983.
4. Angus WM: A commentary on the development of diagnostic imaging technology. RadioGraphics 9:1225-1244, 1989.
5. Moon RB and Richards JH: Determination of intracellular pH by ^{31}P magnetic resonance. J Biol Chem 48:7276-7278, 1973.
6. Hoult DI, Busby SJW, Gadian DG, et al: Observation of tissue metabolites using ^{31}P nuclear magnetic resonance. Nature 252:285-287, 1974.
7. Arnold JT, Dharmatti SS, and Packard ME: Chemical effects on nuclear induction signals from organic compounds. J Chem Phys 19:507-511, 1951.

8. Lauterbur PC: Image formation by induced local interactions: Examples employing nuclear magnetic resonance. Nature 242:190-191, 1973.
9. Damadian R: Tumor detection by nuclear magnetic resonance. Science 117:1151-1153, 1971.
10. Damadian R, Minkhoff L, Goldsmith M, et al: Field focusing nuclear magnetic resonance (FONAR): Visualization of a tumor in a live animal. Science 194:1430-1432, 1976.
11. Damadian R, Goldsmith M, and Minkhoff L: NMR in cancer. XVI. FONAR image of the live human body. Physiol Chem Phys 9:97-108, 1977.
12. Hutchison JMS, Mallard JR, and Goll CC: In-vivo imaging of body structures using proton resonance. In Allen PS, Andrew ER, and Bates CA (eds): Proceedings of the 18th Ampere Congress, University of Nottingham, 1974.
13. Mansfield P and Maudsley AA: Planar and line-scan spin imaging by NMR. Proc XIXth Congress Ampere, Heidelberg, 1976, pp 247-252.
14. Mansfield P, Pykett IL, Morris PG, and Coupland RE: Human whole body line-scan imaging by NMR. Brit J Radiol 51:921-922, 1978.
15. Mallard J: The noes have it! Do they? Br J Radiol 54:831-849, 1981.
16. Hinshaw WS, Bottomley PA, and Holland GN: Radiographic thin-section image of the human wrist by nuclear magnetic resonance. Nature 270:722-723, 1977.
17. Smith FW, Mallard JR, Hutchison JMS, et al: Clinical application of nuclear magnetic resonance. Lancet 1:78-79, 1981.

18. Smith FW, Mallard JR, Reid A, and Hutchison JMS: Nuclear magnetic resonance tomographic imaging in liver disease. Lancet 1:963-966, 1981.
19. Young IR, Hall AS, Pallis CA, et al: Nuclear magnetic resonance imaging of the brain in multiple sclerosis. Lancet 2:1063-1066, 1981.
20. Young IR, Brul M, Clarke GJ, et al: Magnetic resonance properties of hydrogen: Imaging the posterior fossa. AJR 187:895-901, 1981.
21. Hounsfield GN: Computed medical imaging: Nobel lecture, December 8, 1979. J Comput Assist Tomogr 4:665-674, 1980.
22. Steiner RE and Bydder GM: Nuclear magnetic resonance in gastroenterology. Clinics in Gastroenterology 13:265-279, 1984.
23. Kneeland JB: Instrumentation. In Stark DD and Bradley WD (eds): Magnetic resonance imaging. St. Louis, CV Mosby Co, 1988.
24. Runge VM, Stewart RG, Clanton JA, et al: Potential oral and intravenous paramagnetic NMR contrast agents. Radiology 147:789-791, 1983.
25. Edelman RR: MRI angiography: Approaches and strategies. MRI Decisions July/Aug 1989.
26. Alger JR, Frank JA, Bizzi A, et al: Metabolism of human gliomas: Assessment with H-1 spectroscopy and F-18 fluorodeoxyglucose PET. Radiology 177:633-641, 1990.
27. Andrew ER: A historical review of NMR and its clinical applications. Brit Med Bull 40:115-119, 1984.
28. Partain CL, Price RR, Patton JA, et al (eds): Magnetic resonance imaging. Philadelphia, WB Saunders, 1988.

THERAPEUTIC APPLICATIONS

LINES ON AN X-RAY PORTRAIT OF A LADY

She is so tall, so slender; and her bones—
Those so frail phosphates, those carbonates of lime—
Are well produced by cathode rays sublime,
By oscillations, amperes, and by ohms.
Her dorsal vertebrae are not concealed
By epidermis, but are well revealed.

Around her ribs, those beauteous twenty-four,
Her flesh a halo makes, misty in line,
Her noseless, eyeless face looks into mine,
And I but whisper, "Sweetheart, Je t'adore."
Her white and gleaming teeth at me do laugh.
Ah! lovely, cruel, sweet cathodograph!

Lawrence K Russell, *Life*, March 12, 1896

CHAPTER 29

X-Ray Therapy

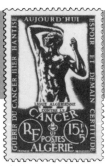
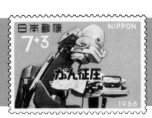
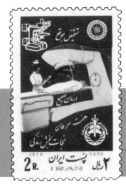
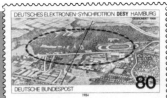

There is no disease that physicians like less to encounter than carcinoma in any of its forms, especially when it has progressed to the stage where the probabilities of its complete removal are slight. Few surgeons today doubt that carcinoma can be cured when it is localized and in a location favorable to operation. More often than not, however, cases are concealed until glandular involvement or widespread dissemination has occurred and the hope of a cure from operation is practically gone. This common and dangerous delay is due to the popular dread of the knife. If, then, we have at hand an agent that will effect a cure without the use of the knife or of painful caustics, one of the most frequent causes for neglect of the disease has been removed. We are firmly convinced that, by means of the proper application of this agent under conditions of no practical discomfort to the patient, we can bring about the painless removal of the slow-growing epitheliomas. These growths, especially when they occur on the face, are very disfiguring; if allowed to progress they produce a condition loathsome in the extreme. Treatment of such cases by the x-rays leaves a remaining defect that is incomparably better in cosmetic results than that which must accompany extirpation by knife or caustic. Furthermore, our experiments lead us to believe that even in inoperable cases of carcinoma attacking superficial parts, we may give great relief from pain and can even prolong life. If we can dispense with the use of opiates in this class of cases and free the patients from pain while leaving the intellect clear and digestion undisturbed, we have made a great improvement in the therapeutics of this condition.

These words, written in 1900 by Wallace Johnson and Walter Merrill,[1] come from the first article in English detailing the favorable results of radiation therapy for cancer of the skin. However, the earliest therapeutic use of radiation was to treat benign rather than malignant disease.

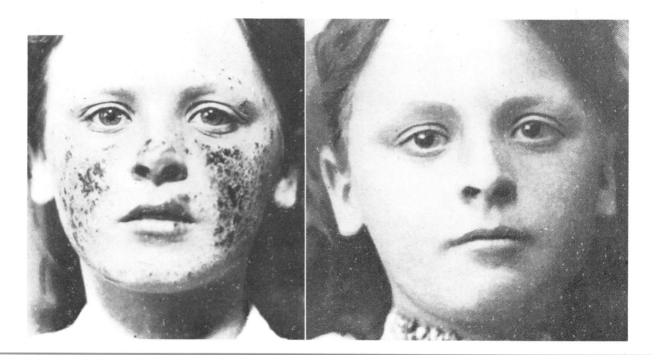

X-ray therapy of eczema (1904). Twelve-year-old girl (*left*) before and (*right*) after treatment.[2]

X-ray therapy of lupus of the nose (1902). "Note the sheet-lead bent around the face with a hole cut for the affected nose. It is being tied behind with two pieces of tape to hold it in place, and the operator is adjusting the tube to position. When the lower pair of ribbons (seen hanging down) are also tied, have the patient drop his hand to his lap, light up the tube and expose."[4]

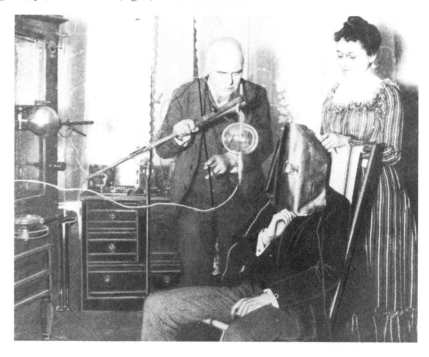

X-ray therapy of tuberculosis of the knee joint (1902). Note the position of the large mask (*left*) and the smaller sheet-lead mask (*right*).[4]

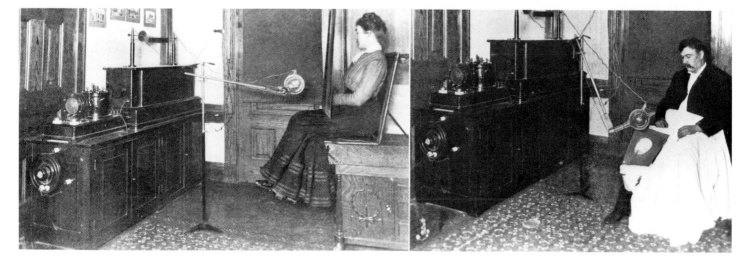

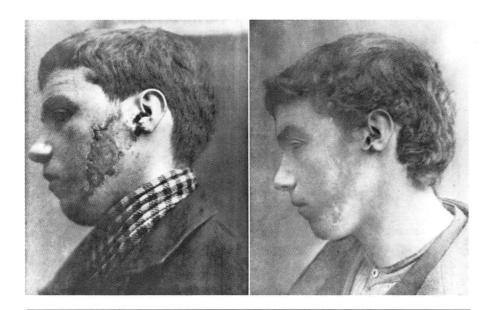

X-ray treatment of lupus of the face (1898). *Left,* Before and (*right*) after 17 treatments of 15 minutes each over 2 months.[5]

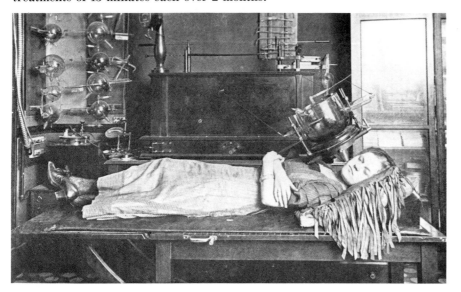

Method of x-ray treatment for cancer of the face (1912).[10]

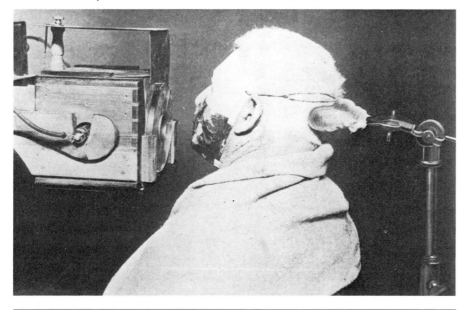

X-ray therapy of cancer of the face (1904).[8]

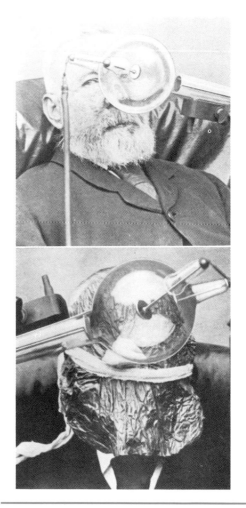

X-ray therapy of epithelioma of the nose (1902). *Top,* "View of the face without the shield demonstrates the relation of the tube to the lesion, the surface of which has been scraped to facilitate the action of the rays." *Bottom,* "When the position of the tube is focused on the lesion with the glass wall a hand-breadth distant, a layer of surgical cotton is placed over the part and the shield tied on."[4]

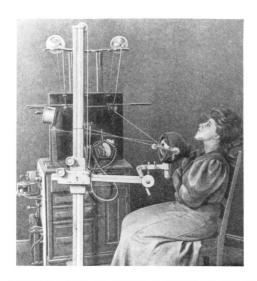

X-ray treatment of exophthalmic goiter (1910). A Friedlander shield is in place and the point of the chin is still further protected by x-ray metal.[6]

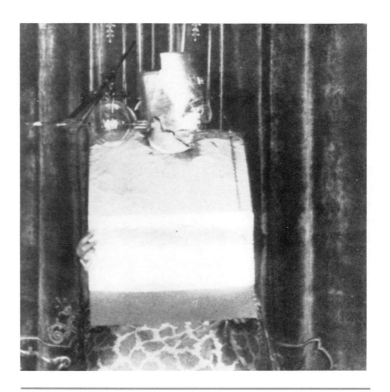

Side view of a foil-covered mask with space cut out for x-ray treatment of side and chin whiskers on a woman's face (1902). "The front shield protects the chest and shoulders during the exposures. The patient is seated on a revolving stool during treatment, the mask and shield grounded by the chain seen at the right, the tube placed with its wall 6 inches from the tissues, and a total exposure of twenty minutes is divided upon the four areas of the two sides of the face and neck by turning the patient on the stool. A medium tube is used with the least current that will excite it properly. Treatment is repeated three times a week, making certain to watch for any signs of irritation. Permanent depilation requires patience and careful treatment."[4]

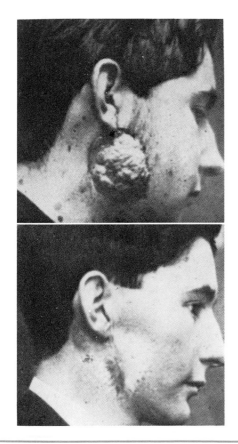

X-ray therapy of recurrent sarcoma (1901). *Left,* Recurrent tumor before therapy. *Right,* Lesion healed 11 months after the beginning of treatment.[11]

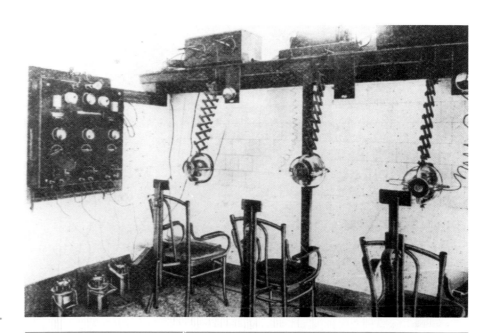

Roentgen-ray therapy room at London hospital in 1905. The barber chair arrangement reflected the main therapeutic use of x-rays at that time—the treatment of ringworm of the scalp.[12]

According to the Brechers, there were three major pathways to the development of radiation for therapeutic purposes. The first was "simple, empirical curiosity: let's try it out and see what happens." A number of investigators decided to experiment with these new rays to see whether they might have some positive effect on patients with inoperable tumors. Indeed, as early as 7 months after Roentgen's discovery of x-rays, a report in the *Medical Record* (August 29, 1896) described the work of V. Despeignes of Lyons, who had described "a case of gastric carcinoma which had appeared to be greatly benefited by the transmission of the rays through the seat of disease."

A second pathway toward the development of radiation therapy was the report by John Daniel in April 1896 that an excessive dose of x-rays caused human hair to fall out (see Chapter 11). Before the end of the year, several investigators in Europe and the United States were actively using x-rays for the treatment of hypertrichosis (excessive growth of hair), especially on the faces of women. By serendipity, this work led to the discovery of other uses. An eminent Chicago dermatologist, William Allen Pusey (later the coauthor of a major radiology textbook), noted that a woman he was treating for excess hair had "on the chin and around the mouth . . . an acne simplex of moderate severity." To his surprise, after the use of x-rays the acne disappeared and did not recur. Similar accidental discoveries probably occurred in Europe, where reports before 1900 included the successful use of x-rays to treat tinea capitis (ringworm of the scalp), favus (a parasitic skin infection), sycosis (inflammation of the hair follicles), and chronic eczema.

The third pathway toward the discovery of the therapeutic usefulness of x-rays was the successful treatment of several skin conditions using ultraviolet light therapy reported by Niels Finsen of Copenhagen in 1900. To obtain a good result with the Finsen lamp, it was necessary to produce a "reaction which might vary in degree from an erythema to a vesicular or bullous dermatitis."[14] Because x-rays produced a reddening of the skin much like sunburn and were considered by some at that time to be merely a variation of ultraviolet light, it probably occurred to many clinicians that x-rays might have similar therapeutic effects.

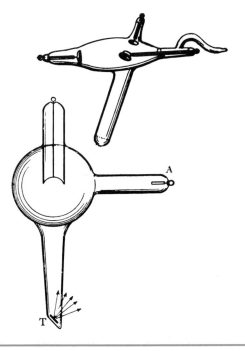

Intracavitary x-ray tubes (1904). *Top,* Cossar's tube for treating carcinoma of the cervix. *Bottom,* Caldwell tube for treating the larynx and other sites such as the cervix or rectum.[13]

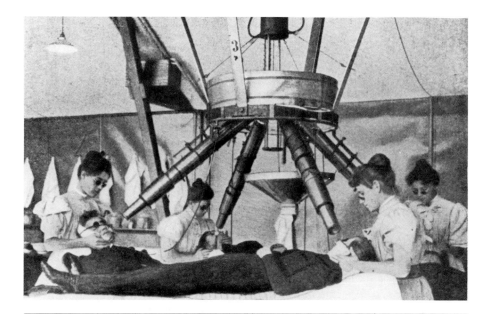

Finsen lamp therapy. This pioneer arc-light "tube" apparatus was capable of treating four patients an hour.[15]

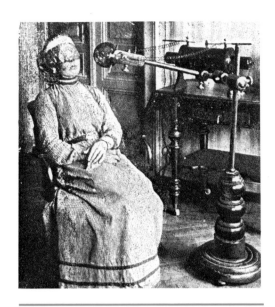

Radiation therapy of the face (1904).[16]

In 1898, Leopold Freund and Eduard Schiff in Vienna successfully treated patients with lupus vulgaris (skin tuberculosis). In the next year, Philip Mills Jones of San Francisco reported similar results. His 55-year-old patient had undergone a variety of treatments, including "cautery, curretting, creosote, silver nitrate, and hydrogen dioxide." Jones selected a "soft" tube and began x-ray exposures of the patient's right forehead.

There were present three ulcerating points and one large, hard nodule which had not yet broken down. A sheet of lead was arranged so as to protect the whole of the head save the lupus area; a hole cut in the lead sheet allowed the x-rays to reach all the diseased areas, with the exception of one of the ulcerating points. This one small point was protected as a sort of control upon the treatment . . . At the end of four weeks the whole area, with the exception of the one ulcer protected, was healed and the nodule had disappeared.

The protected ulceration had meanwhile increased in size. "I then exposed the ulcerated area that had been previously protected by the lead plate. In three weeks this had quite healed."

Today, the use of radiotherapy for treating benign disease is considered quackery and is rigorously avoided. It is worth remembering, however, that years ago, before the introduction of antibiotics, chemotherapeutic agents, and steroids, there were a host of chronic inflammatory and nonspecific lesions that were unsightly, disabling, and even dangerous to life that could be relieved by small, safe, almost homeopathic doses of radiation. Radiation was recommended and widely used in the treatment of pyogenic infections, chronic tuberculous adenitis, and the innumerable nonspecific conditions that plagued the dermatologist and ophthalmologist.[13]

The discovery that x-rays were effective against skin cancer soon followed reports that they were valuable in treating tuberculosis of the skin. Credit for initiating x-ray treatment of skin cancer is often given to two Swedes, Thor Stenbeck and Tage Sjogren, each of whom independently demonstrated a case of epithelioma treated with x-rays at a meeting of the Swedish Medical Society in December, 1899. Johnson and Merrill[1] reported a series of favorable results in five patients. These findings were confirmed by the noted Boston radiologist, Francis H. Williams, who presented his therapeutic work in his classic 1901 textbook. Soon there were many detailed and convincing reports of successful x-ray treatments, generally illustrated by astonishing "before-and-after" photographs.

Perhaps the first report of a deep-lying internal cancer *cured* by x-rays (i.e., no detectable evidence of recurrence after 5 years) was the celebrated case of Clarence E. Skinner of New Haven. The patient was a schoolteacher suffering from a rapidly growing malignant fibrosarcoma of the abdomen and, when referred to Skinner, was "losing flesh, markedly cachectic, very weak, and complaining bitterly of pressure symptoms." The referring physician considered her case "entirely hopeless." After almost 80 x-ray treatments over a span of about 7 months, the tumor had shrunk in volume by about 20%, making it necessary for her "to shorten her waistbands and the fronts of her skirts to keep them from dragging on the ground." A year and a half later after a total of 136 applications of the x-ray, Skinner could proudly report to the referring physician that his "entirely hopeless" patient was feeling well and again teaching school. Ironically, 5 years later she subsequently developed a radiation-induced cancer of the skin (see Chapter 11).

Enthusiastic reports initially appeared extolling the virtues of radiation therapy for a whole host of benign and malignant conditions. Pusey's textbook (1904)[9] contained nearly 475 pages on therapeutics and reported the author's own experience with x-ray therapy in 52 different diseases. Two years previously, Heber Robarts (1902), editor of the *American X-Ray Journal*, had estimated that "there are about 100 named diseases that yield favorably to x-ray treatment."

One reason for the excessive enthusiasm of many early reports may have been the favorable psychological effect of the x-ray treatment on patients.

A visit to the "x-ray doctor" was an impressive occasion indeed. Patients were awed by the hiss or the roar of the equipment, by the tingle of ozone in the air. An aura of something akin to magic surrounded the very word "X-ray" in the public mind. Thus, a patient was almost sure to leave an X-ray seance (as some of the electrotherapeutists called their treatments) psychologically encouraged even though not physically benefited.

X-rays were reported to have impressive success in suppressing pain. As Seabury W. Allen noted (1902),[17] "Not infrequently patients whom I have subjected to x-rays for one cause or another have spoken of the relief of the pain or discomfort which previously existed in the part exposed." He reported a patient with severe chronic rheumatoid arthritis who 5 days after a diagnostic x-ray examination was able to "resume practice on the piano, which she had previously had to abandon." An elderly woman who received x-ray therapy for a chronic foot ulcer of more than 50 years' duration reported that she "knew it would heal, for it had stopped burning and paining."

An intriguing early use of radiation therapy was the relief of blindness. After several investigators had experienced irritation of the eyes while experimenting with x-rays, it was suggested that exposure to x-rays might have a beneficial effect on certain types of blindness, especially those from cataracts. Edison[18] treated two cases and reported "favorable" results. A Havana ophthalmologist, Francis de Astudillo,[19] reported improvement in 11 cases of blindness after treatment with x-rays. Although he gave no details of the method employed, he asserted that all 20 patients treated, each with a different malady of the eye, experienced some kind of modification. However, careful analysis of these and subsequent optimistic articles clearly indicated the futility of radiation therapy to alleviate blindness, and such treatment was soon abandoned.[20]

The initial responses of skin cancers and other superficial neoplasms treated by irradiation were so dramatic that they generated the unrealistic expectation that a miraculous cure for all cancers had been discovered. This unrealistic view was soon followed by a wave of disillusionment and pessimism when reports of tumor recurrence and injuries to normal tissues made it unclear whether the benefits of radiation therapy outweighed the risks. These discouraging experiences should not be surprising, for in the absence of specialized training programs, virtually all the early practitioners in x-ray therapy were dermatologists and surgeons who had no understanding of the physical nature or biological effects of the new and mysterious agents with which they worked. There were no reliable methods for measuring the amount of x-ray therapy given or even a generally agreed unit of dose. The equipment was primitive, temperamental, and too limited in energy to permit any but the most superficial neoplasms to be treated. The early radiation therapists initially adopted

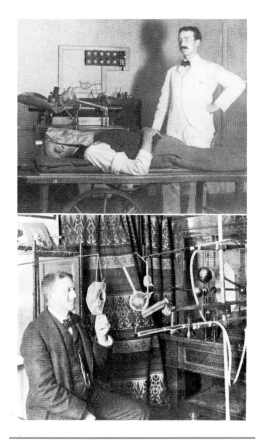

X-ray therapy of two different patients with carcinoma of the face (1902).[4]

treatment techniques involving massive exposures aimed at the eradication of tumors in a single treatment, comparable with the extirpation of tumors by surgery. Therefore it was to be expected that the primary morbidity, and even the acute mortality, of such massive-dose treatment was often comparable with major surgery at that time. Patients who survived the immediate postirradiation period often experienced impressive partial or complete regression of their tumors, but these initial responses were all too often followed by major complications, as well as a high rate of tumor recurrence.[21]

In the October 6, 1906, issue of the *British Medical Journal*, A.R. Robinson, in discussing "Errors in the Treatment of Cutaneous Cancer," stated that roentgen-ray devices had been too widely used, even to the extent that they warranted the designation of "race suicide machines." Attempts were even made to introduce legislation that would outlaw the use of roentgen rays. Nevertheless, the advantages of radiation therapy were recognized, and it was clear that some tumors responded unexpectedly well while others became operable despite initial inoperability.[62] The general consensus was well stated by W.B. Coley, the referring physician in Skinner's case, who concluded that "the amount of success that has been obtained, while less than we had hoped, is sufficient, we feel, to make it strongly advisable to continue the work in selected cases."

A discussion of the early days of radiation therapy would be incomplete without mention of Emil Grubbé, a German emigre living in Chicago who was a manufacturer of incandescent lamps at the time of Roentgen's discovery. After several months of testing the vacuum of his tube by placing his left hand between the tube and fluorescent substance, Grubbé developed a severe dermatitis on the back of his left hand and allegedly, as he wrote, "I happened to be the first person detrimentally affected by these new rays."[22] One of the dermatologists who saw Grubbé's hand was J.E. Gilman, who

> after thinking over the origin of the dermatitis, said that although he would not suggest a remedy for the treatment of my burned hand, he was very much impressed with the power of these new rays, and he concluded with the statement that any physical agent capable of doing so much damage to normal or healthy cells and tissues might offer possibilities, if used as a therapeutic measure in the treatment of pathological conditions . . . As examples of such lesions he mentions cancer, lupus, and indolent ulcers.

Emil Grubbé (1875-1960). *Left,* Photograph obtained in 1951 shows lesions on his right hand and face. His left hand and wrist had been amputated in 1929 after an automobile accident. *Right,* Grubbé's reception room.[22]

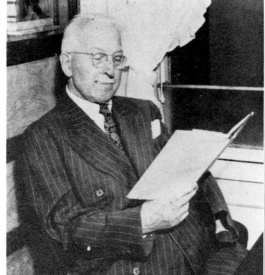

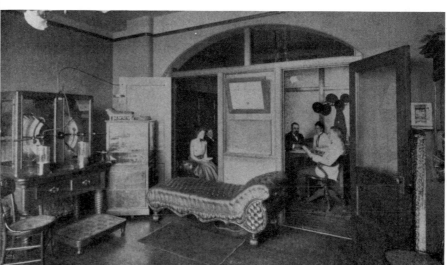

Grubbé reported that he was soon sent two patients, one with carcinoma of the breast and the other with lupus vulgaris, to treat with x-rays. "For the first time in history, x-rays had been used for *treatment*, not diagnostic purposes." Neither patient seems to have responded favorably. Grubbé frankly admitted that

> no dramatic results were obtained. Neither case was reported clini-
> cally by the physicians who sent them to me because both parties
> died within a month after commencing x-ray treatment, and before
> sufficient cumulative effects had been obtained in either case to
> warrant any conclusions as to the value of the new therapeutic
> agent . . . This, briefly, is the story of the origin and birth of the
> treatment of diseases with x-rays.

Grubbé again stressed his role in the conclusion of his autobiography, "I have lived long enough to see the child that I fathered develop into a sturdy, mature, and worthwhile product; and I hope, as I approach the evening of my day, to see even more uses for x-ray therapy in the alleviation of the ills of mankind."

In the absence of any record in a scientific publication, was Grubbé's story true? Undoubtedly, Grubbé had worked with x-rays and he under-went multiple surgical procedures for radiation-induced injury. But did he really play a major role in the development of radiation therapy?

This curious story took an ironic final twist. A prominent radiologist, Paul C. Hodges, was commissioned to write a definitive biography of Emil Grubbé. After prolonged and meticulous research, Hodges un-equivocally established that Grubbé was a publicity seeker who was "vain, boastful, incompletely truthful" and an unreliable witness con-cerning his own accomplishments.[23] Not only was there no contemporary support for Grubbé's story, but all the circumstantial evidence appeared to argue against acceptance of his claims. As the Brechers concluded, "Grubbé's story is so implausible, so lacking in contemporary corrobora-tion, and in such irreconcilable conflict with readily provable facts, and Grubbé's untruthfulness in other respects is so readily demonstrable, as to warrant the inclusion of his claims in this postscript rather than in the body of a history of Amerian radiology."

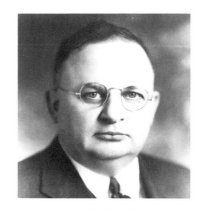

Paul C. Hodges.

ORTHOVOLTAGE THERAPY

The availability of substantial quantities of radium in the early 1910s led to the widespread use of this substance in the treatment of cancer (see Chapter 30). During the second decade of the twentieth century, radium therapy completely overshadowed the therapeutic use of x-rays, except for superficial skin conditions. As James Ewing[24] of New York later recalled, "Roentgenologists who engaged in therapy were looked upon with suspi-cion. It was difficult to enlist the interest of any qualified roentgenologist in this questionable field. Unlike the gamma rays from radium, which penetrated deep into tissues, the 100,000-volt x-rays of that period were for the most part absorbed in the superficial tissues. There was no understanding that this limitation could be overcome by placing the x-ray tube farther away from the body."

With the invention of the hot-cathode tube by Coolidge in 1913 (see Chapter 8), x-rays in the range of 140 keV could be produced under more stable operating conditions. After World War I, when word arrived about remarkable work in Germany using tubes of higher voltage that could emit more penetrating x-rays, Coolidge began to develop a high-voltage hot-cathode tube for General Electric. One of the few reputable radiologists using x-rays for therapy at that time was James T. Case of Battle Creek, Michigan. After seeing Coolidge's new experimental tube in operation at the factory, he described it as "a large tube, nearly a yard long and with a much larger bulb than usual and therefore requiring a much larger lead-glass bowl" to cut off stray rays. Although Case was eager to acquire such a tube, he was told that "it was not on the market and would not be for nearly a year."

As luck would have it, a patient with recurrent breast carcinoma whom Case was requested to treat happened to be the wife of the manager of a nearby General Electric plant. When Case told his visitor about the new Coolidge high-voltage tube, "the gentleman remarked that he would get Doctor Coolidge on the telephone and have one of the tubes for me day after tomorrow." Indeed, the tube arrived 2 days later but immediately burned up Case's high-voltage transformer. "The gentlemen found me almost weeping over the loss of the 196,000-volt transformer, but after listening to my explanation, he assured me that he would have another one of 300,000-volt capacity the day after tomorrow." Three days later Case tried again and his first patient "survived nearly eight years, all but the last few months in comfort and general good health."[25]

Radiation therapy using energies in the 200 keV range was termed *deep roentgen therapy* to indicate that the penetration of the x-rays at this energy level (in contrast to that of superficial x-rays) was such that it could reach any depth of the body to be therapeutically effective. Later this technique was termed *orthovoltage* radiation therapy.

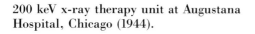
200 keV x-ray therapy unit at Augustana Hospital, Chicago (1944).

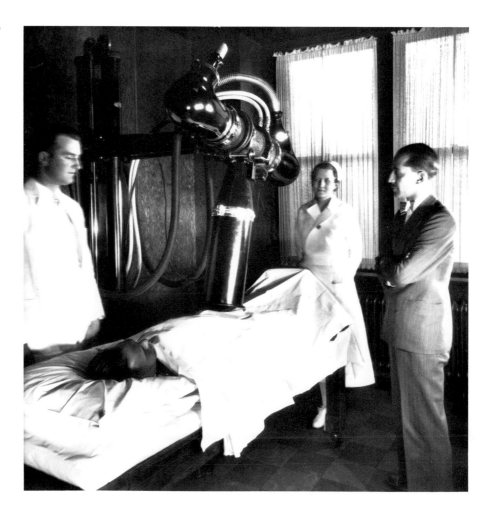

As E. Dale Trout[26] later described,

The usual therapy installation consisted of a room lined with ⅛″ lead. In one end of the room was a large cabinet containing the high-voltage transformer and rectifier. In the center of the room was a wood treatment table on which was mounted a wood tube stand holding the tube in a lead glass bowl. The high-voltage conductors called the "overhead" consisted of ¾″ nickel-plated tubing suspended from the ceiling by 2-foot long insulators. The exposed tube terminals were connected to the overhead by flexible leads. The roar of the rectifying switch, the crackling of the corona and the ozone-filled atmosphere left memories never to be forgotten by those who worked with such equipment. It was soon realized that the noise and ozone produced by the machine should be eliminated from the treatment room, and wall insulators were developed which made it possible to install the machine outside the treatment room. The high-voltage hazard remained. In addition, it was quickly realized that leakage radiation from the lead glass bowl was excessive. The answer came in lead-lined tube housing of two general types, the couch and the drum. The couch was built against the wall of the machine room, permitting the high-voltage conductors to be run from the machine into the back side of the couch. The couch was lined with lead, with the exception of a cutout in the center of the top surface. This opening usually about 12″ square had provision for the placement of filters and lead diaphragms for different field sizes. The drum was usually a ceiling or floor stand–supported steel cylinder lined with lead. Occasionally it took the form of a lead-lined box. The high-voltage leads were carried into the housing through insulators or through the open ends of the container. The port was in the bottom of the drum or box, with provision for the insertion of filters and diaphragms. The treatment table had to provide the vertical adjustment necessary to obtain the treatment distance. These tables usually consisted of the base of a barber or dental chair mounted on a moveable base with a table top replacing the chair.

In the 1920s there was great concern as to the physiological, biological, and histopathological effects of x-rays on normal and diseased tissues. The three most important questions were[14]:

(1) Does the action of the roentgen rays for a given exposure produce in every cell, structure or tissue an effect of the same magnitude;
(2) Does an identical maximal dose, whether administered singly, fractionally, or in a protracted way, produce a lethal effect on every pathologic cell, structure or tissue;
(3) If such a lethal dose is administered to any pathologic process, what reaction is there produced in the surrounding normal structures or the rest of the body?

As early as 1906, Bergonie and Tribondeau[27] had stated that "immature cells and cells in an active stage of division are more sensitive to radiation than are cells which have already acquired their adult morphological and physiologic characters." It soon became evident that each variety of cell had a specific range of sensitivity that, although influenced by extraneous factors, was a dominant feature and was related to the natural life cycle of the cell. For example, the lymphocyte that had the shortest metabolic cycle was the most radiosensitive, whereas the nerve cell with its extremely long life cycle was the most resistant to the effects of x-rays. Tumors tended to have a radiosensitivity roughly similar to that of their primary underlying cellular component.

The question of the most efficacious way of administering therapeutic

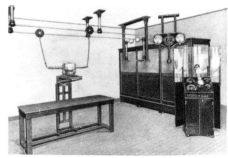

Advertisement for Victor deep roentgen therapy unit (AJR, 1921).

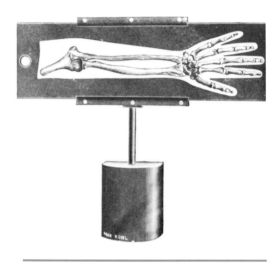

Beck's osteoscope (1904). Use of a skeleton arm fixed to a board eliminated the need for the operator to use his own hand to test the hardness of the x-ray beam.[29]

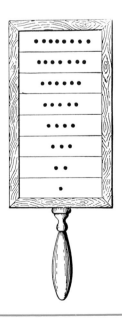

Kolle's x-ray meter (1896).[30]

radiation led to the development of a wide variety of techniques, each of which was of value in specific clinical situations. Initially, there was little concern to the possible adverse effects on normal tissues caused by therapeutically effective dosages to malignant neoplasms. It soon became evident that the large doses required to destroy the most resistant neoplasms often resulted in severe reactions of normal structures that led to prolonged or permanent injury.

Measuring the X-ray Dose

A major problem in therapeutic (as well as diagnostic) radiology was the need to establish a system for measuring the x-ray dose. In the early days of radiotherapy, when equipment was primitive and it was difficult to control the volume of x-rays emitted, little was known or could be learned about dosage. The general practice was to place the x-ray tube at a short distance from the skin or even in contact with it; no filter was used. Focal irradiation alone was considered, and the occurrence of secondary or scattered radiation was not realized. The importance of the inverse square law was not appreciated until the work of Emion G. Williams in 1903. Even after an operator by trial and error had established a technique for his own apparatus, he could not convey any idea of his method to another because of variations in the number and size of windings of coils and rates of interruption, the size and speed of the rotating disks of static machines, and numerous other mechanical factors. In addition, whenever a tube was changed, the intensity became substantially different.[28]

The unreliability of the equipment and the impossibility of reproducing or comparing treatments with any accuracy led to what now appear to be bizarre early attempts to overcome the problems of dosage estimation using photographic and fluoroscopic methods. The Viennese dermatologist, Freund,[16] claimed to have produced epilation of a hairy nevus by x-rays (1897) using radiation of "an intensity that would take a Roentgen photograph of a man's hand at 15 cm distance in a 1 minute exposure." Fluoroscopy was used to determine the hardness or softness of an x-ray tube by viewing the sharpness of the image of the interposed hand of the operator. Once the danger of this procedure was recognized, the hand of the operator was replaced either by the hand of a skeleton fixed to a board (Beck's osteoscope)[29] or by a variety of primitive x-ray meters. Kolle designed a small hand x-ray meter consisting of "a small mahogany frame and handle, grooved to contain eight sections of sheet aluminum, ranging from 1 to 12 mm." These sections had a consecutive number of holes drilled in them and "as the potential or tube efficiency is increased one section after another would become more or less apparent." For example, when the uppermost section containing eight holes was perfectly transparent, this corresponded "to an x-ray efficiency sufficient to make a radiogram of the adult chest and shoulders in from ten to eleven minutes, using the ordinary 60 sensito-meter dry plate and 10 to 12 inch spark coil."[30] Another device for measuring the strength of x-rays by regularly graded resistances was the radiochromometer of Benoist (1902), in which a thin disk of silver, 16 mm in diameter and 0.11 mm thick, was surrounded by 12 steps of aluminum of increasing thicknesses. When the penetrometer was placed behind a fluorescent screen, the luminosity of the central silver circle was compared with that of the spin steps of the aluminum ladder to determine the quality of the x-rays.[31] Tousey[32] proposed a unit named for himself that equalled "the X radiance which produces upon an ordinary Kodak film a photographic effect equal to that of one candle-power of incandescent electric light." Kassabian[33] in his 1907 textbook listed six different principles of dosage estimation on which were based 19 different devices, none satisfactory.

Two of the most popular methods for estimating radiation dose were based on the physicochemical effect of x-rays. Sabouraud and Noiré[34] estimated the x-ray dosage by the degree of discoloration of pastilles of barium platinocyanide when exposed to x-rays. The Sabouraud Radiometer consisted simply of a booklet containing these pastilles and two standard tints, one of which corresponded to the unexposed chemical (Tint A) and the other to the epilation dose (Tint B). The Lovibond Tintometer permitted measurement of the pastille color in terms of fractions and multiples of Tint B. "The light from an 8 candle power carbon filament lamp was allowed to fall on a sheet of white paper and on the exposed pastille. The reflected light from the white paper passed through a tinted glass before reaching the eye of the observer, whereas that from the pastille remained unchanged. A series of tinted glasses provided a range of dose values."[35] The pastille method was extremely popular and continued to be used, particularly by dermatologists, well into the 1930s.

The other x-ray unit that depended on a chemical color change was the H-unit of Holtzknecht, who used a fused mixture of potassium chloride and sodium carbonate. The dose could be calculated using a "chromoradiometer" or by visualizing the discoloration of photographic paper.[36] Holtzknecht proposed using a dose termed H, which was based on the color change induced in his chromoradiometer by the amount of radiation sufficient to produce a light skin erythema. Use of this technique was restricted because the nature of the chemicals employed in the chromoradiometer was kept secret.

For radiation therapy, the erythema and epilation doses were the major determinants in judging treatment progress. A popular measurement was the *threshold erythema dose*, defined as "that quantity of radiation which, when delivered at a single sitting, will produce in 80% of all cases tested, a faint reddening or bronzing of the skin, in from two to four weeks after irradiation, and in the remaining 20% will produce no visible effect." Disadvantages of these measurements included the variation in patient response, the dependence on the interpretation of the therapists, and the occasional idiosyncratic insensitivity. It was necessary to perfect the ionization method of measurement to place x-ray dosimetry on a more

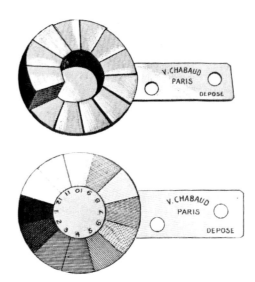

Benoist radiochromometer (1902). *Top,* Variations in thickness of aluminum. *Bottom,* Measurement of x-ray intensity.[31]

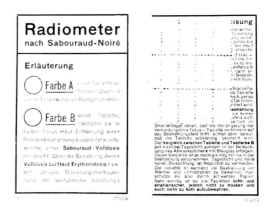

Radiometer of Sabouraud and Noiré (1904).[34]

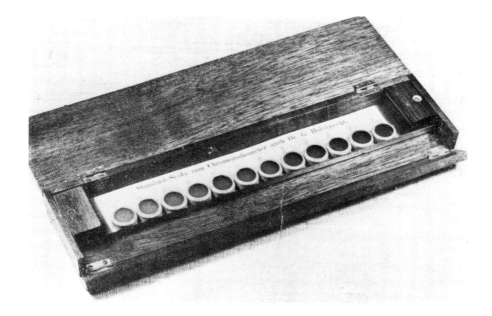

Holzknecht chromoradiometer (1902).[3]

solid scientific basis. The introduction of milliampere meters in the secondary circuit, according to the principle of d'Arsonval (1903), made it possible to control with greater accuracy the mechanical factors influencing x-ray dosage. On the basis of these controllable factors, various formulas were developed by which the intensity output could be determined or calculated. By means of spark-gap measurements, potential was estimated fairly accurately; the milliampere meter gave a control of the current, and therapists could then communicate with each other about dosage for the treatment of diseases with some degree of understanding despite known differences in the output of individual apparatus. Experience taught each therapist how to operate his own apparatus safely and efficiently under fixed conditions.[28]

Not long after the discovery of x-rays, there was discussion concerning the possibility of establishing a "unit measure" for dosage based on ionization of gases. In Roentgen's first communication, he pointed out that the new rays would produce ionization.

Succeeding investigators developed a variety of ionization chambers that eventually could accurately determine the quantity of ions produced in a given quantity of air by a specific beam of x-rays. As early as 1908, Villard designed a combination ionization chamber and electrometer scaled in Holtzknecht units. He also proposed a new unit of the quantity of x-rays, which he defined as "that amount which liberates by ionization one electrostatic unit of charge per cc of air at normal temperature and pressure."[37] Incredibly, this definition was little changed by the International Committee that adopted the definition of the "roentgen" 20 years later.

Experimental arrangement to study the ionization of air produced by x-rays (1896).[38]

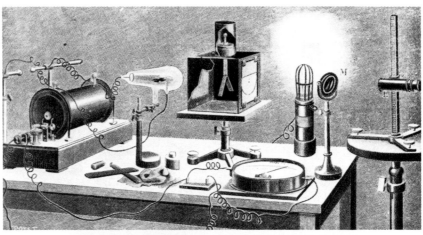

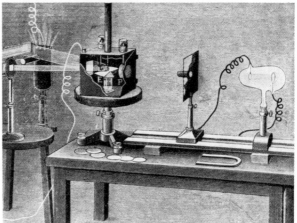

Extensive experiments estimating the ionizing effects of x-rays per unit volume of air under different conditions were performed in physics laboratories with large air chambers that were much too complicated and cumbersome for radiation therapists to use. Therefore it was necessary to devise small, yet dependable, ionization chambers. A major problem was the scattered and characteristic radiation absorbed and created within the metallic walls of the ionization chambers. Eventually, Fricke and Glasser (1924) originated the idea of a small chamber of a material that would not absorb or create more scattered radiation from its walls than air. Their "air wall" chamber, connected by a properly insulated conductor to an electrometer, made it possible to measure radiation more accurately with minimal wall effects.[39]

Investigators in several countries proposed variations in Villard's unit of x-ray dose measurement. This predictably led to substantial confusion, and it became imperative that some standard method of measurement be adopted. Finally, at the Second International Congress of Radiology held in Stockholm in 1928, a dosage unit was established and defined by international agreement. Named for the discoverer of the roentgen rays, the *roentgen* (designated by the letter *r*), was defined as "that dose produced by an amount of Roentgen ray energy which by the radiation of one cubic centimeter of air at 18° Centigrade and a pressure of 760 millimeters of mercury produces such a conductivity, that the quantity of electricity under saturation conditions amounts to one electrostatic unit."

Water-filled "phantoms" were developed to aid in dosage determinations. They were based on the principle that x-rays were absorbed and scattered, and secondary radiation generated, in much the same way whether the medium traversed was water or living tissue. By placing an ionization chamber at a given location in a water-filled phantom at which x-rays were beamed, the amount of radiation (measured in roentgens) reaching a comparable location in the human body under comparable conditions could be determined. "Isodose curves" could be drawn on the basis of these phantom studies to show how the radiation was distributed within the body, and treatments could be planned on the basis of these isodose curves without repeating the measurements in phantoms. Although much of the early work with phantoms was done in Europe, major contributions were provided in the United States by Glasser and Failla.

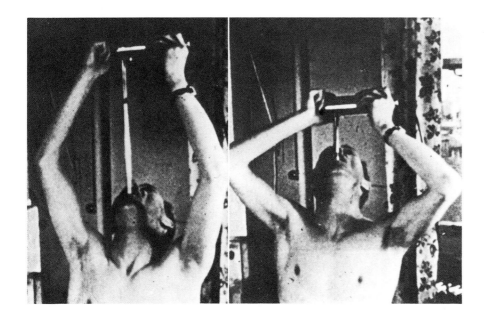

Sword swallower measuring radiation dose.[64]

In addition to the dose of radiation, it was necessary to determine the penetrating character (quality, or "hardness") of x-rays. About 1912, it was learned that the softer rays that penetrated only a short distance into tissue were characterized by relatively long wave lengths and low frequencies. Harder rays, emitted only by tubes operated at a higher voltage, had shorter wave lengths and higher frequencies. Using techniques developed in Europe to directly measure the wave lengths, it became possible to determine what proportion of rays emitted by a given x-ray tube under specific conditions was being emitted in each band of wave lengths.

Although reasonably accurate, these determinations were difficult to perform. A highly practical shortcut, initially proposed by Christen (1912), then came into common use.[40] The amount of radiation reaching a specific region at a given distance from an x-ray tube was first measured in roentgens. Next, the thickness of a filter of a given metal necessary to cut the intensity of the beam in half was determined. For example, if a copper filter 3 mm thick cut the intensity in half, the beam was said to have a *half-value layer* (HVL) of 3 mm of copper. In general, the thicker the layer of filter required to cut the intensity in half, the harder or more penetrating the beam. For practical purposes, the half-value layer could be used instead of the much more cumbersome wave length determination to specify the hardness of x-ray beams.

Combining these two measurements, it became possible for a therapist to specify x-ray dosage with reasonable accuracy by recording the half-value layer of the radiation being used plus the number of roentgens of radiation delivered to the tumor and surrounding tissues as shown by the isodose charts. He could then duplicate the same dosage in other cases, and therapists in other centers could reproduce his method.

An analysis of isodose charts clearly indicated that by increasing the voltage of the x-ray tube and filtering out the softer rays it was possible to increase the dose of radiation that could be delivered to underlying tissues without increasing the skin dose. However, even the heavily filtered beam from an x-ray tube operated at 250 keV could deliver only a relatively small dose to deep tissues without delivering a much larger dose to the skin. Therefore it was necessary to find another mechanism in addition to high-voltage filtration that would increase the relative depth dose without increasing the skin dose.

Quite early it was learned that the simplest way to accomplish this was to increase the distance between the x-ray tube (or radium applicator) and the skin. As the distance between the radiation source and the skin was increased, the number of roentgens that could be delivered to the deeper tissues for a given dose to the skin increased significantly.

A second method of increasing the depth dose without an excessive skin dose was termed *crossfiring*. This technique consisted essentially of beaming radiation at the tumor from two or more angles. For example, the tumor might receive only 40% of the skin dose through one angle, 30% through a second, and 20% through a third. However, when the treatment was completed, the tumor would have received 90% of the skin dose, which might be sufficient to eradicate it without causing substantial damage to the skin. The major disadvantage of crossfiring was the difficulty in limiting the region of overlap (the area receiving radiation from two or more beams) to the tumor itself and to nearby tissues that were not easily damaged. To minimize this limitation, *rotational therapy* was developed. Either the x-ray tube or the radium source was rotated around the patient or, conversely, the patient was rotated in the radiation beam. At least in theory, rotational therapy was roughly the equivalent of crossfiring from an infinite number of angles.

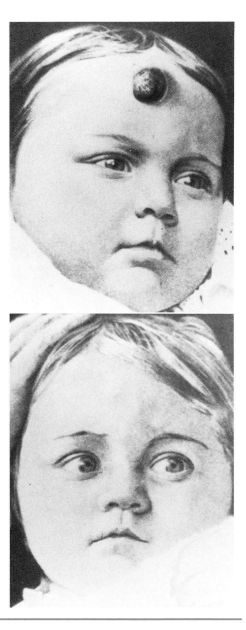

Successful therapy using crossfire technique (1907). *Top,* Initial film shows an erectile angioma projecting 2 cm on the forehead of a 7-month-old infant. *Bottom,* Disappearance of the tumor following therapy.[35]

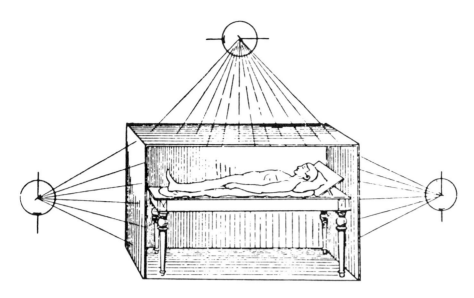

Crossfiring technique. Attempt to deliver homogeneous total body irradiation using a glass box and three x-ray tubes.[35]

Using a culinary example, I. Seth Hirsch (1925)[41] illustrated the theoretical advantages of rotational therapy. If a filtered beam of x-rays was aimed at a roast of beef 8 inches in diameter and the intensity of radiation at the surface (skin) was 118 units, the intensity at the center would be only 5 units. If the tube were rotated around the beef, however, the radiation reaching the center could be doubled (from 5 to 10 units), while simultaneously the radiation to any point on the surface was reduced from 118 units to only 5 units. Although these calculations worked well for slabs of meat, the full advantage of the principles of crossfiring and rotational therapy could not be used in treating living patients until isodose curves became available. By preparing isodose curves for each angle of radiation beamed at the tumor and by using comparable techniques for rotational therapy, the dose of radiation actually delivered to the skin, to each portion of the tumor, and to the nearby organs could be charted on paper in advance.

Dose Fractionation

Even if the physical measurement of x-ray dose could be accurately determined, it still remained difficult to clinically evaluate the biological response to radiation. It soon became apparent that the rate of administration of the radiation was an important consideration. A given dose of radiation delivered in a period of minutes had a quite different effect on both normal and diseased tissue than the same dose delivered more slowly, over a period of many hours. Similarly, a dose delivered in a single day had a different effect than the same dose delivered in small fractions over a period of many days. In general, the slower the rate at which the dose was delivered and the greater the number of days over which it was fractionated, the less damage to skin and other normal tissues and the larger the total dose that could be safely delivered.

Did prolonging and fractionating the dose really improve the results in cancer therapy? Or did the larger total dose made possible by fractionation have less of an effect on cancer cells, just as it did on normal tissues? While this often bitter controversy raged, some therapists delivered massive doses over a short period of time, while others used a prolonged and fractionated dosage schedule.

One theoretical advantage of fractionation was reported by Bergonie and Tribondeau, who in 1906 had shown that immature cells and cells in an active state of division were more sensitive to radiation than other cells. This led to the hypothesis that the damage done to cells by radiation occurred during a particular phase of cell division. If this were true, the problem of killing *all* of the cells in a cancer might resolve itself into the problem of radiating over a long enough period so that all of the cells divided during the time of irradiation.

In 1919, Claude Regaud and co-workers[42] at the Foundation Curie in Paris performed a classic series of experiments in which they convincingly demonstrated that spermatogenesis in the testes of experimental animals could be permanently eradicated by the administration of successive daily doses of fractionated radiotherapy, whereas single massive doses failed to elicit the same biological response without permanent and often intolerable injury to the overlying skin. Regaud hypothesized that the testis, with its high rate of cell turnover, might mimic some aspects of the growth of a malignant neoplasm. Consequently, he and a colleague, Henri Coutard, applied the dose fractionation technique to the treatment of head and neck cancers, while others began using this approach for treating cancer of the cervix. Within a few years, several groups began reporting such impressive 5-year survival rates that dose fractionating became a universally acceptable technique that persists to the present day.[21]

A second rationale for fractionation was well stated by George T. Pack,[43] who wrote (1935) that "the advantages of prolonged irradiation of low intensity or fractionated cumulative treatments are probably explained by the differential recuperation of normal and neoplastic (cancer) tissues. Presumably normal tissues have much greater power of recuperation than do neoplastic tissues, i.e., their rate of recuperation is faster." Therefore if the doses were properly fractionated, normal tissues might be able to recover between treatments while cancer tissues were continually destroyed.

Staging, Grading, and Size of Tumors

As radiation therapy techniques improved, it was difficult to determine which of several various approaches was most effective. At least 5 years were required to determine whether a malignancy would recur following apparently successful radiation therapy. However, during these years changes in equipment and other factors might well make the results of a study irrelevant. In addition, large numbers of patients were required before any firm conclusions could be drawn as to the effectiveness of a specific therapeutic approach. Eventually, it was realized that in addition to the method of therapy and the amount of x-ray dose, the success of radiation treatment depended on characteristics of the tumor itself.

If the cancer were limited to a single, clearly delineated site, the chances of radiation therapy being successful were high. However, if the tumor had already metastasized to other areas, the chances of cure were greatly diminished. Efforts were made to irradiate adjacent lymph nodes and other areas to which cancer cells were most likely to spread. Although these techniques proved successful in some cases, metastatic cancer cells lodged in lymph nodes were usually more resistant to radiation than those in the primary tumor. However, a simple division of tumors into those that had metastasized and those that had not proved inadequate. This led to a system of classifying tumors into four "stages."

Although staging permitted a more realistic appraisal of the effectiveness of a specific therapeutic regimen, it further complicated the evaluation of radiation results. A higher cure rate reported from one medical center did not necessarily mean that its radiation techniques were superior. It might merely reflect that the hospital was treating patients at an earlier stage in their disease. The only valid comparisons were based on the stage of the cancer in each case—but this meant a further delay in evaluation while sufficient cases in each stage were accumulated.

It was soon learned that even those tumors in the same stage of development did not respond uniformly to radiation therapy. This led to the introduction of a grading system for tumors. In general, tumors composed of cells that multiplied only slowly and were unlikely to metastasize were relatively resistant to radiation. Conversely, tumors composed of malignant cells that multiplied rapidly and were likely to spread tended to be most responsive when exposed to even modest doses of x-rays or radium. By examining a group of cells under the microscope, their grade of malignancy could be roughly estimated. This could be used as a major criterion in the choice between surgical and radiation therapy. However, the grading of tumors introduced further problems. An individual tumor could be graded differently depending on which particular group of cells within it happened to be selected for microscopic examination. Similarly, biopsies obtained from different areas could result in different grading on microscopic examination. In addition, some tumors whose microscopic appearance suggested high malignancy, and therefore sensitivity to radiation, proved to be radiation-resistant when therapy was given.

The need to master vast quantities of information concerning the life histories of particular types of tumor at specific sites inevitably led to increased specialization. Radiation therapists tended to devote themselves to treating tumors of a limited area, and textbooks came to be organized in chapters by tumor site. While individual physicians in small hospitals continued to use x-rays and radium in the treatment of malignant conditions, the best results were increasingly achieved in the major cancer centers in which an array of therapists, each specializing in his own anatomical region, had available the ever-widening range of equipment and knowledge relevant to his particular subspecialty.

Another important factor in the success of radiation therapy was the size of the cancer mass. Subclinical disease, which was not necessarily microscopic disease but also included aggregates of cancer cells in accessible areas that could not be palpated, would be expected to be more radiosensitive than gross masses. Studies showed that irradiation was most effective in controlling microscopic disease and small-volume cancer. Indeed, in some clinical situations the use of interstitial or intracavitary x-ray therapy to boost external irradiation doses could permit control of moderately large-volume cancer with radiation alone. Conversely, although surgery was effective in removing gross cancer (provided that the tumor was resectable), it too often failed to remove the diffuse microscopic disease around the primary mass regardless of how radical the procedure. Therefore the two disciplines could often be used in a complementary mode—surgery to remove gross cancer and irradiation preoperatively or postoperatively to eradicate the microscopic disease around the gross mass. Because the surgical goal was to remove only gross disease, there was no longer a need to perform the classic radical surgical procedures, such as radical neck dissection or radical mastectomy. Less radical surgery decreased the probability of forcing viable cancer cells into the bloodstream. When combined with modest doses of irradiation, more conservative surgical procedures could leave the organs and tissues intact, or at least less mutilated, thereby allowing the patient a better quality of life.[44]

SUPERVOLTAGE THERAPY

Throughout the 1920s, the 200,000-volt Coolidge x-ray tube was standard equipment for "deep" radiation therapy. Although radiologists would have preferred x-rays of even higher voltage, these were not easy to produce. As Coolidge explained (1928), "Early in our work on the hot-cathode high-vacuum x-ray tube we were made conscious of a certain limitation. Such a tube behaved consistently only so long as a certain applied voltage was not exceeded. When this voltage *was* exceeded, current flowed through the tube even when the cathode was not heated." This cold-cathode effect "sets a limit to the voltage which can be used on a given tube, for if one attempts to appreciably raise voltage in spite of it, he either punctures the tube, through the local heating attending bombardment of the glass, or gets a runaway arc discharge, through bombardment of the anode."[45]

To solve this problem, Coolidge (1926) developed a new "cascade" tube that was built in sections. An electron leaving the cathode went through several of these sections en route to the anode. With each section operating at 250,000 or even 300,000 volts, a three-section tube might reach 900,000 volts without the need for a potential in excess of 300,000 volts at any single point in its interior.[46]

Coolidge indicated that his new high-voltage tube held promise for nuclear research, as well as for radiology. He claimed that using such a tube it would prove relatively easy to produce x-rays as penetrating as the gamma rays from radium and that it might even be possible to produce electrons at 3 million volts, equivalent to the beta rays from radium. Moreover "the capacity or quantity factor would be tremendously in our favor, as with 12 milliamperes of current we would have as many high-speed electrons coming from the tube as from a *ton* of radium." Neverthe-

Coolidge cascade tube (1928). *Left*, Two-section tube for 600,000 volts attached to exhaust system and connected to a No. 2 unit induction coil, with sphere-gap overhead for measuring voltage. *Right*, Three-section tube for 900,000 volts.[45]

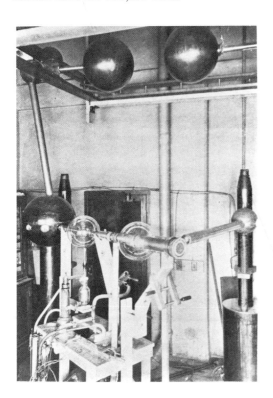

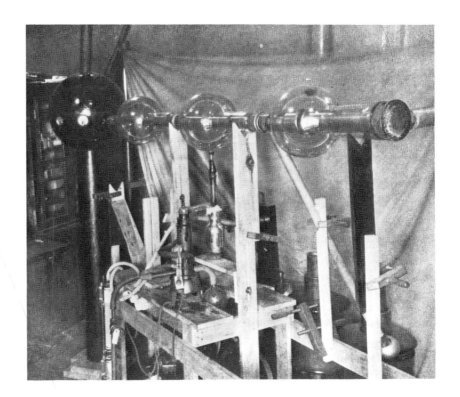

less, there were some practical difficulties. Even though Coolidge's three-section tube was nearly 11 feet long, the glass still was occasionally punctured by runaway cold-cathode currents. To maintain the extremely high vacuum, a vacuum pump attached to the tube had to be kept in continuous operation while the current was on. Because Coolidge used an induction coil producing alternating current as a source of high voltage, the maximum voltage was only achieved at the peak of each cycle. In addition, Coolidge's tube was producing high-voltage *electrons* but not x-rays. Further engineering was needed to focus the electrons on a target and to devise a target capable of withstanding bombardment by 900,000-volt electrons.

At the California Institute of Technology, the Southern California Edison Company had established a high-voltage laboratory to study problems of long-distance electric power transmission. In 1925, an engineer in this laboratory, R. W. Sorenson, had cascaded four 250,000-volt transformers to produce a peak potential of 1 million volts. Using this transformer array, Charles C. Lauritsen (1928) produced 750,000-volt x-rays that "can be observed by means of a fluoroscope at a distance of 100 meters (328 feet)."[47] Unfortunately, this transformer array caused severe problems for the practicing radiologist. It occupied a room 138 feet long and 64 feet wide. Even though the ceiling was 50 feet high, one of the four transformers had to be placed in a pit to get sufficient overhead clearance. The tube was made of four glass cylinders, "each 12 inches in diameter and 28 inches long, of the kind used in gasoline dispensing pumps." To support his tube, Lauritsen found it necessary to erect "a tower 14 feet high and 8 feet square at the base, constructed of redwood timber crossed and braced to give rigidity." As with Coolidge's tube, Lauritsen's tube required continuous pumping to maintain the vacuum and only achieved maximum power during the peak of each alternating-current cycle.

A new approach to supervoltage production was developed by Robert J. Van de Graaff. In preliminary trials, this electrostatic generator produced spark-gap measurements showing a potential of approximately 1,500,000 volts. "The generator has the basic advantage of supplying a direct steady potential, thus eliminating certain difficulties inherent in the application of non-steady (alternating-current or pulsating-current) high potentials. The machine is simple, inexpensive, and portable. An ordinary lamp socket furnishes the only power needed."[48]

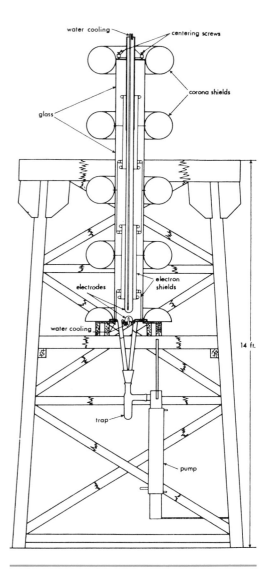

Lauritsen's 750,000-volt unit (1928).[47]

Van de Graaff's supervoltage unit. *Left*, Overview showing relative size of the unit. *Right*, Diagram of internal workings. *P*, Positive spherical terminal; *N*, negative spherical terminal.[48]

ELECTROSTATIC GENERATORS

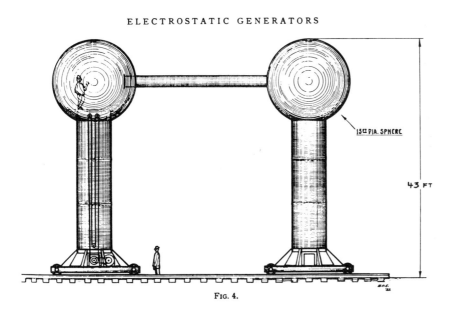

FIG. 4.

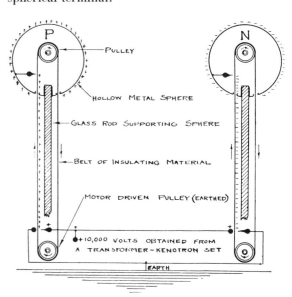

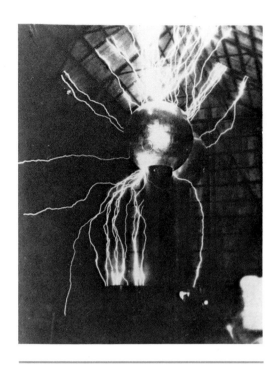

Original Van de Graaff electrostatic generator in a sparkling demonstration (1932).[49]

Van de Graaff's curious device consisted essentially of two hollow copper spheres, each 24 inches in diameter, mounted on two upright Pyrex pedestals 7 feet tall. A continuous silk belt, mounted on two pulleys, ran up and down each pedestal at 3,500 feet per minute. These "conveyer belts" were run by a toy motor. The lower pulleys were grounded. An array of metal points (Van de Graaff used phonograph needles) sprayed electrons and other negatively charged ions onto one of the conveyer belts. The belt carried the negative ions to the top of the pedestal, where another set of points picked them off for storage on the surface of the copper sphere. Simultaneously, a second set of points was spraying protons and other positively charged ions onto the second belt, and these were being simultaneously carried up and stored on the second sphere. Since each sphere could be charged to 750,000 volts, a potential of 1.5 million volts could be built up between them.[48]

As with other supervoltage generators, Van de Graaff's electrostatic generator was soon plagued by growing size and rising costs. For example, a model described for Van de Graaff's new position at the Massachusetts Institute of Technology was too large to be built there and had to be constructed in an air ship hangar 140 feet long, 75 feet wide, and 75 feet high.[50] The "mobility" of the device was a relative term, since it was mounted on wide railroad trucks and a quarter of a mile of track with rails 14 feet apart (donated by the New Haven Railroad) was laid into the hangar so that the device could be wheeled in and out on the trucks. Nevertheless, this generator was completed in 1934 and achieved a potential of 7 million volts. However, there still was need to create an x-ray tube capable of handling that much energy.

The next addition to the supervoltage sweepstakes was the work of Ernest O. Lawrence at the University of California at Berkeley. While browsing casually through some physics journals in the University library, Lawrence in 1929 came across a paper by a European physicist, Rolf Wideroe, that described how a 25,000-volt potential could be used twice to produce 50,000-volt particles in a discharge tube. Like Coolidge, Wideroe divided his tube into sections, but he did not connect his intermediate electrode to the middle tap of his power supply. Instead, he applied the whole voltage twice—once as the particle was moving through the gap between electrodes in the first section and again as it was moving through the gap in the second section. A high-frequency alternating potential was used, and the circuits were arranged so that the electrical potential changed polarity in just the time that it took the particle to pass from gap to gap. Thus the two "pushes" received by the particle were in the same direction.

Lawrence soon developed variations on Wideroe's promising technique and set his graduate students to work on several of them. One student, David H. Sloan, developed a process for accelerating particles through a series of 10 cylindrical electrodes mounted in line inside a discharge tube. In 1930, Sloan and Lawrence reported on a linear accelerator of this kind that accelerated particles by means of 30 successive electrodes.[51] Subsequent technical improvements, mainly at Stanford University after World War II, resulted in the development of linear accelerators of 20 million volts for radiation therapy and 50 million volts for electron beam therapy. In 1966, Stanford placed in operation a huge linear accelerator 2 miles long that accelerated electrons to energies as high as 20 *billion* volts for physical research.

Now that supervoltage x-rays could be produced, it was unknown what effect they would have on tumors and other human tissues. Lauritsen at the California Institute of Technology realized that "the radiation produced by this tube might have some biological effect which could be utilized in the treatment of disease." He invited Albert Soiland, a prominent Los Angeles radiologist, to bring some of his patients to the Institute for experimental clinical tests. The initial results were extremely favorable, but Soiland realized that the cost of equipment and accessories would "be prohibitive for the average radiologist even to consider. It would be more feasible for centralized institutions, geographically selected to serve their respective communities—preferably the larger hospitals having suitable clinical and physical facilities."[52] One year later (1933), patients at the Institute were being treated at 1 million volts using a 30-foot-long tube that was made of porcelain instead of glass and contained four ports through which four different patients could be treated simultaneously.

Meanwhile in New York, General Electric installed a two-section Coolidge cascade tube and associated supervoltage power supply at Memorial Hospital in New York under the joint control of biophysicist, Gioacchino Failla, and radiation therapist, Edith H. Quimby. They performed extensive tests, not only to determine the characteristics of the 700,000-volt x-ray beam from the new apparatus, but also to compare this beam with the beam from conventional 200,000-volt x-ray units and with the gamma-ray beam from a 44-gm pack of radium.

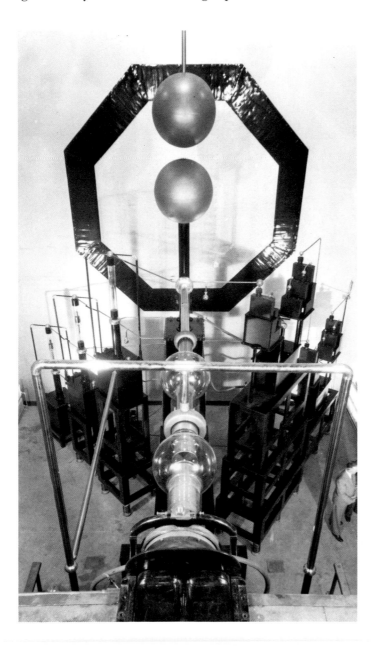

800,000-volt therapy unit at Mercy Hospital in Chicago.

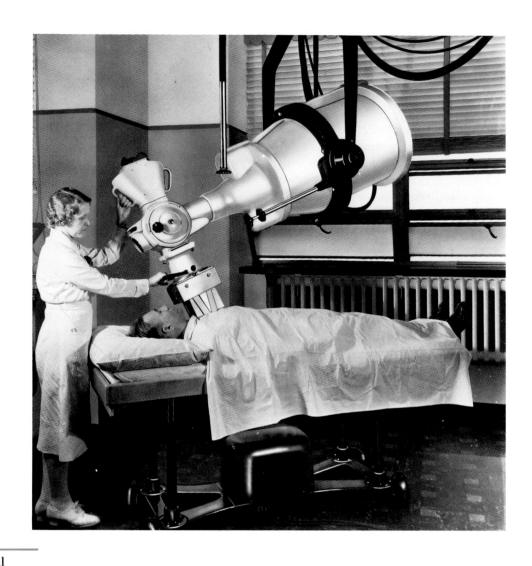

250,000-volt therapy unit at Memorial
Hospital, New York.

The results of the Memorial Hospital experiments clearly indicated
that supervoltage could have an advantage in actual clinical practice.
However, they also threw the entire concept of x-ray dosage into complete
disarray.

Failla, Quimby, and their associates[53] tried to measure in roentgens
the three kinds of radiation. Using several different types of ionization
chambers, they got utterly inconsistent results. The number of roentgens
varied with the size of the chamber and the material of which it was made.
Similarly, when comparing the effects of the three kinds of radiation on
five different radiation-sensitive chemical solutions and on photographic
films with and without intensifying screens, they found that "the *apparent*
radiation emission . . . varies with the chemicals and reactions which
are used to determine it." At least the biological measures of relative
effectiveness were generally consistent. The relative biological effectiveness of 700,000-volt radiation on fruit-fly eggs, wheat seedlings, mouse
tails, and rabbit ears fell somewhere between the effectiveness of
200,000-volt radiation and of gamma radiation from radium. However,
tests on human skin, which also were internally consistent, were quite
inconsistent with the comparison made on other biological substrates.

In summarizing the Memorial Hospital findings, Failla stressed that the question was not whether one kind of ray is more effective than another in killing cancer cells, but whether a wider margin of difference between the effect on cancer cells and on surrounding tissue could be secured at one voltage than at another. Although the results indicated that a wider margin of difference was at least possible with supervoltage radiation, the findings also indicated that it would be much more difficult than expected to precisely determine the margin of difference at various voltages.

As the Brechers[63] concluded:

Thus, far from leading radiation therapy into the promised land, the preliminary Memorial findings in a sense made it seem even more distant. Before the Memorial results were announced, radiologists dealt with what they thought was a complex art, requiring considerations of dose measurement, dose fractionation, filtration, skin-target distance, multiple portals, and other variables. However, the variables were at least *measurable,* and radiologists believed that they had one rock on which to stand: the roentgen. To paraphrase Gertrude Stein, "A roentgen was a roentgen was a roentgen"—until 1932. Now the rock had turned to quicksand. The effect of a 1-roentgen dose delivered to fruit-fly eggs was not the same as one delivered to human skin. A 1-roentgen dose delivered at 700,000 volts differed from one delivered at 200,000 volts. Indeed, a roentgen was seen not to be a measure of dosage at all. Worst of all, a roentgen measured with one device was not the same as a roentgen measured with another. The already complex art of radiation therapy had suddenly become vastly *more* complex. More than a quarter-century was to be required to re-establish firm physical and biological foundations for the art of radiation therapy.

Several modifications of existing supervoltage units were soon made. David Sloan (of Lawrence's laboratory at Berkeley) developed a high-frequency variation of Lawrence's cyclotron that consisted essentially of a cylindrical vacuum tank only 40 inches high and 42 inches in diameter, in which were lodged both the high-energy source and a radiofrequency x-ray generator. The tank itself functioned as the x-ray tube. The lack of high voltage anywhere outside the tank was a major safety factor.

In Boston, John G. Trump[49] developed a relatively small variation of the Van de Graaff generator that was housed in a steel tank filled with compressed nitrogen and carbon dioxide for insulation and could fit in a room only 25 × 23 feet with a ceiling 20 feet high. Traian Leucutia in Detroit was the first to use a radiation therapy unit assembled by the Kelley-Koett Company that was similar in conception to the device with which Cockroft and Walton had first "split the atom" that same year (1932). Subsequently, Leucutia and co-workers produced a series of scholarly papers that not only reported on findings made with this apparatus but also comprehensively reviewed supervoltage developments elsewhere.

The next development in high-voltage technology was the betatron, or *electron accelerator,* first devised by Donald W. Kerst in 1940.[54] This relatively compact device consisted of an evacuated "donut," in which electrons, guided by a carefully shaped, pulsating magnetic field, were accelerated in circular orbits as if they were travelling through the secondary coil of a transformer. Since there was no physical transformer, there were no problems of insulation or heating nor was it necessary first to achieve a high potential and then apply it to the electrons. Instead, the

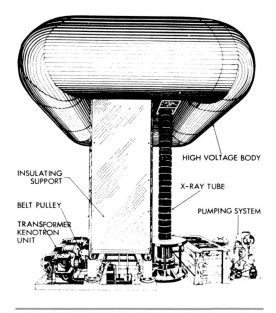

Trump variant of the Van de Graaff generator.[49]

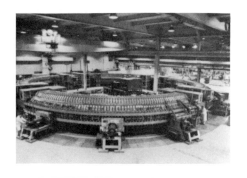

Synchrotron. 3 BeV proton synchrotron, placed in operation in 1952, was surrounded by a row of concrete blocks to protect the operators.

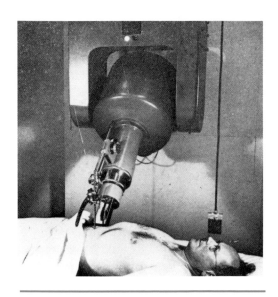

First cobalt-60 radiation therapy unit (1951).

high potential was generated in the circling electrons directly. Within 3 years (1943), Kerst described a 20 million–volt model designed for radiation therapy.

Although the climb toward higher x-ray energies stalled during World War II, it gained a new impetus once the conflict ended. The synchrotron, which resembled the betatron, was a new device in which electrons were brought to high energy by successive applications of radiofrequency energy. The initial synchrotron principle was conceived independently by V. Veksler in the Soviet Union and slightly later by E. N. McMillan at the Los Alamos Laboratory in New Mexico.[55] The chief advantage of the synchrotron was its lesser size and weight. By 1956, a 70 million–volt electron synchrotron was produced by General Electric for Robert Stone at the University of California Hospital in San Francisco.

Following World War II there was renewed interest (especially at Stanford University) in linear accelerators. In 1956, Henry Kaplan[21] treated the first patient using a 6 million–volt unit. Six years later (1962), linear accelerators were produced that were so compact that they could be rotated a full 360 degrees around a reclining patient. The high-energy beams produced their maximal ionization at significant depths below the skin surface, thus effectively eliminating the radiation tolerance of the skin as a dose-limiting factor. The beams had sharply defined, knifelike edges that greatly diminished lateral scatter and permitted treatment of small lesions in the eye, larynx, and other sites in close proximity to vital structures.[58] Because the penetration of these high-energy beams was so much greater than that of orthovoltage x-rays, it became relatively easy to deliver tumoricidal doses to neoplasms deep within the body, even in obese patients. The high-beam intensity also permitted its use at much longer target-patient distances, thus allowing larger fields to be treated in which multiple areas of tumor involvement could be encompassed contiguously. Taken together, all of these advantages greatly increased the versatility and precision of modern radiation therapy, and the linear accelerator has increasingly become the predominant treatment modality.[21,56]

The third major development following World War II was the introduction of radioisotopes, particularly cobalt-60, as sources of powerful gamma-ray beams for radiation therapy. Although cobalt-60 emitted gamma rays at two specific energy levels (1.17 and 1.35 million volts), since the beam from a cobalt-60 radiation therapy unit lacked the "softer" rays present in beams from x-ray tubes, a cobalt-60 beam was roughly equivalent in hardness to the filtered beam from a 2 or even 3 million–volt x-ray tube.[59] Another radioisotope, cesium-137, also was used in therapy units. During the 1950s and 1960s, these isotope-powered units became by far the most popular sources of supervoltage radiation for therapy. They were installed in hospitals of moderate size and even in radiologists' offices, as well as in large medical centers. As William T. Moss[15] of Chicago wrote, the availability of cobalt-60 equipment was "a major stimulus to radiation therapy. For the first time we had a readily available beam with good percentage depth dose, good skin and bone sparing. No longer were intense skin irritations a prerequisite to the adequate irradiation of many of the deeply situated cancers. Thus the reaction was less for the patient and the technique of treating the patient was easier for the radiologist."

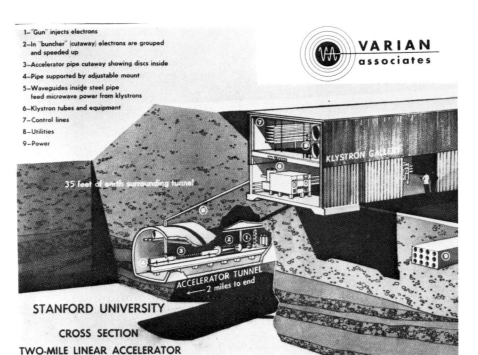

1—"Gun" injects electrons

2—In "buncher" (cutaway) electrons are grouped and speeded up

3—Accelerator pipe cutaway showing discs inside

4—Pipe supported by adjustable mount

5—Waveguides inside steel pipe feed microwave power from klystrons

6—Klystron tubes and equipment

7—Control lines

8—Utilities

9—Power

VARIAN
associates

35 feet of earth surrounding tunnel

KLYSTRON GALLERY

ACCELERATOR TUNNEL
← 2 miles to end

STANFORD UNIVERSITY

CROSS SECTION

TWO-MILE LINEAR ACCELERATOR

Stanford linear accelerator (cutaway view).

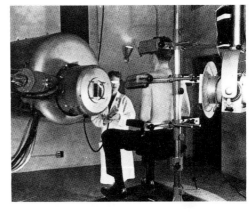

Stanford Medical Linear Accelerator. This 6 MeV unit, shown with rotational stand and image-intensifier beam control, was the first used in the Western Hemisphere.[57]

CLINICAL EFFECTS OF SUPERVOLTAGE

Was supervoltage therapy worth the trouble and expense? Some argued that the larger "depth dose" (i.e., higher dose delivered to a deep-lying tumor as compared with the dose delivered to the skin) of supervoltage units could also be achieved by moving the patient farther away from the conventional x-ray tube and increasing the degree of filtration of "soft" x-rays.

A major problem was that "supervoltage" was not a single entity. Biological effects and clinical results were different, depending on the specific voltage, quality of the beam, and tumor site. It was shown that two machines operating at what appeared to be the same voltage did not necessarily produce an identical beam quality. For example, a unit operating on alternating current produced x-rays of maximum voltage only at the peak of each cycle, whereas even the machine operating on direct

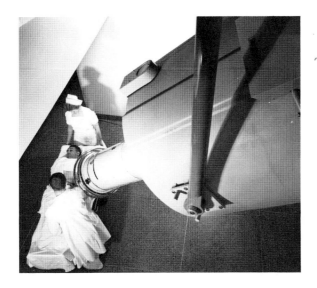

200,000-volt therapy unit at Roswell Park in Buffalo.

current with steady input generated x-rays at all voltages up to the voltage of the electrons striking the target. Thus beams from an x-ray machine could not be compared volt-for-volt with the relatively homogeneous gamma rays from radium, cobalt-60, or other radioisotopes. The specific tumor site was also an important factor. For skin cancer, supervoltage therapy often was substantially poorer than conventional radiation therapy. For deep-seated tumors, the histological type was a critical determinant, and it was necessary to accumulate experience at various voltages for tumors of each type and at each site and for their metastases.

A major problem was the difficulty in comparing doses of various radiation therapy units. The roentgen, which was merely a physical measurement based on the amount of ionization produced in air, proved to be woefully inadequate for evaluating supervoltage dosages, since at these energy levels substantial amounts of radiation might pass right through a tissue with negligible ionizing effect. Consequently, it was necessary to introduce a new unit (the *rad*), which was defined in terms of the energy *absorbed* by a gram of tissue from a given beam of radiation.

Rad for rad, did x-rays at higher voltages have greater biological effects? For most practical purposes, numerous experiments proved that the answer was no. Surprisingly, in some tissues x-rays of several million volts turned out to have a slightly lower biological effect. This made it necessary to introduce the concept of *relative biological effectiveness* (RBE) for each type of radiation. Unfortunately, even RBE was a variable concept. For example, the RBE of one beam might be higher than that of another when measured in terms of the effect on wheat seeds but lower when measured in insect eggs, human skin, human fat, human muscle, or human bone. This led to the development of yet another new unit for comparing radiation effects—the *rem*, defined as the dose in rads multiplied by the RBE for man.

As with conventional radiation therapy, a knowledge of the x-ray dose was not sufficient to predict the clinical results in patients. The rate at which the dose was delivered and the fractionation of the dose over a period of days or weeks were important determining factors.

An unexpected problem with the use of supervoltage was the relative absence of skin effects. When using 200,000-volt x-rays, radiologists had learned to gauge the deeper effects by observing the appearance of reddening, tanning, and other skin effects. As long as the skin was not severely damaged, no irreparable damage to underlying tissues was likely. However, because of the "skin-sparing" effect of supervoltage, serious damage to mucous membranes, nerve cells, intestinal lining, and other deep tissues might develop without prior warning from the skin reaction. As with conventional therapy, this led to an emphasis on the use of multiple fields and rotational therapy so that the tumor could be irradiated as heavily and uniformly as possible without delivering too much of a dose to sensitive neighboring structures.

The availability of supervoltage raised the question of the ultimate aim of cancer therapy. If a complete cure was extremely unlikely, should the x-ray dose be decreased to achieve a good palliative effect with minimal patient discomfort, even at the sacrifice of a small chance of cure? What chance of cure was high enough that higher dosages should be risked even at the expense of patient comfort? And how should the chances be calculated for each patient, each tumor, and each type of radiation?

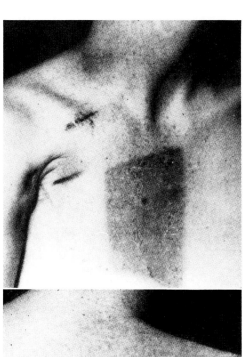
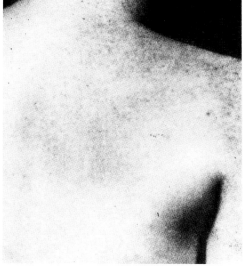

Comparison of skin reactions (1957). Following radical mastectomy for breast cancer, the patient received 140 kVp x-ray therapy to the anterior chest (internal mammary nodes), while the supraclavicular region was treated with the linear accelerator. *Top,* Entry portal shows moist dermatitis with nearly complete denudation of the epithelium in the orthovoltage therapy region. There is essentially no skin reaction at the site of entrance of the beam from the linear accelerator. *Bottom,* First-degree erythema at the exit portal of the linear accelerator beam.[58]

PARTICLES IN THERAPY

High-voltage generating equipment also produced neutrons and protons that could be used for therapeutic purposes.

Neutron beams were produced by Lawrence's cyclotron at Berkeley. It was shown that neutron ionization, in comparison with the effects of x-rays, was far more localized and thus much more intense where it occurred. Initial experiments showed that a dose of neutrons could kill as many tumor cells as an x-ray dose four or five times greater. The crucial question, however, was whether the therapeutic margin between effects on cancer cells and normal tissues was wider for neutrons than x-rays.

The initial experiments on the effect of neutron beam therapy on humans was performed under the clinical auspices of Robert S. Stone in San Francisco. Although the neutron beam clearly had significant tumoricidal properties, instead of widening the therapeutic margin between the effect on cancer cells and the effect on surrounding tissue, when neutrons were used the margin appeared to be almost nonexistent. Stone concluded, "Neutron therapy . . . has resulted in such bad sequelae in proportion to the few good results that it should not be continued."

In an effort to find new treatment modalities with radiobiological properties that may be superior to conventional x-ray and gamma irradiation for the management of certain human cancers, several institutions have initiated clinical trials of fast-neutron therapy. However, this remains an investigational technique.[60]

Because x-ray beams entering living tissue liberate electrons that produce most of the biological effect, perhaps it would be better to beam electrons themselves into tissues. In 1926, Coolidge[45] had reported a cathode-ray tube with an extremely thin metal window (like the Lenard tube), through which electrons at voltages up to 250,000 volts could escape. Although Coolidge noted that these electrons had destructive effects on a variety of insects and plants, subsequent studies showed that electrons of less than 1 million volts did not penetrate deeply enough to be of much practical value. In Germany, Brasch and Lange (1934) performed the first electron-beam therapy. However, this technique was essentially untried in the United States, even though enormous quantities of 1.5 million–volt electrons could readily be extracted from a Van de Graaff machine. These electrons were essentially "monoenergetic"; since they all carried approximately the same energy, they would therefore produce ionization at approximately the same depth and theoretically spare deeper tissues below a tumor from radiation damage.

Subsequent studies at multiple centers using electrons up to 40 million volts produced by betatrons and linear accelerators showed that "advantages of electron radiation include easy manipulation, convenient adjustment of the depth of penetration of radiation, absence of increased bone dose, and satisfactory dose distribution in most cases." However, disadvantages included limitation of field size to 24 × 24 cm and problems in setting up multiple fields without "hot spots," "cold spots," and overlapping. Early studies also demonstrated frequent severe skin reactions, which could be decreased using complex pulsed-scanning beams. Electron beam therapy is currently used in some centers in situations not satisfactorily managed by photon beam therapy alone, such as the irradiation of large areas of potentially infiltrated skin, in lateralized lesions to spare destruction of the opposite side, and in patients who have undergone radical mastectomy or radical neck dissection.[61]

Bibliography

Brecher E and Brecher R: The rays: A history of radiology in the United States and Canada. Baltimore, Williams & Wilkins, 1969.

References

1. Johnson W and Merrill WH: The x-rays in the treatment of carcinoma. Phila Med J 6: 1089-1091, 1900.
2. Gamlen H: Arch Roentgen Ray 9: Plate CXCVIII, 1904.
3. Pizon P: Les origines de la roentgen thérapie en France. Presse Médicale 61:282-283, 1953.
4. Monell HS: A system of instruction in x-ray methods and medical uses of light, hot-air, vibration and high frequency currents. New York, Pelton, 1902.
5. Holland CT: Arch Roentgen Ray 3: Plate LXIII, 1898.
6. Tousey MR: Medical electricity and röntgen rays. Philadelphia, WB Saunders, 1910.
7. Sequeira AB: Arch Roentgen Ray 5: Plate CVI, 1900.
8. Williams FH: The roentgen rays in medicine and surgery. New York, MacMillan, 1901.
9. Pusey WA and Caldwell EW: The practical application of roentgen rays in therapeutics and diagnosis. Philadelphia, WB Saunders, 1904.
10. Martin JM: Practical electro-therapeutics and x-ray therapy. St. Louis, CV Mosby, 1912.
11. Pfahler GE: The early history of roentgenology in Philadelphia. AJR 75:14-22, 1956.
12. Burrows EH: Pioneers and early years: A history of British radiology. Channel Islands, England, Colophon, 1986.
13. Lederman M: The early history of radiotherapy: 1895-1939. Radiation Oncology Biol Phys 7:639-648, 1981.
14. Leucutia T: Roentgen therapy. AJR 76: 1002-1005, 1956.
15. Moss WT: Your radiologist 2:9-10, 1968.
16. Freund L: Elements of general radiotherapy for practitioners. New York, Rebman, 1904.
17. Allen SW: Philadelphia Med J 6:1089-1091, 1900.
18. Edison TA, Morton WJ, Campbell-Swinton AA, and Stanton TW: Discussion: The effect of x-rays upon the eyes. Nature 53:421, 1896.
19. Astudillo F: Los rayos roentgen y los ciegos. Am X-ray J:112-121, November 1897.
20. Case JT: History of radiation therapy. In Buschke F (ed): Progress in radiation therapy. New York, Grune & Stratton, 1958.
21. Kaplan H: Historic milestones in radiobiology and radiation therapy. Semin Oncology 6:479-489, 1979.
22. Grubbé EH: X-ray treatment, its origin, birth and early history. St. Paul, Minn, Bruce Publishing Company, 1949.
23. Hodges PC: The life and times of Emil H. Grubbé. Chicago, University of Chicago Press, 1964.
24. Ewing J: Early experiences in radiation therapy. AJR 31:153-163, 1934.
25. Case JT: Some early experiences in therapeutic radiology: Formation of the American Radium Society. AJR 70:487-491, 1953.
26. Trout ED: History of radiation sources for cancer therapy. In Buschke F (ed): Progress in radiation therapy. New York, Grune & Stratton, 1958.
27. Bergonie J and Tribondeau L: Interpretation of some results of radiotherapy. Compt Rend Acad de Sci 143:983-985, 1906.
28. Portmann UV: Roentgen therapy. In Glasser O (ed): The science of radiology. Springfield, Ill, Charles C Thomas, 1933.
29. Beck C: Roentgen-ray diagnosis and therapy. New York, Appleton, 1904.
30. Kolle FS: A new x-ray meter. Elect Engineer 22:602, 1896.
31. Benoist L: Experimental definition of various types of x-rays by the radiochromator. CR Acad Sciences (Paris) 134:225.
32. Tousey S: A new unit of x-ray power. Arch Roentgen Ray 18:427-433, 1914.
33. Kassabian NK: Electrotherapeutics and roentgen rays. Philadelphia, JB Lippincott, 1908.
34. Sabouraud R and Noire H: Traitement des teignes fondantes par rayons X. Presse Med 12:825-827, 1904.
35. Mould RF: A history of x-rays and radium. 1980.
36. Holzknecht G: A chromo-radiometer. Fortschr Roentgenstr 4:1-4, 1902.
37. Villard P: The radiosclerometer. Arch Elect Med 14:692-699, 1908.
38. Benoist L and Hurmuzescu D: New properties of the x-rays. CR Acad Sci (Paris) 122: 235, 1896.
39. Fricke H and Glasser O: The secondary electrons produced by hard x-rays in light elements. Proc Nat Acad Sci 10:441-443, 1924.
40. Christen T: An absolute measure for the quality of roentgen rays and its use in roentgen therapy. Verhandl Deutsch Roent Gesellsch 13:119-122, 1912.
41. Hirsch IS: Principles and practice of roentgen therapy. New York, American X-ray Publishing Co, 1925.
42. Regaud C: Sur les principes radiophysiologiques de la radiothérapie des cancers. Acta Radiol 11:456-486, 1930.
43. Pack GT: The principles governing the radiation therapy of cancer. AJR 36:233-244, 1936.
44. Fletcher GH: The evolution of the basic concepts underlying the practice of radiotherapy from 1949 to 1977. Radiology 127:319, 1978.
45. Coolidge WD: Cathode-ray and roentgen-ray work in progress. AJR 19:313-321, 1928.
46. Coolidge WD: Use of very high-voltage in vacuum tubes. J Amer Inst Elect Eng 47: 212-213, 1928.
47. Lauritsen CC and Bennett RD: A new high potential x-ray tube. Phys Rev 32:850-857, 1928.
48. Van de Graaff RJ: A 1,500,000 volt electrostatic generator. Phys Rev 38:1919-1920, 1931.
49. Trump JG: Radiation for therapy: In retrospect and prospect. AJR 91:22-30, 1964.
50. Van de Graaff RJ: The electrostatic production of high voltage for nuclear investigations. Phys Rev 43:151-157, 1933.
51. Lawrence EO and Sloan DH: High velocity mercury ions. Phys Rev 38:586, 1931.
52. Soiland A: Experimental clinical research work with X-ray voltages above 500,000. Radiology 20:99-101, 1933.
53. Failla G, Woodard HQ, Henshaw PS, et al: The relative effects produced by 200 KV roentgen rays, 700 KV roentgen rays, and gamma rays. AJR 29:293-367, 1933.
54. Kerst DW: Acceleration of electrons by magnetic induction. Phys Rev 58:841, 1940.
55. McMillan EM: The synchrotron: A proposed high energy particle accelerator. Phys Rev 68:143-144, 1945.
56. Laughlin JS: Development of the technology of radiation therapy. RadioGraphics 9:1245-1266, 1989.
57. Grigg ERN, et al: The RSNA historic symposium on American radiology: Then and now. Radiology 100:1-26, 1971.
58. Kaplan HS and Bagshaw MA: The Stanford medical linear accelerator. III. Application to clinical problems of radiation therapy. Stanford Med Bull 15:141-151, 1957.
59. Tsien KC: World survey of radioisotope teletherapy units. AJR 87:593-599, 1962.
60. Hussey DH, Meyn RE, and Smathers JB: Neutron therapy. In Bleehen NM, Glatstein E, and Haybittle JL (eds): Radiation therapy planning. New York, Decker, 1983.
61. Tapley NV and Almond PR: Treatment planning and techniques with the electron beam. In Bleehen NM, Glatstein E, and Haybittle JL (eds): Radiation therapy planning. New York, Decker, 1983.
62. Krabbenhoft KL: A history of roentgen therapy. AJR 76:859-865, 1956.
63. Brecher E and Brecher R: The rays: A history of radiology in the United States and Canada. Baltimore, Williams & Wilkins, 1969.
64. Roentgen, rads, and riddles. Symposium on Supervoltage Radiation Therapy. United States Atomic Energy Commission, 1959.

CHAPTER 30

Radium Therapy

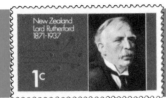
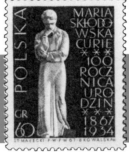
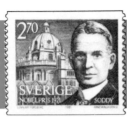
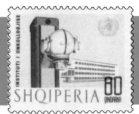

W̲ithin a few years of Becquerel's discovery of radioactivity, Ernest Rutherford and Frederick Soddy showed that the rays emitted by radioactive substances were actually composed of three distinct types of radiation.[1] More than 80% of the energy radiated was due to alpha rays, which were actually not rays but helium nuclei travelling at speeds of 9,000 to 20,000 miles per second. Because all alpha particles from a given substance started with the same velocity, they all travelled the same distance (range), which varied in atmospheric air from 2.7 to 8.6 cm. The penetrating ability of alpha particles was so small that they were stopped by a single sheet of paper.

Like alpha rays, beta rays also were not rays but particles, representing negatively charged electrons travelling at high speeds. Unlike alpha particles, beta particles from a given radioactive substance varied considerably in speed, some reaching almost the velocity of light (186,000 miles per second). They were much lighter than alpha particles but travelled much faster and could penetrate farther into body tissues (up to 1 cm) before their energy was reduced to the point where they could no longer be distinguished from ordinary electrons. Beta particles could pass through thin filters of aluminum but were all stopped by 2 mm of brass or 0.5 mm of gold.

Gamma rays were true rays, which were first identified by P. Villard in 1900. Although accounting for only about 1% of the radiation, they were of high energy and had a short wavelength and great penetrating power. The hardest gamma rays could pass through 25 cm of lead.

The concept of employing radium in medicine traditionally dates back to the famous misadventure of Becquerel, who in 1901 sustained a severe burn after inadvertently carrying a tube of pure radium in his waistcoat pocket for 14 days. After Pierre Curie intentionally produced a similar burn on his arm, he had the idea that radium might be useful in medical work.

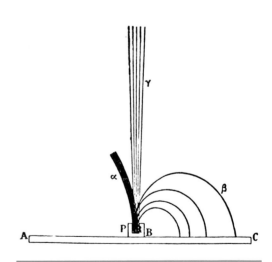

Diagram attributed to the Curies, which demonstrates the three types of radiation released by radium and the influence of an electromagnet (A, negative pole; C, positive pole) on the "rays." Alpha (α) rays were only slightly deviated toward the negative pole, whereas beta (β) rays were extremely susceptible and bent toward the positive pole. The nonparticulate gamma (γ) rays were not at all affected by magnetic forces.

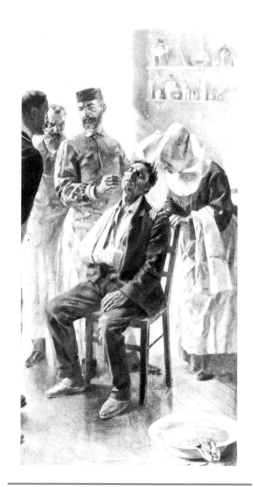

Danlos treating a lupus patient with radium at the Hôpital St. Louis, Paris (1904).

Meanwhile, Becquerel's burn was sufficiently serious that he consulted a dermatologist, Besnier, of the Hôpital St. Louis in Paris. Besnier immediately noted that Becquerel's radium burn resembled an x-ray burn and therefore suggested that radium might have a therapeutic effect similar to that of x-rays. He convinced the Curies to lend a small amount of radium to a hospital colleague, Henri Danlos, who successfully used the radioactive material to treat lupus and other dermatological conditions.

However, the first clinical use of radium therapy was probably the idea of William H. Rollins, the Boston dentist, in conjunction with his brother-in-law physician, Francis H. Williams. After learning of Williams' success in treating the lesions of lupus with x-rays, Rollins speculated that radium, too, might be successful in treating this disease. Accordingly, in late 1900, Rollins placed 500 mg of his radium chloride compound in a sealed capsule and gave it to Williams for clinical trials.

When describing his high hopes for radium therapy, Rollins in early 1902 wrote that

> radioactive substances can be used in sealed capsules held against the body by adhesive plaster, or they can be made to cover larger areas by mixing them with rubber or celluloid to form moisture-proof plasters. These plasters may be still further protected by being coated on the sides nearest the body by aluminum foil and on the opposite sides by lead foil. They could be kept in stock by the yard by druggists and given to patients by prescription with proper directions as to the length of application. They could be worn at night. Their use would prevent the poor from making such frequent visits to a physician as are now required when x-light obtained from a vacuum tube is used. This is a matter of some importance, as the present treatment takes many sittings, which require time and cost money.

As always, Rollins took care to provide protection against the possible harmful effects of the radium. He reported that the capsule he gave to Williams was disk-shaped with a front of aluminum and a back of comparatively nonradiable metal. Thus both the beta and the gamma rays could pass through the front of the disk to the lupus lesion, while stray radiation through the back of the disk would be minimized.

In a discussion of his first 42 cases, Williams[2] (1904) stated that

> the method of using the radiations from radium is simple. If the strongest action of the radium is desired, the metal box containing the salts is placed *on* the part to be treated; in this case the box should be covered with a thin rubber cot, or other suitable substance, which can be readily removed, so that a new cot may be used for each patient and the old one burned up. By this means, the radium capsule does not come into direct contact with the part to be treated, but is separated from it by this new and clean covering. If a weaker action of the radium salts is indicated, the capsule should be placed at a greater or lesser distance, according to the needs of the case, the intensity of the rays diminishing as the square of the distance.

Comparing his radium experience with his years of work in x-ray therapy, Williams concluded that

> the comparison at the present time is greatly to the advantage of radium . . . when radium is employed for healing purposes no cumbersome apparatus is necessary; radium is portable and always

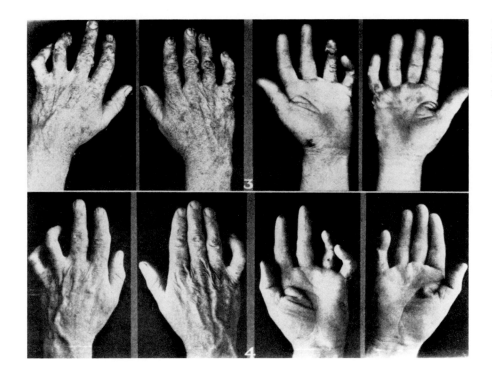

Effect of radium therapy on radiation-induced skin lesions of an x-ray worker. *Top*, Photographs of the hands before radium treatment was begun. *Bottom*, Dramatic improvement 8 months later.[3]

ready for use. Further, the dose from radium is uniform; the strength of the output does not vary, so that the dose depends entirely on the length of exposure and the distance of the radium from the part to be treated. Radium may be applied to parts which are not readily accessible to the x-rays, as the mouth or vagina. Furthermore, the healing action of the radium is more prompt. Treatment, therefore, extends over a shorter period, and fewer exposures are required than when the x-rays are used. Radium has the further advantage of bringing about healing in some cases where the x-rays have failed after careful and long-continued treatment.

Williams emphasized the need for radiation protection when using radium, which "if not properly protected, causes severe burns, which do not manifest themselves for a week or more. These burns are painful and heal slowly." To decrease the chance of injury,

radium, therefore, should be kept in a metal box or capsule with a thin mica front or other suitable covering, so that the radiations may be cut off in all directions except that in which the practitioner desires the rays to proceed. To such a capsule I have attached a long, flexible handle, in order to hold the radium at a distance when applying it. This handle is a protection to the practitioner. When not in use, the capsule should be placed in a thick lead box or tube, so that the radiations may be absorbed.

When treating a small skin lesion, he exposed it to the radium through an opening in a sheet of lead foil to protect the healthy skin nearby.[2]

Williams also described two other uses for radium. One was as a "fluorometer," a device for gauging the quantity of radiation from an x-ray tube.[4] After darkening the room, Williams placed a fluoroscopic screen in the x-ray beam from the tube. He then moved the screen away from the tube until the fluorescence on the screen precisely matched in brightness the fluorescence from a radium sample used as a standard of comparison.

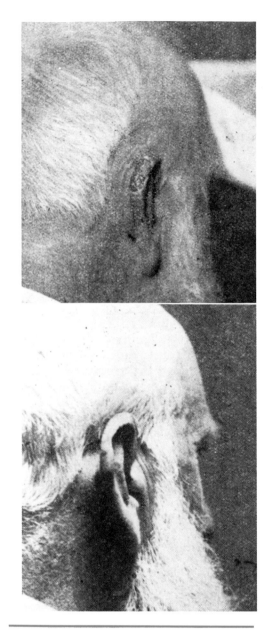

Radium therapy of epithelial cancer of the ear (1904). *Left*, Initial photograph. *Right*, After treatment. The patient was permanently cured.[7]

Apparatus used at the Biological Laboratory of Radium in Paris (1906). The flat applicators were for surface treatments and the cylindrical applicators (nos. 10 and 11) were used for treatment of the urethra, anus, or uterus.[9]

The greater the distance from tube to screen at the point where the screen fluorescence matched the comparison standard, the greater the emanation from the tube. Two tubes whose output matched the radium standard at the same distance were emitting the same quantity of x-rays.

An unusual use of radium was to ensure a minimal x-ray exposure to the patient during a fluoroscopic examination. At that time, physicians were blindfolded or sat in a dark room before fluoroscopy to adapt their eyes to the darkness. This permitted them to clearly see the image on the screen with only a relatively small current to the tube and thus a moderate x-ray dose to the patient. To aid the physician in knowing when his eyes were sufficiently adapted to the dark, Williams secured or made a *spintherascope* (spark viewer). This device, invented by Sir William Crookes in 1903, was a forerunner of the detector used in modern scintillation cameras. A microscope eyepiece was used to visualize flashes of light produced on a zinc sulfide or calcium tungstate screen when it was struck by alpha particles from a radium solution. "If the scintillations appear bright to the practitioner, his eyes are ready for use; if dull, he must wait for awhile longer in the dark room before attempting to make a fluoroscopic examination."[5]

The first successful use of radium therapy for malignant neoplasms came from the Gussenbauer Clinic of Vienna (1902), which reported the complete regression of a massive pharyngeal carcinoma in an elderly man.[6] Similar radium-induced regressions were seen in epithelioma of the lip, psoriasis, rodent ulcer, furunculosis, and lupus vulgaris. However, despite occasional reports of successful radium therapy of superficial cancers, deep-seated malignant growths were unaffected. At the Biological Laboratory of Radium in Paris, Louis-Frederic Wickham argued that the major factor in the success of radium therapy was not the amount of radioactivity in the sealed tube but rather the amount of radiation emerging from it and the proportions of alpha, beta, and gamma rays. He was the first to employ filtration, placing 1-cm-thick cotton wool enclosed in goldbeater's skin and in layers of aluminum between the radium and the tissues that he treated. A co-worker, Henri Dominici, further developed filtration by employing a series of lead and aluminum screens to permit an increased dose to deep tumors while sparing surrounding tissues the necrosing effects of beta rays.

A major improvement in technique was introduced by Robert Abbe of New York, who in 1904 was the first to insert radium tubes directly into tumors (interstitial radium implant).[7] As he reported to the Practitioner's Society of New York,

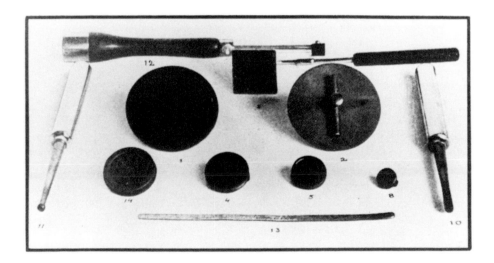

514

Anesthetizing the mucous membrane with a drop of cocaine, I pressed a bistoury through the rim of the tumor and found the soft sarcomatous mass allowed the radium glass tube to be pressed through it down to the lower margin of the jaws, represented by the shell of bone. Two or three times weekly I have thus penetrated the various parts of the tumor, leaving the radium embedded for two to three hours at a time.

Nine years later the patient was still well and without tumor recurrence.[8]

Abbe also was a pioneer in the field of radiobiology. He performed experiments on his own skin, varying the exposure to radium and correlating it to the degree of erythema and necrosis produced. His work with seedlings pointed out the potential dangers of radium effects on germinative tissues.[8]

A well-illustrated account of successful interstitial radium implantation was described by William J. Morton, who in 1914 reported the case of successful treatment of a sarcoma of the humerus with the patient showing no signs of recurrence 9 years later.[10]

The idea of direct radium implantation into tumors is often attributed to Alexander Graham Bell.[11] In 1903, he wrote that

> the Roentgen rays, and the rays emitted by radium have been found to have a marked curative effect upon external cancers, but . . . the effects upon deep-seated cancers have thus far proved unsatisfactory. It has occurred to me that one reason for the unsatisfactory nature of these latter experiments arises from the fact that the rays have been applied externally, thus having to pass through healthy tissue of various depths in order to reach the cancerous matter. The Crookes tube, from which the Roentgen rays are emitted, is, of course, too bulky to be admitted into the middle of a mass of cancer, but there is no reason why a tiny fragment of radium sealed up in a fine glass tube should not be inserted into the very heart of the cancer, thus acting directly upon the diseased material. Would it not be worthwhile making experiments along this line?

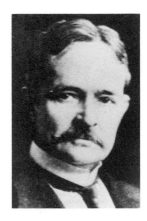

Robert Abbe (1851-1928).

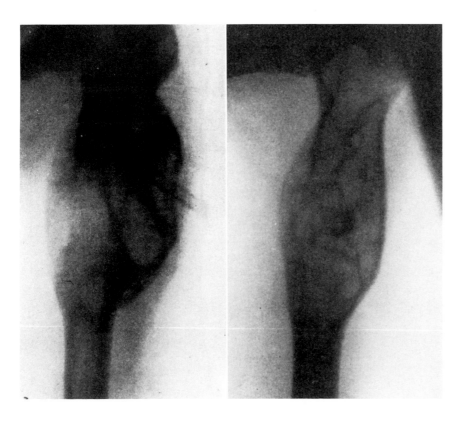

Radium therapy for sarcoma of the humerus (1914). *Left,* Radiograph taken at the beginning of treatment showing the radium tube within the tumor, the radium within the tube, and the state of fracture. *Right,* Radiograph taken more than 9 years later. The patient was in perfect health and had no disability of the arm.

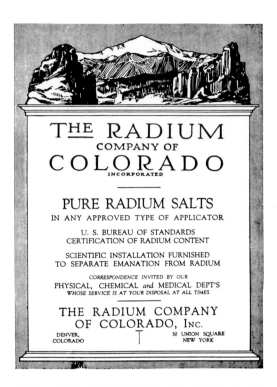

Advertisement for the Radium Company of
Colorado.

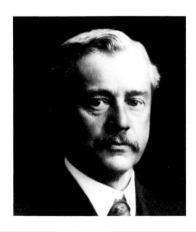

Howard A. Kelly.

Until 1913, the use of radium for therapy continued to expand in
Europe. However, except for a few radium pioneers such as Williams and
Abbe, most American radiologists performed therapy exclusively with
x-rays. The main reason for this lag was an inadequate radium supply
within the United States.

The first radium was produced commercially from the uranium residues obtained from the mines of Joachimsthal, Bohemia. Because the
ores were a government monopoly and the prices astronomical (up to
$180,000 per gram), attempts were made to find sources of radium-
containing ores in other parts of the world. In Colorado, radium was found
in carnotite. The Standard Chemical Company, founded by Joseph Flannery of Pittsburgh, purchased the Colorado mines in 1911 and began to
market radium in 1913. Because neither the *Transactions of the American
Roentgen Ray Society* nor the *American Quarterly of Radiology* made
more than rare casual mention of radium or radium therapy, Flannery
began publishing the monthly journal *Radium* as a means of publicizing
his product. Although a virtual house organ, *Radium* performed a valuable service by abstracting the major European and American literature
on the subject, as well as publishing occasional original articles of merit
until its demise in 1925.

In the mid-1910s, the U.S. Bureau of Mines and the National Radium
Institute (founded by Howard Kelley, a Baltimore gynecologist, and engineer, James Douglas) entered into a joint venture to set up a radium
recovery plant in Denver. This substantially decreased the cost of radium
and made it more widely available in the United States. Until 1922, about
80% of the world's supply of radium was produced in this country. With
the discovery of much cheaper and richer uranium ores in Katanga
Province in the Belgian Congo, American radium production virtually
ceased.[12]

Once sufficient amounts of radium were available, excellent therapeutic results were reported by several major American medical centers. In
Baltimore, Howard A. Kelley (with Curtis Burnam) of the National Radium Institute reported (1915) the highly promising results of radium
therapy in 213 cases of advanced carcinoma of the cervix and vagina
(almost all considered inoperable). With radium as the sole mode of
therapy, there were almost 30% "clinical cures." More than two thirds of
the remaining patients were "markedly improved," which was defined as
"a definite betterment of the patient's condition that included a cessation
of hemorrhage and discharge, or a disappearance of pain which has
resisted all drugs, including morphine."[13]

In Boston, William Duane, a physicist, teamed with physician Robert
B. Greenough in performing radium therapy on 612 patients, about half of
whom "received definite benefit." The results varied widely with the type
of cancer treated. They observed that

> the obviously extravagant claims of some of the earlier exponents of
> radium therapy served to arouse in the more conservative members of
> the profession a natural pessimism, which led them to distrust its
> value altogether. As a fact, the real truth lies somewhere between
> these two extremes. Radium is not a cure for all kinds of cancer.
> There are many cases of cancer in which it can be said to be of no
> material benefit; but there are also many cases where its use pro-
> longs life, relieves distressing symptoms, improves the general con-
> dition and the functional activities of the patient, and mitigates, as
> does no other agent which we have employed, the gradually progres-
> sive symptoms of advanced incurable cancer.[14]

They also noted that patients treated with radium sometimes "suffer pain and inconvenience from the effects of radium burns" that were "of a temporary character." Nausea and depression also occurred. "With continued and excessive doses, very profound constitutional effects may be obtained," including a serious decrease in the white blood cell count.

The third and most important American center for radium therapy was at Memorial Hospital in New York under the direction of surgeon Henry H. Janeway and his brilliant young physicist, Gioacchino Failla. Members of the Memorial group designed many ingenious techniques for interstitial radium implantation. Janeway[15] stressed the difference in sensitivity to radiation between normal and malignant tissues.

> Superficial epitheliomas of the skin can be made to disappear by appropriate exposures to radium without more than the slightest degree of erythema to the surrounding tissues . . . The clearest examples of the selective action of radium on tumor tissue are furnished by the cellular teratomas and lymphosarcomas. These tumors seem to melt away with the greatest rapidity whenever, one might almost say, radium is anywhere in their vicinity.

He noted the difficulty of securing "uniform distribution of the radiation through the affected tissue" so that the cancer cells would receive a maximum fatal dose without at the same time producing an injury to normal tissue.

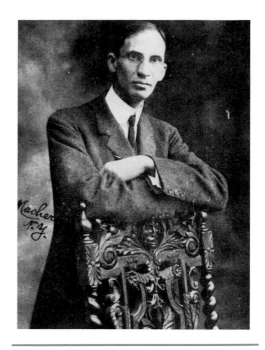

Henry H. Janeway.

MODES OF APPLICATION

The first radium appliances manufactured for clinical use were a variety of containers (rubber bags, ebonite boxes, and glass tubes and capsules) in which the radium salt was enclosed.[2] The earliest pioneers in radium therapy had mostly used flat applicators of one kind or another that were simply strapped close to the lesion being treated. These external devices included plaques of different sizes and shapes covered with special heat-resistant radioactive varnish and a variety of radioactive powders and ointments directly applied to tumor surfaces. Oral ingestion or the intravenous injection of radioactive solutions was found to be extremely toxic.

By 1910, it was clear that although surface applications of radium succeeded in healing over many superficial tumors, most soon recurred. Repeated applications were followed by ulceration and local or general dissemination. Tumors beneath the skin merely regressed temporarily or showed no effect. Efforts to increase the radiation dose led to disastrous results, with much destruction of tissue, prolonged and painful ulceration, and eventual recurrence.[14] This problem led to the development of two different ways to apply radium: by means of containers or applicators inserted into the nose, mouth, rectum, or vagina and uterus (intracavitary radiation) or by means of small seeds or needles inserted directly into the diseased tissue (interstitial radiation).

A major improvement in radium therapy technique was proposed by Duane while an assistant in Marie Curie's laboratory in Paris. Duane knew that radium emitted only alpha particles (nuclei of helium atoms), which were of no therapeutic value because they lacked penetrating power. In the process of emitting an alpha particle, however, a radium atom was transmuted into an atom of a radioactive gas, now called *radon* but known before 1923 as *radium emanation*. Although radon was chemically inert, it was nevertheless radioactive and transmuted itself into

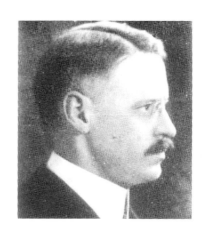

William Duane.

517

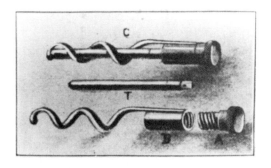

Radioactive corkscrew (1913). In this primitive form of interstitial treatment, a 50 mg tube was secured into the corkscrew, which was then bored into the tissues.[9]

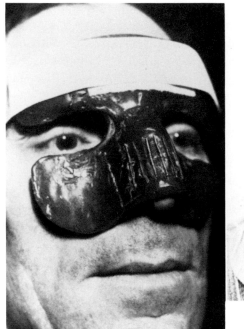
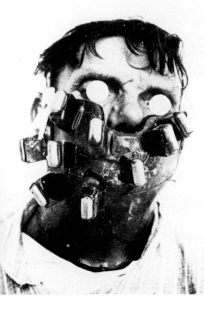

Early radium appliances. *Left*, Radium surface applicator. *Right*, Cervico-mandibular wax mould with embedded radium containers.

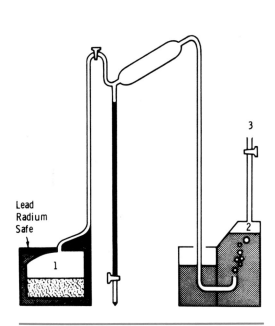

Lead Radium Safe

Early radon extractor. A solution of radium bromide or chloride containing at least 0.5 gm of radium element evolved the heavy gas radon (*1*). It was then pumped off and collected in chamber *2*. Following the selection of a suitable volume, the radon was concentrated by exposure of liquid air and the compressed gas fed into fine capillary tubings surrounded by pure gold (*3*). In this fashion, filtered gold "seeds" were produced.[8]
Redrawn from C.W. Allen.

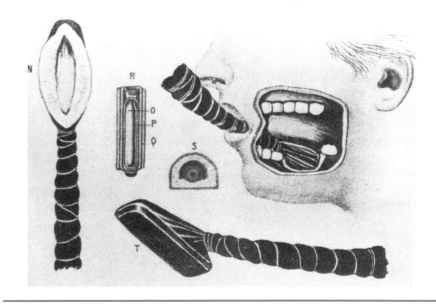

Radium applicator for treating carcinoma of the tongue and floor of the mouth (1913). "A 50 mg tube (*R*) filtered through two half cylinders of 1 mm lead, which were placed on the dorsal side of the tube to protect the overlying structures. The completed tube was then wrapped in tarlatane (*N*) and sheet rubber (*T*)."[9]

radium A, which was transmuted into radium B, and so on through a series of other "daughter elements." In practice, the radium used in therapy was sealed up in a glass or a metal container so that the daughter elements accumulated. Yet, it was the daughter elements, especially radium B and radium C, that emitted the therapeutically useful beta and gamma rays. Duane's ingenious proposal (1908) was to draw off the emanation gas from the radium, seal it into containers, and use these instead of radium containers for therapeutic purposes.

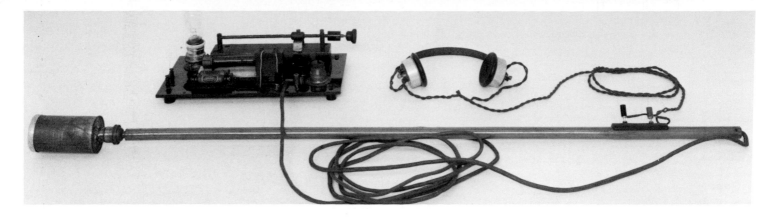

Original portable apparatus for the detection and localization of lost radium.

Radium emanation proved to have many advantages over radium for certain therapeutic purposes. The radium could be kept well shielded in a single large container in the extraction plant instead of risking loss through handling small containers in hospital rooms and doctors' offices. Because the emanation was a gas, it could be sealed in small containers of various shapes and sizes and conveniently handled after sealing. Although the radiations were otherwise identical, a given volume of emanation emitted far more intense radiation than the same volume of radium. Thus tubes, needles, and "seeds" containing emanation could be made small enough to be buried directly in tumor tissue, with a minimum of trauma during the insertion. Because of its long half-life, any radium buried in diseased tissue had to be removed after the treatment was completed. This often required a second operative procedure. Seeds containing emanation lost half of their strength in 3.8 days and almost all of it in a few weeks. Thus they frequently could be left in the tissue permanently. A final advantage was financial. Doctors in hospitals unable to afford radium could buy adequate supplies of emanation as needed from commercial companies at relatively moderate cost.

Initially, radon was administered to patients by inhalation. The apparatus consisted of a closed chamber containing a measured amount of radon and was known as an "Emanatorium" or "Inhalatorium."[16] Later, emanation-activated water (radium water) was reported to have good results in patients with osteoarthritis and gout. Injections of water or Vaseline impregnated with emanation were made; baths and drinks were also administered. Radioactive mud, in which the radioactivity was due to small amounts of radium, was used in the form of poultices.

In 1914, Walter Stevenson[17] of Dublin described a new technique that opened up the whole field of interstitial therapy. In a case of cancer of the tonsil, he inserted a silver serum needle in which was loaded a glass capillary containing radon gas. The sealed glass tube was ⅜ to ½ inch long and less than 0.5 mm in diameter. The emanation tube, which delivered both beta and gamma rays, could be lodged in a body cavity or laid on the surface of the skin. Next came thin tubes of aluminum or silver into which the glass emanation tubes could be inserted. These metal tubes protected the glass tubes from breakage and also filtered out some of the beta rays.

A later development was the introduction of heavier platinum tubes of various sizes and shapes to provide more effective filtration. These tubes filtered out virtually all the beta rays and permitted the emergence of only hard, practically homogeneous gamma rays. Small hooks could be threaded to the ends of these tubes so that they could be "hooked upon almost any ulcer or mucous surface" and be counted on to retain their position. The glass tubes could be lodged in hollow needles, which could

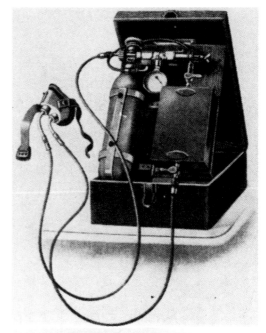

RADIUM EMANATION TREATMENT
— for —
Chronic Rheumatism, Gout, Rheumatoid
Arthritis, Neuralgias, Sciatica, Etc.

RADIO-REM No. 4

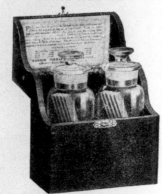

Guaranteed to charge water with 5000 Mache Units per day
Simple, Economical and Dependable
RADIUM THERAPY CO.
Schieffelin & Co., Distributors
270 William Street, New York City
Physicians are asked to send for literature

Radium emanation inhaler treatment. *Top,* Apparatus for inhalation of radium emanation and oxygen, produced by Radium, Ltd. in England about 1907. *Bottom,* Advertisement extolling the value of radium emanation treatment for multiple disorders that appeared in AJR, 1917.

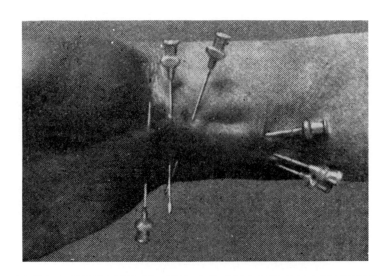

Radium emanation needles positioned in a fibrous scar causing fixation of the wrist (1914). When the needles were removed, the patient stated that her previously constant pain had disappeared.[17]

Glass seeds containing radium emanation (1921). The radon-containing seeds were inserted into malignant tissues by means of a hollow steel needle and plunger. No attempt was made to remove these seeds, because they became "extinct" after a few weeks.

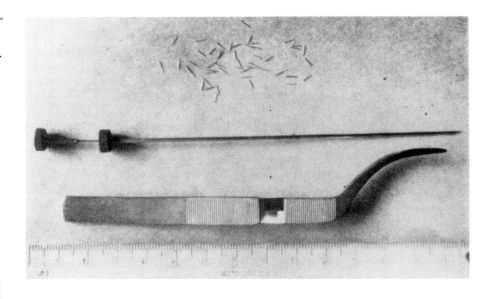

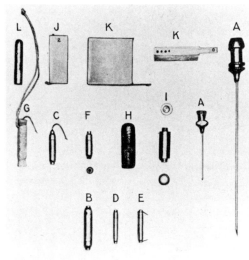

Various forms of tubes and silver plaques for radium application.[13]

be threaded, inserted into tumor tissue, and then withdrawn again at the end of the treatment by pulling on the thread. Also in common use were glass "seeds," tiny emanation-filled containers about 0.1 inch long and 0.01 inch in diameter, which could be implanted directly in tumor tissue and left there permanently.

The radon tubes could be held in place by moulds made of wax or dental compound. For surface radiation, plaques ½- or 1-inch square were designed that contained the emanation tubes placed side by side. These plaques, in turn, could be combined into larger surfaces and used with any desired filter or combination of filters. Initially, the flat plaques were placed directly on the surface to be radiated. However, Janeway and his co-workers[15] at Memorial soon found that holding the plaques 1 or 2 inches away "practically eliminated the radium inflammation, and yet permitted the administration of doses sufficient to produce retrogression of deep-seated tumors."

By the mid-1920s, there were two major methods of burying radiation sources in tumor tissue. One was the Memorial method, using glass seeds containing radium emanation. The other was the Radium Institute of Paris method, developed by Claude Regaud (1920),[18] in which platinum needles filled with radium were sewn into place and then withdrawn.

The major advantage of the Regaud method was that the platinum filtered out the beta rays, resulting in much less painful and hazardous necrosis in the overdosed tissue immediately surrounding the implant. Conversely, with the Memorial method the radon seeds could be left permanently in place. The question was whether a permanent implant could be devised that could also protect the nearby tissues by filtering out the beta rays.

Failla[19] at Memorial initially enclosed the glass radon seeds in a platinum tube and inserted the tube by means of a hollow trocar.

> The results showed that the amount of necrosis could be greatly reduced by using platinum filters. Of necessity, however, the filtered implants were considerably larger than the glass tubes, and the trocar had to be considerably larger in diameter. The question of trauma, therefore, assumed greater importance. In order to make filtered implants of the smallest possible size, it was evident that the radon should be collected directly in a metal tube, and we directed our efforts toward that ideal.

The selection of an appropriate metal became the responsibility of Failla's closest associate, Edith H. Quimby. As Failla[19] related, "Experiments conducted in our laboratory by Quimby to determine the absorption of radium emanation by different metals showed that equal thicknesses of platinum and *pure* gold had the same absorbing power, within the limits of experimental error. This being the case, gold is preferable because it is about one-fifth as expensive as platinum."

It was relatively easy to fill foot-long sections of this tubing with radon gas, using the same equipment used to fill glass seeds. But once a long, thin, gold tube had been filled, how could it be divided into short lengths, each length tightly sealed at both ends to prevent the escape of the radioactive gas? "Pure gold being quite soft, and the bore of the tubing being very small, we found that a gas tight seal could be made by simply pinching the tubing."[19] The gold seeds thus prepared were carefully tested for leakage, and it was found that they could "be boiled for one hour or more without loss of radon." One last detail to be solved was that the last sections to be pinched off contained more than their share of radon. The simple solution was to make the first pinch in the middle of the long tube with each of the two halves then pinched in the middle, and so on—a method assuring equal distribution of the radon.

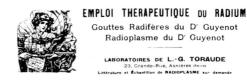

Advertisement for "radium water" (1917). The nurse is carrying an electroscope on a platter.

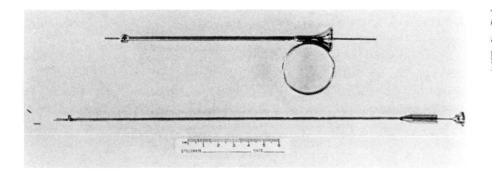

Gold "seeds" containing radon and stylus applicator. These are similar to the ones produced by Failla at Memorial Hospital in New York.[8]

Extensive experimentation was required to determine the optimum thickness of the gold walls of the seeds. Although 0.5 mm of gold was necessary to completely absorb the beta rays, this would require a large trocar for insertion and cause greater damage to the tissues. A convenient test object to measure the amount of radium emanations was ordinary butter. As Failla explained,[20]

> When a tube containing sufficient amount of radon is placed on a smooth surface of a block of butter (which is kept on ice) one can observe an area of discoloration which increases in size for a number of days. The outline of this region is quite sharp and can be measured with fair precision. The physical conditions which determine the distribution of the radiation around the tube are quite comparable when butter and tissue are used as the media. Accordingly, some definite information can be obtained by measuring the area of discoloration around tubes of different strength and different filtration.

The optimal wall thickness proved to be 0.3 mm. Failla's gold seeds were quickly adopted and have remained a part of the modern radiotherapeutic armamentarium.

Once newer and richer radium ores had been discovered following World War I, several institutions that had acquired relatively large amounts (2 to 10 gm) developed the technique of *telecurietherapy* (in contrast to *brachytherapy,* in which the radioactive source was placed in close proximity to the area to be treated). The simplest telecurietherapy apparatus consisted of tubes containing relatively large amounts of radium that were placed several centimeters away from the skin. The radium "pack" was constructed of materials of low density such as wood, celluloid, rubber, or leather to form a base on which the radium was mounted. Other similar devices included the radium bomb, so named because it resembled a small hand grenade, and the radium collar, which was usually made of Columbia paste and could be constructed for individual patients. The most serious disadvantage of this type of apparatus was that much of the radiation was absorbed in superficial tissues and relatively little reached any depth. It also was associated with considerable risk of exposure to both the patient and the operator.[19]

An alternative and safer method was the use of a collimated beam of radiation with a lead container surrounding the exit portal. Military-sounding devices using this technique included the mesothorium cannon and the radium howitzer.[9]

The development of supervoltage x-ray therapy techniques brought the end of telecurietherapy. Years later, however, the availability of artificially radioactive cobalt and cesium, which emit a degree of radiation equivalent to hundreds of grams of radium, revived interest in this type of therapy (see Chapter 29).

The application of artificial radionuclides to brachytherapy was aided by an important innovation that led to reduced radiation exposure of the therapists and their associates. Sources had earlier been moved by pneumatic or cable methods through a flexible tube to a teletherapy head, thus reducing the exposure of the staff and simplifying the shielding of the source head. This same principle was then applied to the development of "afterloading" for radium sources in intracavitary application and, later, for other radionuclides. Widespread adoption of this afterloading technique significantly reduced the staff exposure in brachytherapy procedures. Interstitial iodine-125 (^{125}I) seeds, which were used as a substitute for radon seeds, also reduced staff exposure because of the low

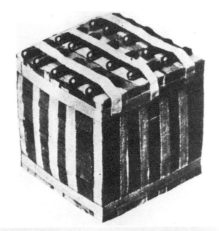

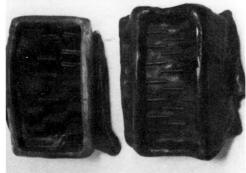

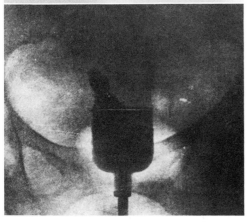

Telecurietherapy devices. *Top,* Radium pack. *Middle,* Radium collar. *Bottom,* Vaginal bomb.[9]

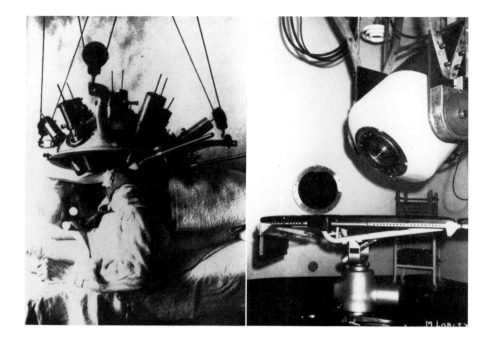

Telecurietherapy devices. *Left*, Sluys-Kessler apparatus. *Right*, Failla's 50-gm radium bomb.

energy of its emission. When used in the form of small encapsulated sources as a permanent implant, ^{125}I was particularly useful for non-resectable malignant lesions of the lung and prostate. For temporary intracavitary applications, radium has now been largely replaced by cesium-137 sources. This radionuclide has a lower energy than that of radium, which allows more effective shielding to reduce personnel exposure and to protect specific organs (e.g., bladder and rectum in treatments of cervical carcinoma).[21] Iridium-192 seeds also have been used for implants in tumors of the head and neck and prostate.

Computer technology has been employed extensively for optimization of brachytherapy. A method devised in 1976 permits the determination of the optimum strength and location of cesium-137 sources in intracavitary applicators. Using the desired range of dose rates determined by the clinician for 16 specific points of interest, a computer program could determine the necessary source strength at each source position.

The determination of the location of the seeds has depended on diagnostic x-ray methods such as the use of orthogonal films or stereoscopic shift films. Sources located in two dimensions on each of the orthogonal films can be localized in space by computer programs that automatically determine their coordinates in three dimensions.

Detailed computer calculations of dose distribution have even permitted the use of low-energy ^{125}I seeds for stereotactic treatment of brain tumors.[21]

RADIUM DOSIMETRY

Measurement of the activity of radium preparations initially was expressed in terms of activity of uranium. Thus pure radium had a "2,000,000 activity." It was soon found that this was a poor way of specifying the activity of radium preparations, especially if they were in sealed containers. When radium salts of high purity were prepared, it was only necessary to state the weight of the salt. But even this notation produced some uncertainty unless the precise chemical formula was given and the amount of water crystallization was known.[22]

Because the activity of a radium preparation depended ultimately on its actual radium content, steps were taken to establish an international radium standard and to base measurements on the gamma ray activity of the standard containing a certain definite quantity of radium element, regardless of the salt used. Marie Curie was asked to prepare an International Radium Standard, which was preserved in the International Bureau of Weights and Measures at Sevres, near Paris. The unit of radiation, named the *curie*, was defined as the amount of radiation emitted by 1 gm of pure radium and its daughter elements under specified conditions. Early radium therapists, who generally used much less than 1 gm of radium, expressed the amount in terms of *millicuries* (thousandths of a curie). Since the length of time to which a tumor was exposed to radiation was as important as the amount of radiation, they spoke in terms of *millicurie-hours*.

Unfortunately, this primitive method of specifying the quantity of radiation was completely inadequate, for it described only the radiation leaving the source and gave no indication of the amount of radiation reaching or absorbed in the tissue being irradiated. Factors that needed to be considered in making this determination included the distance between the source and target tissue, the degree of scattering and secondary radiation, the shape of the source (sphere, needle, or flat plaque), and the type of radiation (alpha, beta, or gamma) and degree of filtration.

Because the primary effect of radiation on living tissue was ionization, an excellent way (in theory) to determine the amount of radiation reaching a given region was to place a small ionization chamber in that area and to determine the number of ions produced within it. Due to the penetrating nature of the secondary rays from a radium source, the standard ionization chambers that had been developed for 200 keV x-rays were unsuitable. As the difficulties began to be understood, it became evident that the basic measurements should be made in large open spaces. In Berlin, Friedrich finally made use of an armory 100 × 50 × 22 m in size to achieve unequivocal results. When the necessary amount of air had been determined, it was evident that the same results should be expected if the air were compressed. Pressure chambers up to 50 atmospheres were tested with satisfactory results. The final step was to replace the air by an "air-equivalent" solid and to use a sufficient thickness of this to make thimble-type chambers. Once the output of 1 mg of radium under specified conditions was known, it was not necessary to calibrate the output of every tube or needle. This could be calculated on the basis of the actual radium content, the geometric size and shape of the source, and the filtration. A large series of measurements in suitable phantoms with adequate ionization chambers was made to define the distribution of radiation within tissues.[23]

In the 1930s, Edith Quimby in the United States and Ralston Paterson and Herbert Parker in England began publishing long series of tables showing the relative amounts of radiation delivered at specified distances from applicators of various sizes, shapes, and strengths and with filters of varying thickness. Separate tables were prepared for surface applications, interstitial applications with buried seeds or needles, and intracavitary applications. These tables transformed radium therapy from an almost wholly intuitive art into a science that permitted precise duplication of dosages from patient to patient and from one laboratory to another.

A discussion of the development of radiation therapy is incomplete

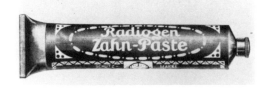

Radon toothpaste (1920). Marketed by the Allgemeine Radiogen-A.G. of Berlin, it contained radium and would release emanation as the teeth were brushed to provide allegedly constant activity. It was said to reduce the decomposition of alimentary residues and thus prevent the deposition of "dental stone."

without at least a brief mention of the dangers from handling the material without proper precautions. There is little doubt that Marie Curie's long illness and death could be attributed largely to the radium with which she worked. Much more common than the fatal cases were damaged fingers, due often to carelessness or foolhardiness in handling tubes and needles, preparing applicators, and making implantations. The development of adequate storage safes, shielded handling tubes, and remote-controlled operations, combined with a large dose of simple common sense, did much to decrease the dangers of working with radium.[23]

The internal administration of radium salts by mouth or intravenously was at one time a popular treatment for anemia and chronic leukemia. However, this technique was abandoned once the severe toxic effects of radium became apparent. Martland and co-workers (1925)[24] reported exhaustive pathological studies of human tissues in patients who had "succumbed to radium poisoning." This included the fascinating study of the occupational poisoning sustained by women employed in painting the dials of watches and clocks with luminous paint containing radioactive substances.

> They painted from 250 to 300 watches a day. It was their practice, for several years and until they were warned to stop, continually to point with their lips the camel's hair brushes which they used. The minimum number of times this was done a day would be about once to a dial, and if the brushes were poor, the maximum might be about 14 times to a dial. If the brush, when loaded, holds about 5 mg of luminous paint, on licking, 1 mg or less, a hardly visible amount, might easily stick to the gums or the roof of the mouth. As the material is mixed with a binder of gum acacia, it is sticky and hard to expectorate.

They calculated that an average worker could ingest "from 125 mg to 1.75 gm daily, which would contain from 3 to 43 micrograms of radioactive substances. Working only six months a year and only five days a week, from 360 micrograms to over 5 mg of radioactive substances could be swallowed in that time."

Victims of this condition suffered severe necrosis of the jaw from local irritative radiation at the point of entry produced by clinging particles of radioactive substances on the gums, teeth, and roof of the mouth. The victims died from severe anemia or, if they survived this, multiple sarcomas developed throughout the bones from the destructive bombardment by the alpha particles.

In an intriguing experiment, they strapped regulation x-ray dental films to portions of femurs obtained from autopsy specimens. Small wire paper clips and pieces of lead were placed between the film surface and the bone. In 6 weeks' time the exposed films showed exact shadowgrams of the interposed metal. When this procedure was repeated on specimens of the inferior maxilla, hazy shadowgrams could be produced in as few as 60 hours, indicating the relatively intense radioactivity in this bone.

RADIUM QUACKERY

As the *Medical Record* observed (1904)[25]:

> The real properties and the alleged properties of radium would seem to have overturned the rational reasoning faculties of a large portion

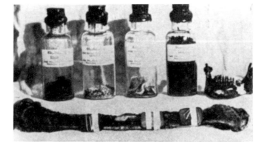

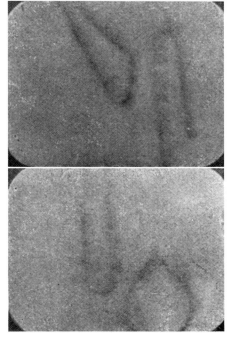

Radium dial painter dying of severe aplastic anemia (1925). *Top*, Specimens of spleen, bones, marrow, and liver used for qualitative electrometer readings. Note the dental films containing metal clips strapped to the split femur and the inferior maxilla. *Bottom*, Dental films removed from the femur after being strapped against the bone for 6 weeks. Note the exact shadowgrams of the metal clips.[24]

Advertisement for preparation of radio-active water.

of the American public and of some of the medical men. Statements for which there is no foundation whatever are being constantly advanced as to the marvelous events that can and will be brought about through the influence of radium. A French scientist has affirmed recently that the heat rays of radium are capable of melting stones, and of disintegrating, with great celerity, iron and steel, so that the effects of the exceeding heat of its rays will destroy fortifications, crumble battleships, and will extinguish human life like dew before the morning sun, thus rendering warfare impossible. In pseudo-scientific articles and in medical literature, to a certain extent, the most extravagant claims have been made for radium.

In Germany, radium emanation was used for a bizarre array of medical problems. Fuerstenberg (1913)[26] stated that "The most important indications for the therapy of radium emanation of today are probably gout and the various forms of rheumatism." Saubermann, in an address to the Röntgen Society of London, listed indications for the use of radium emanation that were virtually a textbook of internal medicine. Radium was said to increase the secretion of urine, stimulate the activity of the digestive tract (thus lessening chronic constipation), dilate blood vessels and diminish blood viscosity (thus lowering blood pressure), soothe the nerves (thus curing insomnia), and increase sexual activity. Neuralgia, sciatica, gout, tabes dorsalis, diabetes, and catarrh of the antrum and frontal sinus were all claimed to be improved by the use of radium emanation. "Several well-known Continental spas, such as Gastein, Baden-Baden, etc., which are now recognized to be markedly radioactive, have for long enjoyed a reputation as 'rejuvenating' waters, while the fact that the use of baths and waters rendered artificially radio-active tends to produce the phenomenon in question has been confirmed by many distinguished and trustworthy physicians."[27]

Bibliography

Brecher E and Brecher R: The rays. A history of radiology in the United States and Canada. Baltimore, Williams & Wilkins, 1964.

Failla G and Quimby EH: Radium physics. In Glasser O: The science of radiology. Springfield, Ill, Charles C Thomas, 1934.

References

1. Rutherford E: Radioactive transformations. New Haven, Conn, Yale University Press, 1906.

2. Williams FH: Some of the physical properties and medical uses of radium salts. Med News 84:241-246, 1904.

3. Williams FH: Reminiscences of a pioneer in roentgenology and radium therapy. AJR 13:253-259, 1925.

4. Williams FH: The roentgen rays in medicine and surgery. New York, MacMillan, 1901.

5. Williams FH: A comparison between the medical uses of the x-rays and the rays from the salts of radium. Boston Med Surg J 150:206-209, 1904.

6. Radium rays for cancer. Medical Record 64:63, 1903.

7. Abbe R: The subtle power of radium. Med Record 66:321-324, 1904.

8. Doss LL: The history of radium. Missouri Med 75:594-599, 1974.

9. Lederman M: The early history of radiotherapy: 1895-1939. Radiation Oncology Biol Phys 7:639-648, 1981.

10. Morton WJ: Imbedded radium tubes in the treatment of cancer. Med Rec 86:913-915, 1914.

11. Bell AG: Letter to the editor. Amer Med 6:261, 1903.

12. Sayers RR: Radium in medical use in the United States. Radiology 20:305-309, 1933.

13. Kelly HA and Burnham CF: Radium in the treatment of carcinomas of the cervix uteri and vagina. JAMA 65:1874-1877, 1915.

14. Duane W and Greenough RB: Methods of preparing and using radioactive substances in the treatment of malignant disease and of estimating suitable dosages. Boston Med Surg J 177:359-365; 787-797, 1917.

15. Janeway HH, Failla G, and Barringer BS: Radium therapy in cancer at the Memorial Hospital. New York, Hoeber, 1917.

16. Mould RF: A history of x-rays and radium. 1980.

17. Stevenson WC: Preliminary clinical report on a new and economical method of radium therapy by means of emanation needles. Brit Med J 9-10, 1914.

18. Regaud C: Some biological aspects of the radiation therapy of cancer. AJR 12:97-101, 1924.

19. Failla G: Dosage study relative to the therapeutic use of unfiltered radon. AJR 15:1-35, 1926.

20. Failla G: The development of filtered radon implants. AJR 16:507-525, 1926.

21. Laughlin JS: Development of the technology of radiation therapy. RadioGraphics 9:1245-1266, 1989.

22. Quimby EH and Failla G: Radium dosimetry. In Glasser O (ed): The science of radiology. Springfield, Ill, Charles C Thomas, 1934.

23. Quimby EH: The background of radium therapy in United States, 1906-1956. AJR 75:443-450, 1956.

24. Martland HS, Cowlan P, and Knef JP: Some unrecognized dangers in the use and handling of radioactive substances. JAMA 85:1769-1776, 1925.

25. Common sense and radium. Medical Record 65:780, 1904.

26. Radium emanation treatment for rheumatism and gout. Radium 1:12-14, 1913.

27. Saubermann J: An address on the progress of radium-therapy. Arch Roentgen Ray 18:99-116, 1913.

CHAPTER 31

Interventional Radiology

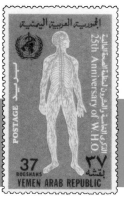

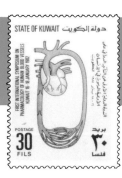

PERCUTANEOUS TRANSLUMINAL ANGIOPLASTY

Despite the frequency and importance of arteriosclerotic obstruction, current (1964) methods of therapy leave much to be desired. Nonsurgical measures, however helpful they may be, provide the patient little more than an opportunity to live with his disease. Consistent success in the use of surgical technics such as endarterectomy, angioplasty, and grafting has largely been confined to highly specialized vascular surgeons of whom there are far too few to cope realistically with literally millions of patients suffering the painful, disabling, or lethal consequences of the disease. Moreover, for practical purposes, surgical success is limited in the management of occlusions in smaller arteries. Thus, while aorto-iliac thromboendarterectomy has been generally successful, gangrene due to femoropopliteal occlusion frequently results in amputation. . . . [This] has led to the development of a safe, simple, and effective technic for directly overcoming arteriosclerotic narrowing and occlusion in the arteries of the leg. Impressive salvages already achieved in otherwise doomed legs amply justify this preliminary report even though long-term follow-up observations are not yet possible.

Thus began the classic report of Charles Dotter and Melvin Judkins,[1] which first described the nonsurgical restoration of normal (or near-normal) hemodynamics in occlusive atherosclerotic disease. After making the incidental observation of recanalization of a totally occluded right common iliac artery by an angiographic catheter during a conventional diagnostic study, Dotter performed the first percutaneous transluminal angioplasty (PTA) on a popliteal artery in an elderly woman with gangrene.[2] Dotter and Judkins used a dilatation system consisting of tapered, radiopaque coaxial Teflon dilators, which were introduced over a guidewire after antegrade puncture of the femoral artery. This technique was

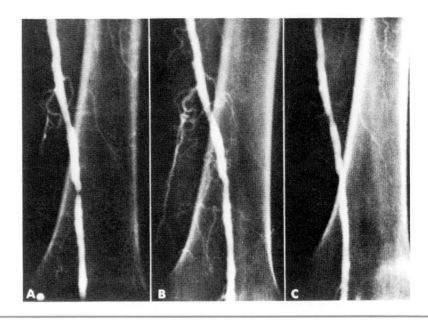

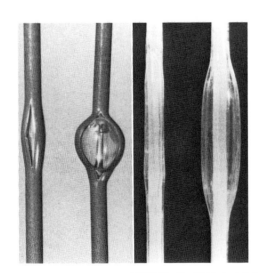

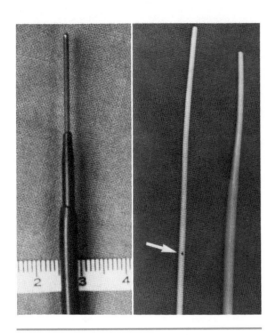

Left, Dotter coaxial Teflon catheter system, consisting of a no. 12 French catheter with a tapered and beveled tip over an inner no. 8 French catheter with an 0.044-inch guidewire.[6] *Right,* Staple-Van Andel catheters nos. 5 and 7 French Teflon catheters with long (5 cm) tapered tips. Proximal side hole (*arrow*) added by Zeitler to permit contrast injections.[6]

First percutaneous transluminal angioplasty (1964). *Left,* Control arteriogram shows segmental narrowing with a threadlike lumen of the left superficial femoral artery in the region of the adductor hiatus. *Middle,* Study immediately after dilatation with a catheter having an outer diameter of 3.2 mm. *Right,* Three weeks after transluminal dilatation, the lumen remains open. Clinical and plethysmographic studies indicated continuing patency over 6 months later.[1]

Balloon catheters for iliac artery dilatation. "*Left,* Caged balloon catheter (Portsmann). *Right,* Polyvinyl balloon catheter (Gruntzig). The polyvinyl balloon catheter, properly handled, is less thrombogenic and easier to use; the caged balloon catheter can provide greater authority but is rarely required."[9]

subsequently modified by Staple (1968),[3] who tapered the end of the outer catheter, and Van Andel (1976),[4] who designed a series of long tapered catheters of increasing size that were introduced one after another. In addition to being less cumbersome to use than the coaxial system, Van Andel's design had the theoretical advantages of a decrease in the undesirable longitudinal shear force on the intima (which predisposed to acute thrombosis of the angioplasty site) and elimination of the possibility of entrapment of the intima between the two coaxial catheters ("snowplow effect") that also predisposed to acute postangioplasty thrombosis. Subsequently, Zeitler[5] added two side holes to the long tapered catheter to permit contrast injection.

Both the Dotter and the Van Andel types of systems were utilized extensively for PTA in Europe but achieved little acceptance in the United States. The main disadvantage of the Teflon dilators was that their small size limited their use to the femoral and popliteal arteries, since larger-diameter dilators needed for the iliac arteries were associated with an unacceptably high frequency of local complications because of the large puncture wounds required in the femoral artery.

The need to produce maximum dilatation of a stenotic lesion in the iliac artery with as small a catheter as possible led to the application of balloon catheters. Latex balloons proved ineffective because they were compressible, could produce only weak lateral forces, and tended to inflate in the direction of least resistance.[6] To overcome these technical limitations, Portsmann (1973)[7] described a "caged" or "corset" balloon catheter. This catheter system consisted of a latex balloon enclosed in a Teflon dilator with strips cut out from the area overlying the balloon to minimize the propensity of the elastic latex to deform around the lesion rather than to dilate it. However, because of fear of excessive damage to the vessel wall, as well as its higher thrombogenicity, the caged balloon catheter was never widely accepted.

The rapid growth and popularity of transluminal angioplasty resulted from the work of Andreas Gruntzig, who with his colleague Hopff,[8] developed a double-lumen balloon catheter made of polyvinyl chloride that produced safe, fast dilatation of narrowed vessel segments by applying radial rather than axial forces against the plaque and arterial wall and thereby minimizing the risk of embolization. Because of its low compliance, the Gruntzig balloon could be inflated to a predetermined diameter (4 to 8 mm), and a pressure of 4 to 5 atmospheres could be applied to an atherosclerotic plaque with no fear of balloon overdistention and potential vessel rupture. Dilatation to the size of a no. 12 French catheter could be accomplished with a no. 7 French catheter, so that vessels as large as the aorta could be dilated while minimizing the size of the puncture needed for catheter insertion and thus reducing the rate of local complications.[6]

Favorable experience with the application of the Gruntzig balloon catheter in atherosclerotic lesions of the iliac, femoral, and popliteal arteries opened the way for angioplasty of other vessels. Within the next few years, Gruntzig reported successful PTA of the coronary and renal arteries[10,11] and treatment of renovascular hypertension by transluminal dilatation of a renal artery stenosis.[12] In addition to developing his own technical expertise, Gruntzig spared no effort to instruct qualified physicians in the correct use of the balloon catheter and initially made balloon catheters available only to these appropriately trained physicians.[6]

The long-term results of percutaneous transluminal angioplasty in properly selected patients are as good as those achieved with traditional surgical techniques. In addition to being safe, simple, and relatively painless, PTA can be performed with the patient in the hospital for little

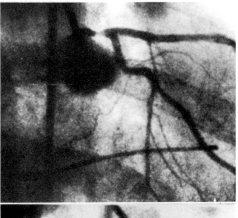

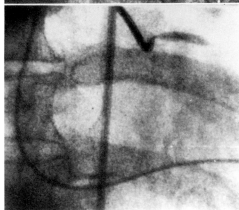

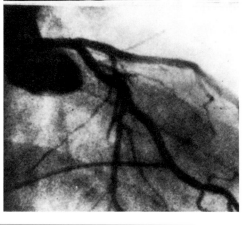

Transluminal dilatation of coronary artery stenosis (1978). *Top,* Initial angiogram of a 43-year-old male with severe angina pectoris reveals severe stenosis of the main left coronary artery. *Middle,* After passage of the dilatation catheter, the distensible balloon segment was inflated twice to a maximum outer diameter of 3.7 mm. *Bottom,* Postprocedure angiogram shows a good result without complications.[10]

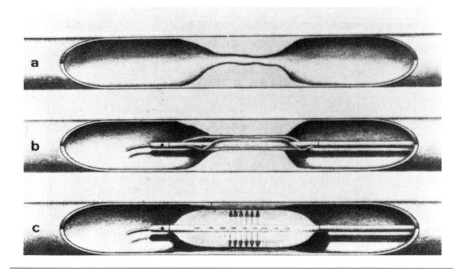

Percutaneous transluminal coronary angioplasty (1979). *Top,* "Stenosis of the coronary artery." *Middle,* "The double-lumen balloon catheter is introduced by use of a guiding catheter positioned at the orifice of the left or right coronary artery. At the tip of the dilating catheter is a short soft wire, which guides the catheter through the vessel. Proximal to the wire is a side hole connected to the main lumen of the dilating catheter. This lumen is used for pressure recording and contrast-material injection. The dilating catheter is advanced through the coronary artery with the balloon deflated." *Bottom,* "The balloon is inflated across the stenosis to its predetermined maximal outer diameter of 3.0 to 3.7 mm at a fluid pressure of 4 to 5 bar (400 to 500 kPa), thereby enlarging the lumen. After balloon deflation, the catheter is withdrawn."[11]

more than a day. Unsuccessful angioplasty does not preclude surgical revascularization, and recurrent or worsening disease after initially successful PTA can be managed with another angioplasty without the necessity of dealing with postoperative scarring. Transluminal angioplasty has been particularly useful in patients with renovascular hypertension, especially those with fibromuscular dysplasia.[13]

More recently, attempts have been made to remove obstructive vascular lesions rather than remodelling and displacing them, as is done with transluminal angioplasty. Several investigative groups have used various types of lasers to ablate atherosclerotic lesions, while others have used a drill or blade mounted on an angiographic catheter and powered by an external source to remove atherosclerotic or thrombotic material at the site of vascular occlusion.[2]

THROMBOLYSIS

Fibrinolytic activity in cultures of Group C beta-hemolytic streptococci related to a bacterial protein termed *streptokinase* was first discovered by Tillett and Garner in 1933.[14] More than a decade later (1947), MacFarlane and Pilling[15] first described thrombolytic activity in human urine. This material, *urokinase*, was initially concentrated from human urine but is now prepared commercially from human renal cell cultures.[16] The subsequent understanding of the interactions of these substances with the human fibrinolytic system resulted in a wide variety of clinical applications. In 1959, Johnson and McCarty[17] reported clinical lysis of clot by the intravenous administration of streptokinase. This report initiated the use of high-dose intravenous systemic infusion of thrombolytic agents to lyse thrombi and thromboemboli. In 1973, a large cooperative therapeutic trial for pulmonary embolism showed greater resolution of thrombi and a more significant improvement in pulmonary artery pressures and clinical status in those patients treated with streptokinase or urokinase than in those receiving heparin therapy.[18] Nevertheless, the use of thrombolytic agents fell into disfavor, mainly because of the fear of systemic complications, particularly hemorrhage.

Lysis of clot by the intravenous administration of streptokinase (1959). To determine the extent of clot lysis and reformation, venograms were made on a patient's right arm (*left*) before the induction of clot, as a control; (*middle*) 48 hours after clot was induced and before infusion of streptokinase, defining the clot; and (*right*) 24 hours after streptokinase infusion, showing that complete lysis occurred without clot reformation. Radiopaque lines at 1 and 2 were made by nichrome wires on the skin surface to define the original area of clot induction. The arrow at 3 indicates the distal portion of the clot. Lysis of the clot occurred after 30 hours of infusion.[17]

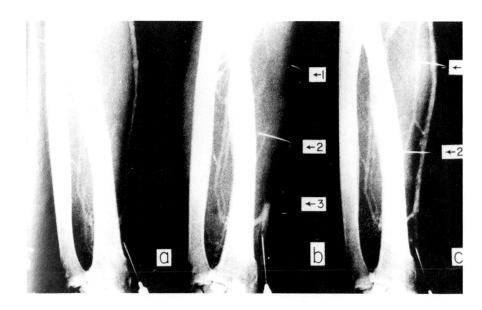

In order to avoid bleeding problems, Dotter and co-workers (1974)[19] suggested delivering streptokinase locally to peripheral vascular occlusions at approximately ⅟20 the systemic dose. Despite good results, this new low-dose method did not become popular. Subsequently, Renthrop (1979) described the use of a high-dose, short-duration infusion of thrombolytic agents in the coronary arterial tree and Katzen (1981) reported the use of local low-dose infusions in the peripheral vasculature. These and subsequent articles attest to the efficacy and increased popularity of local thrombolytic therapy.[2] However, it is important to remember Dotter's[1] words of caution: "Thrombolysis is not curative; it merely restores patency and helps identify a local anatomical obstruction which requires treatment . . . Even in small doses thrombolysis can cause distal systemic complications." Despite clinical successes, continuing severe problems associated with thrombolytic therapy include the incidence of local complications, the high cost of the drugs, and the lengthy hospitalization required for complete resolution of clots.[2]

Some of these problems may be resolved by the development of a new generation of thrombolytic substances, particularly tissue-type plasminogen activator (tPA), which can now be abundantly produced by recombinant genetic techniques. This agent acts only on clots and thus avoids systemic fibrinolytic effects and their associated hemorrhagic complications, as well as reducing the need for intensive and specialized nursing care.[2]

EMBOLOTHERAPY

Whereas angioplasty and thrombolysis have been developed to resolve vascular occlusion, embolotherapy has been developed to produce vascular occlusion. In many situations, embolotherapy has become an alternative to the more conventional techniques of surgery, radiation, and drugs.

Although interest in embolotherapy has been greatest in the past two decades, the principle of vascular embolization dates back to 1904, when Dawbin described the preoperative injection of melted paraffin (Vaseline) into the external carotid arteries of patients suffering from head and neck tumors.[2] Brooks (1930)[20] introduced particulate embolization with the occlusion of a traumatic carotid cavernous fistula by the injection of a muscle fragment attached to a silver clip into an internal carotid artery. Similarly, Luessenhop and Spence (1960)[21] injected spheres of methylmethacrylate into the surgically exposed common carotid artery of a patient suffering from an arteriovenous malformation fed by the middle cerebral artery and achieved clinical improvement. As they noted,

> The major feeding arteries (of the malformation) are greatly enlarged compared to the arteries of the surrounding brain. Because of the reduced peripheral resistance there is a far greater flow of blood to the malformation than to the surrounding brain. The main arterial feeders arborize into considerably smaller, "arteriole-like" vessels before entrance into the larger channels which constitute the bulk of the lesion. Therefore, an embolus of predetermined size and configuration, introduced even far proximal to the malformation, will always find its way to it. By its size, the embolus will be excluded from passage into the smaller branches to the brain and will ultimately come to rest at a site proximal to the malformation where normal and abnormal vessels are seen to be clearly separate.

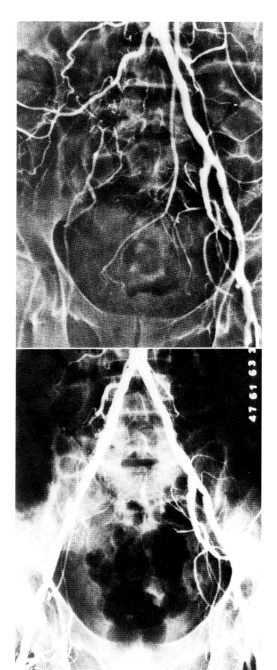

Selective clot lysis with low-dose streptokinase (1974). *Top*, Control angiogram shows occlusion of the upper right common iliac artery. *Bottom*, After 115 hours of a selective infusion of streptokinase, there is good restoration of the occluded artery.[19]

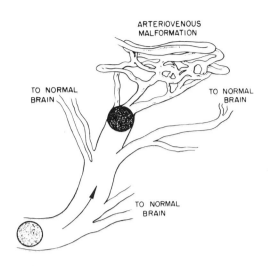

ARTERIOVENOUS
MALFORMATION

TO NORMAL
BRAIN

TO NORMAL
BRAIN

TO NORMAL
BRAIN

Artificial embolization of cerebral arteries
in arteriovenous malformation (1960).
"An embolus placed in the main arterial
channel is excluded by its size from passing
into smaller branches to normal brain
and is forced to become arrested at a point
proximal to the malformation."[21]

Newton and Adams (1968)[22] selectively catheterized the feeding artery of a spinal cord angioma and were able to embolize the malformation and produce noticeable clinical improvement without the need for any surgical intervention. Using a similar percutaneous approach, Kricheff, Madayag, and Braunstein[23] succeeded in embolizing an arteriovenous malformation of the brain itself. They stressed the superiority of catheter embolization to a direct arteriotomy approach, noting that "no surgical incision or general anesthesia is required. There is no damage to the carotid or vertebral arteries. Direct clinical observation of the awake patient may be used as an important guide to the procedure. Repeat embolization can be performed at a later date, if necessary, without sacrifice of an artery or reoperation through a previously scarred site."

Embolotherapy was greatly influenced by a landmark 1963 paper by Nusbaum and Baum,[24] who detected unknown sites of gastrointestinal bleeding by demonstrating the extravasation of contrast material from the bleeding vessel during serial arteriography of visceral arteries. They estimated that bleeding at a rate of 0.5 ml/min could be detected with selective arteriography. In 1967, Nusbaum and Baum[25] introduced the concept of transcatheter selective pharmacoangiography with the injection of various vasoconstrictors in the superior mesenteric artery to reduce portal hypertension while avoiding systemic side effects. Favorable clinical results were reported with mesenteric arterial infusions of vasopressin in variceal bleeding (1971), which led to the use of intraarterial infusion of vasoconstrictors for the control of nonvariceal bleeding as well.[26] This pharmacological success was soon followed by the report of Rosch, Dotter, and Brown (1972)[27] of the control of acute gastric hemorrhage by embolization of the gastroepiploic artery using autologous clot. This material, first used by Doppman in 1968 to occlude a spinal arteriovenous malformation,[28] was later used to control genitourinary bleeding,[29] traumatic hemorrhage from pelvic fractures,[30] and renal arteriovenous fistulas.[31]

A tremendous upsurge of interest in embolization began in the 1970s, fostered by parallel developments in catheter technology and embolic agents. The availability of a wide range of preshaped catheters and the introduction of coaxial systems allowed relatively routine superselective catheter placement and embolic agent delivery.[2] In 1972, the tissue adhesive isobutyl-2-cyanoacrylate (Bucrylate) was introduced as an embolic agent by Zanetti and Sherman.[32] The use of Gelfoam particles as a medium-term embolic agent was first described by Carey and Grace in 1974.[33] For long-term results, the permanent embolic agent Ivalon (polyvinyl alcohol) was first used as a plug for closure of a patent ductus

Transfemoral catheter embolization of
arteriovenous malformation (1972). *Left*,
Initial right carotid angiogram demonstrates a large frontoparietal arteriovenous
malformation fed by middle and anterior
cerebral arteries. *Right*, Following the
introduction of Silastic pellets, about half
the malformation has been obliterated. Several anterior and middle cerebral feeding
arteries are not visualized. An embolus
(*open arrowhead*) can be seen obstructing
the orifice of one of these vessels and
protruding into the lumen of another large
feeding artery (*closed arrowhead*). Note
the Teflon catheter in the internal carotid
artery (*arrow*).[23]

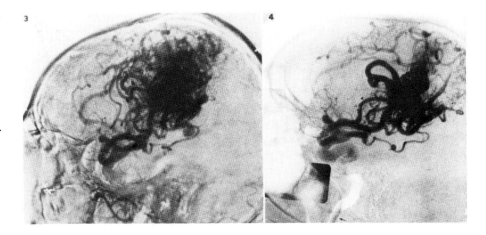

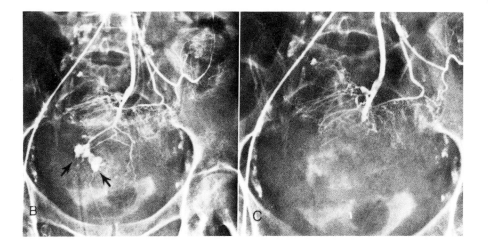

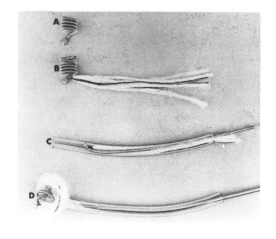

Angiographic control of pelvic bleeding (1976). *Left*, Selective inferior mesenteric arteriogram shows extravasation of contrast material from superior hemorrhoidal branches of the inferior mesenteric artery. *Right*, Following embolization with Gelfoam, a repeat arteriogram shows effective occlusion of the bleeding artery and no further angiographic evidence of bleeding.[29]

arteriosus by Portsmann and co-workers in 1971[34] and then employed in particulate form by Tadavarthy and co-workers 4 years later.[35] Other materials used for embolotherapy have included Silastic spheres, a variety of silicone preparations, and radioactive particles.

The majority of these embolotherapy materials acted as peripheral emboli that became trapped at various levels in the vascular bed into which they were injected. However, the use of many of these materials often gave a variable degree of occlusion, not only because of their inhomogeneous distribution but also because of their nature. Blood clot and Gelfoam, for example, were biodegradable and readily recanalized.[36] The need for a consistently reliable device that could be precisely placed for a more permanent central occlusion of larger vessels and could serve as an internal ligature was satisfied by the stainless steel spring coil embolus devised by Gianturco (1975).[37] Initially, wool strands were attached to the proximal tip of the coil to serve as a nidus for thrombosis. The coil was used with a nontapered-tip 7 French Teflon catheter and was inserted into the catheter with a special, relatively stiff introducer stylette and then passed through the catheter with a modified guidewire. Increased utilization of the original coil created the necessity and demand for design modification. The wool attached to the coil was replaced by Dacron, different sizes of coils were made available, and the long, stiff introducer stylette was reduced in length to avoid inadvertent perforation when in a tortuous vessel.[36]

The use of detachable balloon catheters for embolization of vascular malformations and aneurysms in the cerebral circulation was first described by Serbinenko of the Soviet Union in 1974.[38] This technique was further developed by Debrun and White and their colleagues,[39,40] who produced an injectable flow-directed catheter with a detachable silicone balloon for permanent vascular occlusion. Similarly, Kerber developed a silicone calibrated-leak balloon that allowed highly selective flow-directed placement and then balloon occlusive angiography or embolization using the low-viscosity tissue adhesives.[41]

The use of particulate embolic agents, autologous clot, and coils could be complicated by difficulties in handling the agents, incomplete infarction of target tissue, vascular recanalization, and inadvertent reflux that occluded nontarget vessels.[42] This led Ellman and co-workers[43] to study the potential for transcatheter therapeutic infarction of the kidney

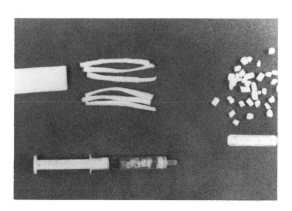

Gelfoam (surgical gelatin). Particles consisting of approximately 3 mm cubes and 3 × 3 × 20 mm segments injected with a 1 to 2 ml syringe. Five to ten particles or one segment is injected at a time.[9]

Gianturco coil (1975). *A*, Stainless steel coil (5-mm helix diameter) with attached wool strands.[9] *B*, The coil with attached woolen strands 6 cm long. *C*, The straightened wool coil within a clear plastic tube. *D*, The reformation of the wool coil, as it emerges from the catheter.[37]

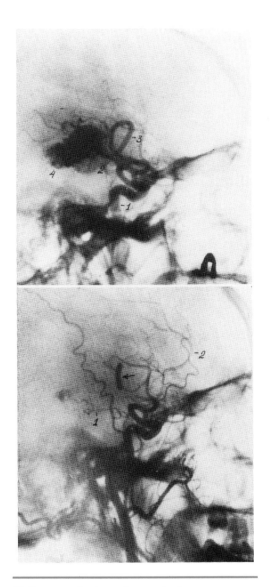

Balloon occlusion of an arteriovenous malformation in the distribution of the middle cerebral artery. *Top*, Preoperative angiogram. *1*, Internal carotid artery; *2*, short afferent vessel; *3*, long looping afferent vessel; *4*, malformation. *Bottom*, Postoperative arteriogram shows that the long, looping afferent vessel has been permanently occluded by the detachable balloon (*arrow*). There is an insignificant blood supply to the malformation from the anterior choroidal artery (*1*).[38]

with absolute ethanol, which in a canine study produced complete renal infarction without damage to the adjacent aorta (1980). In the same year, Klatte reported the first clinical use of absolute ethanol for transcatheter renal artery occlusion in renal cell carcinoma,[42] while Ellman and associates published their success in six patients in the following year.[44]

Endoscopic injection sclerotherapy, the direct injection of a sclerosing agent into distal esophageal varices, was first described by Crafoord and Frenckner in 1939.[45] However, this technique was largely overshadowed by portosystemic shunt surgery until 1979, when it was reintroduced by Terblanche and associates.[46] Advantages of this technique include its relative simplicity, its high success rate (control of acute hemorrhage in about 90% of cases), and the ability to repeat the injections on multiple occasions.

The efficacy of boiling contrast material to occlude veins in laboratory animals was described by Amplatz and associates in 1982.[47] Because of difficulty in finding human volunteers to test the technique, Amplatz volunteered a vein in his own forearm for hot-contrast injection. The vein was subsequently removed, and light microscopy confirmed the angiographic findings of complete obstruction of the venous channel.[2]

TRANSVENOUS INTERRUPTION OF THE INFERIOR VENA CAVA

Anticoagulation therapy is generally considered the procedure of choice in most patients to provide prophylaxis against pulmonary embolism in the presence of deep vein thrombosis. However, when anticoagulation therapy is contraindicated or fails, interruption of blood return via the inferior vena cava is considered an alternative means of preventing pulmonary embolism.[48]

In 1934, Homans[49] observed that

> thrombosis of the veins in and among the muscles of the lower legs—a deep peripheral thrombosis—is a clinical entity, which runs a peculiar course. The number of intermuscular and intramuscular veins, their abundant anastomoses and collateral circulation, cause the thrombosis to present few or no external signs when the leg is not in use. The incidence of fatal pulmonary embolism is high. Ligation of the femoral vein at the groin is recommended, particularly when the thrombosis has become well established.

Although femoral vein ligation was the procedure performed initially, high rates of recurrent embolization (especially from the "normal" leg or pelvic veins) led O'Neil (1945)[50] to describe ligation of the inferior vena cava "when concurrent phlebothrombosis exists in both lower extremities and extends to or above the inguinal ligament, and when pulmonary embolism has occurred and its source is not evident." However, complete occlusion of the inferior vena cava led to acute or chronic stasis in the lower extremities and the development of large, unfiltered collaterals that could permit the passage of peripheral clots to the pulmonary circulation. The solution to this problem was plication of the inferior vena cava with sutures,[51] staples,[52] or external clips,[53] so that it was converted from a single large vessel to a parallel row of several small vessels. Theoretically, this would obstruct emboli of a potentially fatal size while not otherwise seriously interfering with the blood flow from the lower extremities. However, as with surgical ligation, plication of the inferior vena cava required abdominal surgery with general anesthesia, and the rates of operative mortality and recurrent embolization were essentially the same. In addition, preoperative suspension of anticoagulation increased the risk of further thrombus formation.[48]

Interruption of the inferior vena cava by the transvenous placement of an intraluminal device via a local cutdown at the neck or groin was initially developed to avoid the use of general anesthesia in high-risk patients who could not be given anticoagulants. Early attempts to obstruct the vena cava temporarily utilized devices such as the sieve described by Eichelter and Schenk (1968), which remained attached to a coaxial system of catheters, and the triple-lumen catheter with a permanently attached balloon described by Moser and co-workers (1971). However, the potential for embolization of trapped or attached thrombi when these devices were subsequently removed has precluded their use in humans.[48]

The first percutaneously introduced device for sustaining patency and effective filtration without occlusion of the inferior vena cava was the Mobin-Uddin umbrella filter. First commercially available in 1970, this device was a miniature umbrella with six flat stainless-steel spokes radiating from a central hub and covered by a thin, fenestrated Silastic membrane impregnated with heparin.[54] To overcome problems of proximal migration and inferior vena caval thrombosis associated with the Mobin-Uddin umbrella, Greenfield, in collaboration with the Kimray Corporation, designed the Kimray-Greenfield filter.[55,56] This umbrella filter, which could be placed through the femoral or jugular vein, was closed during insertion into the inferior vena cava and sprung open when in place. "Fixation occurs by the recurved hooks which grasp the wall of the vena cava usually without full thickness penetration. This 'fish hook' principle prevents proximal migration and becomes even more secure with capture of a large embolus distending the vena cava."[56] Theoretically, the axial flow of blood should move emboli of 3 mm in diameter or larger into the "trap" of the filter.[48] A more recent inferior vena caval filter is the "bird's nest," named for the appearance of the wires that make up the filtration matrix.

A third transvenous approach introduced by Hunter and co-workers (1977)[57] was the placement via a jugular venous cutdown of a detachable balloon that totally obstructed the inferior vena cava from the moment of its insertion. The originators of this technique concluded that an "intraluminal IVC occluder should not attempt to be a filter and that any foreign body placed in the retroperitoneal space should have a design without sharp edges, pins or points." Although the balloon gradually deflated in about 12 months, it was retained within the vena cava because of the fibrotic reaction occurring in the surrounding vessel wall. "Late results of balloon occlusion are excellent with continued protection from pulmonary emboli; a low incidence of leg problems; and absolute stability of the small, rounded, scar-encased balloon remnant." At present, however, the high cost of the disposable catheter system is a deterrent to the use of this technique.

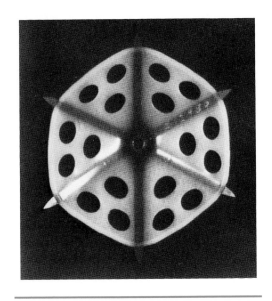

Mobin-Uddin inferior vena caval umbrella filter.[54]

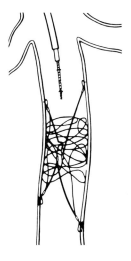

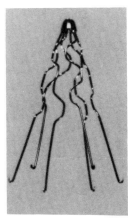

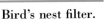

Bird's nest filter.   Kimray-Greenfield filter.[48]

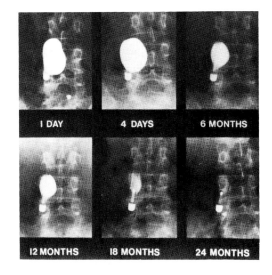

Permanent transvenous balloon occlusion of the inferior vena cava (1977). Sequence of radiographs shows gradual deflation of the balloon. Rounding of the balloon on day 4 occurs as the IVC accommodates to lateral pressure of the balloon. The venogram at 6 months shows the collapsing balloon with a patent IVC above.[57]

PERCUTANEOUS ASPIRATION BIOPSY AND ABSCESS DRAINAGE

Percutaneous aspiration biopsy of suspected neoplasms using an 18-gauge needle was first performed by Hayes Martin and Edward Ellis in 1930.[58] They recommended percutaneous aspiration biopsy of tumor masses in patients in whom a surgical procedure was contraindicated because of technical difficulty or the risk of hemorrhage or infection and whenever there was "lack of justification for any procedure involving physical or mental discomfort or expense to the patient, where the information to be gained may be of doubtful value to the patient or of academic interest only."

For the next 40 years, percutaneous aspiration biopsy was essentially neglected in the United States, mainly because pathologists were reluctant to offer cytological rather than histological interpretation of the material obtained from aspiration and clinicians feared that the procedure would result in dissemination of resectable tumor. In 1960, Franzen and co-workers[59] first described the use of a thin-needle technique (22-gauge) for the cytological diagnosis of prostatic tumors by transrectal aspiration biopsy. With the availability of ultrasound guidance for percutaneous biopsy in the mid-1970s, several groups reported a high degree of accuracy in obtaining and interpreting aspirated material, thus refuting many of the previous objections to this procedure.[60]

Percutaneous fine-needle aspiration biopsy under ultrasound or CT guidance has become a widely accepted technique for rapidly and safely obtaining material for pathological diagnosis. It is of special value in obtaining tissue specimens in high-risk surgical patients, in confirming the presence of a tumor in a patient with unresectable or possibly recurrent disease, and in obviating exploratory surgery by demonstrating the benign nature of some lesions. There are essentially no contraindications to the procedure except for an uncontrollable bleeding diathesis. Even highly vascular lesions such as hepatocellular carcinoma and hemangioma have been safely biopsied percutaneously using fine needles, though great care must be taken and the patient closely observed.[61]

The success of fine-needle aspiration biopsy and the increased availability of cross-sectional imaging (ultrasound and CT) led to the development of percutaneous catheter drainage of abdominal and retroperitoneal abscesses. Combined with systemic antibiotic therapy, the percutaneous placement of relatively small catheters permitted safe mechanical drainage of abscesses without the need for a major surgical procedure. As an early report noted, guided percutaneous aspiration and drainage of abscesses fulfilled the classic surgical criteria suggested in 1938 by Ochsner and DeBakey[62] that "the ideal type of drainage procedure . . . is one characterized by directness, simplicity, and above all, avoidance of unnecessary contamination of uninvolved areas."

References

1. Dotter CT and Judkins MP: Transluminal treatment of arteriosclerotic obstruction. Circulation 30:654-670, 1964.
2. Castaneda-Zuniga WR: Interventional radiology: Yesterday, today, tomorrow. In Castaneda-Zuniga WR and Tadavarthy SM (eds): Interventional radiology. Baltimore, Williams & Wilkins, 1988.
3. Staple TW: Modified catheter for percutaneous transluminal treatment of atherosclerotic obstructions. Radiology 91:1041-1043, 1968.
4. Van Andel GJ: Percutaneous transluminal angioplasty: The Dotter procedure. Amsterdam, Excerpta Medica, 1976.
5. Zeitler E, Gruntzig A, and Schoop W (eds): Percutaneous vascular recanalization: Technology, application, clinical results. Berlin, Springer-Verlag, 1978.
6. Waltman AC, Greenfield AJ, and Athanasoulis CA: Transluminal angioplasty: General rules and basic considerations. In Athanasoulis CA, Greene RE, Pfister RC, and Roberson GH (eds): Interventional radiology. Philadelphia, WB Saunders, 1982.
7. Portsmann W: Ein nur Korsett-Balloon-Ka-

theter zur transluminalen Rekanalisation nach Dotter unter besonderer Berücksichtigung von Obliterationen an den Beckenarterien. Radiol Diag (Berl) 14:239-243, 1973.

8. Gruntzig A and Hopff H: Perkutane Rekanalisation chronischer arterieller Verschlüsse mit einem neuen Dilatations-Katheter. Deutsch Med Wschr 99:2502-2504, 1974.

9. Abrams HL (ed): Vascular and interventional radiology. Boston, Little, Brown, 1983.

10. Gruntzig AR: Transluminal dilation of coronary artery stenosis. Lancet 1:263, 1978.

11. Gruntzig AR, Senning A, and Siegenthaler WE: Non-operative dilation of coronary artery stenosis. Percutaneous transluminal coronary angioplasty. N Engl J Med 301:61-68, 1979.

12. Gruntzig A, Kuhlmann U, Vetter W, et al: Treatment of renal vascular hypertension with percutaneous transluminal dilatation of a renal artery stenosis. Lancet 1:801-802, 1978.

13. Schwarten DE: Aortic, iliac, and peripheral arterial angioplasty. In Castaneda-Zuniga WR and Tadavarthy SM (eds): Interventional radiology. Baltimore, Williams & Wilkins, 1988.

14. Tillett WS and Garner RL: The fibrinolytic activity of hemolytic streptococci. J Exp Med 58:485-488, 1933.

15. MacFarlane RG and Pilling J: Fibrinolytic activity of normal urine. Nature 159:779-785, 1947.

16. Gallant TE and Athanasoulis CA: Regional infusion of thrombolytic enzymes. In Athanasoulis CA, Greene RE, Pfister RC, and Roberson GH (eds): Interventional radiology. Philadelphia, WB Saunders, 1982.

17. Johnson AJ and McCarty WR: The lysis of artificially induced intravascular clots in man by intravenous infusions of streptokinase. J Clin Invest 38:1627-1643, 1959.

18. Urokinase-Streptokinase pulmonary embolism trial (phase II). Results: A co-operative study. JAMA 229:1606-1613, 1974.

19. Dotter CT, Rosch J, and Seaman AJ: Selective clot lysis with low dose streptokinase. Radiology 111:31-37, 1974.

20. Brooks B: The treatment of traumatic arteriovenous fistula. South Med J 23:100-106, 1930.

21. Luessenhop AJ and Spence WT: Artificial embolization of cerebral arteries: Report of use in a case of arteriovenous malformation. JAMA 172:1153-1155, 1960.

22. Newton TH and Adams JE: Angiographic demonstration and nonsurgical embolization of spinal cord angioma. Radiology 91:873-876, 1968.

23. Kricheff II, Madayag M, and Braunstein P: Transfemoral catheter embolization of cerebral and posterior fossa arteriovenous malformations. Radiology 103:107-111, 1972.

24. Nusbaum M and Baum S: Radiographic demonstration of unknown sites of gastrointestinal bleeding. Surg Forum 14:374-375, 1963.

25. Nusbaum M, Baum S, Sakiyalak P, et al: Pharmacologic control of portal hypertension. Surgery 62:299-310, 1967.

26. Baum S and Nusbaum M: The control of gastrointestinal hemorrhage by selective mesenteric arterial infusion of vasopressin. Radiology 98:497-505, 1971.

27. Rosch J, Dotter CT, and Brown MJ: Selective arterial embolization: A new method for control of acute gastrointestinal bleeding. Radiology 102:303-306, 1972.

28. Doppman JL, DiChiro G, and Ommaya A: Obliteration of spinal cord arteriovenous malformation by percutaneous embolization. Lancet 1:477, 1968.

29. Athanasoulis CA, Waltman AC, Barnes AB, et al: Angiographic control of pelvic bleeding from treated carcinoma of the cervix. Gynec Oncol 4:144-150, 1976.

30. Matalon TSA, Athanasoulis CA, Margolies MN, et al: Hemorrhage with pelvic fractures: Efficacy of transcatheter embolization. AJR 133:859-864, 1979.

31. Silber S: Renal trauma: Treatment by angiographic injection of autologous clot. Arch Surg 110:206-207, 1975.

32. Zanetti PH and Sherman FE: Experimental evaluation of a tissue adhesive as an agent for the treatment of aneurysms and arteriovenous anomalies. J Neurosurg 36:72-79, 1972.

33. Carey LS and Grace DM: The brisk bleed: Controlled by arterial catheterization and Gelfoam plug. J Can Assoc Radiol 25:113-115, 1974.

34. Portsmann W, Wierny L, Warnke H, et al: Catheter closure of patent ductus arteriosus: 62 cases treated without thoracotomy. Radiol Clin North Am 9:203-218, 1971.

35. Tadavarthy SM, Moller JH, and Amplatz K: Polyvinyl alcohol (Ivalon): A new embolic material. AJR 125:609-616, 1975.

36. Wallace S, Chuang VP, Anderson JH, and Gianturco C: Steel coil embolus and its therapeutic applications. In Athanasoulis CA, Greene RE, Pfister RC, and Roberson GH (eds): Interventional radiology. Philadelphia, WB Saunders, 1982.

37. Gianturco C, Anderson JH, and Wallace S: Mechanical devices for arterial occlusion. AJR 124:428-435, 1975.

38. Serbinenko FA: Balloon catheterization and occlusion of major cerebral vessels. J Neurosurg 41:125-145, 1974.

39. Debrun G, Lacour P, Caron JP, et al: Inflatable and released balloon technique experimentation in dog: Application in man. Neuroradiology 9:267-271, 1975.

40. White RI, Barth KH, Kaufman SL, et al: Therapeutic embolization with detachable balloons. Cardio Vasc Intervent Radiol 3:239-241, 1980.

41. Kerber C: Balloon catheter with a calibrated leak. Radiology 120:547-550, 1976.

42. Becker GJ, Holden RW, Yune HY, and Klatte EC: Ablation with absolute ethanol. In Castaneda-Zuniga WR and Tadavarthy SM (eds): Interventional radiology. Baltimore, Williams & Wilkins, 1988.

43. Ellman BA, Green EC, Elgenbrodt E, et al: Renal infarction with absolute ethanol. Invest Radiol 15:318-322, 1980.

44. Ellman BA, Parkhill BJ, Curry TS, et al: Ablation of renal tumors with absolute ethanol: A new technique. Radiology 141:619-626, 1981.

45. Crafoord C and Frenckner P: New surgical treatment of varicose veins of the oesophagus. Acta Otolaryngol 27:422-429, 1939.

46. Terblanche J, Northover JMA, Bornman P, et al: A prospective evaluation of injection sclerotherapy in the treatment of acute bleeding from esophageal varices. Surgery 85:239-245, 1979.

47. Cragg AH, Rosel P, Rysavy JA, et al: Renal ablation using hot contrast medium: An experimental study. Radiology 148:683-686, 1983.

48. Dedrick CG and Novelline RA: Transvenous interruption of the inferior vena cava. In Athanasoulis CA, Greene RE, Pfister RC, and Roberson GH (eds): Interventional radiology. Philadelphia, WB Saunders, 1982.

49. Homans J: Thrombosis of the deep veins of the lower leg, causing pulmonary embolism. N Engl J Med 211:993-997, 1934.

50. O'Neil EE: Ligation of the inferior vena cava in the prevention and treatment of pulmonary embolism. N Engl J Med 232:641-646, 1945.

51. Spencer FC, Quattlebaum JK, and Jude JR: Plication of the inferior vena cava for pulmonary embolism. A report of 20 cases. Ann Surg 155:827-837, 1962.

52. Ravitch MM, Snodgrass E, and Rivarola A: Compartmentation of the vena cava with the mechanical stapler. Surg Gynec Obstet 122:561-566, 1966.

53. Adams JT and DeWeese JA: Experimental and clinical evaluation of portal vein interruption in the prevention of pulmonary emboli. Surgery 57:82-102, 1965.

54. Mobin-Uddin K, Callard GM, Bolooki H, et al: Transvenous caval interruption with umbrella filter. N Engl J Med 286:55-58, 1972.

55. Greenfield LJ, McCurdy JR, Brown PP, and Elkins RC: A new intracaval filter permitting continued flow and resolution of emboli. Surgery 73:599-606, 1973.

56. Greenfield LJ, Zocco J, Wilk J, et al: Clinical experience with the Kim-Ray Greenfield vena caval filter. Ann Surg 185:692-698, 1977.

57. Hunter JA, Dye WS, Javid H, et al: Permanent transvenous balloon occlusion of the inferior vena cava. Ann Surg 186:491-499, 1977.

58. Martin HE and Ellis EB: Biopsy by needle puncture and aspiration. Ann Surg 92:169-181, 1930.

59. Franzen S, Giertz G, and Zajicek J: Cytological diagnosis of prostatic tumours by transrectal aspiration biopsy: A preliminary report. Br J Urol 32:193-196, 1960.

60. Holm HH, Pederson JF, Kristensen JK, et al: Ultrasonically guided percutaneous puncture. Radiol Clin North Am 13:493-509, 1975.

61. Doherty FJ: Fine-needle percutaneous aspiration biopsy of abdominal mass lesions. In Athanasoulis CA, Greene RE, Pfister RC, and Roberson GH (eds): Interventional radiology. Philadelphia, WB Saunders, 1982.

62. Ochsner A and DeBakey M: Subphrenic abscess: A collective review and an analysis of 3608 collected and personal cases. Int Abstr Surg 66:426-438, 1938.

NONMEDICAL ASPECTS OF RADIOLOGY

THE CALL TO DINNER

My friends, I hate to seem abrupt
And I deplore to "interrupt,"
To pry your stereoscopic eyes
From off the inner mysteries;
But, sirs, to reason I appeal;
Is there no vacuum you feel?
When the thrice-smitten dinner gong
Falls on deaf ears, there's something wrong.
I view you with an anxious eye—
What if your vacuums run too high
and puncture or collapse befall?
Beware, I cry you, one and all.

Poor souls, unto my warning hark;
The coil that gives the fattest spark
Must guard its precious insulation;
In my opsonic estimation
You're softening down—without your ration!

Do you, by some sad mental hitch
See only when you throw the switch?
Must all appeals to you be sung
In that alluring Roentgen tongue?—
The dinner gong's in English rung.

Where's the transformer of such worth
'Twould firmly step you down to earth?
What prime conductor could assume
To lead you towards the dining-room?
Oh, for a "ground" that should convey
All volts and amperes far away!
Oh, for the luck of burning fuse,
And not another you could use!
Oh, for the minds sane and water-cooled,
By prudent counsels to be ruled!
Ah! did I dare, I would aspire
To be your psychic rectifier
And make the currents of your thought
Face right about the way they ought!
Deluded souls I sweetly pray,
Lead-screen your brains and slip away
From these enthralling rays that cheat
Your days and nights and

Come and Eat!

Caroline Bartlett Crane, *American Quarterly of Roentgenology*
4:238, 1913

CHAPTER 32

Medicolegal and Forensic Radiology

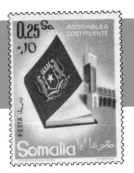
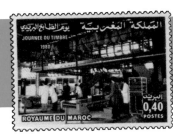
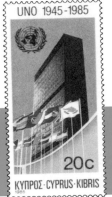
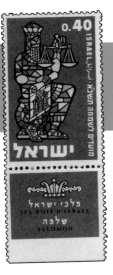

Within a year of Roentgen's discovery, several celebrated cases were reported in which x-ray evidence played an important role. One of the first, from Nottingham, England, involved a suit brought by Miss Gladys Ffolliett, a burlesque and comedy actress, who had injured her foot on a faulty staircase in the theater. Being unable to resume her work after a month's convalescence, she was advised to have radiographs made at a local hospital. The films, produced in court, showed so definite a displacement of the cuboid bone of the left foot that "no further argument on the point was needed on either side, and the only defense, therefore, was a charge of contributory carelessness."[1] As the *Literary Digest*[2] noted,

> Those medical men who are accustomed to dealing with "accident claims"—and such claims are now very numerous—will perceive how great a service the new photography may render to truth and right in difficult and doubtful cases. If the whole osseous system, including the spine, can be portrayed distinctly on the negative, much shameful perjury on the part of a certain class of claimants, and many discreditable contradictions among medical experts will be avoided. The case is a distinct triumph for science, and shows how plain fact is now furnished with a novel and successful means of vindicating itself with unerring certainty against opponents of every class.

Soon afterward, the Court of the Queen's Bench at Montreal, Canada, accepted as evidence a radiograph showing a bullet in a man's leg.[3] In the United States, the first civil case in which x-ray films were presented and admitted as evidence was the Denver case of *Smith v. Grant* (1896), an action for alleged malpractice in the treatment of a fractured femur against a surgeon of national reputation.[3-5] The suit was brought by James Smith, a poor boy who was reading law and doing odd jobs to pay his expenses. While trimming some trees, Smith was injured in a fall from a ladder. After some time he consulted the distinguished surgeon, W. W. Grant, one of the founders of the American College of Surgeons and credited with performing the first appendectomy in the country. Failing to find any signs of fracture, Grant made no attempt to immobilize the thigh but instead advised various kinds of exercises as though treating a contusion.

Smith's attorneys, Lindsey and Parks, realized that their case hinged on demonstrating that their client had indeed suffered a fracture that had been misdiagnosed and incorrectly treated, thus leading to their client's disability. Having seen some early radiographs of Doctor Chauncey Tennant and newspaper photographer H. Buckwalter published in the *Rocky Mountain News*, they convinced Tennant to make several pictures of Smith's hip. The most satisfactory x-ray photograph, which required an exposure of 80 minutes, showed the rough outline of an impacted fracture of the head of the femur.

Could a radiograph be admitted in evidence? To convey the idea of radiographic shadows to the judge and jury, the plaintiff attorneys and the photographers contrived a shadow box with a small hole at one end through which illumination came from a lighted candle casting a shadow on a screen at the opposite end of the box. In succession, they showed the judge and jury the shadow of a hand, an x-ray shadowgraph of a hand, and x-rays of other objects such as small wheels of a clock. Subsequently, they demonstrated the shadow of a normal femur projected onto the screen by the light of the candle followed by a roentgen shadowgraph of such a femur. Finally, the x-ray plate taken of Smith's left femur was presented. This showed that the femoral head was not in normal relation to the greater trochanter and shaft. Lindsey and Parks proposed that this "shadow picture," or "roentgen picture" as it was called, be submitted to the jury as evidence that there had been a fracture of the femur in the region of the greater trochanter, with impaction of the fragments.

The defense attorney, former U.S. Senator Charles J. Hughes, argued that "x-ray photographs" were not admissible under the law and cited several Eastern cases supporting his view. Furthermore, he contended that even should it be admitted that this was a photograph of James Smith's femur, it could not be used as competent testimony under the broad principle of the law concerning the use of photographs as testimony, which required that witnesses must testify to having seen the object that had been photographed and to have identified the photograph as a good likeness of the object. Clearly, no one had ever seen the broken bone that the x-ray photograph purported to reveal.

Judge Owen E. LeFevre rendered the following opinion[6]:

> The defendant's counsel objects to the admission in evidence of exhibits, the same being photographs produced by means of the x-ray process, on the ground that, being photographs of an object unseen by the human eye there is no evidence that the photograph accurately portrays and represents the objects to be photographed. This rule of law is well settled by a long line of authorities and we do not dissent therefrom as applied to photographs, which may be seen by the human eye. The reason for this salutory rule is so apparent to the profession that as a rule of evidence we will not discuss it.
>
> We, however, have been presented with a photograph taken by means of a new scientific discovery, the same being acknowledged in the arts and science. It knocks for admission at the temple of learning; what shall we do or say? Close fast the door or open wide the portals?

These photographs are offered in evidence to show the present condition of the head and neck of the femur bone which is entirely hidden from the eye of the surgeon. Nature has surrounded it with tissues for its protection and there it lies hidden; and cannot, by any possibility be removed nor exposed that it may be compared with its shadow as developed, by means of this new scientific process.

In addition to these exhibits in evidence, we have nothing to do or say as to what they purport to represent; that will, without doubt, be explained by eminent surgeons. These exhibits are only pictures or maps—to be used in explanation of a present condition, and therefore secondary evidence and not primary. They may be shown to the jury as illustrating or making clear the testimony of experts. The law is the acme of learning throughout ages. It is the essence of wisdom, reason and experience. Learned priests have interpreted the law. They classified reasons for certain opinions which, in time, have become precedents, and these ordinarily guide and control especially trial courts. We must not, however, hedge ourselves round about with rule, precept and precedent until we can advance no further. Our field must ever grow as trade, the arts and science seek to enter it.

During the last decade, at least, no science has made such mighty strides forward as surgery. It is eminently a scientific profession alike interesting to the learned and the unlearned. It makes use of all science and learning. It has been of inestimable service to mankind. It must not be said of the law that it is wedded to precedent, and will not lend a helping hand. Rather let the courts throw open the doors to all well considered scientific discoveries. Modern science has made it possible to look beneath the tissues of the human body and has aided surgery in telling of the hidden mysteries. We believe it to be our duty in this case to be the first if you please to so consider it, in admitting in evidence the process known and acknowledged as a determinant science. The exhibits will be admitted in evidence.

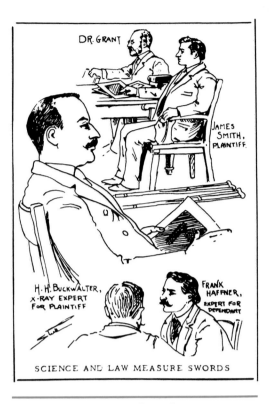

SCIENCE AND LAW MEASURE SWORDS

Illustration of principals and witnesses in the case of Smith v. Grant (*Daily News*, December 3, 1896).[4]

The *Colorado Medical Journal*[7] took a different view.

It is a credit to the profession of this city that they are standing manfully behind Doctor Grant. Damage suits are becoming too numerous. On the stand it was proven that Smith suffered from tuberculosis and specific disease and that he ran from doctor to doctor. Apparently he singled out Doctor Grant because he thought the Doctor's profession would allow a compromise. We are glad to see the Doctor fight the case, and certainly hope that he will win. In our opinion he cannot fail to do so. The value of the x-rays in cases of this kind took up much of the court's time and testimony and was not decisive in either way.

In discussing a paper on the medicolegal aspects of x-rays 2 years later, Grant stated that

no Supreme Court has yet passed upon admission of the x-ray in evidence. Local courts all over the country are divided on the subject. The more experienced and learned judges hesitate to accept it, and until the lawyers and courts ask for its introduction as evidence, surgeons should not try to introduce it, and not then unless we know it is absolutely reliable. It is different from the old photograph, about which long contests were waged in our courts, as to its admission as evidence. Even the photograph of an object, not of the shadow of the object as this is, was not admitted until the photograph itself was verified. That we can never do in the case of the x-ray except by postmortem.[8]

Principal figures in the Orme case (*American X-ray Journal*, March, 1899).[4]

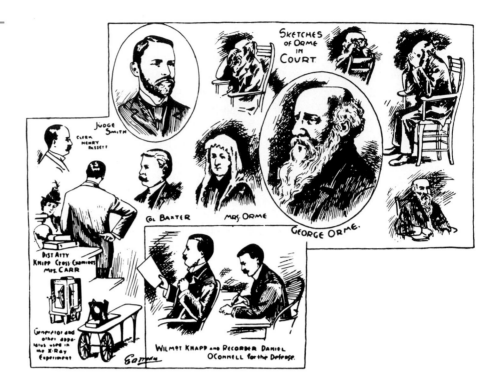

The first criminal case in which x-ray evidence was introduced was the Haynes murder trial (1897). The victim had been struck in the jaw with a 32-caliber bullet. Apparently another bullet was discovered lodged in the back of the head, and it was crucial to the defense to determine whether this was a fragment of the bullet inflicting the jaw wound or whether there was a second intact bullet of another caliber. The defense introduced an x-ray photograph of the victim's neck made by Gilbert Cannon, who said that it was not a 32-caliber bullet. After much haranguing, Judge Wright admitted the radiograph into evidence.[4]

Perhaps the first radiologist to serve as an effective expert witness was James T. Pitkin, who provided pivotal testimony in the Orme murder trial in 1897.[4] Orme was an elderly gentleman who returned home to find his young wife in the embrace of a paramour and immediately shot both of them. His wife promptly recovered, although her lover, James Punzo, fared poorly. After initial probing failed to locate the position of the bullet, it was decided to perform a radiographic examination. A 35-minute exposure with the Crookes tube only 1½ inches from the bullet opening in the skull failed to reveal the foreign body. However, within a few hours after the x-ray exposure the patient's temperature began rising and he became semicomatose before eventually dying.

The defense claimed that Punzo met his death not by the bullet fired into his brain but by the x-ray that was employed to locate the bullet. Pitkin, a radiologist hired by the defense, testified that he regarded "the use of this small apparatus for x-ray purposes extremely dangerous to the subject exposed. I should say that such an examination of a brain already irritated as his was supposed to have been would in my opinion have not only retarded the healing process but cause a distinctive irritation, resulting in a breaking down and softening of the brain tissue and thus cause the death of the sufferer." Thus the tables were turned on the prosecution. Instead of radiography proving their case by identifying the bullet in Punzo's brain, testimony indicating that the x-rays could actually have brought about the death of the victim led to the defendant's acquittal.

The first suit for damages for injury from x-rays was a $10,000 judgment rendered against the owners and operators of the Roentgen X-Ray Laboratory in Chicago. The plaintiff, Frank Balling, was thrown from his buggy and suffered a fractured ankle. When slight stiffness and swelling persisted almost 9 months later, an x-ray examination was recommended. Three photographs were made by exposures ranging from 35 to 40 minutes, during which the tube was placed 5 to 6 inches from the ankle and the top of the foot. As a result of the examination, it was claimed that the patient suffered severe necrosis and ulceration requiring three separate amputations. As a news item in the *Journal of the American Medical Association* noted,[9]

> Experts were employed by both sides and there was probably the usual conflict of testimony, so that, regarding any scientific disposition of the question, nothing practical will have been gained, and as the case will undoubtedly be appealed, its legal status is still in suspense. We already know that some inconvenient symptoms follow x-ray exposures occasionally, but we are very far from having found any constant law of these accidents, and the question of idiosyncrasy, which is only an admission of our ignorance, is always to be considered. Some people endure continued exposures to these rays without danger, others suffer, and this is about the extent of our knowledge. Experts for the prosecution ought, in such cases, it would seem, to be particularly guarded in the utterance of positive opinions or alleged statements of fact.

The first decision of the Supreme Court of the United States dealing with x-rays was handed down on April 7, 1913.[4] It concerned the charge of negligence in the taking of radiographs resulting in an x-ray burn. The plaintiff, Ann Sweeney, underwent an x-ray examination by William Erving to document a fractured rib that she claimed to have suffered through the negligence of a railroad company. Although Erving assured his patient that he and his wife had made a thousand x-ray examinations and had never had an accident, after several exposures over four visits, the part of Sweeney's back that had been exposed was red and itchy and she felt faint. About 2 weeks later, finding her back burned and the injury developing, she instituted suit.

At the trial, Erving "testified to his long experience in the use of such a machine, and to the exact character of its use upon the plaintiff. In addition to this testimony, he introduced six physicians skilled in their particular branch of practice, whose testimony without exception negatived the charge of negligence."

To establish Erving's liability, it was necessary for the plaintiff to prove three elements: that there was an actual injury, that the injury was due to the x-ray exposures made by Erving, and that Erving was negligent in the manner of making the x-ray photographs. The injury and its causation were clear. However, what constituted negligence in the taking of x-ray photographs and how could a patient prove such negligence? Sweeney attempted to invoke the doctrine of *res ipsa loquitur* (the thing speaks for itself). She contended that the burn itself was evidence of negligence because she had been assured by the doctor himself that with due care such burns had never occurred in his practice.

The trial court ruled in favor of Erving. On appeal, the Supreme Court affirmed the judgment and sustained the rule that inflicting a burn on a patient while making an x-ray examination was not in itself evidence of negligence on the part of the physician.

Among the unusual early uses of x-rays for legal purposes was the case of a youth of uncertain age who was arrested for striking and seriously injuring a fellow workman. At the time of his arrest he gave his age as 19; however, when he realized the seriousness of the criminal charge against him, he and his father insisted that he was only 17 years old and thus entitled to the benefits of a law preventing a prisoner under 18 from being tried in a criminal court. As *Scientific American*[10] reported,

> Thoroughly convinced that the youth was at least 18 years old, the juvenile court physician decided to have x-ray photographs made of the epiphyseal bones of his hand, elbow, and hip, and also photos of the same bones of a 17 year old youth. Comparison, it was hoped, would then settle the matter, as it is a known fact in medical circles that when a boy reaches the age of 18 years those bones become hardened. The photographs developed from the x-ray pictures of the bones of the boys showed that those of the 17 year old boy had not hardened but those of the defendant in the case had done so. The physician immediately fixed the age of the prisoner at 18 years or more.

A RADIOLOGIST'S VIEW[11]

A fascinating analysis of "the medicolegal value of the roentgen rays" was offered by Mihran Kassabian in 1904. He observed that "the skiagram, 'the exact picture of the true state of affairs,' will replace in the majority of accident cases the ordinary witnesses; the court and jury arriving at a decision either for plaintiff or defendant in less than half the time previously required." However, it was essential that for a picture to be considered reliable, "it must have been produced by a person who has had sufficient experience and as a result is skilled in the art of skiagraphy." Citing the case of an x-ray equipment salesman who testified as to the presence of fracture lines that really represented a normal spinous process, Kassabian noted that "this illustrates the fact that a skiagram may be unreliable, and should never be permitted to be entered as testimony until passed upon by a person whose expert competence is generally known."

In addition to using radiography to make a proper diagnosis, Kassabian stressed its value "so that the professional man can save himself from malpractice suits. I earnestly urge every physician to early have a skiagram taken of an accident, or other case, i.e. before any treatment has been resorted to, and a second skiagram after treatment has been instituted. Such records will protect the attending physician against any attempts at suits for damages in or out of court."

Radiographs for medicolegal purposes should be obtained using technique that

> does not vary greatly from that in any x-ray examination, except that especial care should be taken to have good, clear negatives. . . Examine carefully first with the closed fluoroscope, in a darkened room, so that the patient himself, or his attendants, may not see the result of the examination. Place the plate in position, in the presence of witnesses, and have a distinguishing mark upon it, such as a key or ring, for purpose of identification. Keep record of such details as the *time* of exposure, distance of the Crookes tube, position of the tube and part, etc. Take negatives from different points of view, and if possible take the injured and normal parts upon the same plate, for the purpose of comparison.

Kassabian recommended that the radiologist

print several copies, light and dark, so you can choose the print that shows the condition the clearer. Write on the negative the names of the bones and try to make the picture intelligible to anyone who examines it. Also make a tracing on the card, which will facilitate a proper understanding of the picture to untrained eyes. Having now made a positive diagnosis, write your expert diagnosis in a clear manner. An x-ray diagnosis will carry more weight in court if made by a physician, than if made by a man who is merely a photographer or a manufacturer of x-ray apparatus.

As to the comportment of the radiologist as an expert witness in a medicolegal case, Kassabian quoted the advice of Sir William Blizzard of London, who said

Be the plainest of men in the world in a court of justice. Never harbor a thought that if you do not appear positive you must appear little and mean. Give your evidence in as concise, plain and yet clear a manner as possible. Be intelligent, candid and just, but never aim at appearing unnecessarily scientific. State all the sources from and by which you have gained your information. If you can, make your evidence a self-evident truth. Thus, though the court may at the time have a mean opinion of your judgment, they must deem you an honest man. Never be dogmatic or set yourself up for judge or jury. Take no side whatever but be impartial and you'll be honest.

RADIOLOGY IN CRIME DETECTION

Several early articles discussed the value of x-rays in crime detection. T. Bordas of France (1896) suggested the possible use of x-rays on suspicious packages "suggestive of being infernal machines" and for identifying persons or bodies by old fractures, bullets, or other peculiarities that might be demonstrated radiographically. One year later (1897), the *Electrical Review* referred to a new technique of French customs authori-

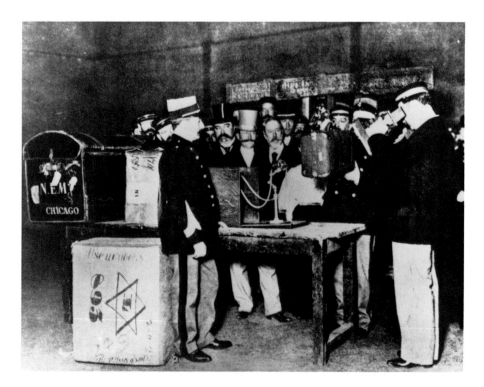

Early baggage inspection procedure using an unprotected gas tube and cryptoscope—there is nothing new under the sun![12]

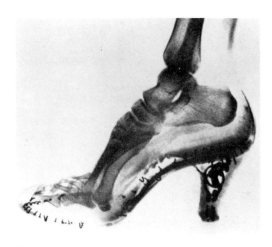

Smuggler's shoe with jewels in the heel.[13]

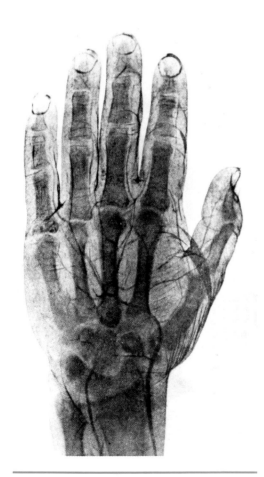

Radiographic dactyloscopy (1920). Impregnation of the skin and injection of the blood vessels with bismuth in a cadaver.[15]

ties to fluoroscope customers' handbags, hats, hair, and so forth. "The custom-house inspector will no longer trample roughshod on our feelings. He will disappear forever, and in his place will cover a mild and innocuous personage with something that looks like an opera glass in his hand. If you have told the truth and have nothing to declare, this newcomer will just take a fluorescent peep at your belongings and will disappear from view like a fleeting shadow."[4]

The same journal reported that "X-rays detect smugglers." As it explained,

The last package . . . examined had been declared to contain "sample of lingerie without value." The x-rays showed that there was a very small collection of underclothes and a very large consignment of Egyptian cigarettes and English matches. This was such a flagrant case (because cigarettes and matches are a government monopoly, and it is second to highway robbery to bring into the country anything that you can smoke and matches that will really burn) that the inspectors hauled before them the consignee of the parcel and showed him the living image of the crime. This is the only case where something serious will happen. The other consignees will merely pay duty.[4]

The forensic use of radiographs first occurred in French courts in 1897. Writing of this initial experience, Fovau d'Courmelles made the suggestion that "knowing of the existence of a fracture in a person, who has been burned or mutilated beyond recognition, we can hope to identify him by the x-ray and conclude therefrom that a member found really belongs to the person supposed to have disappeared."

At the time, the major forensic measurements were those of Bertillon, who had devised a classification of anthropometric indices for rapid personal identification relying principally on surface measurements of the skeleton. In 1899, Levinsohn[14] in Berlin recognized the possibilities for more precise measurement using radiography. Rather than use measurements that could vary with increases or decreases in body fat as well as with pathological changes, he "established numerical values which almost without exception remain constant, and so make possible the very easy recognition of the individual at any time in his life. For the determination of these numerical values, I use roentgen photography."

Henri Béclère (1918)[15,16] developed the technique of "radiographic dactyloscopy."

This simple method permits one to fix on a plate, with the greatest distinctness and without obliteration of the lines, the most minute details of the palmar region of the skin of the digital extremities. The digital grooves appear with all their multiple divisions, and the orifices of the cutaneous glands are quite plainly visible. The clarity of the images obtained permits relatively great photographic enlargement, 30 × 40 for example . . . In order to visualize the boundaries of the nail on the roentgenographic plate, it is only necessary to outline them delicately with the salt of an element of a very high atomic weight. We use lead tetroxide . . . One obtains on the plate, in addition to the image of the skeleton, the finest structural details of the thumbprint.

However, as Collins wrote, "a promising career in crime detection was denied the x-ray by the advent of the fingerprinting system, so much more economical of time and expense." Nevertheless, Béclère's method "was still uniquely useful in cases of drowning or exhumed cadavers in an advanced state of decomposition where the ink and paper technique was not applicable."[4]

Béclère's work was actually anticipated 21 years earlier (1897) by David Walsh[17] of the Western Skin Hospital in England. He reported that "oxide of bismuth, powdered freely over the back of a finger, gave a good tracing of the creases over the knuckles." Noting that "a permanent record might be of value in the identification of criminals," Walsh also observed that this technique could produce "a complete surface map, with numerous lines of longitude and latitude" that could serve "as a guide to the knife of the operator" in those cases in which "the surgeon does not always find it easy to cut down upon a needle or other small object, even when it has been precisely localised by an x ray photograph."

OWNERSHIP OF RADIOGRAPHS

As stated by the Michigan Supreme Court (1935),

> In the absence of agreement to the contrary, such negatives are the property of the physician or surgeon who has made them incident to treating a patient. It is a matter of common knowledge that x-ray negatives are practically meaningless to the ordinary layman. But their retention by the physician or surgeon constitutes an important part of his clinical record in the particular case, and in the aggregate these negatives may embody and preserve much of value incident to a physician's or surgeon's experience. They're as much a part of the history of the case as any other case record made by a physician or surgeon. In a sense they differ little, if at all, from microscopic slides of tissues made in the course of diagnosis or treating a patient, but it would hardly be claimed that such slides are the property of the patient. Also, in the event of a malpractice suit against a physician or surgeon, the x-ray negatives which he has caused to be taken and preserved incident to treating the patient might often constitute the unimpeachable evidence which would fully justify the treatment of which the patient was complaining.

However, while the patient has no right to have his physician's records delivered to him personally, they must be made available to succeeding physicians upon the patient's request.[3]

Twenty-one years previously (1914), a fascinating article by Albers-Schoenberg of Hamburg was reprinted in the *Archives of the Roentgen Ray*.[18] It addressed the ownership of x-ray plates, which "is often claimed by one of two parties—the patient himself or the medical attendant in charge of the case." Regarding the medical attendant, Albers-Schoenberg noted that

> we must bear in mind that the Roentgenologist is applied to in his capacity of consulting medical specialist, not as a mere photographer or lay Roentgenographer who happens to possess the necessary apparatus. He may take a Roentgenogram, make a radioscopic examination, or use the orthodiagraph, according to circumstances. The decision which, if any, of these methods should be used rests with the Roentgenologist alone, neither the patient nor the physician having any voice in the matter. The radiologist then proceeds to give his verdict, basing his diagnosis on the results of his clinical and Roentgenological examinations. This he may give to the physician either verbally or in writing, explaining, if necessary, by demonstration of the skiagram or tracing. This completes the work of the Roentgenologist, and the payment of the fee concludes the business, as in any other medical consultation. The Roentgenologist does not sell one or more skiagrams, but receives his honorarium for scientific opinion on the case.

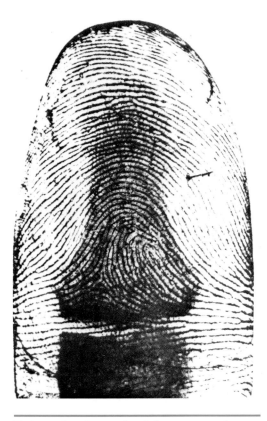

Enlarged radiograph of fingerprint after impregnation of the skin and the ungual grooves with red oxide of lead (1920).

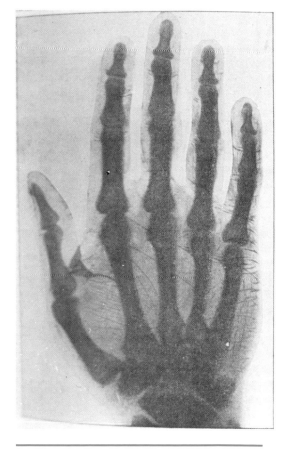

Skin markings of the palmar surface (1897).

Albers-Schoenberg added that "as a general rule it is not advisable to give up the plates, prints, or tracings to the general practitioner, since he is not a specialist, and is therefore not in a position to make a correct diagnosis of the case from the Roentgenographic data." As for the patient,

the possession of the Roentgen plate might even be of actual detriment to the patient, since it might lead to unnecessary anxiety and apprehension. It may, however, be allowed that under certain circumstances the patient may be furnished with a print of the Roentgen plate, on payment of an extra fee; but it should be well understood that the patient has no *right* to this, but receives it only as an act of courtesy from the Roentgenologist.

Of course, "in cases of emergency, accidents, shot-wounds, and the like where surgical aid cannot be delayed, the Roentgen negative itself may be sent directly to the surgeon."

Albers-Schoenberg advised radiologists that

the original plate should be kept, together with the record of the case for future reference. It is often of the highest importance to be able to refer back to the original skiagram. All x-ray plates relating to cases of accidents should be carefully preserved. The granting or otherwise of compensation may depend on the evidence of a Roentgen plate taken many years ago, and if this is missing, because it has passed into the possession of the medical attendant, the subsequent Roentgen examination may prove quite illusory. Many sick-clubs retain their collection of x-ray plates for ten years or more. It is as well that the Roentgen specialist should exercise a similar precaution.

Bibliography

Glasser O: William Conrad Röntgen. Springfield, Ill, Charles C Thomas, 1958.

References

1. Glasser O: William Conrad Röntgen. Springfield, Ill, Charles C Thomas, 1958.
2. Literary Digest, April 11, 1896.
3. Donaldson SW: The roentgenologist in court. Springfield, Ill, Charles C Thomas, 1954.
4. Collins VP: Origins of medico-legal and forensic roentgenology. In Bruwer AJ: Classic descriptions in diagnostic roentgenology. Springfield, Ill, Charles C Thomas, 1964.
5. Withers S: The story of the first roentgen evidence. Radiology 17:99-103, 1903.
6. Smith v. Grant 29, Chicago Legal News 145.
7. Chicago Medical Journal 2:396, 1896.
8. Reed RH: The x-rays from a medico-legal standpoint. JAMA 30:1017-1019, 1898.
9. X-ray dangers. JAMA 32:1006, 1899.
10. Scientific American, December 23, 1896.
11. Kassabian MK: The medico-legal value of the roentgen rays. Am X-Ray J 9:39-43, 1904.
12. Angus WM: A commentary on the development of diagnostic imaging technology. RadioGraphics 9:1225-1244, 1989.
13. Barnard TW: Illustrated notes from the early days of radiography. Radiography 33:234-238, 1967.
14. Levinsohn: Beitrage zur Festellung der Identität. Arch Krim Anthrop Leipzig 2:211-220, 1899.
15. Béclère H: La radiographie anthropométrique du pouce. Compt Rend Acad Sci 167:499-500, 1918.
16. Béclère H: La radiographie cutanée. J Radiol d'Electrol 4:145-149, 1920.
17. Walsh D: Skin pictures by the X rays. Brit Med J 2:797, 1897.
18. Albers-Schoenberg HE: The roentgenologist is a medical specialist, and all roentgen plates, prints, tracing, and other documents which he may prepare are his sole property. Arch Roentgen Ray 19:94-97, 1914.

CHAPTER 33

Radiology of Art, Archeology, and Stamps

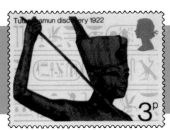

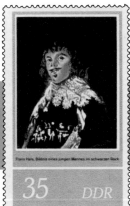

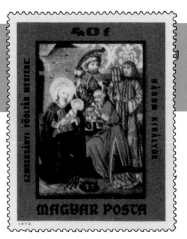

PAINTINGS

Radiographic examination may play a major role in determining the condition and authenticity of a painting. It may provide such information as

(1) stylistic and structural characteristics peculiar to one artist or school; (2) changes in design made by the original artist or alterations by another; (3) damage or loss no longer visible because of restoration; (4) anomalies of structure in the pattern of radiographic densities not usually found in similar paintings, which would tend to indicate forgery or would at least require explanation.[1]

Soon after the discovery of x-rays, Walter Konig, a pupil of Roentgen, radiographed an oil painting to detect alterations made after the painting was finished.[2] In April 1897, the *Electrical Review*[3] described the authentication of a painting of Christ ascribed to Albrecht Dürer by distinctly revealing the artist's monogram *AD* in Gothic characters, as well as the date of 1521. The article concluded, "This application of the Röntgen rays may prove of considerable value to picture dealers and others in detecting fraudulent imitations of valuable paintings."

In 1913, Alexander Faber of Weimar made the first systematic investigation of the absorption characteristics of different pigments. He painted patches of various colors, each of the same thickness, and compared their opacity to x-rays. Faber discovered that there was no relation to the optical densities of the same patches when photographed by normal reflected light.[4] After studying the radiographic effect of superimposed paint layers, Faber (1914) patented in Germany a procedure for the x-ray determination of overpainting in oil paintings and similar objects.[7] In effect, this patent granted Faber a monopoly by prohibiting others from employing x-rays on paintings without a license. Faber clearly demon-

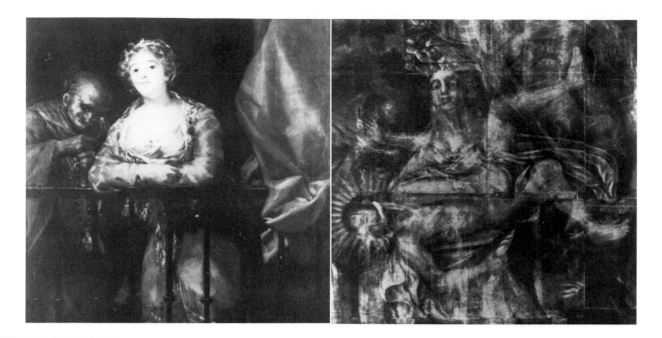

Radiography demonstrating a second picture underneath a famous painting. *Left,* "The Majas on the Balcony" by Goya. *Right,* Radiograph of the painting clearly shows the existence of another picture underneath it that contains various religious scenes.[5]

strated that colors of equal thickness arranged in a sequence according to their physical density gave a scale of gray from white to black on the radiograph; that the colors of the painting were registered on the radiograph according to their weight and thickness, not according to their hue, brightness, or saturation; and that therefore the x-ray photograph and light photograph of a painting rendered quite different phenomena. He also showed that when a dark color of low weight was painted over a pale color of high weight, the color beneath was visible on the radiograph; conversely, when a heavy pale color was applied over the dark color, the lower one was invisible to x-rays.[4]

Meanwhile, André Cheron[8] in France was studying the opacity to x-rays of samples of paint containing pigments traditionally employed by artists and relating this to the atomic number and atomic weight of elements in the pigment. He concluded that two factors were essential for obtaining a good radiographic image of a painting: transparency of both support and ground, and relative opacity of the colors in the paint, or at least of certain colors that could supply the contrasts that form the image. He observed that these factors were generally present in old pictures (fourteenth to mid-eighteenth century), since they were painted with pigments derived from minerals and metals on wood or canvas supports with chalk grounds. However, modern pictures (nineteenth and twentieth

Radiography showing changes in design during the production of a painting. *Left,* "Portrait of a Woman," attributed to Lorenzo Lotto. *Right,* Radiograph of the painting reveals that round-neck and "V"-neck gowns have been hidden by the square-neck dress of the surface paint. This wide variation in design on a single small panel is usually considered of student or "school" origin. Note the cross bars of wood visible on the right that represent the "cradle" applied to the backs of paintings on wood to minimize warping.[6]

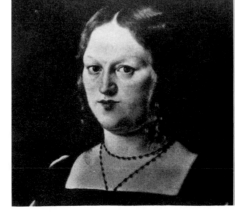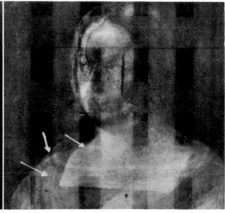

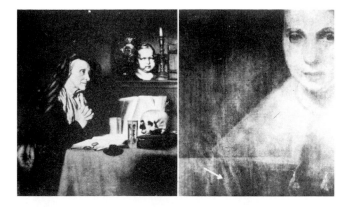

Radiography demonstrating one picture painted over another. *Left*, Life-size study of "An Old Woman at Prayer" by Nicholas Maes. *Right*, Radiograph shows that Maes painted the old woman on a canvas already used for the portrait of a young lady. The thin pigments used to model the old woman are obscured in the radiograph by the heavy impasto of the portrait that will never be seen. Only the folds of the neckerchief and faint outline of neck and face of the old woman are visible in the radiograph (*arrow*).[6]

centuries) commonly have grounds that contain white lead and have colors that are often organic and thus transparent to x-rays. Therefore Cheron argued that the structure revealed by radiography could indicate the age of a painting and be of value in detecting forgeries, especially since in most cases a forger overpainted an old painting using pigments transparent to x-rays.[4]

Radiographs also could reveal damages and losses in the original old paint even if they were invisible to the naked eye.

> Sometimes areas of a picture are discovered in this manner to be by a later hand though the presence of retouching had been absolutely unexpected until the magic rays revealed the evidence of early injury and skillful repair. Possibly some of our public museums and private owners will be none too anxious to submit their more doubtful treasures to the too penetrating vision of this modern mechanical detective of fraud, the x-ray tube. How painful to discover that a cherished Flemish or Italian masterpiece reputed of the fifteenth or sixteenth century in date was really the product of twentieth century skill and fraud in some obscure studio of Paris, Antwerp or Berlin. On the other hand there is at least a possibility that a banal piece representing early Victorian taste, let us say, has been painted on top of a misprized masterpiece of earlier date.[9]

The American pioneer in radiography of paintings was Alan Burroughs. Unlike Faber and Cheron, Burroughs was an art historian rather than a physician or scientist, and he designed a series of experiments to investigate the value and limitations of x-rays in both determining the condition and studying the style of old paintings. After initially showing that x-rays had no physical or other detrimental effect on paintings, Burroughs began forming an extensive collection of radiographs of paintings from major collections throughout the United States and Europe. He indexed the x-ray files alphabetically according to the names of the artists currently credited in catalogues with authorship of the pictures, as well as carefully cross-indexing cases in which works were attributed to several artists. Burroughs' book, *Art Criticism from a Laboratory* (1938), contained almost 3,200 radiographs, and all the great masters were well represented.[10]

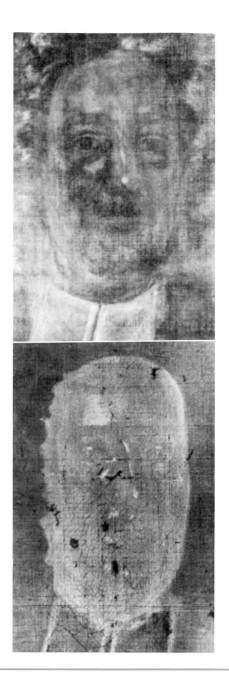

Radiography demonstrating art forgery. *Top*, Radiograph of the original painting of Cotton Mather by Pelham. Note the variety of brush strokes. *Bottom*, Radiograph of a copy of Pelham's portrait, artist unknown. The damaged areas and crackle in the paint surface of the copy are readily visible.[6]

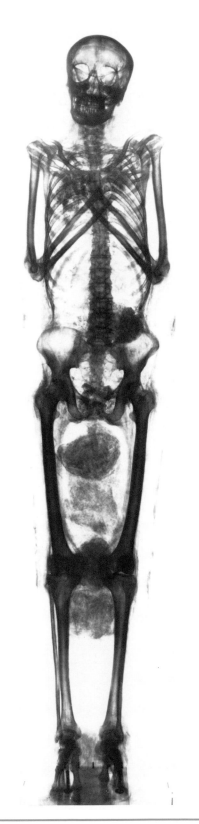

The famed "Harwa" mummy, exhibited at the 1939 World's Fair in New York.

Extensive work on radiography of paintings was also done by Martin De Wild in Holland, Johannes Wilde in Austria, Walter Graff and Kurt Wehlte in Germany, and J.F. Cellerier in France. After submitting samples of paint to 2,000 times the normal radiation doses used in radiography, Wehlte concluded that normal radiographic exposure was harmless to paintings. Nevertheless, he emphasized that they should be exposed only to the extent necessary for research and restoration work. De Wild calculated for a definite wavelength the mass absorption coefficient of various pigments and of the paints made from them. He concluded that paints with a high mass-absorption coefficient were those that contained elements of high atomic number and that the medium in the paint had little influence on total absorption. De Wild also observed that low-energy x-rays generally gave the most satisfactory gradation of shade from black to white and that they also were better for resolving fine details throughout the paint, ground, and support.[4]

At the end of the 1920s, x-ray evidence involving disputes of authenticity began to be introduced into legal proceedings. In the most celebrated case, Mrs. Andree Hahn sued art dealer Sir Joseph Duveen for $500,000 damages. She charged Duveen with public slander of her painting, which she claimed to be by Leonardo da Vinci, because Duveen (who had never seen it) was quoted in the *New York World* as stating that "the Hahn picture is a copy, hundreds of which have been made. The real 'La Belle Ferronier' is in the Louvre." Although radiographs of the two paintings were presented and stressed in court by the defense counsel, the jury failed to agree on a verdict, and the suit was eventually settled out of court.[4]

An interesting observation of the aesthetic aspect of radiography of paintings was Burroughs' subsequent analysis of the radiographic evidence. He wrote:

> Setting aside the question of authorship of the Louvre painting, it is evident that this picture in Paris was modeled like a piece of sculpture with emphasis on the roundness of the forms, and that the modeling extended all over the visible planes of the head without a break. In other words, the artist had made a head upon the knowledge that it is round and had then adjusted the hair, put on the jewelry and ribbons and given the final touches of make-up. The x-ray shadowgraphs of the other (Hahn) version of the portrait told no such story of growth and development. The head was outlined and the details were painted at once upon a surface that had not been modeled. The jewelry was incorporated into the design from the start, the flesh being painted up to the jewels and not beneath them. Briefly, the painter of the second version began—in my opinion, as I must say—with an idea of a pretty girl dressed in jewels and ribbons, instead of with an idea of a head shaped like an egg and a neck as round as a column. It is needless to say which is the original conception, since the point of view of the copyist is explained in the simplest terms, the terms of his procedure.[10]

Another widely publicized trial in which radiographs served as evidence took place in Berlin in 1932. An art dealer named Otto Wacker was indicted for the sale of 30 forged Van Goghs, which he had sold over several years to other dealers and private collectors. Two technical experts testified that the radiographs of the pictures in question were substantially different from those made of genuine Van Goghs. The original Van Goghs showed a direct, strong application of paint and an understructure having a pattern like that on the surface. In contrast, the fraudulent paintings were so loose, weak, and chaotic in the radiographs that the subject was often unrecognizable. Wacker was found guilty and sentenced to a year's imprisonment for fraud and falsification of documents.[4]

With the exception of Burroughs, who had been trained in art history, most art historians were generally skeptical of the value of art radiography. They preferred traditional methods involving stylistic analysis and historical research, combined with the perceptive eye and intuitive reaction of the connoisseur. However, new and improved equipment in the early 1930s led to the establishment of several major museum laboratories and conservation workshops in the United States and Europe. By the end of the decade, art radiography had become a routine procedure, and art historians began to understand its usefulness and limitations.[4]

In 1937, F.I.G. Rawlins[11] of the National Gallery in London published elegant radiographs of paintings using x-rays from a low-voltage tube with a beryllium window. He suggested the use of multiple exposures at varying kilovoltages. Details in thin areas of the painting were demonstrated using lower voltages, whereas details in heavily loaded paint of high atomic number were better penetrated and differentiated by high-kilovoltage x-rays.

One year later (1938), stereoscopic x-ray exposures were applied to medieval illuminated manuscripts by H.F. Sherwood[12] of Rochester, N.Y. This technique permitted visual separation of layers of paint on the front and reverse sides of the parchment. A similar technique was later used not only for panels painted on both sides but also for polychromed wood sculpture to study the structure and method of fabrication.

To demonstrate watermarks in prints, Sheldon Keck[4] of the Brooklyn Museum used x-rays of extremely low kilovoltage (4 to 5 keV). His results were of value in confirming the provenance of the paper, even when the watermarks were visually obscured by the ink of the print.

A major problem in art radiography was the interpretation of the double radiographic image produced by panels, especially wings of altar pieces, painted on both faces. A similar difficulty arose when an unpainted reverse contained plugs of white lead putty filling worm holes and larger areas of wood loss. In both these situations, material on the reverse side cast an obscuring shadow over the portion of the painted design in the path of the x-rays. In 1946, Murray Pease[13] of the Metropolitan Museum in New York published a method of "traverse focus radiography" to eliminate much of the unwanted interference caused by additions to the reverse of paneled paintings. This modification of body-section radiography consisted of mounting the bare x-ray film in close contact with the paint surface. During the exposure, either the x-ray source or panel with the attached film moved in such a way that the source was never in one position relative to the object. This technique resulted in a sharp image of the paint because of its proximity to the film, whereas all material behind the paint was blurred and out of focus.

ARCHEOLOGY

According to Glasser,[2] the first radiograph of an ancient Egyptian mummy was made in March, 1896 by Walter Konig. During that same year, Dedekind of the Vienna Museum discovered by radiography that a mummy, which appeared to be that of a human, was actually a mummy of a large bird, confirming inscriptions on the wrappings that they enclosed

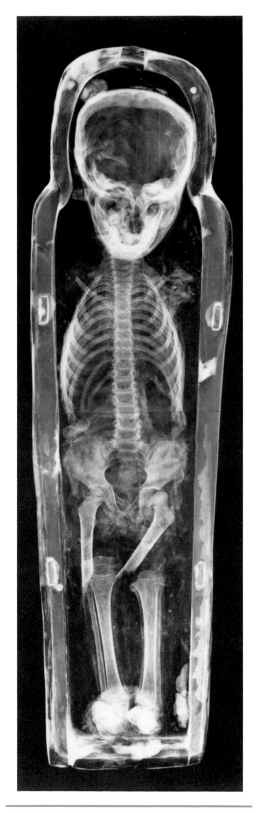

Radiograph of a full-sized Egyptian mummy in a wooden cabinet. Note that the legs have been broken so that the deceased would fit into the space available.

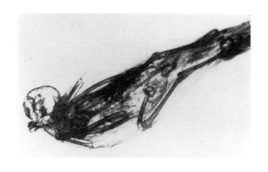

Radiograph of a mummified bird (1896).[15]

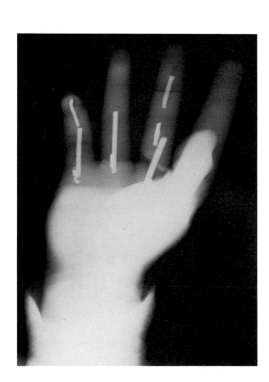

Radiography of Michelangelo's "La Pieta." Coned radiograph of the left hand of the Virgin clearly shows how the fingers, damaged at some unknown time in the past, have been repaired with a number of metal (probably bronze) pins.[17]

an ibis.[2] The next year, W.M.F. Petrie published excellent radiographs of the legs and feet of mummies found during a British expedition.[14]

Before the discovery of x-rays, anatomical studies of mummies were necessarily destructive, requiring the unwrapping and dissection of the specimen. Radiography offered a noninvasive method for the study of mummies both by archeologists, who were interested in precisely dating various cultures and their changes with the passage of time, and by paleopathologists concerned with the diseases that afflicted ancient humans.

Radiography could detect forgeries offered by unscrupulous native dealers by determining the presence or absence of human bones in alleged wrapped mummies. In many instances, travelers were sold modern fakes in which a coffin was empty or perhaps contained only a few bones or a variety of inorganic material. Some small mummies, ostensibly those of children, were in fact the bandaged remains of birds. Although a coffin usually could be dated by its orthography and style, it was dangerous to assume that the coffin contained its original inhabitant. For example, a coffin bearing the names and titles of a man could contain the mummy of a woman, and vice versa. In addition, the period to which the coffin belonged might differ widely from that of its occupant. In one case, radiography demonstrated that a specimen appearing to be the unwrapped mummy of a woman 75 years old was actually that of a teenage girl.[14]

Perhaps the most fascinating use of x-rays by the archeologist has been the correlation of radiographic findings with known embalming techniques. As early as the Fourth Dynasty (2613 to 2494 BC), the "corruptible viscera" (stomach, lungs, liver, intestines) were removed through an incision in the left flank and placed in so-called Canopic jars. During the Twenty-first Dynasty (1085 to 935 BC), the extracted viscera were no longer placed in Canopic jars but were wrapped in four parcels and restored with packing material, such as sawdust, to the body cavity. By the time of the Twenty-sixth Dynasty (664 to 525 BC), the viscera were no longer restored to the body but were packaged and placed between the legs, or were deposited in newly revived Canopic jars. During the Ptolemaic period (332 to 30 BC), the body cavities were filled with masses of solidified resin, and increasing attention was given to the binding and appearance of the wrapped mummy rather than to careful treatment of the body. These various embalming techniques could be clearly demonstrated radiographically, thus aiding in estimating the date of a given mummy.[14]

For religious reasons, amulets made of pottery or metal were frequently incorporated in the wrappings of a mummy. Since they were radiopaque, the amulets could be easily detected and, when desirable, precisely localized and removed through small incisions that did not destroy the overlying wrappings.[14]

Radiographic studies have demonstrated bony conditions such as arthritis and fractures that also plagued ancient humans. Growth arrest lines found in the distal tibias of almost one third of mummies probably reflect the general poor state of health during adolescence in ancient Egypt. A fascinating mummy from the Ptolemaic period was an elderly man whose forearm had been severed a few inches above the wrist during his youth. Radiographs showed that an artificial limb, complete with digits, had been fitted onto the withered limb when he was embalmed many years later.[14]

Radiography also has been applied to pottery and sculpture. For

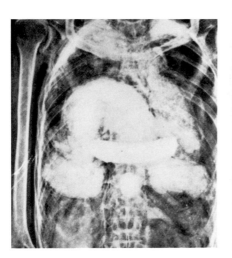 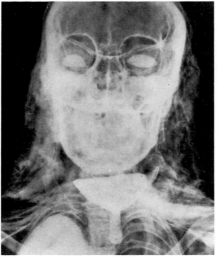 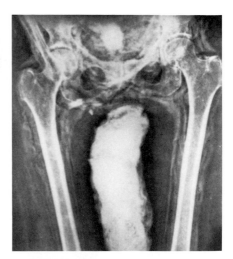

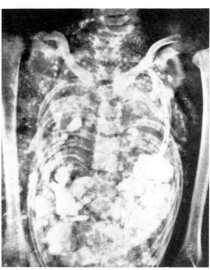

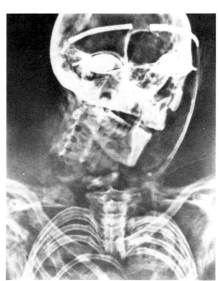

Use of radiography to date Egyptian mummies. *Top left,* Thorax and upper part of the abdomen of a mummy of the Twenty-first Dynasty. Note the visceral packs, containing the stomach, lungs, liver, and intestines, which were restored to the body cavity. *Top middle,* Mummy of a Twenty-first Dynasty woman showing artificial eyes and a mass in the right side of the thorax. Note the amulet about the neck within the bandages. *Top right,* Twenty-sixth Dynasty mummy showing a dense visceral pack between the legs. At this time, the viscera were no longer returned to the body cavity but either were wrapped and placed between the legs or were put in Canopic jars. *Right,* Late-period mummy of a child. The body cavity is filled with rubbish (potsherds, stones, and sand). During the late periods, progressively less care was taken in the treatment of the body. *Bottom right,* Extremely careless treatment of a mummy of the late Ptolemaic or early Roman period. The artificial eyes and eyebrows are set into the cartonnage mask covering the head.[14]

example, in 1958 Pease[16] published the results of a radiographic repair, restoration, and falsification of a Persian ceramic bowl. In 1964, both x-rays and gamma rays were employed in radiographing Michelangelo's magnificent marble sculpture, *La Pieta.* Before shipping the large and heavy sculpture from St. Peter's in Rome to the New York World's Fair, the Vatican requested the Eastman Kodak Company to conduct an x-ray examination to record possible flaws and areas of weakness from former repairs. Cobalt-60 gamma rays were used to study the thicker parts, such as the head and neck of the Virgin. Conventional radiographs (140 keV) of the Virgin's left hand clearly showed that the fingers had at one time been broken off and rejoined to the hand with metal pins for reinforcement.[17]

POSTAGE STAMPS

The x-ray investigation of postage stamps was championed by Herbert Pollack and Charles Bridgman[18] in the United States. As they wrote,

> the philatelic value of a stamp is determined not only by its rarity but also by its condition. Tears, thin spots, damaged areas, and margins that are too narrow will reduce its worth. Unscrupulous artists are able to repair damaged stamps so well that their handiwork sometimes cannot be detected by the naked eye, high magnification, or studies with ultraviolet light. Also, postage stamps have been counterfeited so cleverly that experts have found it extremely difficult to distinguish them from the original. Therefore, a detailed study of such important aspects as design, cancellation, paper, and watermark is often necessary to determine the authenticity of rare stamps.

The x-ray examination of postage stamps makes apparent many of these details that otherwise would be most difficult, if not impossible, to visualize.

To fully analyze printing inks, papers, watermarks, cancellations, repairs, and alterations, Pollack and Bridgman used three techniques: low-voltage radiography, x-ray autoelectronography, and x-ray electronography. As they wrote,

> To make a valid analysis, it is necessary to radiograph together a questionable stamp and one known to be genuine. The early "classic" stamps were generally printed with metallic inks. Cancellations were, and still are, usually printed with a carbon ink of such low effective atomic number that it does not absorb x-rays appreciably. Therefore, a low-voltage radiograph of a stamp printed with an ink containing a metallic pigment and canceled with a carbon ink will show the design of the stamp without superimposition of the cancellation.

In x-ray autoelectronography, electrons rather than the x-rays were employed to create the image on the film. When irradiated with heavily filtered x-rays (160 to 250 kV), the postage stamp itself emitted electrons. The quantity of this emission depended on the atomic number of the elements present in the pigments of the inks used, the amount of ink, and the components of the paper. X-ray electronography was used to show only the details of the paper structure and watermark and not the printed design of the stamp. This was accomplished by placing the stamp in contact with a "metallic material of high atomic number such as lead, which, when radiated with x-rays, produces an electronic emission sufficient to penetrate the stamp." This demonstrated of fine details of paper structure and watermark with no superimposition of the design image.

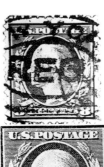
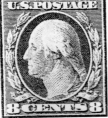
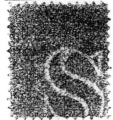
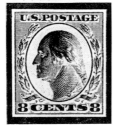

Radiography of postage stamps. *First*, Photograph of a stamp issued by the United States in 1908. *Second*, Low-voltage radiograph (kVp) does not show the carbon ink cancellation because of its lack of x-ray absorption. *Third*, On the electron radiograph, neither the image of the design nor the cancellation are shown. Only the paper structure with the watermark is visible. *Fourth*, Electron emission image shows only the design of the stamp that was printed with a metallic ink. Neither the image of the cancellation nor the paper is visualized. (This was printed as a positive image to facilitate interpretation alongside a standard radiograph.)[19]

References

1. Bridgman CF and Keck S: The radiography of paintings. Med Radiogr Photogr 37:62-70, 1961.
2. Glasser O: Wilhelm Conrad Röntgen. Springfield, Ill, Charles C Thomas, 1934.
3. Testing pictures by the Roentgen rays. Electrical Review 40:607, 1897.
4. Keck S: History of x-ray examination of works of art and archaeology. Unpublished work from American College of Radiology.
5. Padron MD and Recchiuto A: Application of x-rays to the study of some paintings in the Prado Museum. Radiología, 1973.
6. Elliott WJ: The use of the Roentgen ray in the scientific examination of paintings. AJR 50:779-790, 1943.
7. Bridgman CF: The amazing patent on the radiography of paintings. Studies in Conservation 9:135-139, 1964.
8. Cheron A: La radiographie des tableaux. Académie des Sciences 172:57-59, 1920.
9. Tevis M: X-ray tests of old paintings. Scientific American Monthly 165-167, Feb. 3, 1921.
10. Burroughs A: Art criticism from a laboratory. Boston, Little, Brown, 1938.
11. Rawlins FIG: The physics and chemistry of paintings. Royal Society Arts, March 1937.
12. Sherwood HF: Stereoscopic soft x-ray examination of parchment antiphonaries. Technical studies 6:277-280, 1938.
13. Pease M: A note on the radiography of paintings. Metropolitan Museum of Art Bulletin 4:136-139, 1946.
14. Gray PHK: Radiography of ancient Egyptian mummies. Med Radiogr Photogr 43:34-44, 1967.
15. Holland CT: X-rays in 1896. Liverpool Med Chir J 45:61-77, 1937.
16. Pease M: Two bowls in one. Metropolitan Museum of Art Bulletin 16:236-240, 1958.
17. Corney GM: Radiography of La Pieta. Med Radiogr Photogr 41:1-2, 1965.
18. Pollack HC, Bridgman CF, and Splettstosser HR: The x-ray investigation of postage stamps. Med Radiogr Photogr 30-31:75-78, 1955.
19. Bridgman CF: Use of radiation in philately and in examination of paintings. In Etter LE (ed): The science of ionizing radiation. Springfield, Ill, Charles C Thomas, 1965.

CHAPTER 34

Radiological Organizations and Journals

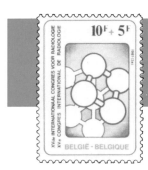
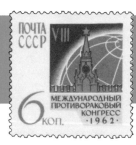
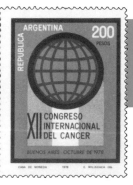
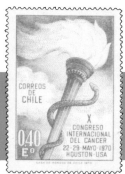

In the development of any new branch of science or medicine, some means must be promptly found to bring investigators and practitioners together and to establish channels of communication among them. In radiology, organizations and periodicals of high quality were established soon after Roentgen's discovery and played an important role in the rapid development of the specialty. Although dynamic radiological societies and prominent journals arose on both sides of the Atlantic, space limitations require that the American and British experience be chronicled as examples of more global activities.

AMERICAN ROENTGEN RAY SOCIETY (ARRS)

The history of the American Roentgen Ray Society began 3 years before its founding with an x-ray pioneer, Heber Robarts of St. Louis. One of his earliest ambitions was to found an American periodical for the rapidly developing specialty. In May, 1897, Robarts launched as a personal venture the *American X-Ray Journal*, which he described as "a monthly journal devoted to practical x-ray work and allied arts and sciences." As Robarts[1] subsequently recalled,

> In starting the *American X-Ray Journal*, I did not consult anyone about the propriety or wisdom of my course. If I had it would have been swallowed up by the historic monster of disapproval. At that time there seemed to come a dearth or spell over the Roentgen world. The lay press had already ceased to print sensational matter about the x-rays and medical journals were not certain that the profession could read skiagraphs.

In an editorial in the first volume, Robarts offered reasons why he thought that physicians were not readily adopting the "new science," even though the public was clamoring for its use. He reviewed the application of the new rays in some surgical conditions, stressing "the ease and certainty of diagnosticating which has advanced more in the past twelve months than any previous hundred years." Robarts[2] promised that

> it is the design of this Journal to give the readers and thinkers a faithful resume of all x-ray work done in any portion of the globe. . . . It is the intention of the promoters of this Journal to give to the world only truthful results, with full credit to the experimenter, in all its relations to the new science.

Concerning the "allied arts and sciences," Robarts wrote that "this field of inquiry [e.g., the "new science"] must have associated with it practical and useful adjuncts. The most essential of which shall occupy space are medical jurisprudence, the therapy of electro-medical science, preventive medicine, hygiene, dentistry and collateral branches."

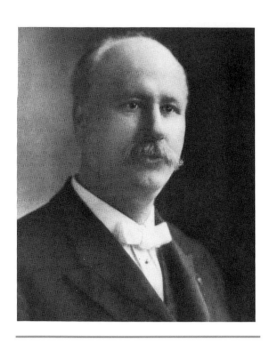

Heber Robarts (1852-1922).

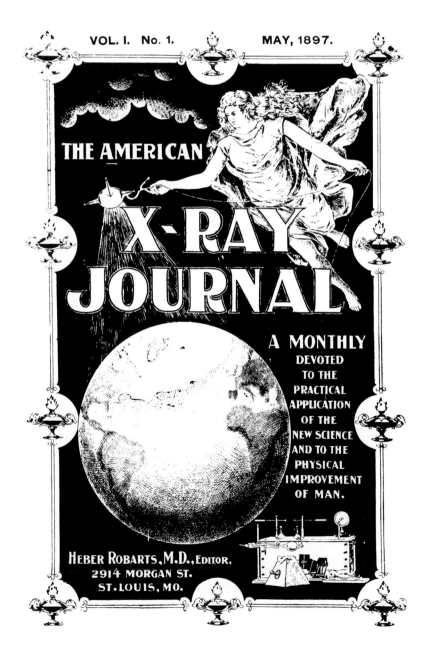

VOL. I. No. 1.   MAY, 1897.

THE AMERICAN

X-RAY JOURNAL

A MONTHLY DEVOTED TO THE PRACTICAL APPLICATION OF THE NEW SCIENCE AND TO THE PHYSICAL IMPROVEMENT OF MAN.

HEBER ROBARTS, M.D., EDITOR,
2914 MORGAN ST.
ST. LOUIS, MO.

Cover of the first issue of the *American X-Ray Journal* (May, 1897).

Concerning advertisements, an essential for any young and struggling medical journal, Robarts asserted that "no advertisements shall appear in this Journal that savour of quackery, deception or fraud." With reference to his own conduct as editor, Robarts[2] declared that:

The conduct of this Journal shall not be arrogant, defiant or bigoted, but it will have the courage of conviction to press forward the truth as we understand the truth. It will be ethical, as the throbbings of every breast should be, regardless of any written code devised by man for another's guidance. There will be no personal venom, as we hold no animus against any man, but false principles will be attacked with all the vigor of our ability. This is a pioneer Journal of x-ray work. We are not imitators. We are casting our hopes among the needs and wants of man. We expect encouragement.

While it cannot be expected or desired that we shall escape just criticism and it may be, contumely, yet our aim shall be to improve each coming Journal, encouraged as we are in the faith and usefulness of our mission.

Unfortunately, most of the leading investigators of the period preferred to report their work initially in the established journals. Thus Robarts was forced to reprint extracts from radiological papers initially published in other periodicals and to fill the journal with materials from the "allied sciences" that were not directly related to radiology.[3] Despite the editor's wholehearted enthusiasm for the new rays, its columns were open to reports of damage resulting from their misuse. This proved to be an important service to the x-ray pioneers.

The first American organization devoted to radiology was founded in 1900. Four years earlier, Samuel H. Monell of New York City had proposed that an x-ray society be formed, but "he found poor encouragement and no meeting was held."[1] The idea was revived 4 years later by John Rudis-Jicinsky of Cedar Rapids, Iowa, in a letter to Robarts. Eventually, on March 26, about 15 persons, mostly physicians, crowded into Robarts' St. Louis office for the purpose of organizing the Roentgen Society of the United States. They elected Robarts president and Rudis-Jicinsky secretary. The group approved a constitution that stated:

The object of this society shall be the advancement of the knowledge of practical x-ray work and allied arts and sciences, the promotion of this branch of surgery and medical science, systematic original research, the uniformity of support to the inventive talent and promotion of harmony and fraternity in the professions devoted to this science, the protection of the interests of its members and the promotion of all measures adapted to the practical application of the x-ray for the benefit of the community and physical improvement of man.

The major issues were (1) whether the new organization should be affiliated with the American Medical Association (AMA) and (2) whether its membership should be limited to physicians in good standing with that organization or whether nonphysicians and physicians at odds with the AMA (e.g., electrotherapeutists) be eligible as well. Robarts and Rudis-Jicinsky decided to go ahead without the blessings of the AMA, explaining that "we need the assistance of physicists in our meetings."[1]

Accordingly, the initial constitution specified that:

This society shall consist of honorary members, permanent members, members by invitation and corresponding members, who shall be physicians and surgeons, dentists, investigators, authors on x-ray topics, inventors, radiographers, or their assistants in hospi-

Application Blank.
ROENTGEN SOCIETY OF THE UNITED STATES. APPLICATION FOR MEMBERSHIP.

I hereby make application for membership in the Roentgen Society of the United States.

Si; ned ....
Full name.

P. O. Address ....

$5.00 must accompany each application. There is no initiation fee. The official organ, "THE AMERICAN X-RAY JOURNAL," free. Send this slip with enclosure to Treasurer and Secretary:

DR. J. RUDIS-JICINSKY,
Cedar Rapids, Iowa.

Application for membership in the Roentgen Society of the United States (1900).

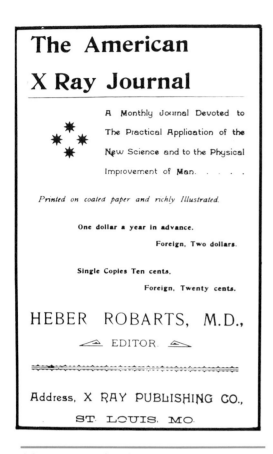

Advertisement for the *American X-Ray Journal.*

tals, military or State institutions, technical electricians, chemists, teachers of chemistry and physics, specialists and experts in electro-technique, qualified by at least one year in experience with radiant matter, its application or therapeutical use.

One of the few limitations was a warning in the *American X-ray Journal* that "no quacks or fakes of whatsoever sort need apply."[4] Unfortunately, these terms were never defined. This lack of membership restriction meant that in addition to serious x-ray workers, there were "those whose interests were merely commercial and who would exploit without compunction a young and struggling scientific body to further their ends."[3] Indeed, Article IX stated that "Subscribers of the Journal may become members of the Society without credentials if they are members of medical or other scientific societies and pay $5.00 dues." It seemed that for many the only qualification for membership was ownership of a static machine.

The first annual meeting of the Roentgen Society of the United States, held in New York City at the Grand Central Palace on December 13 and 14, 1900, drew an enthusiastic audience of about 150 to hear 25 scientific papers and to view extensive commercial exhibits. As Robarts[1] wrote in his review of the meeting,

> Without any doubt there was exhibited in the 2,600 square feet of space devoted to apparatus the finest collection of x-ray appliances yet brought together anywhere in the world. The immense value of comparison as an educational value was here apparent. Side by side were seen competing instruments of the most varied types and construction. The strides that have been taken in mechanical improvements were visible on every hand. Two hours in this room were worth more to the incipient x-ray operator in search of information than two years of price list study.

At the 1901 meeting held in Buffalo, New York, the Society changed its name to the Roentgen Society of America, mainly to encourage Canadian physicians interested in x-rays to join the organization. Both the initial and second annual meetings were described as "chaotic affairs." As Skinner[5] wrote in his history of the Society, "the documentary evi-

First annual meeting of the Roentgen Society of the United States (1900). This room was "filled with exhibits," while a similar one was "seated for 230 members and spectators."

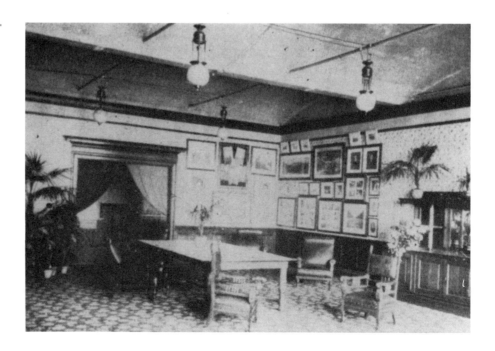

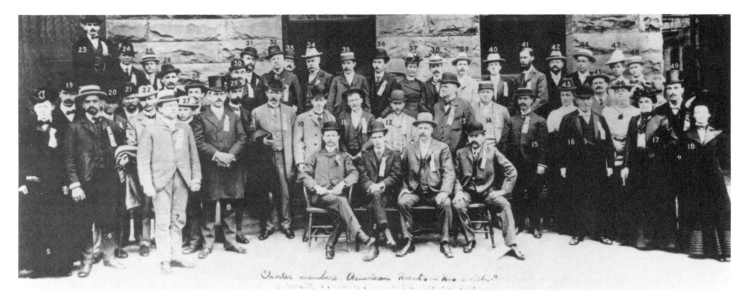

dence, mostly within the columns of the issues of American X-ray Journal, seems to show that a fringe of electro-therapists attempted to either control or sabotage this poorly organized society, much to the embarrassment of Doctor Robarts. They attempted to euchre the editor out of his journal and finally succeeded." Skinner[5] described "the desperate plight in which Doctor Robarts seemed engulfed" at these early meetings, "with electro-therapists to the left of him, jealous x-ray neophytes to the right of him, upstart manufacturers in front of him, and colleagues at home pulling his coat tails."

It soon became apparent to the more far-sighted members that if the Roentgen Society of America were to survive, it was essential to eliminate "undesirable elements" within the membership. It was agreed that:

> Hereafter, members will only be accepted by this Society after being duly recommended by two competent and well known professionals who are members of the Society. . . . It is the intention of this Committee to investigate all such physicians who advertise or seek publicity in daily or other public papers. . . . We may safely say that such members will be expelled so that we may have only the best material in the Society and allow men of good standing only the prestige of membership.[6]

Meanwhile, the *American X-ray Journal* was facing serious financial difficulties. To increase income, the subscription rate was raised from $1 to $3 per year. Robarts offered x-ray books to new subscribers at substantial discounts from retail prices. A new subscriber also could choose a premium, such as a fever thermometer, an albumoscope, or a fountain pen with a 14-carat gold point. Anyone securing 100 new members was offered an x-ray machine worth $100.[6]

After the formation of the Roentgen Society, Robarts expected that its members would enthusiastically support the journal. However, members severely criticized its free-wheeling advertising policy, especially from dubious schools and laboratories of electrotherapeutics. Although Robarts promised to crack down on excesses, advertisements still were cheerfully accepted for various oil and gold mining stocks and patent medicine remedies.

Finally, in 1902 Robarts sold the *American X-ray Journal* to Harry Preston Pratt of Chicago, a physician specializing in electrotherapy. Two years later, the *American X-ray Journal* took over the *Archives of Electrology and Radiology* (formerly the *American Electro-Therapeutic and X-Ray Era*). This joint publication was called the *American Journal of Progressive Therapeutics*, which eventually disappeared in January, 1906.

Charter members of the American Roentgen Ray Society (Buffalo, 1901). Identified attendees include: *1*, Weston Price, D.D.S., Cleveland; *2*, E.A. Florentine, M.D., Saginaw (Michigan); *3*, Heber Robarts, M.D., St. Louis; *4*, J. Rudis-Jicinsky, M.D., Cedar Rapids; *5-6*, Henry Engeln and wife, Cleveland; *8*, Henry Hulst, M.D., Grand Rapids (Michigan); *10*, John McIntosh, Chicago; *15*, Mihran Kassabian, M.D., Philadelphia; *25*, Augustas W. Crane, M.D., Kalamazoo (Michigan); *26*, G.G. Burdick, M.D., Chicago; *32*, H.E. Waite, M.D., New York; *37-38*, Ed Jerman and wife, Indianapolis; *44*, Preston Hickey, M.D., Detroit.

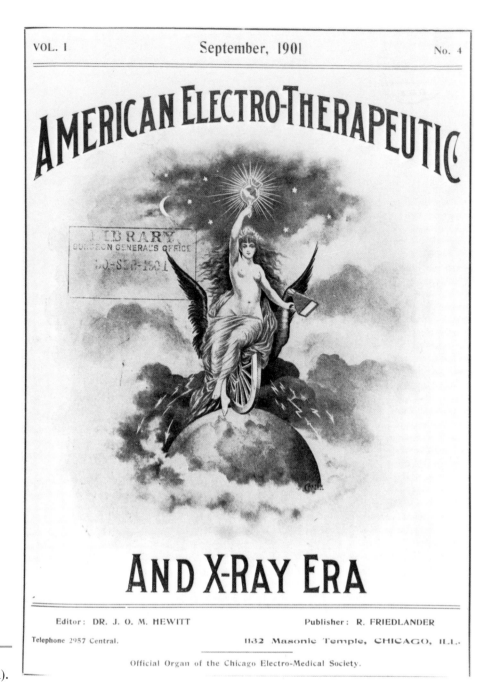

VOL. I   September, 1901   No. 4

AMERICAN ELECTRO-THERAPEUTIC

AND X-RAY ERA

Editor: DR. J. O. M. HEWITT   Publisher: R. FRIEDLANDER

Telephone 2957 Central.   1132 Masonic Temple, CHICAGO, ILL.

Official Organ of the Chicago Electro-Medical Society.

Cover page of an early issue of *American Electro-Therapeutic and X-Ray Era* (1901).

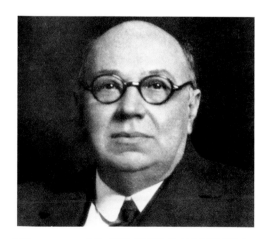

Preston M. Hickey (1865-1930).

Although the electrotherapeutists gained control of the *American X-ray Journal*, by the time of the third annual Society meeting held in Chicago in 1902, the physicians aligned with the American Medical Association had gained control over the organization, which was renamed the American Roentgen Ray Society (ARRS). As Skinner wrote, "Within two years, our Society was rescued from its despoilers and detractors, and the improvement and progress has been constant ever since." The membership list was weeded out. Many Western members, in particular, either resigned or were dropped for nonpayment of dues, so that the ARRS became increasingly an Eastern society.

Beginning with the third annual meeting in 1902, the ARRS began publication of the *Transactions* of the Society. In addition to carrying the full text of scientific papers presented, the *Transactions* carried edited yet remarkably frank versions of the often heated informal discussions that followed. Following the 1906 meeting, the *Transactions* was replaced by the *American Quarterly of Roentgenology* under editor Preston M. Hickey of Detroit. This periodical consisted of a variety of original contributions by American radiologists and others. Many articles were abundantly illustrated despite the fact that authors were required to pay the added cost of publication of illustrations out of their own pockets. Finally, in November 1913, the *Quarterly* expanded into a monthly publication with a new and larger format under the name *American Journal of Roentgenology*. Ten years later (1923), it also became the official organ of the American Radium Society, and its name was extended to become the *American Journal of Roentgenology and Radium Therapy*. In 1952, the publication expanded further to become the *American Journal of Roentgenology, Radium Therapy, and Nuclear Medicine*. Finally, in 1976 the name changed once again to its current title of *American Journal of Roentgenology*.

Since its inception, the *American Journal of Roentgenology* has had only eight editors: Preston M. Hickey (1913), James T. Case (1916), Harry M. Imboden (1918), Arthur C. Christie (1924), Lawrence Reynolds (1930), Traian Leucutia (1961), Melvin M. Figley (1976), and Robert N. Berk (1986).

In 1911, admission standards were raised for prospective members of the ARRS. Applicants were required to have a medical degree, 2 years of x-ray work following graduation, and three letters of recommendation—two from ARRS members in good standing and one from a physician or surgeon residing in the applicant's immediate vicinity. They were also required to "submit a scientific paper to the Executive Committee, which if approved, may be published in the Proceedings of the Society."[5]

As Arthur C. Christie[7] has written,

> One of the traditions of the American Roentgen Ray Society from early years has been its insistence upon the complete integration of radiology into the practice of medicine. This was doubtless due in part to the fact that nearly all of the pioneer radiologists were originally practitioners of medicine, but this ideal has been maintained within the Society and among its members down to the present time. The Society has jealously guarded the idea that the practice of radiology is the practice of medicine; that its practitioners must be broadly trained in general medicine; that they, like other physicians, must maintain a close personal relationship with their patients; that the relationship to physicians referring patients to them is that of a medical consultant; and that in all hospital and clinic relationships the radiologist must preserve his own freedom and autonomy as a practicing physician.

The American Roentgen Ray Society currently has about 7,000 active members.

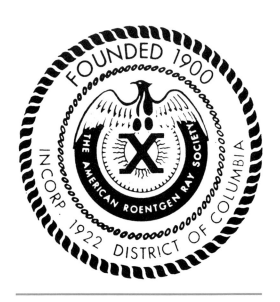

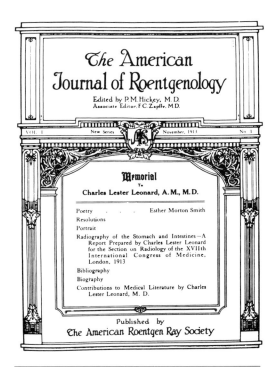

Cover page of the first volume of *American Journal of Roentgenology* (1913).

Seal of the American Roentgen Ray Society.

RADIOLOGICAL SOCIETY OF NORTH AMERICA (RSNA)

By the middle of the second decade of the twentieth century, the ARRS had become largely an Eastern society. The great majority of its members were from Eastern states; most of the meetings were held in that part of the country, and the cost of attendance for those west of the Alleghenies was high in terms of both money and time away from their practices. In addition, the membership requirements made it difficult for Westerners, since many of them did not personally know two active ARRS members in good standing who could sponsor them. Even though the ARRS had made some conciliatory overtures by setting up "Western Section" meetings and establishing a new class of "Associate Members," a schism was developing in the organizational structure of American Radiology.

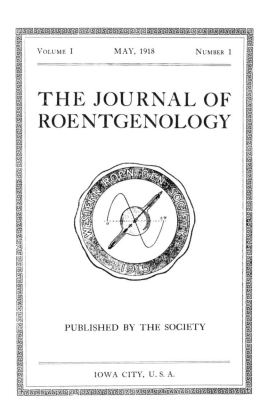

Cover page of first volume of *Journal of Roentgenology* (1918).

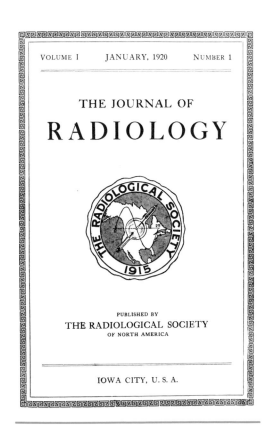

Cover page of first volume of *Journal of Radiology* (1920).

According to A.W. Erskine[8]:

Probably the most compelling reason for forming a new society was the firm belief held by its founders that there should be a place in organized radiology for young men, who should be encouraged to develop within the organization. There was a paragraph in the newly adopted constitution which is still retained. It provides for members-elect, whose qualifications are the same as those of active members except that the applicant need have devoted the major portion of his time to the practice of radiology for only one year instead of three. The founders and the older members have been proud of the fact that no member, regardless of his obscurity or the modesty of his attainments, has ever been denied the right to raise his voice in either the scientific or executive sessions of the Society.

In 1915, after returning from a midwinter meeting of the American Roentgen Ray Society, Edwin C. Ernst, a young St. Louis physician, felt that the time was ripe for the formation of an independent central or western society and decided to arrange a special organizational meeting. George W. Brady, head of the manufacturing company in Chicago making x-ray accessories and Paragon X-ray Plates and who had a wide acquaintance with radiologists, hospitals, and lay technicians, offered to assume the expense of mailing letters to his customers to obtain expressions of opinion for or against the idea of a new organization. These letters went out from Brady's office, although as Howard P. Doub[9] wrote in his history of the RSNA, "It now appears that a communication directly from Doctor Titterington (acting secretary) might have had better primary response, as some prominent roentgenologists at first showed a lack of interest because both physicians and lay workers were approached."

After further discussions and informal meetings, it was decided to hold an organizational meeting in Chicago on December 15 and 16, 1915 (ironically, almost the exact same dates as the first annual meeting of the ARRS 15 years previously). Fred O'Hara of Springfield, Illinois (an associate of Heber Robarts at the time when the latter founded the ARRS!) was chosen as temporary chairman and Miles B. Titterington of St. Louis as secretary. The new organization, with 62 paid-up charter members at $10 each, was named the Western Roentgen Society (WRS) and held its first scientific session in June, 1916, in St. Louis. The *American Journal of Roentgenology* failed to mention the scientific meeting or even note the organization of the WRS.[9]

Although launched as a regional organization in 1915, within 4 years (1919) the WRS with its 472 members from 38 states was more nearly a nationwide organization (although still less prestigious) than the American Roentgen Ray Society. Accordingly, in 1920 the WRS changed its name to the Radiological Society of North America (RSNA).[9]

In 1918, the WRS president, Benjamin H. Orndoff, stressed that the growing Society needed an official publication. Thus was born the *Journal of Roentgenology*, which under the editorship of Bundy Allen of Iowa City, appeared quarterly during 1918 and 1919. However, the publication suffered from severe lack of funds and a name too similar to the ARRS' *American Journal of Roentgenology*. In 1920, when the WRS became the RSNA, the *Journal of Roentgenology* was renamed the *Journal of Radiology* and became a monthly. To provide a stronger financial background, the Radiological Publishing Company was established under RSNA president Albert F. Tyler of Omaha, Nebraska. Many of the officers and members of the RSNA subscribed to stock in this organization, although the Society itself was not a stockholder. Doctor Tyler appointed his brother, H.S. Tyler, as business manager and assumed the duties of editor. The Tylers became increasingly independent and disregarded RSNA directives. As before, finances were a problem. The members of the Society did not subscribe freely, and there was a lack of working capital. The annual dues of members of the RSNA were $10 each, of which half was for a subscription to the *Journal*. However, factional differences arose, and after 1922 the Society did not pay the subscriptions to the publishing company.

As Doub[9] wrote,

> Under these conditions it was not long before the officers and members of the Society realized that they were actually without control of their official Journal. Steps were taken to change this, and after much litigation . . . and added expense to those loyal members who supported the Society's claims with their own money, dissolution of the publishing company was effected and a new journal was started.

Thus Tyler was expelled from the RSNA, and the Society assumed publication of its new monthly publication, renamed *Radiology*, with the September, 1923, issue under editor Maximilian J. Hubeny of Chicago. But the controversy had not ended. Tyler continued to issue the *Journal of Radiology* with the same by-line, "published for the RSNA." He then sued the 1923 slate of RSNA officers, including its president, Russell D. Carman, claiming that the *Journal of Radiology* was the property of the publishing company, which had "permanent and irrevocable right" to publish the official proceedings of the Society. Eventually, the suit reached the U.S. Supreme Court, which affirmed the trial court ruling[10]:

> That the Journal of Radiology is, and always has been, the property of said defendant Society and never at any time became the property of the Radiological Publishing Company. That said defendant Society never intended to give up, turn over or lose the ownership and control of said Journal.
>
> That said Journal has never been in any form or manner turned over or given to said publishing company other than for the purpose of publishing said Journal for said defendant.

In its opinion, the Supreme Court added that restraining the publication of *Radiology*, or other official organs of the Society, would mean that

> the Society be without an official medium of communication with its members and others, unless it chooses to adopt as such the Journal published by the plaintiff; . . . the Society has the right to maintain an official organ responsive to its purposes and subject to its control. The plaintiff does not own the right to publish it nor can it insist rightfully that the Society shall not publish as it chooses.

The *Journal of Radiology* was discontinued with its December, 1925, issue, when it merged with the *American Journal of Electrotherapy and Radiology* to become the *Archives of Physical Therapy*.

Internal dissension regarding the publication of its journal beset the RSNA a few years later. During the annual meeting of the Society in 1929, the Chemical Foundation, a nonprofit organization (controlled by noted cancer specialist Francis Carter Wood) with large assets resulting from seizure of German dye patents during World War I, offered to subsidize the complete publication of original articles and abstracts of the world literature on cancer. Despite some misgivings by the Executive Committee, this proposal was accepted, and the size and scope of *Radiology* were enormously enlarged. It soon became apparent, however, that the officers of the Chemical Foundation intended to have a major voice in the manage-

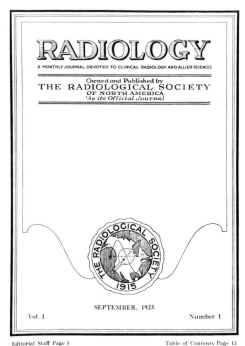

Cover page of first volume of *Radiology* (1923).

SUPREME COURT DECISION
JUDGMENT AFFIRMED FOR "RADIOLOGY"
Filed July 10, 1925
Grace F. Kaercher, Clerk
Albert F. Tyler, et al,
Appellants,
24459   vs.
John R. Bruce, et al,
Respondents.
SYLLABUS
1. The evidence sustains the trial court's finding that the Journal of Radiology, published by the plaintiff publishing company for the defendant society, was the property of the defendant society and not of the plaintiff corporation.
2. The plaintiff publishing company by its arrangement with the defendant society did not have the permanent and irrevocable right to publish the official proceedings of the society, or its journal or official organ.
3. The plaintiff corporation was not entitled to an injunction restraining the defendant society from publishing "Radiology," the name of a journal published by the society after its relations with the plaintiff corporation ceased, nor compelling it to give to the plaintiff for publication in the proceedings of the Society.
Affirmed.

Supreme Court decision in favor of *Radiology* (1925).[10]

THIRTY-FOURTH ANNUAL MEETING, HOTELS FAIRMONT AND MARK HOPKINS
SAN FRANCISCO, DECEMBER 5 TO 10, 1948

Radiology. Cover design changes in 1948 (*left*) and 1962 (*right*).

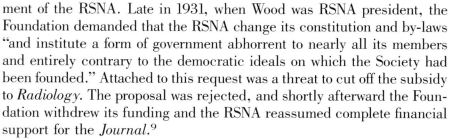

RADIOLOGY

A MONTHLY JOURNAL DEVOTED TO CLINICAL RADIOLOGY AND ALLIED SCIENCES

SILVER ANNIVERSARY NUMBER
1923–1948

OCTOBER · 1948

VOLUME 51   NUMBER 4

Owned and Published as its Official Journal by
THE RADIOLOGICAL SOCIETY OF NORTH AMERICA

VOLUME 79   NUMBER 1   July 1962

Radiology

*a monthly journal devoted to
clinical radiology and allied sciences*

owned and published as its official journal by
THE RADIOLOGICAL SOCIETY OF NORTH AMERICA

Forty-eighth Annual Meeting / Palmer House, Chicago / November 25–30, 1962

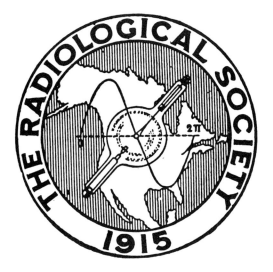

Seal of the Radiological Society.

ment of the RSNA. Late in 1931, when Wood was RSNA president, the Foundation demanded that the RSNA change its constitution and by-laws "and institute a form of government abhorrent to nearly all its members and entirely contrary to the democratic ideals on which the Society had been founded." Attached to this request was a threat to cut off the subsidy to *Radiology*. The proposal was rejected, and shortly afterward the Foundation withdrew its funding and the RSNA reassumed complete financial support for the *Journal*.[9]

Since that time, *Radiology* has thrived and prospered under its four succeeding editors, Leon J. Menville (1931), Howard P. Doub (1941), William R. Eyler (1966), and Stanley S. Siegelman (1985). In 1981, the RSNA introduced a second periodical, entitled *RadioGraphics,* which was primarily designed to capture scientific exhibits from the annual RSNA convention. *RadioGraphics* was edited from its inception by William Tuddenham, who was succeeded in 1989 by William W. Olmsted.

The RSNA currently has 25,000 active members.

AMERICAN COLLEGE OF RADIOLOGY (ACR)

Albert Soiland of Los Angeles, a pioneer in radiation therapy on the West Coast and 1922 president of the RSNA, felt that radiology as a science had not received the recognition that its achievements warranted in American medical circles. He envisioned a new organization that would outstrip the ARRS in eminence and exclusiveness of membership just as the RSNA had outstripped the ARRS in size. The new organization would be limited to 100 outstanding Fellows "who have distinguished themselves in the science of radiology." Each Fellow must be a graduate of a "reputable institution of medicine and surgery" and must have devoted at least 10 years to the science of radiology. In addition to Fellows, there would be an even higher class of Honorary Fellows, composed of "those whose contributions to the science of radiology warrant honorary recognition."[11]

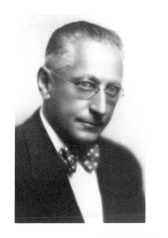

Albert Soiland (1873-1946).

Soiland initially proposed this new organization in a letter to 75 prominent radiologists. On June 26, 1923, at the AMA meeting in San Francisco, 21 of these eminent figures, including Soiland, established the American College of Radiology. (An American College of Surgeons had been founded in 1913 and an American College of Physicians in 1915.) Seventy radiologists initially accepted Fellowships, and the first Convocation of the College was held in Chicago 1 year later, with Soiland as Executive Secretary and George E. Pfahler of Philadelphia as President.

As Soiland[12] wrote, the ACR was established for the purpose of

> selecting a working group of men whose years of successful experience entitle them to respect and the confidence of their colleagues. It is hoped this movement will co-ordinate—more closely than has been possible in the past—the efforts of different groups and thus lessen the burdens incident to attending to a multiplicity of meetings and bring about a closer fellowship among those who stand for the most lofty ideas of humanity, as well as of scientific achievement in this highly specialized branch of medicine.

The ACR should exert a widespread influence in the following respects[12]:

1. Co-ordinating and unifying different groups of men already working in this field in various associations, and also including in its membership isolated workers who would thus receive much help and stimulation;
2. To encourage research in medical schools, private laboratories and, in certain restricted fields, by individual workers;
3. To exchange new ideas as to methods and equipment;
4. To stimulate the younger men in the profession to take up seriously this branch of medicine;
5. To standardize equipment, therapeutic procedure, safeguarding of both patients and operators, the proper keeping of records and reports, so that sufficient uniformity may exist to make them comparable;
6. To see that the proper opportunities are offered for the training of technicians and assistants; and finally, but by no means of the least importance,
7. To guard and uphold the professional status of the radiologist himself by seeking from the medical profession at large such recognition as he has honestly earned, and by discrediting charlatans and ill-prepared operators or self-advertisers.

As if to ward off an expected barrage of criticism, Soiland[13] stressed in an editorial in *Radiology* that:

> The idea of this College was not to place a wreath upon the brows of the older men, or to set them aside as supermen; the writer felt that men who had conscientiously and honestly striven to make radiology a respected and useful branch of general medicine were capable of directing future work of this specialty and laying out a course which the younger members could safely follow. He realizes that probably twice the number called upon are just as eligible to be members as the first list interrogated. He also wants to state that if some feel that they have been overlooked or slighted, such is not the intention or spirit of this organization, but a beginning has to be made and a nucleus formed, around which can be built up a sort of College which will meet the requirements of all those eligible.

In a brief unpublished history of the ACR, Lowell S. Goin of Los Angeles noted that during the 1920s

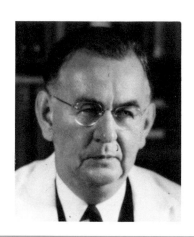

Otto Glasser (1895-1964).

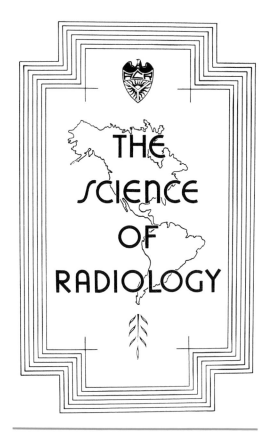

The Science of Radiology, the ACR-sponsored historical survey edited by Otto Glasser.

The College existed as a rather exclusive organization intended primarily to confer distinction upon its members. Lest it be thought that the foregoing constitutes a denigration of the College in its early years, it must be remembered that the decoration of a man with the Order of Chivalry, or the conferring upon him of an honorary Doctorate, serves no purpose other than to honor the recipient and to recognize his distinction. These are, in fact, useful functions. Moreover, in the early years, the existence of the College served to emphasize the fact that Radiology had assumed its rightful place as a medical specialty, and as a peer of the other great branches of Medicine, some of which had Colleges in existence . . .

According to Arthur W. Erskine,[8]

The activities of the College were limited to an annual Convocation, a dinner, and an oration. During that period many radiologists were doubtful that it was useful enough to justify its continued existence, and its death from inanition would not have been surprising. But it did survive, probably because the governing body, the Board of Chancellors, carried out its task of selecting Fellows with conscientious care. Radiologists were indeed rare who could bring themselves to decline the real and implied honor of election to Fellowship.

Once the initial limit of 100 Fellows was reached, the ceiling was raised and then abolished altogether.

It is ironic that the ACR, which originally was almost exclusively an honorary organization emphasizing exclusivity and ritual, soon emerged as a forceful spokesman for its medical specialty. As early as 1927, the ACR became concerned with the economic aspects of radiological practice, and one of its members, Arthur Christie of Washington, D.C., became the voice of radiology on a newly established national committee on the costs of medical care. Thus the ACR tentatively assumed the role of spokesman on the economic front, while the ARRS and RSNA remained the voices of American radiology in professional and scientific matters.

In 1933, the ACR joined with the ARRS, ARS, and RSNA in planning the American Congress of Radiology, a nationwide showcase for the specialty that was held in connection with the Chicago Century of Progress Exposition. To commemorate the event, a historical survey of radiology was prepared by 26 contributors and edited by Otto Glasser of Cleveland. One year later, the ACR launched a *Bulletin* devoted to economic and educational matters. By this time three Commissions had been formed: Medical Economics, Radiological Education, and Public Instruction.

The major growth of the ACR began in 1935 under the leadership of W. Edward Chamberlain of Philadelphia. A new constitution cited "the purpose of advancing the science of radiology by means of the study of the economic aspects of radiology and the encouragement of improved educational facilities for radiologists." However, the constitutional change that had the most influence on the tremendous increase in power of the ACR was the admission of ordinary members, "ethical radiologists who have satisfied the requirements of the American Board of Radiology." Within 5 years, total membership of the ACR increased five times, from about 200 to more than 1,000. Beginning in 1939, all Diplomates of the American Board of Radiology became eligible for membership.

The revitalized ACR plunged into action on the economic front. The rapid rise of Blue Cross and other medical prepayment insurance plans during the years of recovery from the Depression had greatly expanded the role of the hospital on the American medical scene. Hospitals were increasingly demanding that radiologists should be only employees of hospitals and that radiology must be considered a purely ancillary hospital service. There was also a concern among many radiologists that plans for a nationwide health insurance program then under discussion in Washington might impair their traditional fee-for-service relations with patients. In these and many other matters, radiologists needed a strong voice. Because of the continuing rivalry between the ARRS and RSNA, only the ACR could speak for radiology as a whole. Thus in 1937 the Board of Chancellors of the ACR proposed and the ARRS, RSNA, and ARS cooperated in the formation of an Inter-Society Committee for Radiology to speak for the entire specialty on radiologist-hospital relationships, Blue Cross–Blue Shield relationships, compulsory health insurance, and other economic issues. Funds were collected to finance the committee's activities, and Mac F. Cahal was hired as the Executive Secretary of the ACR, probably the first full-time employee of any American radiological organization.

In effect, the Inter-Society Committee became the modern ACR, which gradually transformed itself into today's aggressive, businesslike association that is truly representative of organized American radiology.

The ACR now has about 16,000 active members and engages in a wide range of activities through its Board of Chancellors, Council, Commissions, and Committees. Major areas of interest include standards in radiological practice, radiation protection, and radiological units; education, public health, health insurance, and technologist affairs. Most recently, the ACR developed a Professional Bureau to assist residents and young radiologists in finding suitable positions.

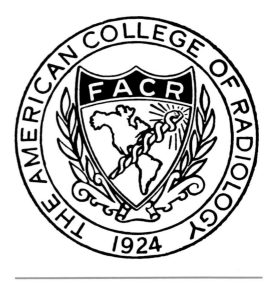

Seal of the American College of Radiology.

SECTION ON RADIOLOGY OF THE AMERICAN MEDICAL ASSOCIATION

At the June, 1923 meeting of the AMA, where the initial nucleus of the American College of Radiology was formed, Soiland also pressed intensively for AMA recognition of Radiology as a full-fledged medical specialty. The annual AMA meeting was potentially an excellent showplace where radiologists could display their new advances to fellow physicians, on whom they depended for patient referrals. Yet as far back as the 1912 meeting in Atlantic City, radiologists had complained that "the space for Roentgen plates was confined to an out-of-the-way gallery with absolutely no conveniences provided for those who might desire to exhibit." At the next AMA meeting in Minneapolis in 1913, the radiological exhibit "was placed upon the top floor of the scientific building and it required a maximum of enthusiasm to climb the long flights of stairs." Thus an editorial in the *American Journal of Roentgenology* for March, 1913 urged that ". . . one member of the (AMA) committee of scientific exhibits . . . be a man interested in roentgenology . . . who would see that better accommodations were provided." A radiologist was indeed appointed to the AMA exhibit committee for the next year, but still there was no provision on the program for radiologists to present scientific papers. Therefore Soiland, as the delegate from California, presented a resolution urging that the 15 official "Sections" of the AMA be expanded to 16 to make room for a new "Section on Radiology." Soiland pointed out that 1,000 members of the AMA were engaged full-time or part-time in the practice of radiology, and he warned that various state bodies were

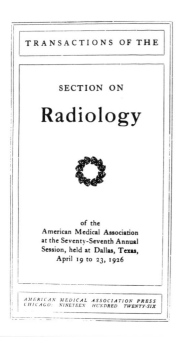

Cover page of first volume of *Transactions of the Section on Radiology of the American Medical Association* (1926).

attempting to legalize and license the practice of radiology by laymen. Creation of an AMA Section on Radiology would recognize the specialty as an integral part of the science of medicine and surgery. As a compromise, the AMA House of Delegates recommended that each of the 15 Sections include in its program at least one paper pertaining to some other specialty such as radiology. However, it refused to create a sixteenth Section.

During the following year, the AMA was inundated (perhaps at Soiland's suggestion) with "numerous communications from all parts of the country requesting one or more sessions on radiology" at the next AMA meeting. In a rare show of unity, the RSNA, ARRS, and ARS sponsored a resolution supporting the new section. Although these efforts were unsuccessful in 1924, the AMA formally approved establishment of a Section on Radiology in 1925. Since that time, the Section has arranged radiological programs and exhibits at various AMA meetings and has served as a spokesman representing the interests of radiology in the AMA House of Delegates.

BRITISH INSTITUTE OF RADIOLOGY

The complex history of organized radiology in Britain began with the inaugural issue of *Archives of Clinical Skiagraphy*, the world's first radiological journal, which appeared in April or early May, 1896, only 4 months after the news of Roentgen's discovery reached London. The *Archives* has remained continuously in print to the present day, being known since 1924 as the *British Journal of Radiology*. The title page of the first number carried these subtitles, "A Series of Collotype Illustrations with Descriptive Text, Illustrating Applications of the New Photography to Medicine and Surgery." The first number of the *Archives* consisted of 16 printed pages, six plates of radiographs, and several other illustrations. It was issued in green wrappers in a quarto format, and the back wrapper carried advertisements for a variety of x-ray apparatus.

The major force behind the development of the *Archives* was its youthful editor, Sydney D. Rowland, who provided all 16 pages of copy in the first number and most of the radiographs. Rowland coined the word *skiagraphy* and was a 24-year-old medical student when he began serving as editor of the world's first radiological journal. His interest in radiology did not last long beyond his undergraduate years, and in 1897 he began a career in laboratory medicine.

Two more issues of the *Archives* were published in 1896, though both were substantially thinner, probably because Rowland was preparing for his final examinations and could devote limited time to his editorial duties. The fourth number (April, 1897) bore the abbreviated title, *Archives of Skiagraphy*, dropping the word *clinical* to reflect a deliberate change in editorial policy and the presence of several articles dealing with nonclinical aspects of x-ray work.

The mounting interest provoked in London medical circles by the new photography led to the establishment of the Röntgen Society, which held its first annual meeting on June 3, 1897, with physicist Silvanus P. Thompson as President. The objects of the Society were:

1. to discuss the Röntgen rays in relation to Medicine, the Arts and Sciences.
2. to discuss and exhibit apparatus and methods in connection with the rays.

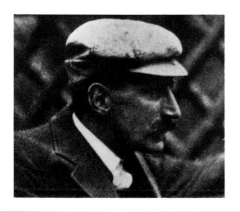

Sydney D. Rowland (1872-1917).

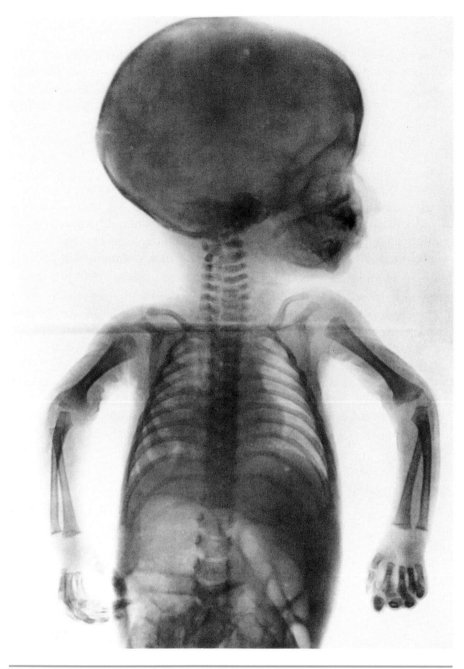

First radiograph in *Archives of Clinical Skiagraphy* (1896). Full-grown child 3 months of age. Exposure of 14 minutes.

Archives
— of —
Clinical Skiagraphy.

BY

SYDNEY ROWLAND, B.A., CAMB.,

LATE SCHOLAR OF DOWNING COLLEGE, CAMBRIDGE, AND SHUTER SCHOLAR OF
ST. BARTHOLOMEW'S HOSPITAL.
SPECIAL COMMISSIONER TO "BRITISH MEDICAL JOURNAL" FOR INVESTIGATION OF
THE APPLICATIONS OF THE NEW PHOTOGRAPHY TO MEDICINE AND SURGERY.

*A SERIES OF COLLOTYPE ILLUSTRATIONS WITH DESCRIPTIVE
TEXT, ILLUSTRATING APPLICATIONS OF THE NEW
PHOTOGRAPHY TO MEDICINE AND SURGERY.*

London:
THE REBMAN PUBLISHING COMPANY, LIMITED,
11, ADAM STREET, STRAND.
1896.

Cover page of first volume of *Archives of Clinical Skiagraphy* (1896).

3. to hold periodical meetings for the reading of papers and discussions thereon; with exhibition of clinical cases, skiagrams and all matters bearing on Röntgen Rays.
4. to provide a museum, library and Röntgen Ray appliances.
5. to publish transactions in a convenient form.

One of the first acts of the new Society was to reach agreement with the publisher of *Archives of Skiagraphy* to publish its proceedings quarterly and to provide each member with a copy of the journal. This agreement was a lifesaver for the ailing journal, which was suffering from a shortage of contributions as well as its editor's impending departure into another specialty. In keeping with the fashion of the moment to honor the discoverer of the new rays, the title was changed to *Archives of the Roentgen Ray.* Although the *Archives* was never the official journal of the Röntgen Society and remained a separate commercial enterprise, the special relationship that had been established was defined in a phrase that became the subtitle of the journal: "The Only Journal in Which the

ARCHIVES
— OF —
THE ROENTGEN RAY

(*Formerly* ARCHIVES OF SKIAGRAPHY).

THE ONLY JOURNAL IN WHICH THE TRANSACTIONS OF THE ROENTGEN
SOCIETY OF LONDON ARE OFFICIALLY REPORTED.

VOLUME II.

EDITED BY

W. S. HEDLEY, M.D.,   SYDNEY ROWLAND, M.A.,
M.R.C.S., in charge of the Electro-Therapeutic   M.R.C.S., &
Department, the London Hospital.

London:
THE REBMAN PUBLISHING COMPANY, LIMITED,
129, SHAFTESBURY AVENUE, CAMBRIDGE CIRCUS, W.C.

AMERICAN AGENT:
W. B. SAUNDERS, 925, WALNUT STREET, PHILADELPHIA, PA.
1898.

Cover page of *Archives of the Roentgen Ray* (1898).

Transactions of the Röntgen Society of London are Officially Reported." For the first time, the *Archives* began to assume the appearance of a true scientific journal. Original articles began to appear that were written by physicists and early manufacturers of x-ray apparatus, in addition to practicing radiologists. Regular features were book reviews, summaries of articles written by early Continental and American pioneers, and detailed reports of meetings of the Röntgen Society. The senior coeditor (Rowland agreed to continue as junior coeditor) was W.S. Hedley, the medical electrician of the London Hospital.

A bitter controversy that had beset the Röntgen Society even before its establishment was whether nonmedical men were to be admitted. How could confidentiality be preserved if doctors were obliged to discuss clinical matters before an audience of apparatus makers and photographers? The crucial decision was not to restrict membership of the Society to medical men, but instead to offer membership to any scientist or layman who wished to join and had shown "some scientific interest in the Roentgen Rays." An inability to maintain a balance between medical and lay interests led inevitably to a schism that affected both the Society and its journal.

The papers read at the first session of the Röntgen Society had a strong nonmedical slant, and this did not alter in succeeding years. For the doctors, the problem of discussing patients' diseases and radiographs before a mixed audience proved to be an insurmountable barrier to wholehearted medical participation. Consequently, in 1901 some of the prominent medical members announced their wish for a society devoted exclusively to medical matters. Fifteen members, who collectively formed the radiological "establishment" of London, resigned from the Röntgen Society, and in 1902 the dissident doctors formed the British Electrotherapeutic Society.

A second setback befell the Röntgen Society early in 1904 when its directors disagreed with the publishers of the *Archives of the Roentgen Ray* over editorial control of the journal. At the root of the matter was the secession of the doctors, whose new society had become an immediate success. The Röntgen Society decided to terminate its agreement with the publishers of the *Archives* and to publish its own house journal, the *Journal of the Röntgen Society.*

Cover page of *Archives of the Roentgen Ray and Allied Phenomena: An International Monthly Review of the Practice of Physical Therapeutics* (1908).

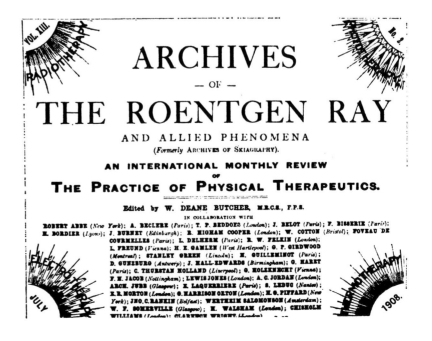

With the departure of the radiologists, the *Archives* expanded to appeal to readers interested in aspects of electrotherapeutics apart from radiology. In July, 1904, the name changed to the *Archives of the Roentgen Ray and Allied Phenomena: an International Monthly Review of the Practice of Physical Therapeutics.* Each of the four corners of the title page had one of the following words inserted diagonally across it: Electrotherapy, Radiotherapy, Phototherapy, Thermotherapy. The new editor was William Deane Butcher, who developed the *Archives* into an international journal for electrotherapeutics.

Roentgen's wholehearted support of the German effort in World War I, especially his decision to donate his Rumford Medal when the German Red Cross Society appealed for gold objects in 1914, had incensed his British colleagues. This gesture, which Roentgen viewed as a patriotic one, was seen by the British as provocative and led to the dispensing of the words *Roentgen Ray* from the Archives, which now became *Archives of Radiology and Electrotherapy.*

Meanwhile, the new *Journal of the Röntgen Society* began publication as a quarterly and, as the mouthpiece of the scientific and commercial following of the new science, attracted strong financial support from x-ray apparatus makers and other suppliers. Edited by the physicist, James H. Gardiner, the journal stressed physics and x-ray apparatus and contained few clinical papers. Gardiner was succeeded by physicist, G.P.C. Kaye (see Chapter 11), who remained the editor until the complicated merger that produced the *British Journal of Radiology.*

The inaugural meeting of the British Electrotherapeutic Society was held on July 10, 1902. Within a few years, virtually all British physicians working with x-rays belonged to this first national association for clinical radiologists in Britain. The Society decided to publish a journal of its own and accordingly took over the *Journal of Physical Therapeutics*, a quarterly potpourri designed to "embrace all the various physical therapies

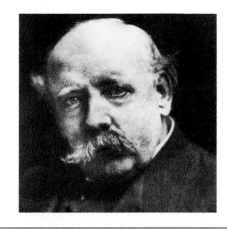

William Deane Butcher.

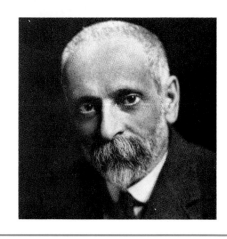

James H. Gardiner.

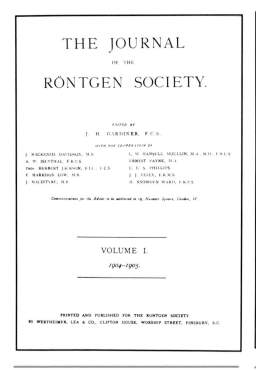

Cover page of *Archives of Radiology and Electrotherapy* (1917).

Cover page of *Journal of the Röntgen Society* (1904-1905).

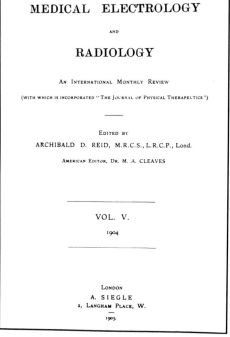

First new cover page of *Journal of Medical Electrology and Radiology* (1904).

then practiced, namely electro-, hydro-, vibro-, photo-, radio-, balneo- and aerotherapy." Thus was born the *Journal of Medical Electrology and Radiology* (1903).

The British Electrotherapeutic Society was one of the 22 medical groups in London that chose in 1907 to unite to form the Royal Society of Medicine. Ironically, the Electro-Therapeutic Section, which included radiology, was the sixteenth established—the identical number as the Section on Radiology of the AMA that began 18 years later. At the end of the 1930-1931 session, an internal arrangement within the Royal Society of Medicine brought into being a true Section on Radiology.

The amalgamation of the British Electrotherapeutic Society into the Royal Society of Medicine led to the demise of the *Journal of Medical Electrology and Radiology*, which from 1907 onward was effectively replaced by the Electro-Therapeutic Section of the Proceedings of the Royal Society of Medicine. Ironically, the *Proceedings* slowly lost its position as the leading radiological journal to its competitor, *Archives of Radiology and Electrotherapy*, which turned from its previous course and began printing more articles on subjects relevant to clinical radiologists.

The third major society of British radiologists was formed in 1917 with the single aim of protecting the status of radiologists and electrotherapists. As stated in the preamble of the organization, it was designed "to promote the advancement of radiologists and physiotherapists on scientific lines under the direct control of the medical profession." To understand the reason for establishing this new society, it is essential to review the position of the medical electrician at the outset and during the course of the First World War, before radiology had come into its own as a specialized branch of the medical profession.

Before 1914, anyone who purchased an x-ray apparatus became ipso facto a radiologist. Radiologists were regarded as glorified technicians, and the legacy of the basement origins of hospital x-ray work bred an inferiority complex in the early workers.[15] Outside the teaching hospitals, many persons in charge of x-ray departments were untrained and unqualified. With the advent of World War I, which suddenly placed radiology in the limelight as an urgently needed specialty, anyone with a nodding acquaintance of electricity, photography, or physics was pressed into service as a radiologist. Professional concern at the use of unqualified radiologists was voiced as early as 1915 in an editorial in the *Archives:*

> New departments have sprung into existence, as it were with the wave
> of a hand, and men to work these departments are urgently required.
> The demand exceeds the supply, and must continue to do so unless
> steps are taken at once to meet the need. The employment of men
> who have had no medical training and no special instruction is to be
> deprecated.

The editorial recommended "(1) the need for teaching facilities and the appointment of lecturers; (2) the creation of the chairs of radiology in universities; and (3) the full recognition of the radiologist and electrotherapeutist as consultants in the Army and Navy."

At a meeting in the house of Sir James MacKenzie Davidson, the only pioneer radiologist to be knighted for services to medicine, it was decided that one of the universities be urged to institute a diploma course for radiologists and that a new and purely medical society be instituted to deal with clinical teaching. This second conclusion was implemented immediately with the development of the British Association of Radiology and Physiotherapy (BARP) in April, 1917. Despite its proximity to the major sources of clinical material in the country, London University refused to undertake the diploma course. Thus BARP set up its diploma course in radiology at Cambridge University, where Sir Ernest Rutherford was soon to succeed J. J. Thomson as Cavendish Professor of Experimental Physics. BARP also began to undertake other functions for the radiological profession, including the establishment of a subcommittee to deal with political and ethical affairs involving radiologists. In 1918, the *Archives of Radiology and Electrotherapy* became the official organ of the British Association of Radiology and Physiotherapy.

The early convoluted history of British radiology came to a conclusion when representatives of the Röntgen Society, the Electro-Therapeutic Section of the Royal Society of Medicine, and the British Association of Radiology and Physiology joined to develop the British Institute of Radiology, a professional focal point in London in which teaching, research, and other activities could be undertaken under one roof. In 1924, the Institute attached its plate to the door of 32 Welbeck Street, a house which had formerly been the Imperial Russian Embassy.

In the same spirit of professional unity, the Röntgen Society and the British Association of Radiology and Physiotherapy slowly worked to merge their publications. A joint editorial committee was established to advise both editors. The name of the journal of the Röntgen Society was changed to the *British Journal of Radiology* (Röntgen Society Section), while the *Archives of Radiology and Electrotherapy* was changed to the *British Journal of Radiology* (British Association of Radiology and Physiotherapy Section/British Institute of Radiology Section). Finally, in January, 1928 the two publications officially merged with the initial volume of the *British Journal of Radiology, New Series.*

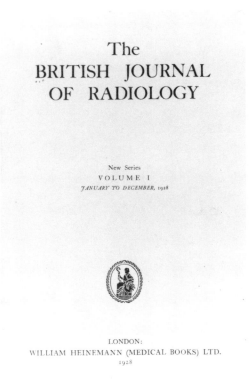

Cover page of first volume of *British Journal of Radiology, New Series* (1928).

OTHER EARLY RADIOLOGICAL JOURNALS AND SOCIETIES

The first radiological publication in continental Europe was *Fortschritte auf dem Gebiete der Röntgenstrahlen*, which appeared in Hamburg, Germany, in 1897 under the editorship of Henrich Albers-Schoenberg. Three

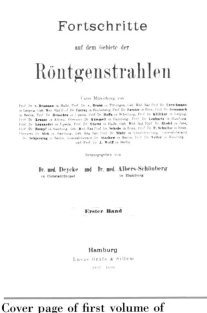

Cover page of first volume of *Fortschritte auf dem Gebiete der Rontgenstrahlen* (1897).

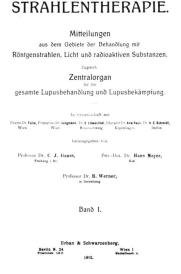

Cover page of first volume of *Strahlentherapie* (1912).

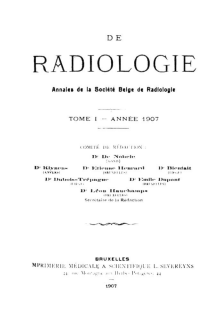

Cover page of first volume of *Journal Belge de Radiologie* (1907).

Left, Cover page of first volume of *Journal de Radiologie et d'Electrologie* (1914). *Right*, Cover page of first volume of *Acta Radiologica* (1921).

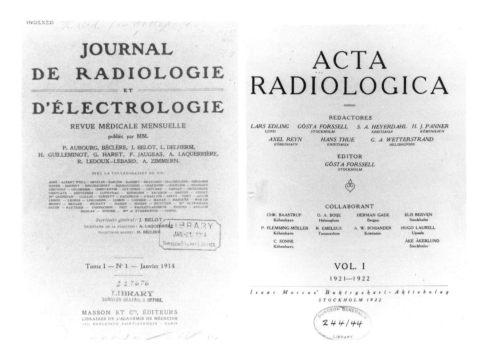

years later, the German Radiological Society (Deutsche Röntgen-Gesellschaft) was founded. The second major German radiological periodical, *Strahlentherapie*, began publication in 1912. In Belgium, the *Journal Belge de Radiologie* debuted in 1907 as the official organ of the Société Belge de Radiologie, which had been founded 1 year previously. The French Radiological Society (Société de Radiologie Médicale de Paris) held its first official session in 1909 under the presidency of Henri Béclère. The organization soon expanded to include several affiliated branches throughout France, and in 1912 this nationwide coverage led to the organization being renamed the Société de Radiologie Médicale de France. Two years later, its *Journal de Radiologie et d'Electrologie* was first published. *La Radiologia Medica*, the official organ of the Società Italiana di Radiologia Medica, published its first volume in 1914. Seven years later (1921), *Acta Radiologica*, under the editorship of Gosta Forssell, became the official organ of the Society of Radiologists of the four Scandinavian countries (Denmark, Finland, Norway, and Sweden).

Bibliography

Brecher E and Brecher R: The rays: A history of radiology in the United States and Canada. Baltimore, Williams & Wilkins, 1969.

Burrows EH: Pioneers and early years: A history of British radiology. Channel Islands, England, Colophon, 1986.

References

1. Robarts H: Editorial. Amer X-ray J 7:12-13, 1900.
2. Robarts H: Editorial. Amer X-ray J 1:1-3, 1897.
3. Brown P: American martyrs to science through the Roentgen rays. Springfield, Ill, Charles C Thomas, 1936.
4. Amer X-ray J 7:10-11, 1900.
5. Skinner EH: The American Roentgen Ray Society (1900-1950). Springfield, Ill, Charles C Thomas, 1950.
6. Nelson PA: History of the once close relationship between electro-therapeutics and radiology. Arch Phys Med Rehabil 54:608-640, 1973.
7. Christie AC: The American Roentgen Ray Society. AJR 76:1-6, 1956.
8. Erskine AW: Organized roentgenology in America. Radiology 45:549-554, 1945.
9. Doub HP: The Radiological Society of North America. Radiology 83:771-784, 1964.
10. Supreme Court decision: Judgment affirmed for "Radiology." Radiology 3:264-267, 1925.
11. del Regato JA: The American College of Radiology. Radiology 107:1-13, 1973.
12. Soiland A: American College of Radiology. Radiology 6:122-124, 1926.
13. Soiland A: The American College of Radiology. Radiology 1:122, 1923.
14. Burrows EH: Pioneers and early years: A history of British radiology. Channel Islands, England, Colophon, 1986.
15. Barclay AE: The history and future of British radiology. Brit J Radiol (Röntgen Society Section) 21:3-20, 1925.

CHAPTER 35

Radiology Education

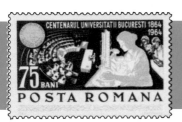

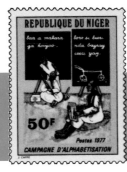

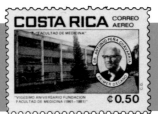

EARLY INSTRUCTION IN RADIOLOGY[1]

Although the first x-ray workers were physicists and photographers, within a few years the performance and interpretation of clinical images "soon found its way into the hands of medical men with more or less genius for things mechanical." The early physician-radiologists gained their practical experience at a time when there was no organized teaching of any kind on the subject. Individual radiologists improved their diagnostic abilities by correlating their plates with operative and autopsy findings. Radiologists learned from one another at conventions, by extensive travel to other medical centers, and by careful examination of the rapidly expanding literature. As described by James T. Case, the relation of these early radiologists to each other was "much like that of a group of widely separated research workers devoted to problems of common interest." Young physicians interested in radiology had the great privilege of learning firsthand from pioneers of the specialty, who were eager to share the knowledge and experience they had acquired. Many American radiologists, often at great personal sacrifice, visited the various radiologic centers of Europe in order to further widen their educational horizon.

As late as the 1930s, few American universities offered a diploma for the completion of postgraduate work in radiology. These universities were hesitant to give anything less than a master's degree in radiology, and few physicians were willing to put in the 2 or 3 years of carefully directed study and research under rigid university regulations that were necessary to procure this degree.

A number of teaching centers offered 1- or 2-year fellowships in radiology, though they were not nearly sufficient to meet the demand. These courses lacked uniformity and proper scope and were given to physicians who did not possess the essential preliminary grounding in the basic principles of physics and radiologic technique. Many postgraduate

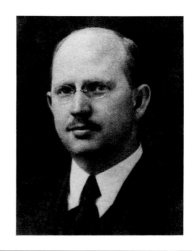

James T. Case.

courses were designed to teach that part of radiology that was especially applicable to certain specialties, such as gastroenterology, urology, and industrial surgery.

A majority of physicians seeking special instruction in radiology were content with a brief course of instruction, which often could be obtained in an x-ray department of dubious distinction or simply by spending a few weeks looking over the shoulder of a practicing radiologist. Many radiologists began practical work without the necessary fundamental basic training. Indeed, a number of these physicians had not even received adequate training in basic medicine or surgery.

Writing in 1933, Case decried "the vicious tendency on the part of incompetent or dishonest laymen, and even by unscrupulous physicians, to commercialize radiology [which] is a natural danger of too rapid expansion of the specialty of radiology and a consequent faulty and insufficient training of physicians entering it." He cited Feodor Haenish, who when speaking of the rapid expansion of the specialty of radiology stated,

> Incompetent and dishonest elements have grasped this specialty. . . . These, in some instances, were unscrupulous physicians who were guided merely by the expected pecuniary advantages and who, unhampered by clinical and roentgenological knowledge and experience, sold "x-ray pictures," paying the referring physician rebates or commissions . . . In other instances, laymen, with or without connivance of dishonest physicians, saw in the purchase of x-ray equipment a get-rich-quick scheme at the expense of innocent patients.

This state of affairs set the stage for the development of an organization that would set educational standards and administer examinations designed to certify physicians qualified to practice radiology.

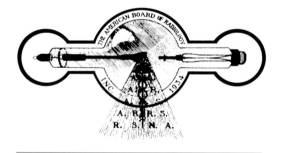

Early official seal of the American Board of Radiology.[3]

AMERICAN BOARD OF RADIOLOGY (ABR)[2]

Although the basic qualification of a physician in the United States was generally an M.D. degree from a recognized medical school plus a license to practice issued by his state government, prior to 1917 there was no similar requirement for recognition as a medical specialist. In that year, the American Board of Ophthalmology was established to set examinations and issue certificates to those individuals who were fully qualified in the specialty. Over the next 15 years, three additional boards were established: Otolaryngology (1924), Obstetrics and Gynecology (1932), and Dermatology and Syphilology (1932).

In the absence of a certifying board, any licensed physician who so desired, regardless of his qualifications or lack of them, could limit his practice to any specialty he chose and hold himself out as a specialist in that field. Any Doctor of Medicine was entitled to a listing in the Directory of the American Medical Association as specializing in the field in which he considered himself qualified.

In Radiology, as in other specialties, it became clear that a certifying board was needed to separate fully trained and qualified specialists from others merely claiming to be so. Also, many feared that if the various specialties did not organize their own certifying boards, each of the states might enact laws regulating entrance into the specialties, just as they already controlled the granting of licenses for the general practice of medicine. The only practical solution was for each specialty to establish a mechanism for placing its mark of approval on those qualified to practice predominantly in that particular field.

In 1932, the five nationwide radiologic societies (ARRS, ARS, RSNA, ACR, and AMA Section on Radiology) each sent three delegates to an organizing session held in connection with the 1933 AMA meeting in Milwaukee. This resulted in the formal incorporation of the American Board of Radiology (ABR) on January 31, 1934. The first candidates for board certification were examined in June of that year.

Initially, the field was divided into five sections for the purpose of certification: (1) Diagnostic Roentgenology; (2) Roentgenology; (3) Therapeutic Roentgenology; (4) Therapeutic Radiology; and (5) Radium Therapy. In 1959, these divisions were reduced to three: Radiology, Diagnostic Roentgenology, and Therapeutic Radiology. The initial cost of examination was $35 per candidate, and this remained in effect until the first increase to $50 in 1948. As of 1990, the fee was $1,050.

Candidates for examination were originally divided into three classes. Class A consisted of outstanding radiologists of long experience, associated for the most part with medical schools or directors of departments of radiology in large hospitals. Class B were radiologists of less experience, usually associated with hospitals and holding lesser teaching ranks in medical schools. Class C were younger radiologists who had recently completed their training. At the initial meeting, only those in Class A were certified, most without examination. At present, all applicants for certification must face examination, although the Class A rule is still occasionally invoked.

The methods of grading have changed over the years. Originally, the candidate was graded using the word X-RAY (X = 90-100; R = 90-80; A = 70-80; Y = below 70, and a failure). After a few years this method of grading was dropped, and numbers were used. Each question was and still is graded individually, with an average representing the candidate's final grade with the examiner. Candidates who fail one or two subjects may be conditioned and be reexamined in only these areas at a subsequent date. Failure in three or more areas necessitates a complete reexamination.

Before 1956, candidates applying for examination in Radiology were required to complete 3 years of formal residency training in an approved department of Radiology. Thereafter, 3 years of formal training plus an additional year of further training or practice was required. In 1984, the rules for Diagnostic Radiology were changed to require 4 years of formal residency training, of which the equivalent of 6 months must be in Nuclear Medicine.

At an early meeting, it was decided that the qualifying examination would be oral. When some older candidates complained that they might be at a disadvantage in taking an oral examination because of nervousness, it was suggested that a candidate might be given a written examination on request. The possibility of a screening written examination was proposed, but it was considered too complicated and thus was not accepted by the Board of Trustees. The advisability of having a written examination as an integral part of the Board's examination was discussed at many meetings, but it was concluded that "a tremendous amount of money and a large expenditure of time on the part of the members of the Board to provide a written examination is unlikely to improve the results of the present oral examination." However, in 1967, in view of the rapid expansion in the scope of knowledge required of a diagnostic radiologist, the Board reversed this position and instituted a rigorous written examination that now serves as a prerequisite before a candidate is eligible to take the oral examination.

In 1947, the ABR expanded its activities to provide for the certification of radiological physicists. In 1974, a special competence examination in nuclear medicine was established.

UNDERGRADUATE MEDICAL EDUCATION[1]

The teaching of radiology to undergraduate medical students was somewhat slow in developing, perhaps because of the need for a familiarity with electrophysics and the technical knowledge and experience required for manipulating relatively intricate apparatus. Nevertheless, as Case noted,

> There are many reasons in favor of instruction of undergraduates in medical radiology, although few of them anticipate practicing radiology as a specialty or even using it directly even in a small way. Radiology must serve all physicians. Whether or not it will be either desirable or practical for any given student to utilize radiology to any considerable extent in his future practice is questionable; nevertheless one must recognize the necessity of including as part of his medical education the fundamental principles of radiology and its general application. He must be able to appreciate the normal and pathologic x-ray appearances as they are demonstrated to him . . . he cannot acquire a knowledge of a means of diagnosis and treatment upon which he must call frequently for assistance unless he has some familiarity with anatomy and physiology as they are expressed in the roentgenograms and on the screen. At every turn he will find the literature abounding with references to important uses of the x-ray in diagnosis and treatment in practically every specialty of medicine . . . Another very important reason for undergraduate instruction lies in the enormous amount of mediocre roentgenologic work being done these days by undertrained and inexperienced physicians, and especially by non-medically trained individuals usurping the field which should be occupied exclusively by medical practitioners. A large part of this great volume of work is valueless and misleading. The student should learn the difference between dependable and valueless roentgenologic work.

MEDICAL ELECTRICITY

AND

RÖNTGEN RAYS

WITH CHAPTERS ON PHOTOTHERAPY AND RADIUM

BY

SINCLAIR TOUSEY, A.M., M.D.

CONSULTING SURGEON TO ST. BARTHOLOMEW'S CLINIC, NEW YORK CITY

CONTAINING 750 PRACTICAL
ILLUSTRATIONS, 16 IN COLORS

PHILADELPHIA AND LONDON
W. B. SAUNDERS COMPANY
1910

Title page of Tousey's *Medical Electricity and Röntgen Rays* (1910).[9]

A SYSTEM OF INSTRUCTION

IN

X-RAY METHODS AND MEDICAL USES
OF LIGHT, HOT-AIR, VIBRATION
AND HIGH-FREQUENCY
CURRENTS

A PICTORIAL SYSTEM OF TEACHING BY CLINICAL INSTRUCTION
PLATES WITH EXPLANATORY TEXT. A SERIES OF PHOTO-
GRAPHIC CLINICS IN STANDARD USES OF SCIENTIFIC
THERAPEUTIC APPARATUS FOR SURGICAL
AND MEDICAL PRACTITIONERS

PREPARED ESPECIALLY FOR THE POST-GRADUATE HOME STUDY
OF
SURGEONS, GENERAL PHYSICIANS, DENTISTS, DERMATOLOGISTS
AND SPECIALISTS IN THE TREATMENT OF CHRONIC
DISEASES, AND SANITARIUM PRACTICE

BY

S. H. MONELL, M.D.

NEW YORK

Professor of Static Electricity in the International Correspondence Schools; Founder
and Chief Instructor of the New York School of Special Electro-Therapeutics;
Member of the New York County Medical Society; Member of Kings County
Medical Society; Charter Member of the Roentgen Society of the United
States; Formerly Editor of the Electro-Therapeutic Department of
the Medical Times and Register, 1894-8; Author of "The
Treatment of Disease by Electric Currents," "Manual of
Static Electricity in X-Ray and Therapeutic Uses,"
"Elements of Correct Technique," "Rudiments
of Modern Medical Electricity," etc., etc.

NEW YORK
E. R. PELTON, PUBLISHER
19 EAST SIXTEENTH STREET

All rights reserved

Title page of Monell's *A System of Instruction in X-ray Methods and Medical Uses of Light, Hot-air, Vibration and High-frequency Currents* (1902).[5]

ROENTGEN DIAGNOSIS

OF

DISEASES OF THE HEAD

BY

DR. ARTHUR SCHÜLLER

HEAD OF THE CLINIC FOR NERVOUS DISEASES AT THE
FRANZ-JOSEPH AMBULATORIUM, VIENNA

AUTHORIZED TRANSLATION BY

FRED F. STOCKING, M.D., M.R.C.

WITH A FOREWORD BY ERNEST SACHS, M.D.
ASSOCIATE PROFESSOR OF SURGERY IN WASHINGTON UNIVERSITY.

Title page of Stocking's 1918 English translation of Schuller's *Roentgen Diagnosis of Diseases of the Head* (1912).[10]

In a 1930 survey of the teaching of radiology in undergraduate medical schools in America, Preston Hickey found that undergraduate teaching of radiology began before 1900 in one college; before 1910 in 15 additional colleges, and between 1910 and 1928 in 37 additional colleges. Thus, by 1930, 53 American medical schools were teaching radiology. Of these, 36% gave instruction during the first year, generally in connection with the Department of Anatomy. During the second year, 46% gave instruction in radiology, usually amounting to 10 hours given in connection with the departments of Anatomy and Physiology. About 80% gave instruction in radiology during the third year, averaging 30 hours' time and usually devoted to the general aspects of the specialty. In the fourth year, 98% of schools gave instruction averaging 25 hours that stressed the clinical applications of radiology. Nevertheless, Case noted that "The average graduate in practice, as we find him today, cannot boast of great familiarity with the conduction or interpretation of roentgen examinations, or of adequate comprehension of the possibilities of diagnostic aid to be obtained from x-ray studies."

RADIOLOGY TEXTBOOKS

The earliest books in radiology were popular "how-to" guides aimed at rapidly informing the interested reader from any background of the fundamental principles of x-ray production. These books combined a wealth of technical illustrations with examples of the few images available in the first several months following the discovery of the x-ray. Many images were of nonhuman subjects or of human hands and feet. A few published figures were experimental images of thicker parts of the body. Of the 87 illustrations in William J. Morton's *The X-ray*,[4] for example, 54 were technical and 3 were of nonhuman subjects. Of the remaining 30 illustrations of human subjects, 23 were images of bones and joints.

The first truly comprehensive American textbook was *The Roentgen Rays in Medicine and Surgery*, published by Francis Williams in 1901.[5] This and subsequent books in English by such authors as Monell,[6] Pusey and Caldwell,[7] Tousey,[8] and Kassabian,[9] dealt with the entire spectrum of the applications of x-rays to clinical problems. They were written to serve as overall reference sources for physicians who were actively engaged in x-ray practice. Most of the books began with a discussion of the nature and properties of x-rays, followed by a description of various types of x-ray equipment and practical hints for positioning the patient. They then described the classic imaging findings in a variety of disorders of the bones and joints, heart and lungs, and even the abdomen and pelvis. In Williams' 632-page text, after 100 pages of physics and technique, 257 pages were devoted to the heart and lungs and about 170 to the bones and joints. In later textbooks, radiation therapy received as much if not more consideration as diagnostic radiology.

After 1910, textbooks begin to appear that were devoted to specific areas in diagnostic imaging. Examples included *Roentgen Diagnosis of Disease of the Head* by Schuller (1912; English translation 1918),[10] *Pyelography* by Braasch (1915),[11] *The Roentgen Diagnosis of Diseases of the Alimentary Canal* by Carman and Miller (1917),[12] and *Injuries & Diseases of the Bones and Joints* by Baetjer and Waters (1921).[13] These monumental literary efforts were designed to be used by radiologists, either those in training or in full-time practice.

Title page of Braasch's *Pyelography* (1915).[11]

Title page of Carmen and Miller's *The Roentgen Diagnosis of Diseases of the Alimentary Canal* (1917).[12]

SUBSPECIALIZATION[14]

Subspecialization in radiology initially began in neuroradiology, with Cornelius Dyke at the Neurological Institute of New York (see Chapter 18) and in pediatric radiology, under John Caffey at Babies Hospital of Columbia in New York. After the Second World War, the pace of subspecialization accelerated with the application of radioisotopes to medicine and the development of nuclear medicine. Since that time, subspecialty societies have developed in chest, gastrointestinal, urologic, skeletal, cardiac, vascular, and head and neck radiology as well as in ultrasound, computed body tomography, and MR imaging.

Subspecialization has become increasingly more widespread in current radiology practice. This trend has been noted by the American Board of Radiology, which now divides its certifying examination into 10 diagnostic specialties: chest, gastrointestinal, genitourinary, musculoskeletal, cardiovascular/interventional, pediatrics, neuroradiology, mammography, nuclear medicine, and sonography.

A lively debate has been engendered concerning the advantages and disadvantages of subspecialization in radiology. As M. Paul Capp noted in his Presidential Address for the American Roentgen Ray Society in 1990, subspecialization improves the level of patient care, increases the credibility of radiologists among referring physicians and thus helps decrease turf problems, improves the quality of residency programs, is conducive to research and continued advancement of the field, and may encourage third-party insurance carriers to increase reimbursement of radiologists in contrast to physicians who practice radiology without adequate training. Disadvantages of subspecialization include possible reduction of hospital privileges for general radiologists, fragmentation of radiology if subspecialists tend to become more allegiant to their national subspecialty group rather than to broad-based organizations, and the danger of biased decisions in patient care by technology-based subspecialists who may be unaware of the value of other imaging modalities.

At present, most university hospitals are highly subspecialized. In large community hospitals, subspecialization is becoming more widespread, though virtually all subspecialists do some general work and many generalists perform subspecialty tasks.

References

1. Case JT: Teaching of radiology. In Glasser O (ed): The science of radiology. Springfield, Ill, Charles C Thomas, 1933.
2. Jenkinson EL: A history of the American Board of Radiology (1934-1964). Unpublished.
3. Editorial: The American Board of Radiology: Its 50th anniversary. AJR 144:197-200, 1985.
4. Morton WJ and Hammer EW: The x-ray. New York, American Technical Book, 1896.
5. Williams FH: The roentgen rays in medicine and surgery. New York, MacMillan, 1901.
6. Monell SH: A system of instruction in x-ray methods and medical uses of light, hot-air, vibration and high-frequency currents. New York, Pelton, 1902.
7. Pusey WA and Caldwell EW: The practical application of the Röntgen rays in therapeutics and diagnosis. Philadelphia, WB Saunders, 1903.
8. Tousey S: Medical electricity and Röntgen rays. Philadelphia, WB Saunders, 1910.
9. Kassabian MK: Rontgen rays and electrotherapeutics, with chapters on radium and phototherapy. Philadelphia, JB Lippincott, 1907.
10. Schuller A: Roentgen diagnosis of disease of head (1912) (Translated by F.F. Stocking). St. Louis, CV Mosby, 1918.
11. Braasch WF: Pyelography. Philadelphia, WB Saunders, 1915.
12. Carman RD and Miller A: The roentgen diagnosis of diseases of the alimentary canal. Philadelphia, WB Saunders, 1917.
13. Baetjer FH and Waters CA: Injuries & diseases of the bones and joints. New York, Hober, 1921.
14. Capp MP: Subspecialization in radiology. AJR 155:451-454, 1990.

CHAPTER 36

Anecdotes and Vignettes

 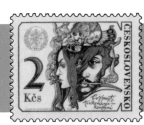 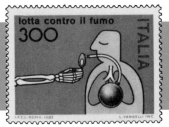 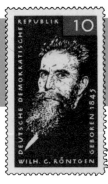

After the sensational reports of the discovery of a mysterious new ray that appeared in the popular press, a large number of stories, poems, and caricatures were published that reflected the underlying popular belief that roentgen photography was identical to ordinary photography except that it made possible the penetration through clothes, flesh, and all opaque bodies. Among the early jokes and anecdotes are several cited in Glasser's classic text:

Studies in Anatomy

Dealer (pointing towards a thin horse): "There, sir! That's what I call a picture!"

Prospective buyer: "H'm, yes, he does rather suggest one of those Röntgen-ray photographs!"[1]

Guest (to waiter who has brought him chops with a large bone and little meat): "Waiter, is this a chop à la Röntgen?"[2]

Strange Discovery

Shah Kal-Y-Jula had all of his court officials photographed with Roentgen rays. In spite of one hour's exposure, no backbone could be detected in any one of them.[3]

The New Rays

Professor of Physics to weak student: "You must have a board in front of your brain through which even the roentgen rays cannot penetrate."[4]

The X-rays

A lady who knows still less about algebra than about Roman numerals, recently asked us something about those wonderful "Ten rays."[5]

New Properties of Roentgen Rays

The recent increase in the price of Crookes tubes and of barium platino-cyanide might be termed the "Roentgen Raise."[6]

A study in anatomy (April 25, 1896).[1]

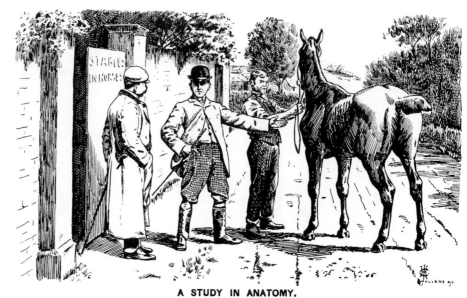

A STUDY IN ANATOMY.
Dealer. "THERE, SIR! THAT'S WHAT I CALL A PICTURE!"
Prospective Buyer. "H'M—YES—HE DOES RATHER SUGGEST ONE OF THOSE RÖNTGEN-RAY PHOTOGRAPHS!"

The latest photographic discovery. "By Professor Röntgen's process we shall soon be able to verify the above surmises as to the contents of certain bodies." (*Literary Digest*, February 15, 1896).[8]

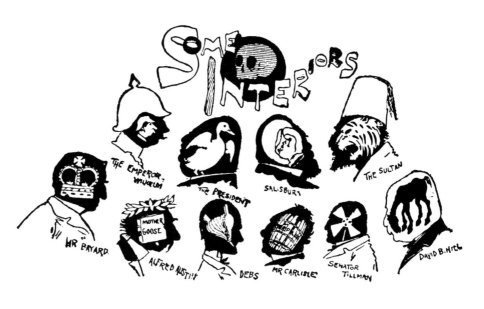

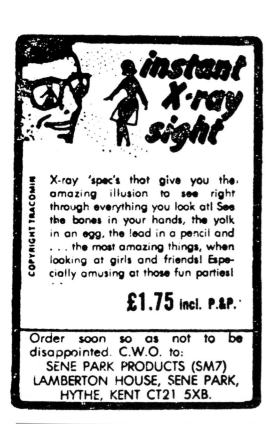

Advertisement for x-ray glasses.

The Wonderful Ray

Apropos of the wonderful penetrating powers of the cathodic ray, a young lady at a recent dinner party in New York ventured to remark that she understood that these new cathartic rays could go through anything.[7]

As a well-known figure working with the new rays, Thomas A. Edison received numerous unusual requests. One individual sent Edison the hollow eyepieces of a pair of opera glasses with the request that he "fit them with the X-rays" and return them. Another "seeker after the unattainable" wrote: "Dear Sir: Will you please send me one pound of X-rays and bill as soon as possible?"[10]

The *Electrical World*[11] reported the receipt of

the following interesting letter to be forwarded to Prof. Röntgen, which it takes the liberty of sending in this manner, as the Professor's mail must be very large at the present time:

586

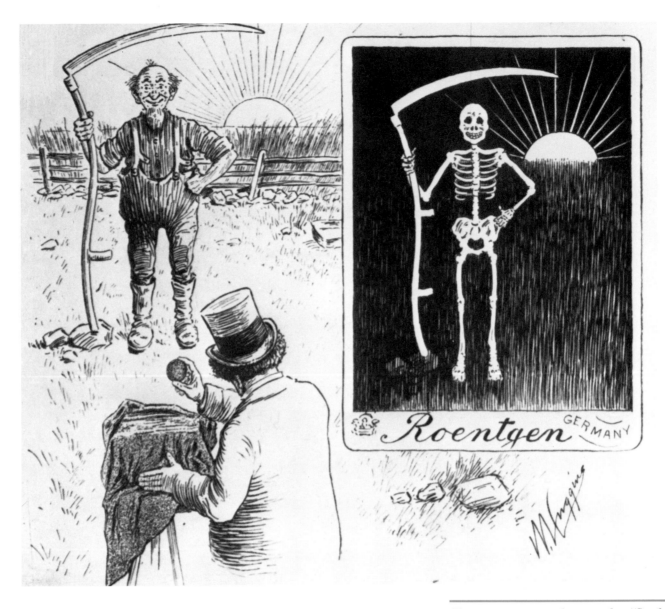

The new roentgen photography. "Look pleasant, please." (*Life*, February, 1896).[8]

Prof. Röntgen,

My Dear Professor: I have been greatly interested in your discovery, and congratulate you on having jumped Edison's claim of being the only original Wizard (of the Nile). Your discovery is very interesting from a scientific point of view, but will you be kind enough to tell me if I can apply it so as to get an "X raise" out of my boss? As I am the humble recipient of the magnificent salary of $9.50 per week, even a V raise would be most acceptable, but I do not know how to apply the process to him.

Shall I induce an "electrical resistance" on the part of the office cat to having her tail squeezed in the letter press by the errand boy, then continue to cause a "current" of envy in the entry clerk by flirting with the typewriter girl to prevent her from "sparking?" I could give the bookkeeper a "laden-jar" on the elbow while he is writing in his ledger, and then cause a "vacuum" by handing in my resignation. Would it work? I am afraid I might get an "electrical discharge." Please give exact directions in your reply.

That delicious moment when you find you are to take into dinner the girl who yesterday refused you (*Life*, April 6, 1896).[9]

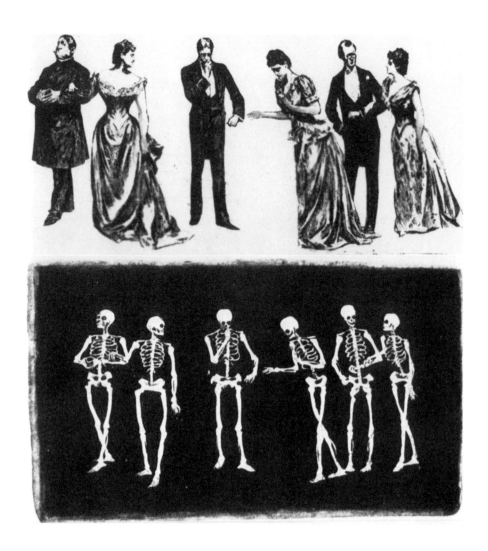

A New York newspaper[12] reported seriously "that at the College of Physicians and Surgeons the roentgen rays were used to reflect anatomic diagrams directly into the brains of the students, making a much more enduring impression than the ordinary methods of learning anatomic details." A report from London described the experience of a correspondent who was assisting at a large bazaar by holding a small roentgen ray gallery.

> An elderly gentleman of prosperous appearance objected that the show was not "up to date," as he had read somewhere in a newspaper that now you can see "the liver palpitating and the heart circulating." Two elderly ladies entered the small room and, solemnly seating themselves, requested me to close and fasten the door. Upon my complying, they said they wished to "see each other's bones," but I was not to expose them below the waist-line, each wishing to view the apparently dismantled osseous structure of her friend first! A young and anxious mother asked me to see if her little boy had really swallowed a threepenny bit, as he was uncertain himself. She had read in the papers that a great doctor, Sir Something Blister, in a speech in a large meeting in Liverpool a little while ago, said that a half-penny had been seen in a boy's "sarcophagus!" A young girl of the domestic servant class, taking advantage of her opportunity, as she thought, and my sex, asked me in confidence if I would "look through her young man unbeknown to him while he looked at the picture, to see if he was quite healthy in his internals."

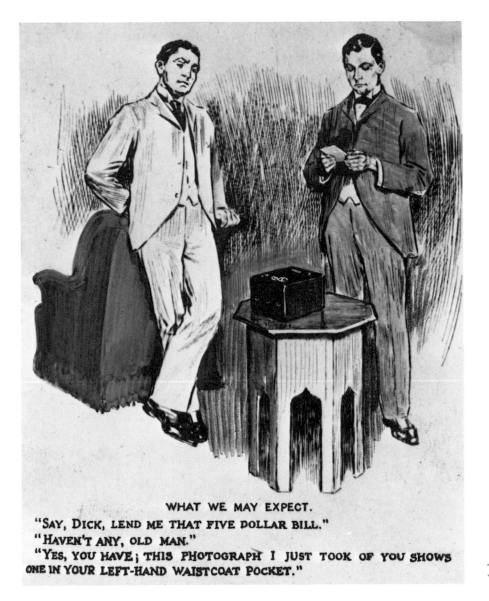

What we may expect.

"Say, Dick, lend me that five dollar bill."

"Haven't any, old man."

"Yes, you have; this photograph I just took of you shows one in your left-hand waistcoat pocket."

What we may expect.

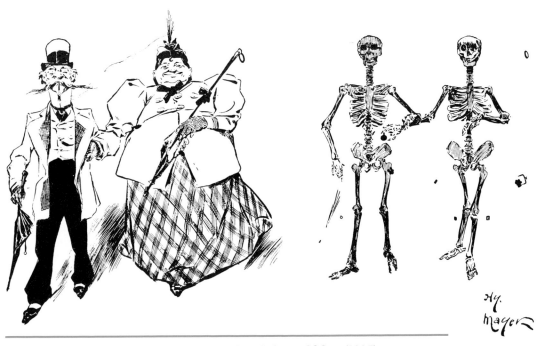

Whether stout or thin, the x-ray makes the whole world kin (1897).

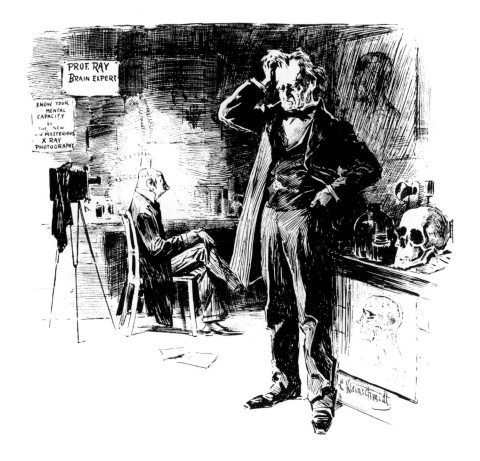

Empty. Professor Ray (after a vain search, musingly)—"How shall I break it to him?" (1897).

On the political front, "a loud laugh went over the State of New Jersey on February 19, when Assemblyman Reed, of Somerset County, introduced a bill in the House at Trenton, prohibiting the use of x-rays in opera glasses in theaters."[13]

Glasser[9] noted that "the newly discovered rays were soon associated with many mysterious hoaxes and fads which have continued to occupy human fancy through many centuries, such as the discovery of the magic stone, the discussions on vivisection, temperance, and prohibition movements, spiritualism, and soul photography." For example, a Cedar Rapids, Iowa, newspaper reported a young student's discovery of the magic stone. "By means of what he called the X-rays he is enabled to change in three hours' time a cheap piece of metal worth about 13 cents to $153 worth of gold. The metal so transformed has been tested and pronounced pure gold."[14] In an editorial, *Life Magazine* suggested that the use of x-rays could solve the problem of vivisection, which had been heatedly discussed at the end of the nineteenth century. "If the Röntgen method of seeing through things pans out anywhere near as its friends expect, we are entitled to hope that it will almost put an end to vivisection. There will be no need to put a knife into a living animal when a ray will make its inner workings visible."[15]

Francis E. Willard, a well-known protagonist of the temperance movement in the United States, was convinced that the newly discovered x-rays "are going to do much for the temperance cause. By this means drunkards and cigarette smokers can be shown the steady deterioration in their systems which follows the practice, and seeing is believing."[16] Baraduc, a French scientist who championed the theory of "soul photography," exhibited 400 cases purporting to show the effect of a series of discharges of the human soul on light-sensitive plates. He also stated that he made photographic exposures by a transmission of thought with a friend more than 300 km away.[17] However, as the skeptical Paris correspondent of the *London Daily Telegraph* noted, "the pictures of Dr. Baraduc are equally as unsafe as his theories."

C. Thurston Holland, the famed British radiologist, recalled a series of sensational stories in the July, 1896 issue of *Strand Magazine*, which illustrated "The Adventures of a Man of Science." In one, a man suspected of having stolen and swallowed a diamond was lured into the laboratory of a scientist, who narrated that "he followed me into the laboratory without a word. I desired him to strip, and then, after some difficulty, arranged him in such a position that the rays should pass through his body. I turned off the light in the room, my electrical battery worked well, the rays played admirably in the vacuum tube. I removed the cap from the CAMERA . . ." and so on. The result was an excellent plate showing the diamond just below the region of the ileocaecal valve! But, as Holland pointed out, the real tragedy in this comedy of errors was of course that if the "diamond" were shown, then it could not have been a real one, as real diamonds are transparent to x-rays.[18]

Articles recounted unusual properties of the new rays. In the *Boston Medical and Surgical Journal* (September 3, 1896), M.H. Richardson described a stout woman of 50 who had been complaining of episodic pain in the left ankle. His x-ray examination revealed healing of a previous fracture of the distal tibia with some angulation and only mild impairment of the movements of the joint. After examining with the fluoroscope, he took photographs of the ankle using an exposure of about 5 minutes. He reported the following letter, which suggested a new use for the x-rays:

> My dear Doctor Richardson:
> I feel that I should write and tell you the splendid effect the x-rays had on my foot. It is now three weeks since I was at your office, and I have not had one particle of pain since. The swelling and soreness have disappeared also. My family thinks it is all imagination, but that is impossible, because all that I expected from the rays was what you might discern . . .
>
> Yours gratefully,

As Richardson wrote, "The remarkable improvement in the case reminds me of the occasional cures which are by some patients attributed to the use of the clinical thermometer twice daily."

The *Electrical Engineer*[19] noted in 1899 that

> Paris doctors declared that x-rays produced violent palpitations of the heart. Doctors Seguy and Quenisset have experimented on their students and on themselves, and declared that when continued the palpitations are unendurable. They stopped them by placing a metal plate between the heart and the rays. They advised people who are not in perfect health to keep out of the way of the x-rays, or, at any rate, to protect their vital organs against them.

The x-rays were also said to have some effect on vision. As Fredrick S. Kolle wrote (1897),

> Of seven persons with amaurosis subjected to the Röntgen rays, six observed the Sternschuppenlicht, a peculiar shooting-star light. Four of the patients could count the individual stars, ranging between six and thirty-two in number . . . The patient who did not respond to the rays had been injured early in life, and both globes had been removed. It is needless to say that none of the patients was able to

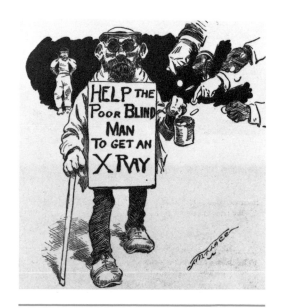

The latest (1897).

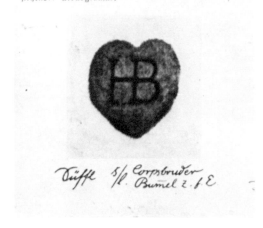

Heart. "Student Suffl, one of the regular visitors of the Huf-Brau-Haus had his heart photographed with Röntgen's rays and one discovered in it the following initials: H.B. (the famous Munich beer cellar)" (May 26, 1896).[2]

A grinning skeleton sat beside her (*Chicago Tribune*, February, 1896).[8]

see with the aid of the rays, although by cutting off the rays by the interposition of a steel plate an eighth of an inch thick, no such sensation was experienced. From the foregoing, I infer that this peculiar sensation depends, as regards its activity, that is, an increase in the number of Schuppen, upon the better or less atrophied or otherwise affected retina. That the lenses are not opaque, or rather impervious, is shown by the same phenomena appearing in the normal eye after a lengthy exposure, attended by headaches, supraorbital and deep-seated pain in the globes of the eyes.[20]

Unusual physiological effects of x-rays were noted in a dispatch[21] from Berlin describing the case of

Dr. Markuse whose "interior" has been photographed thirty times within the past 20 days by the roentgen process, has lost all of his hair as a result and his face has assumed a brownish color. The skin has peeled off his breast where the Hittorff instrument nearly touched it, and on his back what was first a sore finally developed into a bleeding wound, surrounded by burnt looking cuticle. The victim is exhausted.

Use of the roentgen rays could lead to embarrassing situations. Thurston Holland recalled the time when he was giving a popular lecture on x-rays. After the lecture, during which the translucency of real gem stones to x-rays was mentioned, the audience had the opportunity of

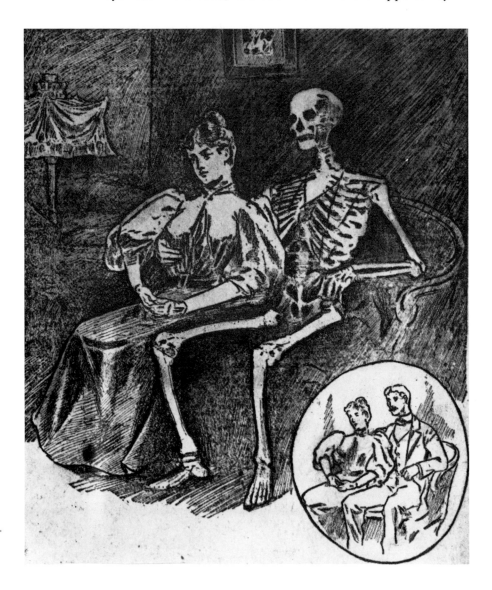

viewing several items on a fluoroscopic screen. An overdressed lady looked carefully at one of her hands on the screen, obviously examining a large ring, the stones of which were densely opaque to x-rays. As Holland noted, "From the quite unprintable and vitriolic remarks she made in an undertone as she took her departure, it was quite evident that I had done someone a very bad turn."[22]

X-rays were also used for a variety of nonmedical purposes. Ferdinand Ranvez reported the ability of x-ray photography to detect evidence of the addition of mineral substances into vegetable articles of food.

> This method offers manifold advantages; it requires only small quantities of the substances; it leaves the specimen completely intact; it allows us to affect in a very short time a great number of examinations (about a quarter of an hour sufficing for a series of specimens). Lastly, the proof obtained is a piece of convictive evidence quickly demonstrated, easily understood even by persons strangers to any analytical operation. Samples of falsified saffron (taken in trade) consisted of mixtures in different proportions of pure saffron and saffron coated with barium sulfate. The adulteration was very skillfully masked, and could not be suspected on a mere inspection of the merchandise. The pure (saffron) allowed itself to be traversed by the x-rays and produced on the proof merely shadows scarcely visible . . . The three falsified samples acted strongly upon the sensitive plate, marking very distinctly the filaments coated with barium sulfate, while the stigmati of the pure product, which was mixed with it, appeared only as scarcely perceptible shadows analogous to those of the former product.[23]

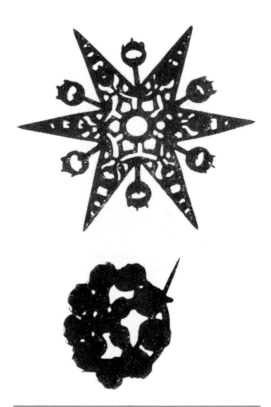

Radiography of jewelry (August 7, 1896). *Top*, Diamond star; *bottom*, paste brooch.[18]

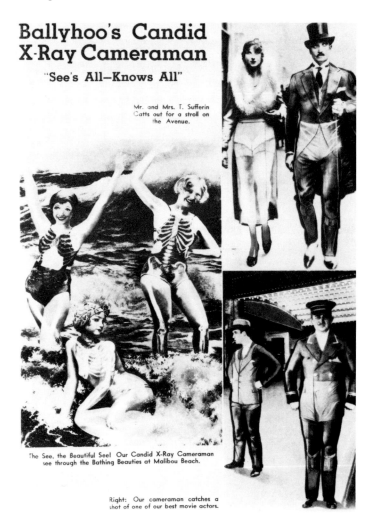

Cartoon from October, 1934.

Grin and Bear It
By LICHTY

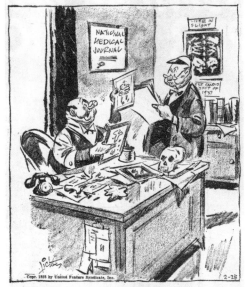

"We gotta have more X-rays, Fisbee! Readers these days demand pictures, pictures and more pictures!"

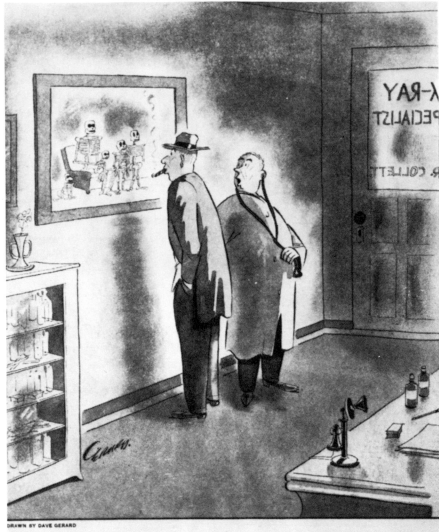

"I Took That Picture This Spring of the Wife and Kiddies"

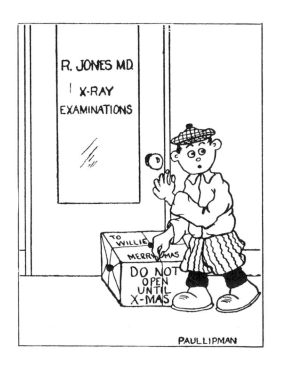

R. JONES M.D.

X-RAY EXAMINATIONS

TO WILLIE

MERRY XMAS

DO NOT OPEN UNTIL X-MAS

PAUL LIPMAN

Marangani[27] attempted to use x-rays to detect the larvae of insects that infested grapes and other fruits. "They can be photographed inside the fruit or, better still, observed with the cryptoscope." And speaking of insects, George Batten of London unpacked a new x-ray tube he had bought and found a moth sealed inside the bulb. Full of indignation, he wrote a strong letter of complaint to the maker, who sent him a "moth ball" by return post![24]

The *Electrical Engineer*[25] described experiments made by William Shrader testing the effect of the roentgen rays on various disease germs.

> In nearly every instance they are reported to have met with success and proved conclusively that the rays are invaluable in the treatment of these diseases. Among the first experiments were those made with the diphtheria bacilli; tubes were inoculated with the germs, one exposed to the rays and the other not exposed. In the former the germs were destroyed, while in the latter they lived. Following these tests two guinea pigs were inoculated with a solid culture of diphtheria . . . One was exposed to the rays for four hours in a wooden box, having a rubber cover, and is alive today after eight weeks, and no trace of the disease can be found. The other pig, not exposed to the rays, died within 28 hours after the injection of a poison. The post-mortem examination showed that his death was due to the diphtheria germs.

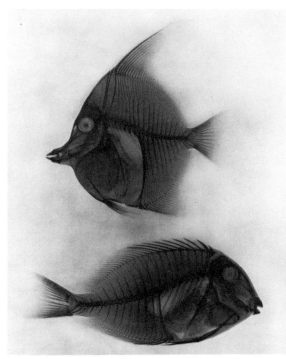

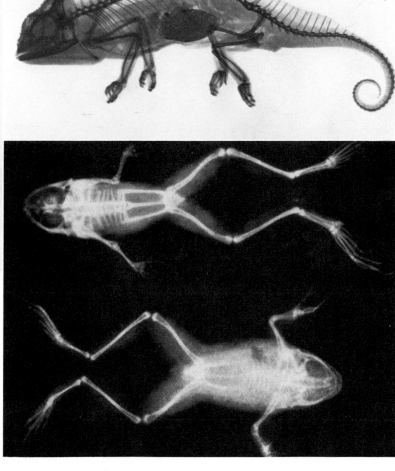

Roentgen pictures by J.N. Eder and E. Valenta of Vienna (January and February, 1896). *Above*, Tropical fish (*top*, Zanclus Cornutus; *bottom*, Acanthurus nigros). *Above right*, Chamaleon cristatus. *Right*, Frogs, dorsal and ventral positions.[8]

Starfish in Chicago Natural History Museum (*left*). Nautilus (*right*).

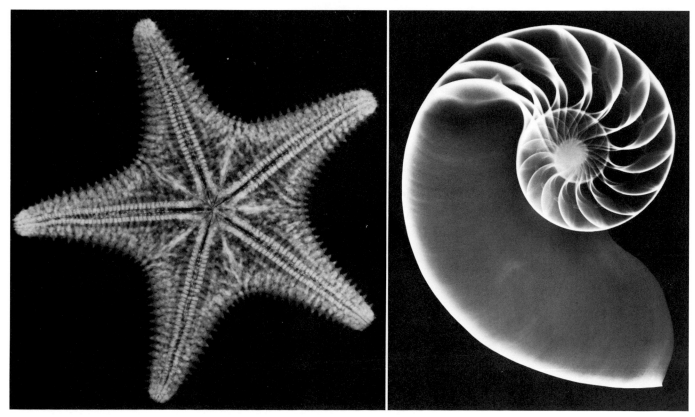

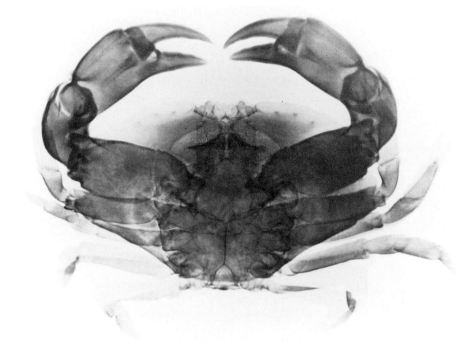

Cancer pagurus (the edible crab). (From Wolfenden RN: Archives of Clinical Skiagraphy, 1896.)

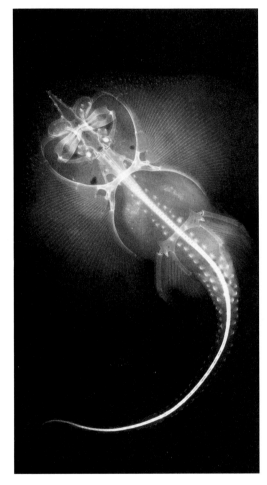

Stingray.

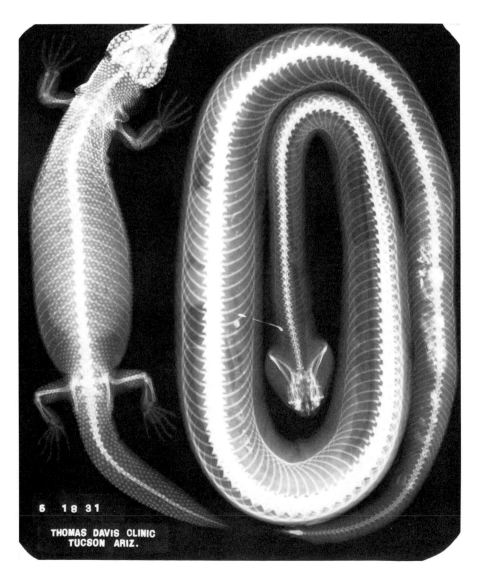

Gila monster and rattlesnake.

Could the mysterious new x-rays be used to thwart "those more crafty witted gentlemen established in the art of smuggling?" As the *Globe*[26] reported under the title "Roentgen rays and French customs,"

> The Roentgen rays, which have been employed to examine the interior of bombs with success by M. Girad, are now enlisted in the service of French customs by M. Palliam. We are afraid that some of the newspapers have exaggerated the dread importance of this latest application. No doubt some contraband articles may be detected in this way, but certainly others cannot. Might not a smuggler of lace, for instance, be able to stow as much as he likes of it in his bag and without fearing detection by the rays? We hear of cigars and cigarettes being discovered by this new Ithuriel, but probably the metal box containing them was the cause of it. Cigars as well as lace, are vegetable matter, more or less transparent to the rays, and one could easily select and pack them so as to escape the vigilance of the "douanier." Perhaps we shall presently see tobaccos and other articles ordered for sale warranted x-ray proof. Professional smugglers may also subscribe to the Roentgen Society.

Could roentgen rays be produced by other sources?

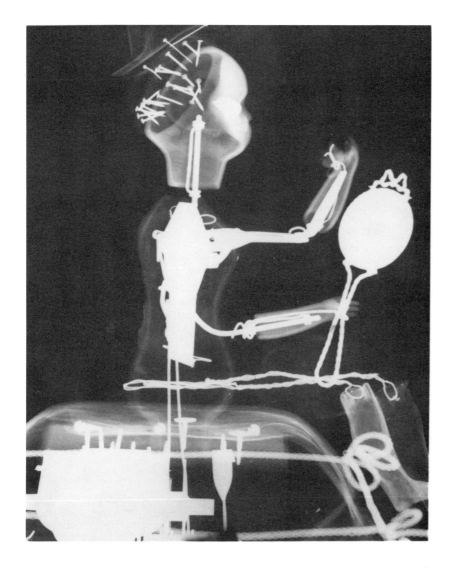

Mechanical doll.

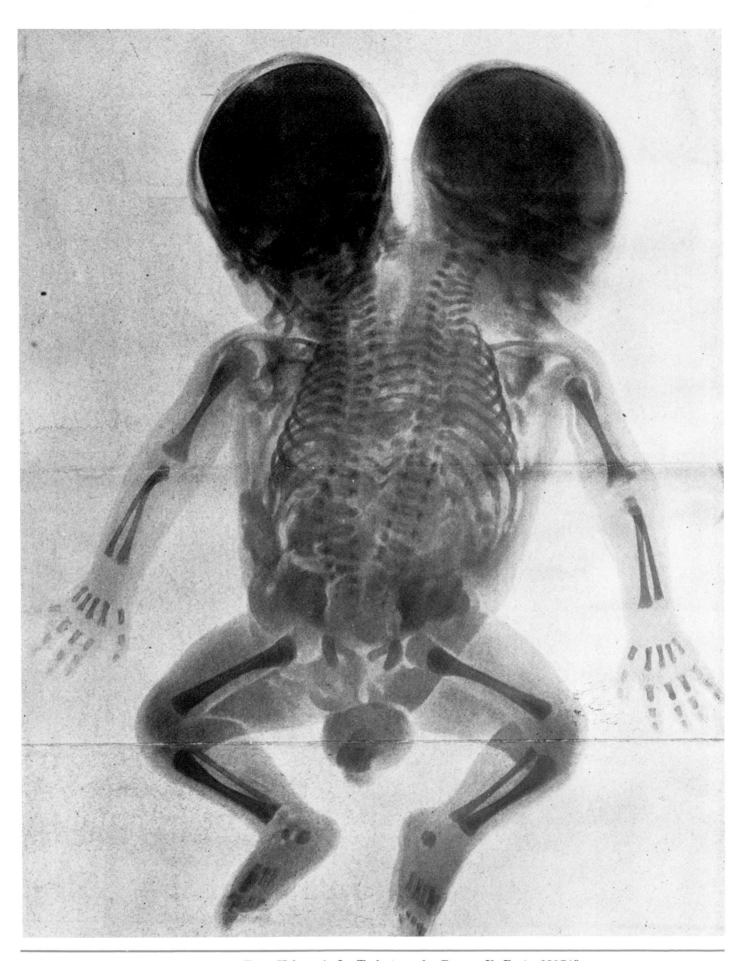

French Roentgen picture of a monster. (From Hebert A: La Technique des Rayons X, Paris, 1897.)[8]

Professor H. Muraoka, who holds the Chair of Physics at Kyoto, Japan, has been making investigations into the properties of the light emitted by fireflies. His method was to place from 30 to 1,000 of these insects in a small flat box under a net made of hemp. The box also contained a photographic dry plate between which and the fireflies Prof. Muraoka placed various substances composed of metal, paper and wood. After wrapping the box carefully with several thicknesses of black paper he would leave it for two nights in a photographic darkroom, from which all sunlight and artificial light were carefully excluded. From his experiments the Japanese professor found that the light of fireflies possesses all the properties of ordinary light. In addition he found that rays are given out which resemble those of the Rontgen ray in their power to penetrate paper, wood, metals and similar substances. However carefully he wrapped the sensitized plate before placing it in contact with the fireflies, it was always more or less blackened by their light. A very marked resemblance was found in these rays to the light of fluorescent bodies, as shows by recent investigations by M. Becquerel.[8]

Several respected scientists voiced skepticism regarding the value of the new x-rays. In opening the discussion on a paper by Francis H. Williams of Boston, before the Boston Medical Library in 1899, the famous Professor of Clinical Medicine, F.C. Shattuck, stated

I have been much interested in the development of x-ray and have seen something of its uses as demonstrated by Mr. Walter Dodd at the Massachusetts Hospital. I will admit that I can see broken bones; that I can see metallic foreign bodies in the extremities, but when it comes to x-rays of the chest and to some extent of the abdomen, I am much less clear. Frank Williams has just shown you some plates and tells you that the heart is here and that the lung is here. Now I can't see a thing in these plates and to be truthful, I don't think he can.

A.E. Dobaer of Tufts College wrote in the *Electrical World* that

It must seem like a ghostly experiment to photograph the skeleton of a living person as though it was dissected out and articulated with wires. But the same process has its threatening aspect. If one can photograph through wood, blank walls, and in the dark too, then privacy is impossible; for it will be light everywhere but to one's eyes, and for these there will be substitutes.

Radium also was the subject of some unusual press coverage. In a 1907 communication to the *Archives of the Röntgen Ray*, Robert Abbe related a conversation he had with a friend while sitting on his porch one recent summer night.[28]

In answer to the question, "What difference is there between the light from the stars and radium rays?" . . . I said to a friend: "Radium rays move in absolutely straight lines without deviation by atmosphere, water lenses or prisms, and nothing is opaque to them; they would even penetrate the stone column near you, which light does not." To his incredulity I replied: "Bring me a stone and I will demonstrate it." He brought me a smooth granite boulder. I cut a strip of lead wire into bits and twisted them into letters, which I laid upon the thick light-proof envelopes enclosing a photographic plate. On these I laid a board, and on this the stone. On top of the stone I placed a small glass tube containing a bit of radium about the size of a grain of rice (60 milligrams). On developing the plate after three days' exposure, a strong picture of the relatively denser lead was seen [see Chapter 30].

Some of the early reports describing the value of radium were exceedingly effusive. A 1904 article stated that

> Radium is worth three times its weight in gold ($2,700,000 a pound). I believe that radium represents in its atoms the primordial elements of matter which God first charged with light, when He said, "Let there be light." In the aggregating of these elements to form the earth, radium was condensed from the rarefied ultra-gouous state into solid masses, and with an immense amount of latent heat was packed away down in the mines of the earth. So soon as brought to the surface, and the pressure on its atoms lessened, the latter begins to disintegrate, and the internal heat is liberated. The particles at and near the surface rapidly fly off in every direction until the underlying more compact part is reached, the particles of which in their turn become gradually detached, and fly off in rapidly increasing quantities. Thus the atoms in one zone after another undergo disintegration with the liberation of energy.

> God *created* the primordial elements of matter before He made *atoms*, and molecules, and suns, and moons, and stars; and God created the primordial energy of motion before He made light, and heat, and electricity, and other energies . . . Radium shoots its myriads of fiery missiles through tumors, indurations, plastic deposits, etc., cuts them to pieces and renders them absorbable. It also shoots to death bacteria and protozoa by riddling them with its fast-flying projectiles and shattering them into a thousand fragments. This self-loaded and self-discharging engine of destruction keeps up its continuous but noiseless work with no appreciable evidence of exhaustion. Another remarkable fact is that the projectiles sent out from radium, wherever they may lodge, explode and scatter their fragments in all directions, dealing death and destruction to microbes.

All cartoons and animal photographs courtesy Eastman Kodak.

Bibliography

Glasser O: William Conrad Röntgen and the early history of the roentgen rays. Springfield, Ill, Charles C Thomas, 1934.

References

1. Punch 110:195, April 25, 1896.
2. Fliegende Blatter 104:163, May 26, 1896.
3. Fliegende Blatter 104:155, April 19, 1896.
4. Meggendorfer Humoristische Blatter 24:100, March 1896.
5. Electrical World 27:308, March 21, 1896.
6. Electrical World 27:315, March 21, 1896.
7. JAMA 26:892, May 2, 1896.
8. Electrical Engineer 23:464, 1897.
9. Glasser O: William Conrad Röntgen and the early history of the roentgen rays. Springfield, Ill, Charles C Thomas, 1934.
10. Literary Digest 13:305, July 4, 1896.
11. Electrical World 27:281, March 14, 1896.
12. Science (New York) 3:436, March 3, 1896.
13. Electrical Engineer 21:216, February 26, 1896.
14. Electrical Engineer 21:472, May 6, 1896.
15. Life 27:152, February 27, 1896.
16. Electrical Review 38:737, June 5, 1896.
17. Brit J Photogr 43:396, June 19, 1896.
18. Holland CT: X-rays in 1896. Liverpool Med-Chir J 45:61-77, 1937.
19. Electrical Engineer 23, 1897.
20. Electrical Engineer 23:241, 1897.
21. Electrical Engineer 22:126, August 5, 1896.
22. Brit J Radiol 11:15, 1938.
23. Electrical Engineer 22:87, July 22, 1896.
24. Jupe, 1961.
25. Electrical Engineer 22, August 19, 1896.
26. Globe, July 16, 1896.
27. Marangani C: The study of larvae of insects in plants by means of the Roentgen rays. Atti Accad Georgofili Florenz, September 19, 1896.
28. Abbe R: Illustrating the penetrating power of radium. Arch Roent Ray 11:247, 1907.

Index